PEDIATRIC CARDIOLOGY FOR PRACTITIONERS

PEDIATRIC CARDIOLOGY FOR PRACTITIONERS

THIRD EDITION

Myung K. Park, MD

Professor of Pediatrics,
Head, Division of Cardiology,
University of Texas Health Science Center,
San Antonio, Texas

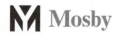 Mosby

St. Louis   Baltimore   Boston   Carlsbad   Chicago   Naples   New York   Philadelphia   Portland
London   Madrid   Mexico City   Singapore   Sydney   Tokyo   Toronto   Wiesbaden

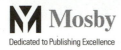
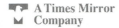

Editor: Laurel Craven
Developmental Editor: Dana Battaglia
Project Manager: Linda McKinley
Production Editor: Aimee E. Loewe
Manufacturing Manager: Theresa Fuchs
Design Coordinator: Elizabeth Fett

THIRD EDITION

Printed in the United States of America
Composition by Graphic World, Inc.
Printing/binding by Maple-Vail Book Manufacturing Group

Mosby–Year Book, Inc.
11830 Westline Industrial Drive
St. Louis, MO 63146

Library of Congress Cataloging in Publication Data

Park, Myung K. (Myung Kun), 1934-
    Pediatric cardiology for practitioners / Myung K. Park.—3rd ed.
        p.   cm.
    Includes bibliographical references and index.
    ISBN 0-8151-6632-X
    1. Pediatric cardiology.   I. Title.
    [DNLM: 1. Heart Diseases—in infancy & childhood.   2. Heart
Defects, Congenital.   WS 290 P235p 1995]
RJ421.P37 1995
618.92′12—dc20
DNLM/DLC
for Library of Congress   95-7530
                                                                              CIP

96 97 98 99 00 / 9 8 7 6 5 4 3 2 1

To my wife, Issun, and our sons
Douglas, Christopher, and Warren.

Foreword to the First Edition

I was very honored by Dr. Park's request that I review his manuscript and write a foreword. Having carefully read it, I am even more pleased to be able to write a foreword with unqualified praise and to recommend this book to my colleagues in pediatrics and family medicine. I think that it is so well organized and logical that serious students and even pediatric cardiologists in training will find it useful.

One of the more obvious difficulties encountered by a busy house officer or a practitioner is that most textbooks are organized to be useful to the individual who already knows the diagnosis. This "Catch-22" is resolved by Dr. Park's presentation, which permits scanning and rapid identification of the problem area, and then stepwise progresses to the clinical diagnosis, the medical management of the problem, and the general potential of surgical assistance.

This book is both concise and thorough, a relatively rare combination in the medical literature. It spares the practitioner the great detail usually found in a cardiology textbook on esoteric details of the echocardiogram, catheterization, angiocardiogram, and surgical procedures. The presentations are practical, giving drug dosages, intervals, and precautions. Although he presents alternative views where appropriate, Dr. Park is courageous in presenting his own recommendations, which are well thought out and, above all, logical.

It is easy for me to see the impact of Dr. Park's career in this excellent book. He had a thorough general pediatric training, followed by several years in pediatric cardiology and cardiovascular physiology in this country. After some years in academic pediatric cardiology in Canada, he returned to this country and served as a family practitioner in a small community in the state of Washington. He learned well the problems of practicing in an area where consultants were not convenient for the practitioner, nor was it easy to transport a patient quickly to a major center. He returned to a research fellowship in pharmacology, and consequently knows more about the dynamics of cardiovascular drugs than anyone I can think of in the field of pediatric cardiology. For the past several years he has actively taught and practiced pediatric cardiology in a university setting and learned the process of transmitting the information and the skills that he has acquired in his career. This book reflects all of these experiences, and the balance between science and practical considerations is reflected in every page, with the particular clarity of a natural teacher.

I am proud of my earlier association with Dr. Park, and particularly proud of his present contribution to pediatric cardiology.

Warren G. Guntheroth, MD
Professor of Pediatrics,
Head, Division of Pediatric Cardiology,
University of Washington School of Medicine,
Seattle, Washington

Preface to the First Edition

Since I started teaching pediatric cardiology, I felt that there was a need for a book that was written primarily for noncardiologists, such as medical students, house staff, and practitioners. Although many excellent pediatric cardiology textbooks are available, they are not very helpful to the noncardiologist, since they are filled with many details that are beyond the need or comprehension of practitioners. In addition, these books are not very effective in teaching practitioners how to approach children with potential cardiac problems; they are usually helpful only when the diagnosis is known. This book is intended to meet the need of noncardiologist practitioners for improving their skills in arriving at clinical diagnosis of cardiac problems, using basic tools available in their offices and community hospitals. This book will also serve as a quick reference in the area of pediatric cardiology. Although echocardiograms, cardiac catheterization, and angiocardiograms provide more definite information about the problem, these tools are not discussed at length in this book, since they are not routinely available to practitioners, and their use requires special skills.

In writing a small, yet comprehensive book, occasional oversimplification was unavoidable. Major emphasis was placed on the effective utilization of basic tools: history taking, physical examination, ECGs, and chest roentgenograms. Significance of abnormal findings in each of these areas is discussed, with differential diagnosis whenever applicable. A section is provided for pathophysiology for in-depth understanding of clinical manifestations of cardiac problems. Accurate but succinct discussion of congenital and acquired cardiac conditions is presented for quick reference. Indications, timing, procedures, risks, and complications for surgical treatment of cardiac conditions are also briefly discussed for each condition. Common cardiac arrhythmias are presented, with brief discussion of description, causes, significance, and management of each arrhythmia. A special section addresses cardiac problems of the neonate; another is devoted to special problems, such as congestive heart failure, systemic hypertension, pulmonary hypertension, chest pain or syncope, etc.

I would like to thank my teachers and my colleagues, past and present, who directly and indirectly influenced me and taught me how to teach pediatric cardiology, and those students and house staff who gave me valuable suggestions during the early stages of this book. My special thanks are due Dr. Warren G. Guntheroth, who encouraged me to write this book, read the entire manuscript, and gave me many helpful suggestions. I gratefully acknowledge Mrs. Linda Barragan for the expert secretarial assistance, Mr. Ronald Reif for careful proofreading, and the Department of Educational Resources, University of Texas Health Science Center at San Antonio, for their superb art and photographic works, especially Mrs. Deborah Felan for her excellent art work.

Finally, it is impossible to express adequately my debt to my brother, Young Kun, and my sister Po Kun, who provided me with powerful stimulus, encouragement, and hearty support throughout my schooling and who maintained confidence in me. Most of all, I am deeply indebted to my lovely wife and our wonderful boys, who accepted with understanding the inconvenience associated with my long preoccupation with this book.

Myung K. Park, MD

Preface to Third Edition

Important advances have been made in the diagnosis and management of children with congenital and acquired heart diseases since the publication of the second edition of this book. Advances made in infant cardiac surgery in particular have been extraordinary for correction and palliation of many defects, including the most complex lesions. These advances make it necessary to update the book. *The Pediatric Cardiology Handbook,* written by this author in 1991, provides practitioners with brief practical information only. To fill the void between bulky standard pediatric cardiology textbooks and the handbook, this new edition is expanded in depth and updated to serve as a small reference book. Despite the major updating and expansion, the book maintains the original goal of providing pediatricians, family practitioners, and medical students with practical information. Thus the general layout of the book has been preserved to serve as a quick information source, avoiding excessive theoretical details and literature review.

Extensive updating and revisions have been made throughout the book, and many chapters have been rewritten. In addition, a large number of new tables and new figures have been added to facilitate in-depth understanding for the readers. Specifically, several important tables have been added to the chapters on history taking and physical examination. Chapters on echocardiography, exercise tests, ambulatory electrocardiography, and cardiac catheterization have been substantially expanded. Individual congenital and acquired heart defect has been updated or rewritten with incorporation of the most recent diagnostic and therapeutic advances, especially the surgical advances in terms of timing, indications, type of surgeries, and the results. A number of new diagrams depicting pathology and surgical procedures have been added for most conditions. A new section of postoperative follow-up has been added for each condition.

Cardiovascular infections, including Kawasaki's disease, and cardiomyopathy have been updated. The chapters on cardiac arrhythmias have been expanded beyond the format of this book to include a more detailed discussion on supraventricular tachycardia and premature ventricular contractions, the two most common arrhythmias encountered by practitioners. Part IV, Neonates with Cardiac Problems, has been extensively rewritten and updated, especially sections on cardiomyopathy of infants of diabetic mothers, persistent pulmonary hypertension of the newborn, and neonatal congestive heart failure. Arrhythmias and atrioventricular conduction disturbances have been rewritten to include immediate management, as well as the natural history of these disturbances. Chapters on chest pain, syncope, and hyperlipidemia in Part VIII, Special Problems, have been rewritten. R. George Troxler, MD, MPH, Director, Cardiovascular Risk Reduction Clinic, Department of Family Practice, University of Texas Health Science Center at San Antonio, was kind enough to collaborate in Hyperlipidemia in Children, bringing his expertise to the book.

In the section of the appendix, drug dosages has been appropriately expanded and revised. In addition, normal echocardiographic data, materials related to hyperlipidemia, and other information have been added.

I wish to acknowledge the contributions of the following individuals. Nancy Place, CMI, MS, and Nick Lang, CMI, MS, have been instrumental in producing superb artwork for the new edition. April Cox, RBP, and Dieter Karkut, RBP, provided their expertise in photography. Dae-Hwan Shin, a personal friend and a doctoral candidate in Bioengineering, University of Texas at Austin, taught me how to use the Microsoft

Windows program and helped me whenever I had problems with the computer. I would also like to thank Da-Hae Lee, my colleague in the division of pediatric cardiology, for her constructive advice; Glory Ann Johnson, RN, for her enthusiastic effort to find good illustrations; Diane Halim for typing and editing; and Warren, my son, for his help in editing. Most of all, I thank my wife for understanding my long period of preoccupation with the project.

Myung K. Park, MD

Frequently Used Abbreviations

AR	Aortic regurgitation
AS	Aortic stenosis
ASD	Atrial septal defect
CHD	Congenital heart disease or defect
CHF	Congestive heart failure
COA	Coarctation of the aorta
ECD	Endocardial cushion defect
echo	Echocardiography or echocardiographic
HOCM	Hypertrophic obstructive cardiomyopathy
IHSS	Idiopathic hypertrophic subaortic stenosis
IVC	Inferior vena cava
LA	Left atrium or left atrial
LAD	Left axis deviation
LAH	Left atrial hypertrophy
LBBB	Left bundle branch block
LICS	Left intercostal space
LLSB	Lower left sternal border
LPA	Left pulmonary artery
LPLs	Left precordial leads
LRSB	Lower right sternal border
LSB	Left sternal border
LV	Left ventricle or left ventricular
LVH	Left ventricular hypertrophy
MLSB	Mid-left sternal border
MPA	Main pulmonary artery
MR	Mitral regurgitation
MRSB	Mid-right sternal border
MS	Mitral stenosis
MVP	Mitral valve prolapse
PA	Pulmonary artery
PAC	Premature atrial contraction
PAPVR	Partial anomalous pulmonary venous return
PAT	Paroxysmal atrial tachycardia
PBF	Pulmonary blood flow
PDA	Patent ductus arteriosus
PR	Pulmonary regurgitation
PS	Pulmonary stenosis
PVC	Premature ventricular contraction
PVM	Pulmonary vascular markings
PVOD	Pulmonary vascular obstructive disease
PVR	Pulmonary vascular resistance
RA	Right atrium or right atrial
RAD	Right axis deviation

RAH	Right atrial hypertrophy
RBBB	Right bundle branch block
RICS	Right intercostal space
RPA	Right pulmonary artery
RPLs	Right precordial leads
RV	Right ventricle or right ventricular
RVH	Right ventricular hypertrophy
S1	First heart sound
S2	Second heart sound
S3	Third heart sound
S4	Fourth heart sound
SEM	Systolic ejection murmur
SVC	Superior vena cava
SVR	Systemic vascular resistance
TAPVR	Total anomalous pulmonary venous return
TGA	Transposition of the great arteries
TOF	Tetralogy of Fallot
TR	Tricuspid regurgitation
TS	Tricuspid stenosis
ULSB	Upper left sternal border
URSB	Upper right sternal border
VSD	Ventricular septal defect
WPW	Wolff-Parkinson-White

Contents

PART III Pathophysiology

PART IV Specific Congenital Heart Defects

PART VI   Electrocardiography II

PART I

Basic Tools in Routine Evaluation of Cardiac Patients

Initial cardiac evaluation of a child in an office practice is usually accomplished by history taking; physical examination (PE) that includes inspection, palpation, and auscultation; electrocardiogram (ECG); and chest roentgenogram.

The weight of the information gained from these different techniques varies with the type and severity of the disease. For example, if a mother had German measles early in her pregnancy, congenital heart defects (CHDs) and other malformations (e.g., rubella syndrome) are usually present. Patent ductus arteriosus (PDA) and peripheral pulmonary artery stenosis are the most common cardiovascular defects. The physician should look for these defects when examining the child. Auscultation may be the most important source of information in the diagnosis of acyanotic heart disease such as ventricular septal defect (VSD) or PDA. However, auscultation is rarely diagnostic in cyanotic congenital heart disease (CHD) such as transposition of the great arteries (TGA) in which the heart murmur is often absent. Careful palpation of the peripheral pulses is more important than auscultation in the detection of coarctation of the aorta (COA). Measurement of blood pressure is the most important diagnostic tool in the detection of hypertension. The ECG and chest x-ray films have strengths and weaknesses in their ability to assess the severity of heart disease. The ECG detects hypertrophy well and therefore detects conditions of pressure overload, but it is less reliable at detecting dilatation from volume overload. The chest x-ray films are most reliable in establishing volume overload but they demonstrate hypertrophy without dilatation poorly.

The next five chapters discuss these basic tools in depth (i.e., history, physical examination, ECG, chest roentgenogram) and provide flow diagrams, which help to correctly diagnose pediatric cardiac problems.

1 / History Taking

As in the evaluation of any other system, history taking is a basic step in cardiac evaluation. Maternal history during pregnancy is often helpful in the diagnosis of congenital heart disease (CHD) because certain prenatal events are known to be teratogenic. Past history, including the immediate postnatal period, provides more direct information relevant to the cardiac evaluation. Family history also helps link a cardiac problem to other medical problems that may be prevalent in the family. Box 1-1 lists important aspects of history taking for children with potential cardiac problems.

GESTATIONAL AND NATAL HISTORY

Infections, medications, and excessive smoking or alcohol intake may cause CHD, especially if they occur early in pregnancy.

Infections

Maternal rubella infection during the first trimester of pregnancy commonly results in multiple anomalies, including cardiac defects. Infections by cytomegalovirus, herpesvirus, and coxsackievirus B are suspected to be teratogenic if they occur in early pregnancy. Infections by these viruses later in pregnancy may cause myocarditis.

Medications, Including Alcohol and Smoking

Several medications are suspected teratogens. Amphetamines have been associated with ventricular septal defect (VSD), patent ductus arteriosus (PDA), atrial septal defect

---

BOX 1–1

Selected Aspects of History Taking

Gestational and Natal History

Infection, medications, excessive smoking or alcohol intake during pregnancy
Birth weight

Postnatal (or Past) History

Weight gain and development, including feeding pattern
Cyanosis, "cyanotic spells," and squatting
Tachypnea, dyspnea, puffy eyelids
Frequency of respiratory infection
Exercise intolerance
Heart murmur
Chest pain
Joint symptoms
Neurologic symptoms
Medications

Family History

Hereditary disease
CHD
Rheumatic fever
Sudden unexpected death
Diabetes mellitus, arteriosclerotic heart disease, hypertension, and so on

---

(ASD), and transposition of the great arteries (TGA). Other medications suspected of causing CHD include anticonvulsants (hydantoin has been associated with pulmonary stenosis [PS], aortic stenosis [AS], coarctation of the aorta [COA], and PDA, and trimethadione with TGA, tetralogy of Fallot [TOF], and hypoplastic left heart syndrome [HLHS]), progesterone/estrogen (VSD, TOF, TGA), and alcohol (fetal alcohol syndrome, in which VSD, PDA, ASD, and TOF are common). Although cigarette smoking has not been proved to be teratogenic, it does cause intrauterine growth retardation.

Maternal Conditions

There is a high incidence of cardiomyopathy in infants born to diabetic mothers. In addition, these babies have a higher incidence of structural heart defects (e.g., TGA, VSD, PDA). Maternal lupus erythematosus and mixed connective tissue disease have been associated with a high incidence of congenital heart block in offspring. The incidence of CHD increases from about 1% in the general population to as much as 15% if the mother has CHD, even if it is postoperative (see Table A-2 in Appendix A).

Birth Weight

Birth weight provides important information about the nature of the cardiac problem. If an infant is small for gestational age, this may indicate intrauterine infections. Rubella syndrome is a typical example. Infants with high birth weight, often seen in offspring of diabetic mothers, show a higher incidence of cardiac anomalies. Infants with TGA often have a birth weight higher than average; of course, these infants are cyanotic.

POSTNATAL HISTORY

Weight Gain and Development, Including Feeding Pattern

Weight gain and general development may be delayed in infants and children with congestive heart failure (CHF) or severe cyanosis. Weight is affected more significantly than height. If weight is severely affected, physicians should suspect a more general dysmorphic condition. Poor feeding of recent onset may be an early sign of CHF in infants, especially if the poor feeding is the result of fatigue and dyspnea.

Cyanosis, "Cyanotic Spells," and Squatting

If the parents think that their child is cyanotic, the physician should ask them about the onset of cyanosis (e.g., did it occur in the nursery, shortly after coming home), its severity, permanent or paroxysmal nature, and whether the cyanosis becomes worse after feeding.

A true "cyanotic spell" is seen most frequently in infants with TOF and requires immediate attention. Physicians should ask about the time of its appearance (e.g., in the morning on waking, after feeding), duration of the spell, and frequency of the spells. Most important is whether infants were breathing *fast* and *deep* during the spell or were holding their breath. This helps differentiate between a true cyanotic spell and a breath-holding spell. The physician should ask whether the child squats when tired or has a favorite position (such as knee-chest position) when tired. A history of squatting strongly suggests cyanotic heart disease, particularly TOF.

Tachypnea, Dyspnea, and Puffy Eyelids

These are signs of CHF. Left-sided heart failure produces tachypnea with or without dyspnea. Tachypnea becomes worse with feeding and eventually results in poor feeding and poor weight gain. A sleeping respiratory rate of more than 40 breaths/min is noteworthy. A rate of more than 60 breaths/min is abnormal, even in a newborn. Wheezing or persistent cough at night may be an early sign of CHF. Puffy eyelids and sacral edema are signs of systemic venous congestion. The ankle edema, which is commonly seen in adults, is not found in infants.

Frequency of Respiratory Infections

CHDs with large left-to-right shunts and an increased pulmonary blood flow (PBF) predispose to lower respiratory tract infections. Frequent upper respiratory tract infections are not related to CHD, although children with vascular rings may sound as if they have a chronic upper respiratory tract infection.

Exercise Intolerance

Decreased exercise tolerance may result from any significant heart disease, including large left-to-right shunt lesions, cyanotic defects, valvular stenosis or regurgitation, and arrhythmias. Obese children may be inactive and have decreased exercise tolerance in the absence of heart disease. An excellent assessment of exercise tolerance may be obtained by asking the following questions: Does the child keep up with other children? How many blocks can the child walk or run? How many flights of stairs can the child climb without fatigue? Does the weather or the time of day influence the child's exercise tolerance?

With infants who do not walk or run, an estimate of exercise tolerance may be gained from the infant's history of feeding pattern. The parents often say that their child takes naps; however, many normal children nap regularly.

Heart Murmur

If a heart murmur is the chief complaint, the physician should obtain information about the time of its first appearance and the circumstances of its discovery. A heart murmur heard within a few hours of birth usually indicates a stenotic lesion (AS, PS) or small left-to-right shunt lesions (VSD, PDA). The murmur of large left-to-right shunt lesions, such as VSD or PDA, may be delayed because of slow regression of pulmonary vascular resistance (PVR). In the case of stenotic lesion, the onset of the murmur is not affected by the PVR, and the murmur is usually heard shortly after birth. A heart murmur that is first noticed on a routine examination of a healthy-looking child is more likely to be innocent, especially if the same physician has been following the child's progress. A febrile illness is often associated with the discovery of a heart murmur.

Chest Pain

If chest pain is the primary complaint, the physician asks whether the pain is activity related (e.g., Do you have chest pain only when you are active, or does it come even when you watch television?) The physician also asks about the duration (e.g., seconds, minutes, hours), nature of the pain (e.g., stabbing, squeezing), and radiation to other parts of the body (e.g., neck, left shoulder, left arm). The physician needs to determine whether the pain was accompanied by syncope or palpitation. Chest pain of cardiac origin is not sharp but rather a deep, heavy pressure or the feeling of choking or a squeezing sensation, and it is usually triggered by exercise. The physician should ask whether deep breathing improves or worsens the pain. Pain of a cardiac origin, except for pericarditis, is not affected by respiration. The physician should also ask whether the patient has experienced a recent trauma to the chest or has engaged in activity that may have resulted in a pectoralis muscle soreness. Parents should be asked whether there has been a recent cardiac death in the family. The three most common noncardiac causes of chest pain in children are costochondritis, trauma to the chest wall or chest muscle strain, and respiratory disease (bronchitis, pneumonia, pleuritis, and so on) (see Chapter 34).

Cardiac conditions that may cause chest pain include severe AS (usually associated with activity), pulmonary vascular obstructive disease (PVOD), and mitral valve prolapse (MVP), which is not necessarily associated with activity, but there may be a history of palpitation. There is increasing doubt as to the causal relationship between chest pain and MVP in children. Less common cardiac conditions that can cause chest pain include severe PS, pericarditis of various etiology, and Kawasaki's disease (in which stenosis or aneurysm of coronary artery is common). Most children complaining of chest pain do not have a cardiac condition (see Chapter 34).

Palpitation

Palpitation is a subjective feeling of rapid heart beats. Some children incorrectly report an irregularity in heart rate as palpitation. Paroxysms of tachycardia or single premature beats commonly cause palpitation. Children with MVP may first be taken to the physician for the complaint of palpitation.

Joint Symptoms

When joint pain is the primary complaint, rheumatic arthritis is a possibility. The physician should ask about the number of joints involved, duration of the symptom, and migratory or stationary nature of the pain. Arthritis of acute rheumatic fever typically involves large joints, either simultaneously or in succession, with characteristic migratory nature. If the patient has recently had a sore throat the physician should ask whether a throat culture was taken. The parents should be asked whether the child had rashes suggestive of scarlet fever and can (or could) walk. If the child can walk, then the child probably does not have rheumatic arthritis in the leg. Pain in rheumatic joints is so severe that children refuse to walk. Also, if rubbing the joint alleviates the pain, it is probably not a rheumatic joint. It is important to ask the parents about aspirin or other analgesics administered (i.e., dose, number, timing), since even small doses of salicylates may suppress the full manifestation of joint symptoms of rheumatic fever or may abolish joint pain completely. The physician also asks whether the joint was swollen, red, hot, or tender. Abdominal pain, chest pain (pericarditis), and nosebleeds, all of which may be seen in rheumatic fever, should also be discussed (see Chapter 20).

Neurologic Symptoms

A history of stroke suggests embolization or thrombosis secondary to cyanotic CHD with polycythemia or infective endocarditis. A history of headache may be a manifestation of cerebral hypoxia with cyanotic heart disease, severe polycythemia, or brain abscess in cyanotic children. Although it is claimed in adults, hypertension with or without COA rarely causes headaches in children. Choreic movement strongly suggests rheumatic fever. A history of syncope may suggest arrhythmias, particularly ventricular arrhythmias, and may be seen in long QT syndrome (e.g., Jervell and Lange-Nielsen syndrome, Romano-Ward syndrome) and MVP. Syncope related to exercise may result from severe AS. It should be pointed out, however, that vasodepressor syncope without underlying cardiac disease is the most common syncope in children (see Chapter 35).

Medications

Physicians should note the name, dosage, timing, and duration of cardiac and noncardiac medications. Medications may be responsible for chief complaints or certain physical findings. Tachycardia and palpitation may be caused by cold medications or antiasthmatic drugs such as aminophylline and related drugs.

FAMILY HISTORY

Hereditary Disease

Some hereditary diseases may be associated with certain forms of CHDs. For example, Marfan's syndrome is frequently associated with aortic aneurysm or with aortic and/or mitral insufficiency. PS, which is secondary to dysplastic pulmonary valve, is common in Noonan's syndrome. Lentiginous skin lesion (LEOPARD syndrome) is often associated with PS and cardiomyopathy. Table 1-1 lists selected hereditary diseases in which cardiovascular disease is frequently found.

Congenital Heart Disease

The incidence of CHD in the general population is about 1% or, more precisely, 8 to 12 of 1000 live births. This does not include PDA in premature infants. The recurrence risk of CHDs associated with inherited diseases or with chromosomal abnormalities is related to the recurrent risk of the syndromes.

TABLE 1–1.

Hereditary Diseases Associated with Cardiovascular Abnormalities

Hereditary Diseases	Mode of Inheritance	Common Cardiac Disease	Important Clinical Features
Apert's syndrome	AD	Occasional; VSD, TOF	Irregular craniosynostosis with peculiar head and facial appearance, syndactyly of digits and toes
Carpenter's syndrome	AR	Occasional; PDA, VSD, PS, TGA	Variable craniosynostosis, mild facial hypoplasia, severe syndactyly ("mitten hands")
Cockayne's syndrome	AR	Accelerated atherosclerosis	Dwarfing, microcephaly, prominent nose and sunken eyes, visual loss
Crouzon's disease (craniofacial dysostosis)	AD	Occasional; PDA, COA	Ptosis with shallow orbits, craniosynostosis, maxillary hypoplasia
Cutis laxa	AR	Occasional; pulmonary hypertension, peripheral PA stenosis	Loose, pendulous skin; pulmonary emphysema
Ehlers-Danlos syndrome	AD	Frequent; aneurysm of aorta and carotids	Hyperextensive joints, hyperelasticity; fragility and bruisability of skin
Ellis-van Creveld syndrome (chrondroectodermal dysplasia)	AR	Frequent (50%); single atrium	Neonatal teeth, short distal limbs, polydactyly, nail hypoplasia
Friedreich's ataxia	AR	Frequent; cardiomyopathy	Late onset ataxia, skeletal deformities
Glycogen storage disease II (Pompe's disease)	AR	Very common; cardiomyopathy	Large tongue and flabby muscles, cardiomegaly; LVH and short PR interval on ECG, normal FBS and GTT
Holt-Oram syndrome (cardiac-limb)	AD	Frequent; ASD, VSD	Defects or absence of thumb or radius
Homocystinuria	AR	Frequent; medial degeneration of aorta and carotids, arterial or venous thrombus	Subluxation of lens, malar flush, osteoporosis, arachnodactyly with pectus excavatum or carinatum, mental defect
Hypertrophic obstructive cardiomyopathy	AD	Hypertrophic obstructive subaortic stenosis	
Kartagener's syndrome	AR	Dextrocardia	Situs inversus, chronic sinusitis and otitis media, bronchiectasis, abnormal respiratory cilia and immotile sperm
Laurence-Moon-Biedle syndrome	AR	Occasional; VSD, other CHDs	Obesity, retinitis pigmentosa, polydactyly, hypoplastic genitalia, diabetes mellitus, renal disease, mental retardation
LEOPARD syndrome	AD	Very common; PS, long PR interval, cardiomyopathy	*L*entiginous skin lesion, *E*CG abnormalities, *O*cular hypertelorism, *P*ulmonary stenosis, *A*bnormal genitalia, *R*etarded growth, *D*eafness

AD, Autosomal dominance; *AR,* autosomal recessive; *PA,* pulmonary artery; *LVH,* left ventricular hypertrophy; *FBS,* fasting blood sugar; *GTT,* glucose tolerance test; *MR,* mitral regurgitation; *AV,* atrioventricular; ±, may be present; *XR,* sex-linked recessive. *VSD,* ventricular septal defect; *TOF,* tetralogy of Fallot; *PDA,* patent ductus arteriosus; *PS,* pulmonary stenosis; *TGA,* transposition of the great arteries; *COA,* coarctation of the aorta; *ASD,* atrial septal defect; *CHD,* congenital heart disease or defect; *PR,* pulmonary regurgitation.

Continued.

TABLE 1–1. *Continued*

Hereditary Diseases	Mode of Inheritance	Common Cardiac Disease	Important Clinical Features
Long QT syndrome		Very common; Long QT interval on ECG, ventricular tachyarrhythmia	Congenital deafness (not in Romano-Ward syndrome), syncope resulting from ventricular dysrhythmias, family history of sudden death ($\pm$)
Jervell and Lange-Nielsen syndrome	AR		
Romano-Ward syndrome	AD		
Marfan's syndrome	AD	Frequent; aortic aneurysm, AR and/or MR	Arachnodactyly, subluxation of lens
MVP	AD	Frequent; MR, dysrhythmias	Thoracic skeletal anomalies (80%)
Mucopolysaccharidosis		Frequent; AR and/or MR, coronary artery disease	Coarse features, large tongue, depressed nasal bridge, kyphosis, retarded growth, hepatomegaly, corneal opacity (not in Hunter's syndrome), mental retardation
Hurler's syndrome (type I)	AR		
Hunter's syndrome (type II)	XR		
Morquio's syndrome (type IV)	AR		
Muscular dystrophy (Duchenne's type)	XR	Frequent; cardiomyopathy	Waddling gait, "pseudohypertrophy" of calf muscle
Neurofibromatosis (von Recklinghausen's disease)	AD	Occasional; PS, COA, pheochromocytoma	Café-au-lait spots, acoustic neuroma, variety of bone lesions
Noonan's syndrome	AD	Frequent; PS (dystrophic pulmonary valve), LVH (or anterior septal hypertrophy)	Similar to Turner's syndrome but may occur in phenotypic male and without chromosomal abnormality
Rendu-Osler-Weber syndrome	AD	Occasional; pulmonary arteriovenous fistula	Hepatic involvement, telangiectases, hemangioma or fibrosis
Osteogenesis imperfecta	AD/AR	Occasional; aortic dilatation, AR, MVP	Excessive bone fragility with deformities of skeleton, blue sclera, hyperlaxity of joints

MVP, Mitral valve prolapse.

Most CHDs are caused by genetic-environmental interaction (i.e., multifactorial inheritance). History of CHDs in close relatives increases the chance of CHD in a child. When one child is affected, the risk of recurrence in siblings is about 3%, which is a threefold increase. However, the risk of recurrence is related to the incidence of particular defects. In general, lesions with higher incidence (e.g., VSD) tend to have a higher risk of recurrence. Lesions with lower incidence (e.g., tricuspid atresia, persistent truncus arteriosus) have a lower risk of recurrence. Table A-1 in Appendix A lists the suggested recurrence risk figures for various CHDs, which can be used for counseling. Recently, the importance of cytoplasmic inheritance has been shown in some families based on the observation that the recurrence risk is substantially higher if the mother is the affected parent (See Table A-2 in Appendix A), which can also be used for counseling when a prospective parent had a CHD.)

Rheumatic Fever

Rheumatic fever frequently occurs in more than one family member. There is a higher incidence among relatives of rheumatic children. Although the knowledge of genetic factors involved in rheumatic fever is incomplete, it is generally agreed that there is an inherited susceptibility to acquiring rheumatic fever. A single autosomal-recessive gene may cause rheumatic fever.

TABLE 1–1. *Continued*

Hereditary Diseases	Mode of Inheritance	Common Cardiac Disease	Important Clinical Features
Progeria (Hutchinson-Gilford syndrome)	AR	Accelerated atherosclerosis	Alopecia, atrophy of subcutaneous fat, skeletal hypoplasia and dysplasia
Shprintzen's syndrome (velocardiofacial syndrome)	AD?	Very common (85%); VSD, right aortic arch, TOF	Conductive hearing loss, auricular anomalies, prominent nose with squared nasal root and narrow alar base, vertical maxillary excess with long face
Smith-Lemli-Opitz syndrome	AR	Occasional; VSD, PDA, others	Short statue, microcephaly, ptosis, anteverted nose, micrognasia, syndactyly toes, mental retardation
Thrombocytopenia-absent radius (TAR) syndrome	AR	Occasional (33%); ASD, TOF, dextrocardia	Thrombocytopenia, hypoplastic radius, normal thumb
Treacher Collins syndrome	AD	Occasional; VSD, PDA, ASD	Mandibular and maxillary hypoplasia, downslanting eyes, ear malformation, cleft palate
Tuberous sclerosis	AD	Frequent; rhabdomyoma	Triad of adenoma sebaceum (2 to 5 years of age), convulsion, and mental defect
von Hippel Lindau disease	AD	Frequent; hemangiomas, pheochromocytoma with hypertension	Asymptomatic till late adolescence; hemangiomatosis of cerebellum, retina, and skin
Williams syndrome	AD	Frequent; supravalvar AS, PA stenosis	Mental retardation, peculiar "elfin" facies, hypercalcemia of infancy?
Zellweger syndrome	AR	Frequent; PDA, VSD or ASD	Hypotonia, high forehead with flat facies, hepatomegaly

Hypertension and Atherosclerosis

Essential hypertension and coronary artery disease show a strong familial pattern. Therefore when a physician suspects hypertension in a young person, the family history is important to obtain. Atherosclerosis results from a complex process in which hereditary and environmental factors interact. The most important risk factor of atherosclerosis is onset of CHD before the age of 55 in male parents or grandparents and before the age of 60 in female parents or grandparents (see Chapter 33).

2 / Physical Examination

As with the examination of any child, the order and extent of a physical examination of infants and children with potential cardiac problems should be individualized. The more innocuous procedures, such as inspection, should be done first, and the more frightening or uncomfortable parts should be delayed until later in the examination.

Supine is the preferred position for examination of the patient in any age group. However, if older infants and young children between 1 and 3 years of age refuse to lie down, they may be examined initially while sitting on their mothers' laps.

The growth chart should reflect height and weight in terms of absolute values and also in percentiles. Accurate plotting and following of the growth curve is an essential part of initial and follow-up evaluations.

INSPECTION

Much information can be gained by simple inspection without disturbing a sleeping infant or frightening a child with a stethoscope. Inspection should include the following: general appearance and nutritional state; any obvious syndrome or chromosomal abnormalities; color (i.e., cyanosis, pallor, jaundice), clubbing, respiratory rate, dyspnea, and retraction; sweat on the forehead; and the chest.

General Appearance and Nutritional State

The physician should note whether the child is in distress, well-nourished or undernourished, and happy or cranky.

Chromosomal Syndromes

Obvious chromosomal abnormalities known to be associated with certain congenital heart defects (CHDs) should be noted by the physician. For example, about 50% of children with Down syndrome have a CHD; the two most common defects associated with this syndrome are endocardial cushion defect (ECD) and ventricular septal defect (VSD). A newborn with trisomy 18 syndrome usually has a CHD. Table 2-1 shows cardiac defects associated with selected chromosomal abnormalities.

Hereditary or Nonhereditary Syndromes and Other Systemic Malformations

A high incidence of congenital cardiovascular anomalies are associated with a number of hereditary or nonhereditary syndromes and malformations of other systems. For example, a child with a missing thumb or deformities of a forearm may have an atrial septal defect (ASD) or a VSD (e.g., Holt-Oram syndrome, cardiac-limb syndrome). Newborns with CHARGE association (coloboma, heart defects, choanal atresia, growth/mental retardation, genitourinary anomalies, ear anomalies) show a high incidence of conotruncal abnormalities (e.g., tetralogy of Fallot (TOF), double-outlet right ventricle [DORV], persistent truncus arteriosus). For a list of cardiac anomalies in selected hereditary diseases see Table 1-1. Nonhereditary syndromes and diseases in which cardiovascular abnormalities are known to occur are shown in Table 2-2. Congenital malformations of certain organ systems are associated with an increased incidence of CHDs (Table 2-3).

10

TABLE 2–1.

CHD in Selected Chromosomal Aberrations

Conditions	Incidence of CHD (%)	Common Defects in Decreasing Order of Frequency
5p−(Cri du chat syndrome)	25	VSD, PDA, ASD
Trisomy 13 syndrome	90	VSD, PDA, dextrocardia
Trisomy 18 syndrome	99	VSD, PDA, PS
Trisomy 21 (Down syndrome)	50	ECD, VSD
Turner's syndrome (XO)	35	COA, AS, ASD
Klinefelter's variant (XXXXY)	15	PDA, ASD

VSD, ventricular septal defect; *PDA*, patent ductus arteriosus; *ASD*, atrial septal defect; *PS*, pulmonary stenosis; *ECD*, endocardial cushion defect; *COA*, coarctation of the aorta; *AS*, aortic stenosis; *CHD*, congenital heart disease.

TABLE 2–2.

Nonhereditary Syndromes with Cardiovascular Anomalies

Syndromes	Frequency and Type of Cardiovascular Anomalies	Important Clinical Features of Syndromes
CHARGE association	Common (65%); conotruncal anomalies (e.g., TOF, truncus arteriosus), aortic arch anomalies (e.g., vascular ring, interrupted aortic arch)	*C*oloboma, *h*eart defects, choanal *a*tresia, growth/mental *r*etardation, *g*enitourinary anomalies, *e*ar anomalies, genital hypoplasia
Congenital diaphragmatic hernia	Occasional (25%); VSD, TOF	Diaphragmatic hernia, pulmonary hypoplasia
Cornelia de Lange's (de Lange's) syndrome	Occasional (30%); VSD	Prenatal growth retardation, microcephaly, hirsuitism, synophrys, anteverted nares, downturned mouth, mental retardation
DiGeorge syndrome	Frequent; interrupted aortic arch, truncus arteriosus, VSD, PDA, TOF	Hypertelorism, short philtrum, downslanting eyes, hypoplastic thymus and parathyroid, hypocalcemia, deficient cell-mediated immunity
Fetal alcohol syndrome	Frequent (25% to 30%); VSD, PDA, ASD, TOF	Prenatal growth retardation, microcephaly, short palpebral fissure, mental deficiency, irritable infant or hyperactive child
Fetal hydantoin syndrome	Occasional (<5%); PS, AS, COA, PDA, VSD, ASD	Prenatal growth retardation; mild mental retardation; hypertelorism; broad, depressed nasal bridge; hypoplastic nails and phalanges
Fetal trimethadione syndrome	Frequent (15% to 30%); TGA, VSD, TOF	Ear malformation, hypoplastic midface, unusual eyebrow configuration, mental deficiency, speech disorder
Fetal warfarin syndrome	Occasional (15% to 45%); TOF, VSD	Facial asymmetry and hypoplasia, microtia, ear tags, cleft lip or palate, epitubular dermoid, hypoplastic vertebrae

PPHN, Persistent pulmonary hypertension of newborn; *PFC*, persistent fetal circulation; *TOF*, tetralogy of Fallot; *VSD*, ventricular septal defect; *PDA*, patent ductus arteriosus; *ASD*, atrial septal defect; *COA*, coarctation of the aorta; *TGA*, transposition of the great arteries; *CHD*, congenital heart disease or defect.

TABLE 2–2.   *Continued*

Syndromes	Frequency and Type of Cardiovascular Anomalies	Important Clinical Features of Syndromes
Infant of diabetic mother	CHDs (3% to 5%); TGA, VSD, COA; cardio-myopathy (10 to 20%); PPHN (PFC syndrome)	Macrosomia; hypoglycemia and hypocalcemia; polycythemia; hyperbilirubinemia; other congenital anomalies
Pierre Robin syndrome	Occasional (29%); VSD, PDA; less commonly ASD, COA, TOF	Deafness, cataracts, CHDs, mental deficiency, hepato-splenomegaly, jaundice, thrombocytopenia, anemia
VATER association (VATER/VACTERL syndrome)	Frequent (>50%); VSD, other defects	*V*ertebral defects, *a*nal atresia, *c*ongenital heart defects, *tr*a-cheoesophageal fistula, *r*enal dysplasia, *l*imb anomalies (e.g., radial dysplasia)

TABLE 2–3.

Incidence of Associated CHDs in Patients with Other System Malformations

Organ System and Malformations	Frequency Ranges (%)	Specific Cardiac Defects
CNS		
Hydrocephalus	6 (4.5 to 14.9)	VSD, ECD, TOF
Dandy-Walker syndrome	3 (2.5 to 4.3)	VSD
Agenesis of corpus callosum	15	No specific defects
Meckel-Gruber syndrome	14	No specific defects
Thoracic Cavity		
TE fistula and/or esophageal atresia	21 (15 to 39)	VSD, ASD, TOF
Diaphragmatic hernia	11 (9.6 to 22.9)	No specific defects
Gastrointestinal		
Duodenal atresia	17	No specific defects
Jejunal atresia	5	No specific defects
Anorectal anomalies	22	No specific defects
Imperforate anus	12	TOF, VSD
Ventral Wall		
Omphalocele	21 (19 to 32)	No specific defects
Gastroschisis	3 (0 to 7.7)	No specific defects
Genitourinary		
Renal agenesis		
Bilateral	43	No specific defects
Unilateral	17	No specific defects
Horseshoe kidney	39	No specific defects
Renal dysplasia	5	No specific defects

CNS, Central nervous system; *TE*, tracheoesophageal, *CHD*, congenital heart disease or defect; *VSD*, ventricular septal defect; *ECD*, endocardial cushion defect; *TOF*, tetralogy of Fallot; *ASD*, atrial septal defect.
Modified from Copel JA et al: *Am J Obstet Gynecol* 154:1121, 1986.

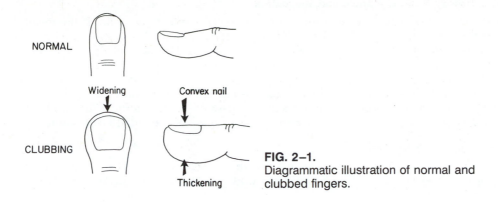

NORMAL

Widening   Convex nail

CLUBBING

Thickening

FIG. 2–1.
Diagrammatic illustration of normal and clubbed fingers.

Color

The physician should note whether the child is cyanotic, pale, or jaundiced. In cases of cyanosis, the degree and distribution should be noted (e.g., throughout the body, only on the lower or upper half of the body). Mild cyanosis is difficult to detect. The arterial saturation is usually 85% or lower before cyanosis is detectable in patients with normal hemoglobin levels (see Chapter 11). Cyanosis is more noticeable in natural light than in artificial light. Cyanosis of the lips may be misleading, particularly in children who have deep pigmentation. The physician should also check the tongue, buccal mucosa, nail beds, and conjunctiva. Children with cyanosis do not always have cyanotic CHD. Cyanosis may result from respiratory diseases or central nervous system disorders. Cyanosis that is associated with arterial desaturation is called *central cyanosis*. Cyanosis associated with normal arterial saturation is called *peripheral cyanosis*. Even mild cyanosis in a newborn requires thorough investigation (see Chapter 29).

Peripheral cyanosis may be noticeable in newborns who experienced exposure to cold, congestive heart failure (CHF) because of sluggish peripheral blood flow, or polycythemia. Circumoral cyanosis describes cyanosis around the mouth, which is found in either normal children with fair skin or children with cyanotic CHD. Isolated circumoral cyanosis is not significant. Acrocyanosis is a bluish or red discoloration of the fingers and toes in the presence of normal arterial oxygen saturation. Normal newborns often experience acrocyanosis. Cyanosis should be checked against the hematocrit. Polycythemic infants may look cyanotic without arterial desaturation.

Pallor may be seen in infants with vasoconstriction from CHF or circulatory shock or in severely anemic infants. Newborns with severe CHF and those with congenital hypothyroidism may have prolonged physiologic jaundice. Patent ductus arteriosus (PDA) and pulmonary stenosis (PS) are common in newborns with congenital hypothyroidism. Hepatic disease with jaundice may cause arterial desaturation because of pulmonary arteriovenous fistula (e.g., arteriohepatic dysplasia).

Clubbing

Long-standing arterial desaturation (usually longer than 6 months), even if too mild to be detected by an inexperienced person, results in clubbing of the fingernails and toenails. When fully developed, clubbing is characterized by a widening and thickening of the ends of the fingers and toes, as well as by convex fingernails and loss of angle between the nail and nail bed (Fig. 2-1). Reddening and shininess of the terminal phalanges are seen in the early stage of clubbing. Clubbing appears earliest and most noticeably in the thumb. It may also be associated with lung disease (e.g., abscess), cirrhosis of the liver, and subacute bacterial endocarditis (SBE). Occasionally, clubbing occurs in normal people. This is called *familial clubbing*.

Respiratory Rate, Dyspnea, and Retraction

The physician should note the respiratory rate of every infant and child. If the infant breathes irregularly, the physician should count for a minute. The respiratory rate is faster in children who are crying, upset, eating, or feverish. The most reliable respiratory rate is that taken during sleep. After finishing a bottle of formula, an infant may breathe faster than normal for 5 to 10 minutes. A resting respiratory rate of more than 40 breaths/min is unusual and more than 60 breaths/min is abnormal at any age. Tachypnea, along with tachycardia, is the earliest sign of left-sided heart failure. If the child has dyspnea or retraction, this signals a more severe degree of left-sided heart failure.

Sweat on the Forehead

Infants with CHF often have a cold sweat on their foreheads. This is an expression of sympathetic overactivity as a compensatory mechanism for the decreased cardiac output.

Inspection of the Chest

Precordial bulge, with or without actively visible cardiac activity, suggests *chronic* cardiac enlargement. Acute dilatation of the heart does not cause precordial bulge. Pigeon chest (i.e., pectus carinatum) in which the sternum protrudes on the midline is usually not a result of cardiomegaly.

Pectus excavatum (i.e., undue depression of the sternum) rarely, if ever, causes cardiac embarrassment. Rather, it may be a cause of a pulmonary systolic ejection murmur (SEM) or a large cardiac silhouette on a posteroanterior view of a chest roentgenogram, which compensates for the diminished anteroposterior (AP) diameter of the chest.

Harrison's groove, a line of depression in the bottom of the rib cage along the attachment of the diaphragm, indicates poor lung compliance of long duration such as that seen in large left-to-right shunt lesions.

PALPATION

Palpation should include the peripheral pulses (e.g., their presence or absence, the pulse rate, the volume of the pulses) and the precordium (e.g., the presence of a thrill, the point of maximal impulse [PMI], precordial hyperactivity). Although ordinarily palpation follows inspection, auscultation may be more fruitful on a sleeping infant who might wake up and become uncooperative.

Peripheral Pulses

1. The physician should count the pulse rate and note any irregularities in the rate and volume. The normal pulse rate varies with the patient's age and status. The younger the patient, the faster the pulse rate. Increased pulse rate may indicate excitement, fever, CHF, or arrhythmia. Bradycardia may mean heart block, digitalis toxicity, and so on. Irregularity of the pulse suggests arrhythmias, but sinus arrhythmia (an acceleration with inspiration) is normal.

2. The right and left arm and an arm and a leg should be compared for the volume of the pulse. Every patient should have palpable pedal pulses, either dorsalis pedis, tibialis posterior, or both. It is often easier to feel pedal pulses than femoral pulses, particularly on sleeping infants. Attempts at palpating a femoral pulse often wake up a sleeping infant or upset a toddler. If a good pedal pulse is felt, coarctation of the aorta (COA) is effectively ruled out, especially if the blood pressure in the arm is normal.

   Weak leg pulses and strong arm pulses suggest COA. If the right brachial pulse is stronger than the left brachial pulse, then this finding is associated with COA proximal to or near the origin of the left subclavian artery or supravalvular aortic stenosis.

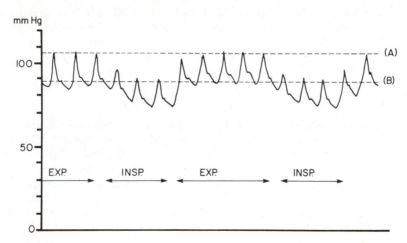

FIG. 2–2.
Diagrammatic drawing of pulsus paradoxus. Note the reduction of systolic pressure of more than 10 mm Hg during inspiration. *EXP,* Expiration; *INSP,* inspiration.

3. Bounding pulses are found in aortic run-off lesions such as PDA, aortic regurgitation (AR), large systemic arteriovenous fistula, or persistent truncus arteriosus (rarely). Pulses are bounding in premature infants because of the lack of subcutaneous tissue and because many have a PDA.

4. Weak, thready pulses are found in cardiac failure or circulatory shock or in the leg of a patient with COA. Systemic-to-pulmonary artery shunt (either classic Blalock-Taussig shunt or modified Gore-Tex shunt) or the subclavian flap angioplasty for repair of COA may result in an absent or a weak pulse in the arm affected by surgery. Arterial injuries resulting from a previous cardiac catheterization may cause a weak pulse in the affected limb.

5. Pulsus paradoxus (i.e., paradoxical pulse) is suspected when there is marked variation in the volume of arterial pulses with respiratory cycle. The term *pulsus paradoxus* does *not* indicate a phase reversal; rather, it is an exaggeration of normal reduction of systolic pressure during inspiration. Accurate evaluation requires sphygmomanometry (Fig. 2-2). This condition may be associated with cardiac tamponade secondary to pericardial effusion or constrictive pericarditis or to severe respiratory difficulties seen with asthma or pneumonia. It is also seen in patients who are on ventilators with high pressure settings, but then the blood pressure increases with inflation.

   The presence of pulsus paradoxus is confirmed by the use of sphygmomanometer as follows:

   a. The cuff pressure is raised about 20 mm Hg above the systolic pressure.

   b. The pressure is lowered slowly until Korotkoff sound I is heard for some but not all cardiac cycles and the reading is noted (line *A* on Fig. 2-2).

   c. The pressure is lowered further until systolic sounds are heard for all cardiac cycles and the reading is noted (line *B* on Fig. 2-2).

   d. If the difference between readings *A* and *B* is greater than 10 mm Hg, pulsus paradoxus is present.

Chest

Palpate the following: apical impulse, point of maximal impulse (PMI), hyperactivity of the precordium, and palpable thrill.

Apical impulse. Palpation of the apical impulse is usually superior to percussion in detection of cardiomegaly. Its location and diffuseness should be noted. Percussion in infants and children is inaccurate and adds little. The apical impulse is normally at the 5th intercostal space (5ICS) in the midclavicular line after age 7. Before this age, the apical impulse is in the fourth intercostal space (4ICS) just to the left of the midclavicular line. The apical impulse displaced laterally and/or downward suggests cardiac enlargement.

Point of maximal impulse. The PMI is helpful in determining whether the right ventricle (RV) or left ventricle (LV) is dominant. With RV dominance, the impulse is maximal at the lower left sternal border (LLSB) or over the xiphoid process; with LV dominance, the impulse is maximal at the apex. Normal newborns and infants have RV dominance and therefore more RV impulse than older children. If the impulse is more diffuse and slow rising, it is called a *heave*. If it is well localized and sharp rising, it is called a *tap*. Heaves are more often associated with volume overload. Taps are associated with pressure overload.

Hyperactive precordium. The presence of a hyperactive precordium characterizes heart disease with volume overload such as that seen in CHD with large left-to-right shunts (e.g., PDA, VSD) or in heart disease with severe valvular regurgitation (e.g., AR, mitral regurgitation [MR]).

Thrills. Thrills are vibratory sensations that represent palpable manifestations of loud, harsh murmurs. Palpation for thrills is often of diagnostic value. A thrill on the chest is felt better with the palm of the hand than with the tips of the fingers. However, the fingers are used to feel a thrill in the suprasternal notch (SSN) and over the carotid arteries.

1. Thrills in the upper left sternal border (ULSB) originate from the pulmonary valve or pulmonary artery (PA) and therefore are present in PS, PA stenosis, or PDA (rarely).

2. Thrills in the upper right sternal border (URSB) are usually of aortic origin and are seen in aortic stenosis (AS).

3. Thrills in the LLSB are characteristic of a VSD.

4. Thrills in the SSN suggest AS but may be found in PS, PDA, or COA.

5. The presence of a thrill over the carotid artery or arteries accompanied by a thrill in the SSN suggests diseases of the aorta or aortic valve (e.g., COA, AS). An isolated thrill in one of the carotid arteries without a thrill in the SSN may be a carotid bruit.

6. Thrills in the intercostal spaces are found in older children with severe COA that has extensive intercostal collaterals.

BLOOD PRESSURE MEASUREMENT

When possible, every child should have a blood pressure measurement as part of the physical examination. However, there are problems associated with indirect blood pressure measurement in infants and children. Unacceptably wide ranges of normative blood pressure levels have been reported. A new set of normal blood pressure data recommended by the National Institutes of Health Task Force on Blood Pressure Control in Children (1987) created further confusion because it is considerably lower than that reported in 1977. The methodology used in both recommendations is problematic (see Chapter 31).

Before taking a blood pressure measurement, the physician must select the correct size of cuff. Cuffs that are too narrow overestimate the true blood pressure, cuffs that are too wide underestimate the true pressure. To determine the correct size of cuff, in 1977 the NIH Task Force recommended that the width of the cuff's air bladder be

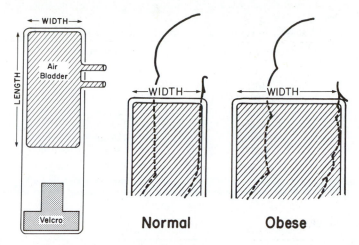

FIG. 2–3.
Diagram showing a method of selecting an appropriate-sized BP cuff. The selection is based on the thickness rather than the length of the arm. The end of the cuff is at the top, and the cuff width is then compared with the circumference or diameter of the arm. The width of the inflatable part of the cuff (bladder, *cross-hatched areas*) should be 40% to 50% of the circumference (or 125% to 155% of the diameter) of the arm. *BP,* Blood pressure.

two-thirds the length of the upper arm. In 1987 the same task force recommended that the cuff width be three-fourths the length of the upper arm. Selecting the cuff solely on the length of the arm is scientifically unsound, and doing so violates the physical principles underlying the indirect measurement. Studies in which indirect blood pressures were compared with intraarterial blood pressures also do not support this selection process. A committee of the American Heart Association recently recommended that the width of the cuff's bladder be 40% to 50% of the circumference (i.e., 125% to 155% of the diameter) of the limb on which the blood pressure is being measured (Fig. 2-3). This recommendation is scientifically sound and has been confirmed by numerous studies involving infants, children, and adults. Such studies proved that this standard applies for children and adults, and that it is important for the continuity of blood pressure levels from childhood to adulthood. The cuff selected by the American Heart Association criterion compensates for variation in arm thickness. Thickness of the arm is the most important factor in determining the compression of the underlying artery and therefore ensures the accuracy of the indirect auscultatory pressure. The air bladder should be long enough to completely or almost encircle the limb.

Some confusion still exists as to which should be taken as the diastolic signal—the point of muffling (phase IV) or the point of disappearance (phase V) of the Korotkoff sounds. In general, the point of muffling is closer to the true diastolic pressure than the point of disappearance in children. When the points of muffling and of disappearance are more than 6 mm Hg apart, both values should be noted; for example, 110/75/50 mm Hg, where 110 mm Hg is systolic pressure (i.e., the phase I of Korotkoff sound), 75 mm Hg is the point of muffling, and 50 mm Hg is the point of disappearance. When the points of muffling and of disappearance are less than 6 mm Hg apart, the physician should record phase V as the diastolic pressure.

Although there is no single, reliable set of normative blood pressure values, a working guide of normal values is needed until more reliable data become available. Table 2-4 shows values adapted from well-conducted, large epidemiologic studies that based the selection of the cuff on the thickness of the arm.

TABLE 2–4.

Suggested Normal BP Values (mm Hg) by Auscultatory Method (systolic/diastolic K5)

Age (in years)	Mean BP Levels	90th Percentile	95th Percentile
6 to 7	104/55	114/73	117/78
8 to 9	106/58	118/76	120/82
10 to 11*	108/60	120/77	124/82
12 to 13*	112/62	124/78	128/83
14 to 15 boys	116/66	132/80	138/86
girls	112/68	126/80	130/83
16 to 18 boys	121/70	136/82	140/86
girls	110/68	125/81	127/84

Modified from Goldring et al: *J Pediatr* 91:884, 1977; Prineas et al: *Hypertension* suppl 1:18, 1980.
*Values for ages 10 to 13 years have been extrapolated from these two studies using age-related increments from other studies.
BP, Blood pressure.
K5, the phase V of Korotkoff sound.

TABLE 2–5.

Normative BP Levels (systolic/diastolic/[mean]) by Dinamap Monitor in Children 5 Years Old and Younger

Age	Mean BP Levels (in mm Hg)	90th Percentile	95th Percentile
1 to 3 days	64/41 (50)	75/49 (50)	78/52 (62)
1 mo to 2 yr	95/58 (72)	106/68 (83)	110/71 (86)
2 to 5 yr	101/57 (74)	112/66 (82)	115/68 (85)

Modified from Park MK, Menard SM: *Am J Dis Child* 143:860, 1989.
BP, Blood pressure.

Recently, accuracy of indirect measurement by an oscillometric method (e.g., Dinamap) has been demonstrated. The American Heart Association's cuff width recommendation is also appropriate for the Dinamap method. The oscillometric method is not only accurate but also provides advantages over the auscultatory method: it eliminates observer-related variations, it can be successfully used in infants and small children, it eliminates controversies over the diastolic signals, and it provides mean pressure and heart rate. Normative blood pressure levels obtained by the Dinamap method for newborns and children 5 years old and younger are presented in Table 2-5.

The same selection criterion applies for the leg pressure determination (i.e., 40% to 50% of the leg's circumference or 125% to 155% of the diameter). Even when a considerably wider cuff is selected for the thigh, the systolic pressure in the thigh is 10 to 20 mm Hg higher than that obtained in the arm by the auscultatory method. By the Dinamap method, the systolic pressure in the thigh or calf is about 5 to 10 mm Hg higher than that found in the arm. Thus the systolic pressure in the thigh should be at least equal to that in the arm when using the appropriate cuffs. If the systolic pressure is lower, COA is likely. Thigh blood pressure determinations are mandatory in a child with hypertension in the arm. The presence of a femoral pulse does not rule out a coarctation.

AUSCULTATION

Although auscultation of the heart requires more skill, it also provides more valuable information than other methods of heart examination. The bell-type chest piece is better suited for detecting low-frequency events, whereas the diaphragm selectively picks up the high-frequency events. When the bell is firmly pressed against the chest wall, it acts like the diaphragm by filtering out low-frequency sounds or murmurs and by picking up high-frequency events. Physicians should not limit examination to the four traditional auscultatory areas. The entire precordium, as well as the sides and the back of the chest, should be explored with the stethoscope. Systematic attention should be given to the following aspects:

1. Heart rate and regularity: Heart rate and regularity should be noted on every child. Extremely fast or slow heart rates or irregularity in the rhythm should be evaluated by an ECG and a long rhythm strip (see Chapters 24 and 25).

2. Heart sounds: Intensity and quality of the heart sounds, especially the second heart sound (S2), should be evaluated. Abnormalities of the first heart sound (S1) and the third heart sound (S3) and the presence of a gallop rhythm or the fourth sound (S4) should also be noted.

3. Systolic and diastolic sounds: Systolic and diastolic sounds (e.g., an ejection click in early systole and midsystolic click) provide important clues to the diagnosis. An opening snap should be noted, but it is extremely rare in pediatrics.

4. Heart murmurs: Heart murmurs should be evaluated in terms of intensity, timing (systolic or diastolic), location, transmission, and quality.

Heart Sounds

The heart sound should be identified and analyzed before the analysis of heart murmurs.

First heart sound. The S1 is associated with closure of the mitral and tricuspid valves. It is best heard at the apex or LLSB. Splitting of the S1 may be found in normal children, but it is infrequent. Abnormally wide splitting of S1 may be found in right bundle branch block (RBBB) or Ebstein's anomaly. Splitting of S1 should be differentiated from:

1. Ejection click, which is more easily audible at the ULSB in PS; in bicuspid aortic valves the click may be louder at the LLSB or apex than at the URSB.

2. S4, which is rare in children.

Second heart sound. The S2 in the ULSB (i.e., pulmonary valve area) is of critical importance in pediatric cardiology. The S2 must be evaluated in terms of the degree of the S2's splitting and the relative intensity of the pulmonary closure component of the second heart sound (P2) in relation to the intensity of the aortic closure component of the second heart sound (A2). Although best heard with the diaphragm of a stethoscope, both components are readily audible with the bell. Abnormalities of splitting of the S2 and the intensity of the P2 are summarized in Box 2-1.

Splitting of the S2. In every normal child, with the exception of occasional newborns, two components of the S2 should be audible in the ULSB. The first is the A2; the second is the P2.

Normal splitting of the S2. The degree of splitting of the S2 varies with respiration, increasing with inspiration and decreasing or becoming single with expiration (Fig. 2-4).

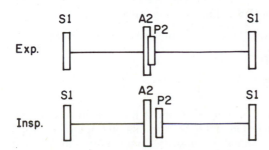

FIG. 2–4.
Diagram showing relative intensity of A2 and P2 and the respiratory variation in the degree of splitting of the S2 at the ULSB (pulmonary area). *Exp.,* Expiration; *Insp.,* inspiration.

BOX 2–1
Summary of Abnormal S2

Abnormal Splitting

Widely split and fixed S2
  Volume overload (e.g., ASD, PAPVR)
  Pressure overload (e.g., PS)
  Electrical delay (e.g., RBBB)
  Early aortic closure (e.g., MR)
  Occasional normal child
Narrowly split S2
  Pulmonary hypertension
  AS
  Occasional normal child
Single S2
  Pulmonary hypertension
  One semilunar valve (e.g., pulmonary atresia, aortic atresia, persistent truncus arteriosus)
  P2 not audible (e.g., TGA, TOF, severe PS)
  Severe AS
  Occasional normal child
Paradoxically split S2
  Severe AS
  LBBB, WPW syndrome (type B)

Abnormal Intensity of P2

Increased P2 (e.g., pulmonary hypertension)
Decreased P2 (e.g., severe PS, TOF, TS)

PAPVR, Partial anomalous pulmonary venous return; *MR*, mitral regurgitation; *LBBB*, left bundle branch block; *WPW*, Wolff-Parkinson-White; *TS*, tricuspid stenosis; *ASD*, atrial septal defect; *PS*, pulmonary stenosis; *RBBB*, right bundle branch block; *AS*, aortic stenosis; *TGA*, transposition of the great arteries; *TOF*, tetralogy of Fallot.

Although a new theory regarding the cause of normal respiratory variation in the splitting of the S2 is based on the vascular impedance of systemic and pulmonary circuits, the traditional explanation relates these events to the closure of the aortic and pulmonary valves. During inspiration, because of a greater negative pressure in the thoracic cavity, there is an increase in systemic venous return to the right side of the heart. This increased volume of blood in the RV prolongs the duration of RV ejection time, which delays the closure of the pulmonary valve resulting in a wide splitting of the S2. The absence of splitting (i.e., single S2) or a widely split S2 usually indicates an abnormality.

ABNORMAL SPLITTING OF THE S2. Abnormal splitting may be in the form of wide splitting, narrow splitting, a single S2, or paradoxical splitting of the S2 (rarely).

1. A widely split and fixed S2 is found in conditions that prolong the RV ejection time or that shorten the LV ejection. Therefore it is found in:

    a. ASD or partial anomalous pulmonary venous return (PAPVR) (conditions in which the amount of blood ejected by the RV is increased; *volume overload*).

    b. PS (the valve stenosis prolongs the RV ejection time; *pressure overload*).

    c. RBBB (a delay in *electrical* activation of the RV).

    d. MR (a decreased forward output seen in this condition shortens the LV ejection time).

    e. Occasional normal child, including "prolonged hangout time" seen in children with dilated PA (i.e., "idiopathic dilatation of the PA"). In dilated PA, the increased capacity of the artery produces less recoil to close the pulmonary valve, which delays closure.

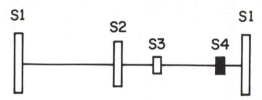

FIG. 2–5.
Diagram showing the relative relationship of the heart sounds. Filled bar shows an abnormal sound.

2. A narrowly split S2 is found in conditions in which the pulmonary valve closes early (e.g., pulmonary hypertension), or the aortic valve closure is delayed (e.g., AS). This is occasionally found in a normal child.

3. A single S2 is found when only one semilunar valve is present (e.g., aortic or pulmonary atresia, persistent truncus arteriosus), the P2 is not audible (e.g., transposition of the great arteries [TGA], TOF, severe PS), aortic closure is delayed (e.g., severe AS), and the P2 occurs early (e.g., severe pulmonary hypertension). This is also occasionally found in a normal child.

4. A *paradoxically split* S2 is found when the aortic closure (A2) follows the pulmonary closure (P2) and therefore is seen when the LV ejection is greatly delayed (e.g., severe AS, left bundle branch block (LBBB), sometimes Wolff-Parkinson-White (WPW) syndrome.

Intensity of the P2. The *relative* intensity of the P2 compared with the A2 must be assessed on every child. In the pulmonary area, the A2 is usually louder than the P2 (Fig 2-4). The A2 is *not* the S2 at the aortic area, rather the first (or aortic closure) component of the S2 at the pulmonary area (i.e., ULSB). Judgment as to normal intensity of the P2 is based on experience. There is no substitute for listening to the heart of many normal children.

Abnormal intensity of the P2 may suggest a pathologic condition. Increased intensity of the P2, compared with that of the A2, is found in pulmonary hypertension. Decreased intensity of the P2 is found in conditions with decreased diastolic pressure of the PA (i.e., severe PS, TOF, tricuspid atresia, and so on).

Third heart sound. The S3 is a somewhat low-frequency sound in early diastole and is related to rapid filling of the ventricle (Fig. 2-5). It is best heard at the apex or LLSB. It is commonly heard in normal children and young adults. A loud S3 is abnormal and is audible in conditions with dilated ventricles and decreased compliance (e.g., large-shunt VSD, CHF). When tachycardia is present, it forms a "Kentucky" gallop.

Fourth heart sound or atrial sound. The S4 is a relatively low-frequency sound of late diastole (i.e., presystole) and is rare in infants and children (Fig. 2-5). When present, it is always pathologic and is seen in conditions with decreased ventricular compliance or CHF. With tachycardia, it forms a "Tennessee" gallop.

Gallop rhythm. A gallop rhythm is a rapid triple rhythm resulting from the combination of a loud S3, with or without an S4, and tachycardia. It generally implies a pathologic condition and is commonly present in CHF. A summation gallop represents tachycardia and a superimposed S3 and S4.

Systolic and Diastolic Sounds

1. An ejection click (or ejection sound) follows the S1 very closely and occurs at the time of the ventricular ejection's onset. Therefore it sounds like a splitting of the S1. However, it is usually audible at the base (usually either side of the upper sternal border), whereas the split S1 is usually audible at the LLSB (exception with aortic click in later section). If the physician hears what sounds like a split S1 at the upper sternal border, it may be an ejection click (Fig. 2-6).

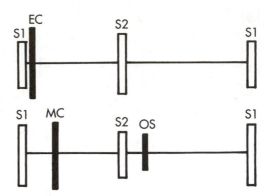

FIG. 2–6.
Diagram showing the relative position
of ejection click *(EC)*, midsystolic click
(MC), and diastolic opening snap
(OS). Filled bars show abnormal
sounds.

The pulmonary click is heard at the second left intercostal space (2LICS) and third left intercostal space (3LICS) and changes in intensity with respiration, being louder on expiration. The aortic click is best heard at the second right intercostal space (2RICS), but may be louder at the apex or mid-left sternal border (MLSB). It usually does not change its intensity with respiration.

The ejection click is most often associated with:

  a. Stenosis of semilunar valves (e.g., PS or AS).

  b. Dilated great arteries seen in systemic or pulmonary hypertension, idiopathic dilatation of the PA, TOF (in which the aorta is dilated), and persistent truncus arteriosus.

2. Midsystolic click with or without a late systolic murmur is heard at the apex in mitral valve prolapse (MVP) (Fig. 2-6 and Chapter 21).

3. Diastolic opening snap is rare in children and is audible at the apex or LLSB. It occurs somewhat earlier than the S3 during diastole and originates from a stenosis of the atrioventricular (AV) valve such as mitral stenosis (MS) (Fig 2-6).

Extracardiac sounds

1. A pericardial friction rub is a grating, to-and-fro sound produced by friction of the heart against the pericardium. This sounds similar to sandpaper rubbed on wood. Such a sound usually indicates pericarditis. The intensity of the rub varies with the phase of the cardiac cycle, rather than the respiratory cycle. It may become louder when the patient leans forward. Large accumulation of fluid (pericardial effusion) may result in disappearance of the rub.

2. A pericardial knock is an adventitious sound associated with chronic (i.e., constrictive) pericarditis. It rarely occurs in children.

Heart murmur. Each heart murmur must be analyzed in terms of intensity (i.e., grade 1 to 6), timing (i.e., systolic or diastolic), location, transmission, and quality (i.e., musical, vibratory, blowing, and so on).

Intensity. Intensity of the murmur is customarily graded from 1 to 6.

Grade 1   Barely audible
Grade 2   Soft, but easily audible
Grade 3   Moderately loud, but not accompanied by a thrill
Grade 4   Louder and associated with a thrill
Grade 5   Audible with the stethoscope barely on the chest
Grade 6   Audible with the stethoscope off the chest

The difference between grades 2 and 3 or grades 5 and 6 may be somewhat subjective. The intensity of the murmur may be influenced by the status of cardiac output. Thus any factor that increases the cardiac output (i.e., fever, anemia, anxiety, or exercise) intensifies any existing murmur or may even produce a murmur that is not audible at basal conditions.

Classification of heart murmurs. Based on the timing of the heart murmur in relation to the S1 and S2, the heart murmur is classified into three types:

1. Systolic murmur, further classified into an ejection type and a regurgitant type

2. Diastolic murmur, further classified into an early diastolic, middiastolic, and presystolic

3. Continuous murmur

Systolic murmurs

TYPES. Most heart murmurs are systolic in timing, in that they occur between the S1 and S2. A systolic murmur is usually classified as one of two types, ejection or regurgitant, depending on the timing of the *onset* of the heart murmur in relation to the S1.

In ejection murmurs (also called stenotic, diamond-shaped, crescendo-decrescendo murmurs), there is an interval between the S1 and the onset of the murmur. These murmurs are generally crescendo-decrescendo or "diamond-shaped" in contour (Fig. 2-7, A) and usually end before the S2. The murmur may be short or long. All systolic murmurs that are not regurgitant (see below) may be classified as ejection-type murmurs. These murmurs are caused by the flow of blood through stenotic or deformed semilunar valves or by increased flow through normal semilunar valves. Therefore ejection murmurs are found at the 2LICS or 2RICS. One source of confusion may be a soft S1 followed by an ejection click; only the latter may be heard. Consequently, the murmur appears to start immediately after the "S1." However, this situation usually occurs at the 2LICS or 2RICS where systolic regurgitant murmurs do not occur.

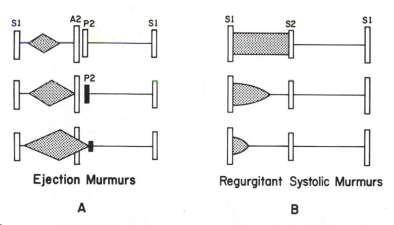

Ejection Murmurs   **Regurgitant Systolic Murmurs**

A   B

FIG. 2–7.
Diagram of ejection and regurgitant systolic murmurs. Classification of systolic murmurs is based primarily on the relationship of the S1 to the onset of the murmur. Both types of systolic murmurs may be long or short. **A,** Short ejection-type systolic murmur with its apex of the "diamond" in the early part of systole is seen with mild stenosis of semilunar valves *(top).* With increasing severity of obstruction to flow, the murmur becomes longer, and its apex moves toward the S2 *(middle).* In severe PS, the murmur may go beyond the A2 *(bottom).* **B,** Regurgitant systolic murmur in children is most often due to VSD and is usually holosystolic, extending all the way to the S2 *(top).* However, the regurgitation murmur may end in middle or early systole (not holosystolic) in some children, especially those with small-shunt VSD and in some newborn infants with VSD *(middle* and *bottom).* Regardless of the length or intensity of the murmur, all regurgitant systolic murmurs are pathologic.

Regurgitant systolic murmurs begin *with* the S1. No gap exists between the S1 and the onset of the murmur and usually, but not always, the murmur last throughout systole (i.e., pansystolic or holosystolic). Therefore analysis of the presence or absence of a gap between the S1 and the onset of the systolic murmur is of utmost importance; the length or the termination of the murmur in relation to the S2 is unimportant (Fig. 2-7, *B*). Regurgitant systolic murmurs are caused by the flow of blood from a chamber that is at a higher pressure throughout systole than the receiving chamber. These murmurs are associated with *only* the following three conditions: VSD, MR, and tricuspid regurgitation (TR). None of these ordinarily occur at the base (i.e., 2LICS or 2RICS). One exception to the early onset of a regurgitant systolic murmur is the late systolic murmur at the apex, which follows a midsystolic click in MVP (see Chapter 21).

LOCATION. In addition to the type of murmur (i.e., ejection vs. regurgitant), the location of the maximal intensity of the murmur is important to making a clinical diagnosis of the heart murmur's origin. For example, a regurgitant systolic murmur heard maximally at the LLSB is characteristic of a VSD. An ejection systolic murmur maximally audible at the 2LICS is usually pulmonary in origin. The location of the heart murmur often helps clarify situations when it is difficult to differentiate between an ejection murmur and a regurgitant murmur. For example, a long PS murmur may sound like a regurgitant systolic murmur of a VSD; however, since the maximum intensity is at the ULSB, it is unlikely that a VSD caused the murmur. Although rare, a subarterial infundibular VSD murmur may be maximally heard at the ULSB (Tables 2-6 to 2-9, Fig. 2-8).

TRANSMISSION. The transmission of systolic murmurs from the site of maximal intensity may help determine the murmur's origin. For example, an apical systolic murmur that transmits well to the left axilla and lower back is characteristic of MR, whereas one that radiates to the URSB and the neck is more likely to originate in the aortic valve. A systolic ejection murmur at the base that transmits well to the neck is more likely to be aortic in origin; one that transmits well to the back is more likely to be of pulmonary valve or pulmonary artery origin.

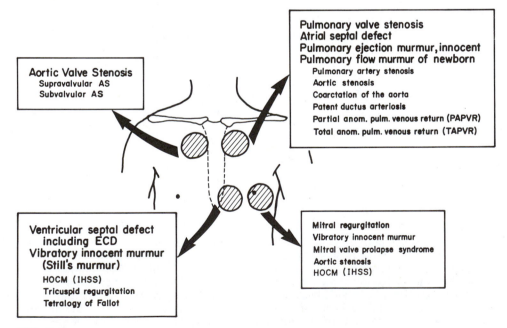

FIG. 2–8.
Diagram showing systolic murmurs audible at various locations. Less common conditions are shown in smaller type (see Tables 2-6 through 2-9). *IHSS,* Idiopathic hypertrophic subaortic stenosis; *AS,* aortic stenosis, *ECD,* endocardial cushion defect; *HOCM,* hypertrophic obstructive cardiomyopathy.

QUALITY. The quality of a murmur may help diagnose heart disease. Systolic murmurs of MR or of a VSD have a uniform, high-pitched quality, often described as blowing. Ejection systolic murmurs of AS or PS have a rough, grating quality. A common innocent murmur in children, which is best audible between the LLSB and apex, has a characteristic "vibratory" or humming quality.

DIFFERENTIAL DIAGNOSIS AT VARIOUS LOCATIONS. Systolic murmurs that are audible at the various locations are presented in Fig. 2-8. More common conditions are listed in larger type and less common conditions in smaller type. For quick reference, characteristic physical, ECG, and x-ray findings that are helpful in differential diagnoses are listed in Tables 2-6 through 2-9.

1. ULSB or pulmonary area: In many conditions, both pathologic and physiologic (i.e., innocent murmur), a systolic murmur is most audible at the ULSB. Audible systolic murmurs at this location are usually an ejection type and may be the result of one of the following:

    a. PS

    b. ASD

    c. Innocent pulmonary flow murmur of newborn

    d. Innocent pulmonary flow murmur of older children

    e. Pulmonary artery stenosis

    f. AS

    g. TOF

    h. COA

    i. PDA with pulmonary hypertension. (A continuous murmur of a PDA is usually loudest in the left infraclavicular area.)

    j. Total anomalous pulmonary venous return (TAPVR)

    k. PAPVR

    Conditions *a* through *d* are more common than the rest of the listed conditions. Table 2-6 summarizes other clinical findings that are useful in differential diagnosis.

2. URSB or aortic area: Systolic murmurs at the URSB are also an ejection type. They are caused by the narrowing of the aortic valve or its neighboring structures. The murmur transmits well to the neck. Often it transmits with a thrill over the carotid arteries. The ejection murmur of AS may be heard just as well at the ULSB (i.e., "pulmonary area"), as well as at the apex. However, the PS murmur does not transmit well to the URSB and the neck; rather, it transmits well to the back and the sides of the chest. The systolic murmurs in the URSB are caused by the following:

    a. AS

    b. Subvalvular aortic stenosis (subaortic stenosis)

    c. Supravalvular aortic stenosis

    Characteristic physical, ECG, and x-ray findings that help in differential diagnosis of these conditions are presented in Table 2-7.

3. LLSB: Systolic murmurs that are maximally audible at this location may be of the regurgitant or ejection type and may result from one of the following conditions:

    a. VSD (small muscular VSD may be heard best between the LLSB and apex)

    b. Vibratory or musical innocent murmur (e.g., Still's murmur)

TABLE 2–6.

Differential Diagnosis of Systolic Murmurs at the Upper Left Sternal Border (Pulmonary Area)

Condition	Important Physical Findings	Chest X-ray Films	ECG Findings
Pulmonary valve stenosis	SEM, grade 2 to 5/6, *Thrill (±) S2 may be split widely when mild *Ejection click (±) at 2LICS Transmit to the back	*Prominent MPA (poststenotic dilatation) Normal PVM	Normal if mild, RAD *RVH RAH if severe
ASD	SEM, grade 2 to 3/6 *Widely split and fixed S2	*Increased PVM *RAE & RVE	RAD RVH *RBBB (rsR′)
Pulmonary flow murmur of newborn	SEM, grade 1 to 2/6 No thrill *Good transmission to the back and axillae Newborns	Normal	Normal
Pulmonary flow murmur of older children	SEM, grade 2 to 3/6 No thrill Poor transmission	Normal Occasional pectus excavatum or straight back	Normal
PA stenosis	SEM, grade 2 to 3/6 Occasional continuous murmur P2 may be loud *Transmits well to the back and both lung fields	Prominent hilar vessels (±)	RVH or normal
AS	SEM, grade 2 to 5/6 *Also audible in 2RICS *Thrill (±) at 2RICS and SSN *Ejection click at apex, 3LICS, or 2RICS (±) Paradoxically split S2 if severe	Absence of prominent MPA Dilated aorta	Normal or LVH
TOF	*Long SEM, grade 2 to 4/6, louder at MLSB Thrill (±) Loud, single S2 (=A2) Cyanosis, clubbing	*Decreased PVM *Normal heart size Boot-shaped heart Right aortic arch (25%)	RAD *RVH or CVH RAH (±)
COA	SEM, grade 1 to 3/6 *Loudest at left interscapular area (back) *Weak or absent femorals Hypertension in arms Frequent associated AS, bicuspid aortic valve, or MR	*Classic "3" sign on plain film or "E" sign on barium esophagogram Rib notching (±)	LVH in children RBBB (or RVH) in infants
PDA	*Continuous murmur, at left infraclavicular area Occasional crescendic systolic only Grade 2 to 4/6 Thrill (±) Bounding pulses	*Increased PVM *LAE, LVE	Normal, LVH, or CVH
TAPVR	SEM, grade 2 to 3/6 Widely split and fixed S2 (±) *Quadruple or quintuple rhythm	*Increased PVM RAE and RVE Prominent MPA "Snowman" sign	RAD RAH *RVH

TABLE 2–6. *Continued*

Condition	Important Physical Findings	Chest X-ray Films	ECG Findings
PAPVR	*Diastolic rumble at LLSB *Mild cyanosis ($\downarrow$ Po$_2$) and clubbing ($\pm$) Physical findings similar to those of ASD *S2 may not be fixed unless associated with ASD	*Increased PVM *RAE and RVE "Scimitar" sign ($\pm$)	Same as in ASD

*Findings that are more characteristic of the condition.
MPA, Main pulmonary artery; *PVM*, pulmonary vascular marking; *RAD*, right axis deviation; *RVH*, right ventricular hypertrophy; *RAH*, right atrial hypertrophy; *RVE*, right ventricular enlargement, *CVH*, combined ventricular hypertrophy; *LAE*, left atrial enlargement; *LVE*, left ventricular enlargement; *LVH*, left ventricular hypertrophy; *TAPVR*, total anomalous pulmonary venous return; *RAE*, right atrial enlargement; *SEM*, systolic ejection murmur; *RBBB*, right bundle branch block; *2RICS*, second right intercostal space; *3LICS*, third left intercostal space; *AS*, aortic stenosis; *MR*, mitral regurgitation; *LLSB*, lower left sternal border; *ASD*, atrial septal defect; *PAPVR*, partial anomalous pulmonary venous return; *PDA*, patent ductus arteriosus; *TOF*, tetralogy of Fallot; *PA*, pulmonary artery.

TABLE 2–7.

Differential Diagnosis of Systolic Murmurs at the URSB (Aortic Area)

Condition	Important Physical Findings	Chest X-ray Films	ECG Findings
Aortic valve stenosis	SEM, grade 2 to 5/6, at 2RICS, may be loudest at 3LICS *Thrill ($\pm$), URSB, SSN, and carotid arteries *Ejection click *Transmits well to neck S2 may be single	Mild LVE ($\pm$) Prominent ascending aorta or aortic knob	Normal or LVH with or without "strain"
Subaortic stenosis	SEM, grade 2 to 4/6 *AR murmur almost always present in discrete stenosis No ejection click	Usually normal	Normal or LVH
Supravalvular aortic stenosis	SEM, grade 2 to 3/6 Thrill ($\pm$) No ejection click *Pulse and BP may be greater in right than left arm *Peculiar facies and mental retardation ($\pm$) Murmur may transmit well to the back (PA stenosis)	Unremarkable	Normal, LVH or CVH

*Findings that are more characteristic of the condition.
LVE, Left ventricular enlargement; *LVH*, left ventricular hypertrophy; *AR*, aortic regurgitation; *BP*, blood pressure; *CVH*, combined ventricular hypertrophy; *URSB*, upper right sternal border; *SEM*, systolic ejection murmur; *SSN*, superasternal notch; *PA*, pulmonary artery.

    c. Hypertrophic obstructive cardiomyopathy (HOCM) (formerly known as idiopathic hypertrophic subaortic stenosis [IHSS])

    d. TR

    e. TOF

Characteristic physical, ECG, and x-ray findings that help in differential diagnosis of these conditions are presented in Table 2-8.

TABLE 2–8.

Differential Diagnosis of Systolic Murmurs at the LLSB

Condition	Important Physical Findings	Chest X-ray Films	ECG Findings
VSD	*Regurgitant systolic, grade 2 to 5/6 May not be holosystolic Well-localized at LLSB *Thrill often present P2 may be loud	*Increased PVM *LAE and LVE (cardiomegaly)	Normal LVH or CVH
ECD, complete	Similar to findings of VSD *Diastolic rumble at LLSB *Gallop rhythm common in infants	Similar to large VSD	*Superior QRS axis, LVH or CVH
Vibratory innocent murmur (Still's)	SEM, grade 2 to 3/6 *Musical or vibratory with midsystolic accentuation *Maximum between LLSB and apex	Normal	Normal
HOCM or IHSS	SEM, grade 2 to 4/6 Medium-pitched Maximum LLSB or apex Thrill (±) *Sharp upstroke of brachial pulses May have MR murmur	Normal or globular LVE	LVH Abnormally deep Q waves in leads V5 and V6
TR	*Regurgitant systolic, grade 2 to 3/6 *Triple or quadruple rhythm (in Ebstein's) Mild cyanosis (±) Hepatomegaly with pulsatile liver and neck vein distention when severe	Normal PVM RAE if severe	RBBB, RAH and 1° AV block in Ebstein's
TOF	Murmurs can be louder at ULSB (see Table 2–5)		

*Findings that are more characteristic of the condition.
PVM, Pulmonary vascular marking; *LAE,* left atrial enlargement; *LVE,* left ventricular enlargement; *LVH,* left ventricular hypertrophy; *CVH,* combined ventricular hypertrophy; *RAE,* right atrial enlargement; *RAH,* right atrial hypertrophy; *AV,* atrioventricular; *ULSB,* upper left sternal border; *LLSB,* lower left sternal border; *VSD,* ventricular septal defect; *ECD,* endocardial cushion defect; *SEM,* systolic ejection murmur; *HOCM,* hypertrophic obstructive cardiomyopathy; *IHSS,* iodiopathic hypertrophic subaortic stenosis; *MR,* mitral regurgitation; *TR,* tricuspid regurgitation; *TOF,* tetralogy of Fallot; *RBBB,* right bundle branch block.

4. Apical area: Systolic murmurs that are maximally audible at the apex may be of the regurgitant or ejection type and result from one of the following conditions:

   a. MR

   b. MVP

   c. AS

   d. HOCM or IHSS

   e. Vibratory innocent murmur

Characteristic physical, ECG, and x-ray findings are summarized in Table 2-9.

Diastolic murmurs. Diastolic murmurs occur between the S2 and S1. Based on their timing and relation to the heart sounds, they are classified into the following three types: early diastolic, middiastolic, and presystolic (Fig. 2-9).

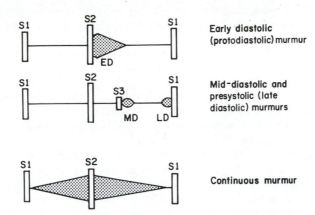

FIG. 2–9.
Diagrammatic drawing of diastolic murmurs and the continuous murmur. *ED,* Early diastolic or protodiastolic murmur; *LD,* late diastolic or presystolic murmur; *MD,* middiastolic murmur.

TABLE 2–9.

Differential Diagnosis of Systolic Murmurs at the Apex

Condition	Important Physical Findings	Chest X-ray Films	ECG Findings
MR	*Regurgitant systolic, may not be holosystolic, grade 2 to 3/6 Transmits to left axilla (less obvious in children) May be loudest in the midprecordium	LAE and LVE	LAH or LVH
MVP	*Midsystolic click with/without late systolic murmur *High incidence of thoracic skeletal anomalies (pectus excavatum, straight back) (85%)	Normal	Inverted T wave in lead aVF
Aortic valve stenosis	The murmur and ejection click may be best heard at the apex rather than at 2RICS	(See Table 2–7)	
HOCM or IHSS	The murmur of IHSS may be maximal at the apex (may represent MR) (See Table 2–8)		
Vibratory innocent murmur	This innocent murmur may be loudest at the apex (See Table 2–8)		

*Findings that are more characteristic of the condition.
LAE, Left atrial enlargement; *LVE,* left ventricular enlargement; *LAH,* left atrial hypertrophy, *LVH,* left ventricular hypertrophy; *MR,* mitral regurgitation; *MVP,* mitral valve prolapse; *HOCM,* hypertrophic obstructive cardiomyopathy; *IHSS,* iodiopathic hypertrophic subaortic stenosis.

Early diastolic (or protodiastolic) decrescendo murmurs occur early in diastole, immediately after the S2, and are caused by incompetence of the aortic or pulmonary valve (see Fig. 2-9).

Because the aorta is a high-pressure vessel, aortic regurgitation (AR) murmurs are high pitched and best heard with the diaphragm of a stethoscope at the 3LICS. The AR murmur radiates well to the apex because the regurgitation is directed toward the apex. Bounding peripheral pulses may be present if the AR is significant. AR murmurs are associated with congenital bicuspid aortic valve, subaortic stenosis, postoperative AS (i.e., postvalvotomy), and rheumatic heart disease with AR and, occasionally, a subarterial infundibular VSD with prolapsing aortic cusps.

Pulmonary regurgitation (PR) murmurs also occur early in diastole. They are usually medium pitched but may be high pitched if pulmonary hypertension is present. They are best heard at the 3LICS and radiate along the left sternal border (LSB). These murmurs are associated with postoperative TOF (because of surgically induced PR); pulmonary hypertension; postoperative pulmonary valvotomy for PS; and mild, isolated deformity of the pulmonary valve.

Middiastolic (ventricular filling or inflow) murmurs start with a loud S3 and are heard in early or middiastole, but are not temporally midway through diastole (see Fig. 2-9). These murmurs are always low pitched and best heard with the bell of the stethoscope applied lightly to the chest. These murmurs are caused by turbulence in the mitral or tricuspid valve secondary to anatomic stenosis or relative stenosis of these valves.

Mitral middiastolic murmurs are best heard at the apex and often referred to as an *apical rumble,* although frequently they sound more like a hum than a rumble. These murmurs are associated with MS or a large left-to-right shunt VSD or PDA, which produce relative MS secondary to a large flow across the normal-sized mitral valve.

Tricuspid middiastolic murmurs are best heard along the LLSB. These murmurs are associated with ASD, partial or total anomalous pulmonary venous return, ECD, because they all result in relative tricuspid stenosis [TS]). Anatomic stenosis of the tricuspid valve is also associated with these murmurs, but such cases are rare.

Presystolic (or late diastolic) murmurs are also caused by flow through the AV valves during ventricular diastole. They result from active atrial contraction that ejects blood into the ventricle, rather than a passive pressure difference between the atrium and ventricle. These low-frequency murmurs occur late in diastole or just before the onset of systole (see Fig. 2-9) and are found with true MS or TS.

Continuous murmur. Continuous murmurs begin in systole and continue without interruption through the S2 into all or part of diastole (see Fig. 2-9). Continuous murmurs are caused by the following:

1. Aortopulmonary or arteriovenous connection (e.g., PDA, AV fistula, after systemic-to-PA shunt surgery, persistent truncus arteriosus [rarely])

2. Disturbances of flow patterns in veins (e.g., venous hum)

3. Disturbance of flow pattern in arteries (e.g., COA, PA stenosis)

The murmur of PDA has a machinery-like quality, becoming louder during systole (crescendo), peaking at the S2, and diminishing in diastole (decrescendo). This murmur is maximally heard in the left infraclavicular area or along the ULSB. With pulmonary hypertension, only the systolic portion can be heard, but it is crescendic during systole.

Venous hum is a common innocent murmur that is audible in the upright position, in the infraclavicular region, unilaterally or bilaterally. The murmur's intensity changes with the position of the neck. When the child lies supine, the murmur usually disappears. It is usually heard better on the right side.

Less common continuous murmurs of severe COA may be heard over the intercostal collaterals. The continuous murmurs of PA stenosis may be heard over the right and left anterior chest, the sides of the chest, and in the back.

The combination of a systolic murmur (e.g., VSD or PS) and a diastolic murmur (e.g., AR or PR) is referred to as a *to-and-fro murmur* to distinguish it from a machinery-like continuous murmur.

Innocent heart murmurs. Innocent heart murmurs, also called *functional murmurs,* arise from cardiovascular structures in the absence of anatomic abnormalities. Innocent heart murmurs are common in children. Over 80% of children have innocent murmurs of one type or another sometime during childhood, usually beginning around ages 3 and 4. All innocent heart murmurs are accentuated or brought out in a high-output state, usually as a fever. A left ventricular false tendon has been found often in children and adults with innocent heart murmurs.

Probably the only way a physician can recognize innocent heart murmurs is to become familiar with the more common forms of these murmurs. Physicians can become more familiar by auscultating many innocent murmurs under the supervision of pediatric cardiologists. All innocent heart murmurs are associated with normal ECG and x-ray findings. When one or more of the following are present, the murmur is more likely pathologic and requires cardiac consultation:

1. Symptomatic

2. Abnormal cardiac size and/or silhouette or abnormal pulmonary vascularity on chest roentgenograms

3. Abnormal ECG

4. Diastolic murmur

5. A systolic murmur that is loud (i.e., grade 3/6 or with thrill), long in duration, and transmits well to other parts of the body

6. Cyanosis

7. Abnormally strong or weak pulses

8. Abnormal heart sounds

CLASSIC VIBRATORY MURMUR (I.E., STILL'S MURMUR). Although occasionally detected in infancy, Still's murmur is not common before the age of 2 years. Most vibratory murmurs are detected between 3 and 6 years of age. It is maximally audible at the MLSB or between the LLSB and the apex. The murmur is midsystolic (i.e., not regurgitant) in timing and of a grade 2 to 3/6 in intensity. It has a distinctive quality, described as a "twanging string," groaning, squeaking, buzzing, musical, or vibratory sound. It is generally of low frequency and best heard with the bell with the patient in the supine position. The vibratory quality may disappear and the murmur becomes softer when the bell is pressed harder, thereby proving its low frequency. This murmur is not accompanied by a thrill or ejection click. The intensity of the murmur increases during febrile illness or excitement, after exercise, or in anemic states. The murmur may disappear briefly at a maximum Valsalva maneuver. The ECG and chest x-ray films are normal (Table 2-10; Fig. 2-10).

An inexperienced examiner may confuse it with the murmur of a VSD. The murmur of a VSD is usually harsh, grade 2 to 3/6 in intensity, regurgitant in timing (starting with the S1), and often accompanied by a palpable thrill. The ECG and x-ray films are often abnormal.

PULMONARY EJECTION FILMS MURMUR (I.E., PULMONARY FLOW MURMUR OF CHILDREN). It is common in children between the ages of 8 and 14 years old, but most frequent in adolescents. The murmur is maximally audible at the ULSB. The ejection type murmur is early to midsystolic in timing, slightly grating (rather than vibratory) in quality, with relatively little radiation. The intensity of the murmur is usually a grade 1 to 3/6. The S2 is normal, and there is no associated thrill or ejection click (see Table 2-10; Fig. 2-10).

This murmur may be confused with the murmur of pulmonary valve stenosis or an ASD. In pulmonary valve stenosis, there may be an ejection click, systolic thrill, widely

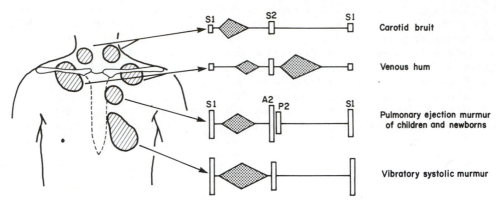

FIG. 2–10.
Diagrammatic illustration of innocent heart murmurs in children.

TABLE 2–10.

Common Innocent Heart Murmurs

Type (Timing)	Description of Murmur	Age Group
Classic vibratory murmur (Still's murmur) (systolic)	Maximal at MLSB or between LLSB and apex Grade 2 to 3/6 Low-frequency vibratory, "twanging string," groaning, squeaking, or musical	3 to 6 yr Occasionally in infancy
Pulmonary ejection murmur (systolic)	Maximal at ULSB Early to midsystolic Grade 1 to 3/6 in intensity Blowing in quality	8 to 14 yr
Pulmonary flow murmur of newborn (systolic)	Maximal at ULSB Transmits well to the left and right chest, axillae, and back Grade 1 to 2/6 in intensity	Prematures and full-term newborns Usually disappears by 3 to 6 mo of age
Venous hum (continuous)	Maximal at right (or left) supraclavicular and infraclavicular areas Grade 1 to 3/6 in intensity Inaudible in the supine position Intensity changes with rotation of the head and compression of the jugular vein	3 to 6 yr
Carotid bruit (systolic)	Right supraclavicular area and over the carotids Grade 2 to 3/6 in intensity Occasional thrill over a carotid	Any age

MLSB, mid-left sternal border; *ULSB*, upper left sternal border.

split S2, right ventricular hypertrophy (RVH) on ECG, and poststenotic dilatation of the main pulmonary artery (MPA) segment on chest x-ray films. Important differential points of ASD include a widely split and fixed S2; diastolic flow rumble of relative TS at the LLSB; at the LLSB if the shunt is large; RBBB or mild RVH on ECG, manifested by rsR′ in lead V1; and chest x-ray films revealing increased pulmonary vascular markings (PVMs) and enlargement of the right atrium (RA), right ventricle (RV), and MPA.

PULMONARY FLOW MURMUR OF NEWBORN. This murmur is commonly present in newborns, especially those with low birth weight. The murmur usually disappears by 3 to

6 months of age. If it persists beyond this age, a structural narrowing of the PA tree (i.e., PA stenosis) must be suspected. It is best audible at the ULSB. Although the murmur is only a grade 1 to 2/6 in intensity, it transmits impressively well to the right and left chest, both axillae, and the back. There is no ejection click. The ECG and chest x-ray film are normal (see Table 2-10; Fig. 2-10).

This murmur originates from the relatively hypoplastic right and left PAs at birth. This relative hypoplasia results from the small amount of blood flow through these vessels during fetal life (only 15% of combined ventricular output goes to these vessels). The turbulence created in these small vessels near the bifurcation is transmitted along the smaller branches of the PAs. Therefore this murmur is heard well around the chest wall.

The murmur resembles the murmur of organic PA stenosis, which may be seen as a component of rubella syndrome or Williams syndrome. Characteristic noncardiac findings in children with these syndromes lead physicians to suspect an organic nature of the PA stenosis murmur. Organic PA stenosis is frequently associated with other cardiac defects (e.g., VSD and pulmonary valve stenosis) or is seen occasionally as an isolated anomaly. The heart murmur of organic PA stenosis persists beyond infancy, and the ECG may show RVH if the stenosis is severe.

VENOUS HUM. This murmur is commonly audible in children between the ages of 3 and 6 years. It originates from turbulence in the jugular venous system. This is a continuous murmur in which the diastolic component is louder than the systolic component. The murmur is maximally audible at the right and/or left infraclavicular and supraclavicular areas (see Table 2-10; Fig. 2-10). The venous hum is only heard in the upright position and disappears in the supine position. It can be obliterated by rotating the head or by gently occluding the neck veins with the fingers.

It is important to differentiate a venous hum from the continuous murmur of a PDA. The murmur of a PDA is loudest at the ULSB or left infraclavicular area with bounding peripheral pulses and wide pulse pressure. The systolic component is louder than the diastolic component. The x-ray films show increased PVMs and cardiac enlargement. The ECG may be normal or show left ventricular hypertrophy (LVH) or combined ventricular hypertrophy (CVH).

CAROTID BRUIT. This is an early systolic ejection murmur, best heard in the supraclavicular fossa or over the carotid arteries (see Table 2-10; Fig. 2-10). It is produced by turbulence in the brachiocephalic or carotid arteries. The murmur is a grade 2 to 3/6 in intensity. Although it rarely occurs, a faint thrill is palpable over a carotid artery. This bruit may be found in children of any age.

The murmur of AS often transmits well to the carotid arteries with a palpable thrill, requiring differentiation from the carotid bruits. In AS, the murmur is louder at the URSB, and a systolic thrill is often present in the URSB and SSN, as well as over the carotid artery. An ejection click is often present in aortic valve stenosis. The ECG and chest x-ray film may appear abnormal.

3 / Electrocardiography I

In the clinical diagnosis of congenital or acquired heart disease, the presence of ventricular and atrial hypertrophy and ventricular conduction disturbances is often helpful. These ECG abnormalities are presented in a flow diagram for diagnosis of congenital heart defects (CHDs) that is found in Chapter 5. This chapter emphasizes hypertrophy of ventricles and atria and ventricular conduction disturbances. A brief discussion of a normal pediatric ECG and the basic measurements necessary for routine interpretation of an ECG are also presented. Other ECG abnormalities such as atrioventricular conduction disturbances, arrhythmias, and ST-segment and T-wave changes are discussed in Part VI, Electrocardiography II.

NORMAL PEDIATRIC ELECTROCARDIOGRAMS

ECGs of normal infants and children are quite different from those of normal adults. The most remarkable difference is right ventricular (RV) dominance in infants. RV dominance is most noticeable in newborns, and it gradually changes to left ventricular (LV) dominance in adults. The ECG reflects anatomic differences; the RV is thicker than the LV in newborns and infants, and the LV is much thicker than the RV in adults.

RV dominance of infants is expressed in the ECG by right-axis deviation (RAD) and large RV forces (i.e., tall R waves in lead aVR and the right precordial leads (RPLs) such as V4R, V1, and V2, and deep S waves in lead I and the left precordial leads (LPLs), such as V5 and V6).

An ECG from a 2-week-old infant (Fig. 3-1) is compared with that of a young adult (Fig. 3-2). The infant's ECG demonstrates RAD (+ 160 degrees) and dominant R waves in the RPLs (V4R, V1, and V2). The T wave in V1 is usually negative. Upright T waves in V1 in this age group suggest right ventricular hypertrophy (RVH). Adult-type R/S progression in the precordial leads (deep S waves in V1 and V2 and tall R waves in V5 and V6; see Fig. 3-2) is rarely seen in the first month of life; instead, there may be *complete reversal* of the adult-type R/S progression with tall R waves in V1 and V2 and deep S waves in V5 and V6. *Partial reversal* is usually present with dominant R waves in V1, V5, and V6 in children between the ages of 1 month and 3 years.

The normal adult ECG shown in Fig. 3-2 demonstrates the QRS axis near +50 degrees and LV dominance manifested by dominant R waves in the LPLs and dominant S waves in the RPLs, the adult R/S progression. The T waves are usually anteriorly oriented, resulting in upright T waves in V2 through V6, and sometimes in V1.

ROUTINE INTERPRETATION

The following sequence is one of many approaches that can be used in routine interpretation of an ECG.

1. Rhythm (sinus or nonsinus) by considering the P axis

2. Heart rate (atrial and ventricular rates, if different)

3. The QRS axis, the T axis, and the QRS-T angle

4. Intervals: PR, QRS, and QT

5. The P wave amplitude and duration

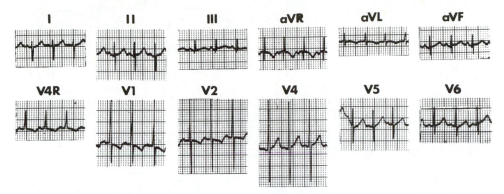

FIG. 3–1.
ECG from normal 2-week-old infant.

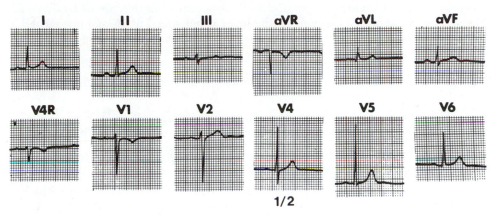

FIG. 3–2.
ECG from normal young adult.

6. The QRS amplitude and R/S ratio; also abnormal Q waves

7. ST-segment and T-wave abnormalities

Basic measurements that are necessary for routine interpretation are briefly discussed.

Rhythm

Sinus rhythm is the normal rhythm at any age and is characterized by P waves preceding each QRS complex and a regular but not necessarily normal PR interval and normal P axis (0 to +90 degrees).

Since the sinoatrial (SA) node is located in the right upper part of the atrial mass, the direction of atrial depolarization is from the right upper part toward the left lower part, producing the P axis in the left lower quadrant (0 to +90 degrees) (Fig. 3-3, *A*). This second requirement of a normal P axis is important in discriminating sinus from nonsinus rhythm. Some atrial rhythm (nonsinus) may have P waves preceding each QRS complex but with an abnormal P axis (Fig. 3-3, *B*). For the P axis to be between 0 and +90 degrees, P waves must be upright in leads I and aVF; simple inspection of these two leads suffices. A normal P axis also results in upright P waves in lead II and inverted P waves in aVR. A method of plotting axes is presented later for the QRS axis.

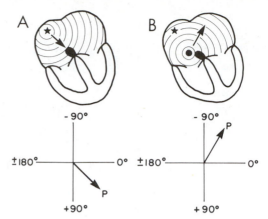

FIG. 3–3.
Comparison of P axis in sinus rhythm
(A), and low atrial rhythm **(B).** In
sinus rhythm, the P waves are upright
in leads I and aVF. In low atrial
rhythm, the P wave is inverted in lead
aVF.

Heart Rate

There are many different ways to calculate the heart rate, but they are all based on the
known time scale of ECG papers. At the usual paper speed of 25 mm per second, 1
mm = 0.04 second, and 5 mm = 0.20 second (Fig. 3-4). The following methods are
often used to calculate the heart rate.

1. Count the R-R cycle in six large divisions (1/50 minute) and multiply it by 50
   (Fig. 3-5).

2. When the heart rate is slow, count the number of large divisions between two R
   waves and divide that into 300 (1 minute = 300 large divisions) (Fig. 3-6).

3. Count the R-R cycles between two markers (3 seconds) on the upper edge of an
   unmounted tracing, and multiply them by 20.

4. Measure the R-R interval (in seconds) and divide 60 by the R-R interval. The R-R
   interval is 0.36 second in Fig. 3-5: 60 ÷ 0.36 = 166.

5. Use a convenient ECG ruler.

6. An approximate heart rate can be determined by memorizing heart rates for
   selected R-R intervals (Fig. 3-7). When R-R intervals are 5, 10, 15, 20, and 25 mm,
   the respective heart rates are 300, 150, 100, 75, and 60 beats/min.

   When the ventricular and atrial rates are different, as in complete heart block or atrial
flutter, the atrial rate can be calculated using the same methods as described for the
ventricular rate; for the atrial rate, the P-P interval rather than the R-R interval is used.
   Because of age-related differences in the heart rate, the definition used for adults of
bradycardia (i.e., less than 60 beats/min) or tachycardia (i.e. in excess of 100 beats/min)
do not help distinguish normal from abnormal heart rates in pediatric patients.
Operationally, tachycardia is present when the heart rate is faster than the upper range
of normal for that age, and bradycardia is present when the heart rate is slower than the
lower range of normal. According to age, normal resting heart rates per minute are as
follows:

Newborn	110 to 150 beats/min
2 years	85 to 125 beats/min
4 years	75 to 115 beats/min
Older than 6 years	60 to 100 beats/min

QRS Axis, T Axis, and QRS-T Angle

The QRS axis. The most convenient way to determine the QRS axis is to use the
hexaxial reference system (Fig. 3-8, A). The hexaxial reference system gives information
about the left-right and superoinferior relationship, as in the *frontal* plane of

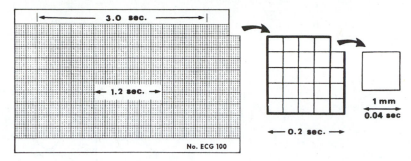

FIG. 3–4.
ECG paper. Time is measured on the horizontal axis. Each 1 mm = 0.04 second, and each 5 mm (a large division) = 0.20 second; 30 mm (or 6 large divisions) = 1.2 second or ⅟₅₀ minute. Every 7.5 cm marked on the top margin of the paper = 3.0 second or ⅟₂₀ minute. (From Park MK, Guntheroth WG: *How to read pediatric ECGs,* ed 3, St Louis, 1992, Mosby.)

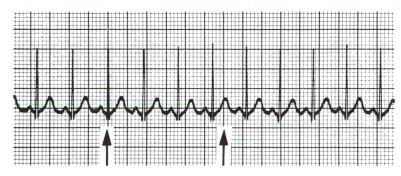

FIG. 3–5.
Heart rate of 165 beats/min. There are about 3.3 cardiac cycles (R-R intervals) in six large divisions. Therefore the heart rate is 3.3 × 50 = 165.

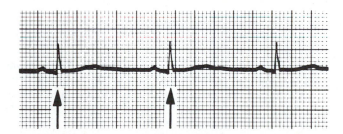

FIG. 3–6.
Heart rate of 52 beats/min. There are 5.8 large divisions between the two *arrows.* Therefore the heart rate is 300 ÷ 5.8 = 52.

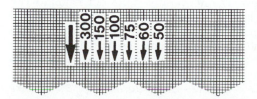

FIG. 3–7.
Quick estimation of heart rate. When the R-R interval is 5 mm, the heart rate is 300 beats/min. When the R-R interval is 10 mm, the rate is 150 beats/min, and so on.

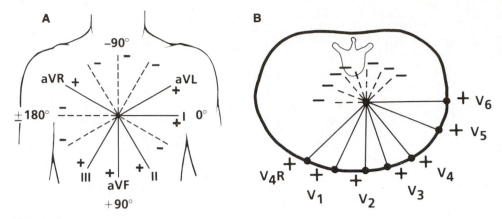

FIG. 3–8.
Hexaxial **(A)** and horizontal **(B)** reference systems. (From Park MK, Guntheroth WG: *How to read pediatric ECGs,* ed 3, St Louis, 1992, Mosby.)

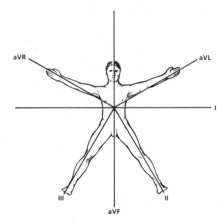

FIG. 3–9.
An easy way to memorize the hexaxial reference system. (From Park MK, Guntheroth WG: *How to read pediatric ECGs,* ed 3. St Louis, 1992, Mosby.)

vectorcardiography. The R wave in lead I represents the leftward force; the S wave in lead I represents the rightward force. The R in aVF is a downward force; the S wave is the upward force (see Fig. 3-8, *A*).

An easy way to memorize the system is shown in Fig. 3-9 by superimposing a body with outstretched arms and legs on the X and Y axes. The right and left hands are the positive poles of the aVR and aVL respectively. The left and right feet are the positive poles of lead II and lead III respectively. The bipolar limb leads I, II, and III are clockwise in sequence for the positive electrode.

Successive approximation method
Step 1: Locate a quadrant, using leads I and aVF (Fig. 3-10).
From the top panel of Fig. 3-10, the net QRS deflection of lead I is positive. This means that the QRS axis is in the left hemicircle (i.e., from −90 degrees through 0 to +90 degrees) from the lead I point of view. The net positive QRS deflection in aVF means that the QRS axis is in the lower half of the circle (i.e., from 0 through +90 degrees to +180 degrees) from the aVF point of view. To satisfy the polarity of both leads I and aVF, the QRS axis must be in the left lower quadrant (i.e., 0 to +90 degrees). Four quardants can be easily identified based on the net deflections of the QRS complexes in leads I and aVF (Fig. 3-10).
Step 2: Find a lead with an equiphasic QRS complex in which the height of the R wave and the depth of the S wave are equal.

The QRS axis is perpendicular to the lead with an equiphasic QRS complex in the predetermined quadrant.

Example: Determine the QRS axis in Fig. 3-11.

Step 1: The axis is in the left lower quadrant (i.e., 0 to +90 degrees), since the R waves are upright in leads I and aVF.

Step 2: The QRS complex is equiphasic in aVL. Therefore the QRS axis is +60 degrees, which is perpendicular to aVL.

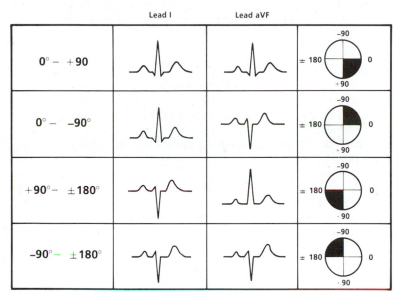

FIG. 3–10.
Locating quadrants of mean QRS axis from leads I and aVF. (From Park MK, Guntheroth WG: *How to read pediatric ECGs,* ed 3, St Louis, 1992, Mosby.)

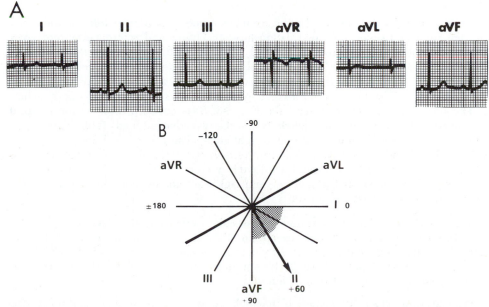

FIG. 3–11.
Examples of the ECG strip **(A)** and the hexaxial reference system **(B).**

TABLE 3–1.
Mean and Ranges of Normal QRS Axes

Age	Range
1 wk–1 mo	+110° (+30 to +180)
1–3 mo	+70° (+10 to +125)
3 mo–3 yr	+60° (+10 to +110)
Older than 3 yr	+60° (+20 to +120)
Adults	+50° (−30 to +105)

Normal QRS Axis:

Normal ranges of QRS axis vary with age. Newborns normally have RAD compared with the adult standard. By 3 years of age, the QRS axis approaches the adult mean value of +50 degrees. The mean and ranges of a normal QRS axis according to age are shown in Table 3-1.

The QRS axis outside normal ranges signifies abnormalities in the ventricular depolarization process.

1. Left-axis deviation (LAD) is present when the QRS axis is less than the lower limit of normal for the patient's age. Left axis deviation (LAD) occurs with left ventricular hypertrophy (LVH), left bundle branch block (LBBB), and left anterior hemiblock.

2. RAD is present when the QRS axis is greater than the upper limit of normal for the patient's age. RAD occurs with RVH and right bundle branch block (RBBB).

3. "Superior QRS" axis is present when the S wave is greater than the R wave in aVF. The overlap with LAD should be noted. It may occur with left anterior hemiblock (in the range of -30 degrees to -90 degrees, seen in endocardial cushion defect [ECD] or tricuspid atresia) or with RBBB. It is rarely seen in otherwise normal children.

Horizontal reference system. The hexaxial reference system gives information about the left-right and superoinferior relationships; the horizontal reference system gives information about the anteroposterior and left-right relationship (e.g., the *horizontal* plane of a vectorcardiogram). The horizontal reference system uses the precordial leads. This system is not used routinely in calculating the QRS axis, but understanding it is important in the diagnosis of ventricular hypertrophy based on vectorial approaches.

The horizontal reference system (see Fig. 3-8, *B*) is not as precise as the hexaxial reference system in which the angle between the two adjacent leads is 30 degrees (see Fig. 3-8). The leads V2 and V6 cross at a right angle. The R wave in V2 represents the anterior force, and the S wave in V2 represents the posterior force. The R wave in V6 represents the leftward force, and the S wave in V6 represents the rightward force. The R wave in V1 represents the anterior and rightward forces, and the S wave in V1 represents the posterior and leftward forces.

T axis. The T axis can be determined by the same methods used to determine the QRS axis. In normal children, with the exception of the newborn, the mean T axis is +45 degrees, with a range of 0 degree to +90 degree, the same as normal adults. The T axis outside of the normal quadrant suggests conditions with myocardial dysfunction similar to those listed for abnormal QRS-T angle.

QRS-T angle. The QRS-T angle is the angle formed by the QRS axis and the T axis. A QRS-T angle of greater than 60 degrees is unusual, and that of greater than 90 degrees is certainly abnormal. An abnormally wide QRS-T angle with the T axis outside the

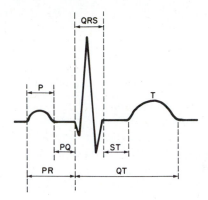

FIG. 3–12.
Diagram illustrating important intervals (or durations) and segments of an ECG cycle.

TABLE 3–2.

PR Interval, With Rate and Age (and ULN)*

Rate	0–1 mo	1–6 mo	6 mo–1 yr	1–3 yr	3–8 yr	8–12 yr	12–16 yr	Adult
< 60						0.16 (0.18)	0.16 (0.19)	0.17 (0.21)
60–80					0.15 (0.17)	0.15 (0.17)	0.15 (0.18)	0.16 (0.21)
80–100	0.10 (0.12)				0.14 (0.16)	0.15 (0.16)	0.15 (0.17)	0.15 (0.20)
100–120	0.10 (0.12)			(0.15)	0.13 (0.16)	0.14 (0.15)	0.15 (0.16)	0.15 (0.19)
120–140	0.10 (0.11)	0.11 (0.14)	0.11 (0.14)	0.12 (0.14)	0.13 (0.15)	0.14 (0.15)		0.15 (0.18)
140–160	0.09 (0.11)	0.10 (0.13)	0.11 (0.13)	0.11 (0.14)	0.12 (0.14)			(0.17)
160–180	0.10 (0.11)	0.10 (0.12)	0.10 (0.12)	0.10 (0.12)				
> 180	0.09	0.09 (0.11)	0.10 (0.11)					

*From Park MK, Guntheroth WG: *How to read pediatric ECGs,* ed 3, St Louis, 1992, Mosby. Used by permission.
ULN, Upper limits of normal.

normal quadrant (i.e. 0 degrees to +90 degrees) is seen in severe ventricular hypertrophy with "strain," ventricular conduction disturbances, and myocardial dysfunction of a metabolic or ischemic nature.

Intervals

Three important intervals are routinely measured in the interpretation of an ECG: PR interval, QRS duration, and QT interval. The duration of the P wave is also inspected (Fig. 3-12).

PR interval. Normal PR interval varies with *age* and *heart rate* (Table 3-2). Prolongation of the PR interval (e.g., first-degree AV block) is seen in myocarditis (rheumatic or viral), digitalis toxicity, CHD (ECD, atrial septal defect [ASD], Ebstein's anomaly), and other myocardial dysfunctions. A short PR interval is present in preexcitation (e.g., Wolff-Parkinson-White [WPW] syndrome and Lown-Ganong-Levine syndrome).

QRS duration. The QRS duration varies with age (Table 3-3). It is short in the infant and increases with age. Conditions grouped as ventricular conduction disturbances have increased QRS duration in common. They include the following: RBBB and LBBB, preexcitation (e.g., WPW) syndrome, intraventricular block (as seen in hyperkalemia, toxicity from quinidine or procainamide, myocardial fibrosis, myocardial dysfunction of metabolic or ischemic nature), and ventricular rhythm (e.g., premature ventricular contractions [PVCs], ventricular tachycardia, implanted ventricular pacemaker, and so on). Since the QRS duration varies with age, the definition of bundle branch block or other ventricular conduction disturbances should vary with age (see section on ventricular conduction disturbances).

TABLE 3–3.

QRS Duration: Average (and Upper Limits) for Age*

	0–1 mo	1–6 mo	6 mo–1 yr	1–3 yr	3–8 yr	8–12 yr	12–16 yr	Adult
Seconds	0.05	0.05	0.05	0.06	0.07	0.07	0.07	0.08
	(0.07)	(0.07)	(0.07)	(0.07)	(0.08)	(0.09)	(0.10)	(0.10)

*Modified from Guntheroth WG: *Pediatric electrocardiography,* Philadelphia, 1965, Saunders.

QT interval. The QT interval varies primarily with heart rate. The heart rate corrected QT (QTc) interval can be calculated by the use of Bazett's formula:

$$QTc = \frac{QT \text{ measured}}{\sqrt{RR \text{ interval}}}$$

According to Bazett's formula, the QTc interval should not exceed 0.44 second, except in infants. A QTc interval up to 0.49 second may be normal for the first 6 months of age. Lead II (usually with a visible q wave) is the best lead to measure the QT interval.

Long QT intervals may be seen in hypocalcemia, myocarditis, diffuse myocardial diseases (including hypertrophic and dilated cardiomyopathies), long QT syndrome (e.g., Jervell and Lange-Nielsen syndrome, Romano-Ward syndrome), head injury, severe malnutrition, and so on. A number of drugs are also known to prolong the QT interval. Among these are antiarrhythmic agents (especially class IA and III), antipsychotic phenothiazines (e.g., Mellaril, Thorazine), tricyclic antidepressants (e.g., imipramine, amitriptyline), arsenics, organophosphates, antibiotics (e.g., ampicillin, erythromycin, trimethoprim-sulfa, amantadine) and antihistamine Seldane (terfanadine). A short QT interval is a sign of a digitalis effect or of hypercalcemia.

P Wave Duration and Amplitude

The P wave duration and amplitude are important in the diagnosis of atrial hypertrophy. Normally, the P amplitude is less than 3 mm. The duration of P waves is shorter than 0.09 second in children and shorter than 0.07 second in infants (see section on criteria for atrial hypertrophy).

QRS Amplitude, R/S Ratio, and Abnormal Q Waves

The QRS amplitude and R/S ratio are important in the diagnosis of ventricular hypertrophy. These values also vary with age (Tables 3-4 and 3-5). Because of normal dominance of RV forces in infants, R waves are taller in the RPLs (i.e., V4R, V1, V2). S waves are deeper in the LPLs (i.e., V5, V6) in infants and small children than they are in adults. Accordingly, the R/S ratio is large in the RPLs and small in the LPLs in infants and small children.

Abnormal Q waves may manifest themselves as deep and/or wide Q waves or as abnormal leads in which they appear. Deep Q waves may be present in ventricular hypertrophy of "volume overload" type. Deep and wide Q waves are seen in myocardial infarction. The presence of Q waves in the RPLs (e.g., severe RVH or ventricular inversion) and/or the absence of Q waves in the LPLs (e.g., LBBB or ventricular inversion) are abnormal. Normal mean Q voltages and upper limits are presented in Table 3-6. The average Q wave duration is 0.02 second and does not exceed 0.03 second.

ST Segment and T Waves

The normal ST segment is isoelectric. However, in the limb leads, elevation or depression of the ST segment up to 1 mm is not necessarily abnormal in infants and children. A shift of up to 2 mm is considered normal in the precordial leads. Abnormal shift of ST segment occurs in pericarditis, myocardial ischemia or infarction, digitalis effect, and so on (see Chapter 27). Associated T wave changes are commonly present.

TABLE 3–4.

R and S Voltages According to Lead and Age: Mean (and ULN)*

	Lead	0–1 mo	1–6 mo	6 mo–1 yr	1–3 yr	3–8 yr	8–12 yr	12–16 yr	Young Adults
R voltage*	I	4 (8)	7 (13)	8 (16)	8 (16)	7 (15)	7 (15)	6 (13)	6 (13)
	II	6 (14)	13 (24)	13 (27)	13 (23)	13 (22)	14 (24)	14 (24)	9 (25)
	III	8 (16)	9 (20)	9 (20)	9 (20)	9 (20)	9 (24)	9 (24)	6 (22)
	aVR	3 (7)	3 (6)	3 (6)	2 (6)	2 (5)	2 (4)	2 (4)	1 (4)
	aVL	2 (7)	4 (8)	5 (10)	5 (10)	3 (10)	3 (10)	3 (12)	3 (9)
	aVF	7 (14)	10 (20)	10 (16)	8 (20)	10 (19)	10 (20)	11 (21)	5 (23)
	V4R	6 (12)	5 (10)	4 (8)	4 (8)	3 (8)	3 (7)	3 (7)	
	V1	15 (25)	11 (20)	10 (20)	9 (18)	7 (18)	6 (16)	5 (16)	3 (14)
	V2	21 (30)	21 (30)	19 (28)	16 (25)	13 (28)	10 (22)	9 (19)	6 (21)
	V5	12 (30)	17 (30)	18 (30)	19 (36)	21 (36)	22 (36)	18 (33)	12 (33)
	V6	6 (21)	10 (20)	13 (20)	12 (24)	14 (24)	14 (24)	14 (22)	10 (21)
S voltage*	I	5 (10)	4 (9)	4 (9)	3 (8)	2 (8)	2 (8)	2 (8)	1 (6)
	V4R	4 (9)	4 (12)	5 (12)	5 (12)	5 (14)	6 (20)	6 (20)	
	V1	10 (20)	7 (18)	8 (16)	13 (27)	14 (30)	16 (26)	15 (24)	10 (23)
	V2	20 (35)	16 (30)	17 (30)	21 (34)	23 (38)	23 (38)	23 (48)	14 (36)
	V5	9 (30)	9 (26)	8 (20)	6 (16)	5 (14)	5 (17)	5 (16)	
	V6	4 (12)	2 (7)	2 (6)	2 (6)	1 (5)	1 (4)	1 (5)	1 (13)

From Park MK, Guntheroth WG; *How to read pediatric ECGs,* ed 3, St Louis, 1992, Mosby. Used by permission.
*Voltages are measured in millimeters, when 1 mV = 10 mm paper.
ULN, Upper limits of normal.

TABLE 3–5.

R/S Ratio According to Age: Mean, LLN, and ULN

Lead		0–1 mo	1–6 mo	6 mo–1 yr	1–3 yr	3–8 yr	8–12 yr	12–16 yr	Adult
V1	LLN	0.5	0.3	0.3	0.5	0.1	0.15	0.1	0.0
	Mean	1.5	1.5	1.2	0.8	0.65	0.5	0.3	0.3
	ULN	19	S = 0	6	2	2	1	1	1
V2	LLN	0.3	0.3	0.3	0.3	0.05	0.1	0.1	0.1
	Mean	1	1.2	1	0.8	0.5	0.5	0.5	0.2
	ULN	3	4	4	1.5	1.5	1.2	1.2	2.5
V6	LLN	0.1	1.5	2	3	2.5	4	2.5	2.5
	Mean	2	4	6	20	20	20	10	9
	ULN	S = 0	S = 0	S = 0	S = 0	S = 0	S = 0	S = 0	S = 0

From Guntheroth WB: *Pediatric Electrocardiography,* Philadelphia, 1965, Saunders. Used by permission.
LLN, Lower limits of normal; *ULN,* upper limits of normal.

TABLE 3–6.

Q Voltages According to Lead and Age: Mean (and ULN)*†

Lead	0–1 mo	1–6 mo	6 mo–1yr	1–3 yr	3–8 yr	8–12 yr	12–16 yr	Adult
III	2 (5)	3 (8)	3 (8)	3 (8)	1.5 (6)	1 (5)	1 (4)	0.5 (4)
aVF	2 (4)	2 (5)	2 (6)	1.5 (5)	1 (5)	1 (3)	1 (3)	0.5 (2)
V5	1.5 (5)	1.5 (4)	2 (5)	2 (6)	2 (6)	2 (4.5)	1 (4)	0.5 (3.5)
V6	1.5 (4)	1.5 (4)	2 (5)	2 (4.5)	1.5 (4.5)	1.5 (4)	1 (2.5)	0.5 (3)

*From Guntheroth WG: *Pediatric Electrocardiography,* Philadelphia, 1965, Saunders. Used by permission.
†Voltages measured in millimeters, when 1 mV = 10 mm paper.
ULN, Upper limits of normal.

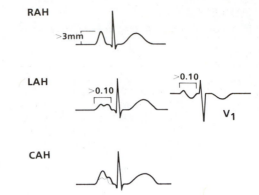

FIG. 3–13.
Criteria for atrial hypertrophy. (From Park MK, Guntheroth WG: *How to read pediatric ECGs,* ed 3, St Louis, 1992, Mosby.)

Tall peaked T waves may be seen in hyperkalemia and LVH (of the "volume overload" type). Flat or low T waves may occur in normal newborns or with hypothyroidism, hypokalemia, pericarditis, myocarditis, myocardial ischemia, and so on.

ATRIAL HYPERTROPHY

Right Atrial Hypertrophy

Tall P "waves" (≥ 3 mm) indicate right atrial hypertrophy (RAH) ("p-pulmonale") (Fig. 3-13).

Left Atrial Hypertrophy

Wide P wave duration (≥ 0.10 second in children; ≥ 0.08 second in infants) is seen in left atrial hypertrophy (LAH) (or "p-mitrale") (see Fig. 3-13).

Combined Atrial Hypertrophy

In combined atrial hypertrophy (CAH), a combination of an increased amplitude and duration of the P wave is present (see Fig. 3-13).

VENTRICULAR HYPERTROPHY

General Changes Seen in Ventricular Hypertrophy

Ventricular hypertrophy produces abnormalities in one or more of the following areas: the QRS axis, the QRS voltages, the R/S ratio, the T axis, and miscellaneous areas.

Changes in the QRS axis. The QRS axis is usually directed toward the ventricle that is hypertrophied. Although RAD is present with RVH, marked LAD is rare with LVH. A marked LAD usually indicates ventricular conduction disturbances (e.g., left anterior hemiblock or "superior" QRS axis).

Changes in QRS voltages. Anatomically the RV occupies the right and anterior aspect, and the LV occupies the left and posterior aspect of the ventricular mass. With ventricular hypertrophy, the voltage of the QRS complex increases in the direction of the respective ventricle.

In the frontal plane (Fig. 3-14, *A*), LVH shows increased R voltages in leads I, II, aVL, aVF, and sometimes III, especially in small infants. RVH shows increased R voltages in aVR and III and increased S voltages in lead I (see Table 3-4 for normal QRS voltages).

In the horizontal plane (Fig. 3-14, *B*), tall R waves in V4R, V1, and V2 or deep S waves in V5 and V6 are seen in RVH. With LVH, tall R waves in V5 and V6 and/or deep S waves in V4R, V1, and V2 are present (see Table 3-4).

Changes in R/S ratio. The R/S ratio represents the relative electromotive force of opposing ventricles in a given lead. In ventricular hypertrophy a change may only be seen in the R/S ratio without an increase in the absolute voltage. An increase in the R/S ratio in the RPLs suggests RVH; a decrease in the R/S ratio in these leads suggests LVH. Likewise, an increase in the R/S ratio in the LPLs suggests LVH and a decrease in the ratio suggests RVH (see Table 3-5).

Changes in the T axis. Changes in the T axis are seen in severe ventricular hypertrophy with relative ischemia of the hypertrophied myocardium. In the presence of other criteria of ventricular hypertrophy, a wide QRS-T angle (i.e., 90 degrees or greater) with the T axis outside the normal range indicates a "strain" pattern. When the T axis remains in the normal quadrant (i.e., 0 degrees to +90 degrees), a wide QRS-T angle alone indicates a *possible* "strain" pattern.

Miscellaneous nonspecific changes

RVH

1. A true q wave in V1 (qR, qRs pattern) suggests RVH. Physicians should make sure that it is not an rsR' with a very small or isoelectric r wave that is giving an erroneous appearance of a qR pattern.

2. An upright T wave in V1 after 3 days of age is a sign of probable RVH.

LVH. Deep Q waves (≥ 5 mm) and/or tall T waves in V5 and V6 are said to be signs of LVH of "volume overload" type. These may be seen with a large-shunt ventricular septal defect (VSD).

Criteria for Right Ventricular Hypertrophy

In RVH, some or all of the following criteria are present. In general, the greater the number of positive, independent criteria, the greater the probability of an abnormal degree of RVH.

1. RAD for the patient's age (see Table 3-1)

2. Increased rightward and anterior QRS voltages (in the presence of a normal QRS duration)

    a. R in V1, V2, or aVR greater than the upper limits of normal for the patient's age (see Table 3-4)

    b. S in I and V6 greater than the upper limits of normal for the patient's age (see Table 3-4)

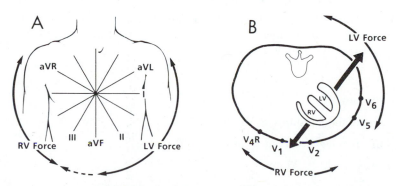

FIG. 3–14.
Diagrammatic representation of left and right ventricular forces on the frontal projection or hexaxial reference system **(A)** and the horizontal plane **(B)**. (From Park MK, Guntheroth WG: *How to read pediatric ECGs,* ed 3, St Louis, 1992, Mosby.)

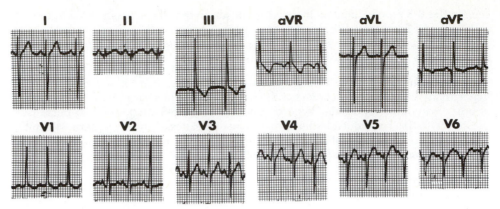

FIG. 3–15.
Tracing from a 10-month-old infant with severe TOF.

3. Abnormal R/S ratio in favor of the RV (in the absence of bundle branch block) (see Table 3-5)

   a. R/S ratio in V1 and V2 greater than the upper limits of normal for age

   b. R/S ratio in V6 less than 1 after 1 3 days of age, provided that the T is upright in the LPLs (V5, V6); upright T in V1 is not abnormal in patients 6 years or older

5. A q wave in V1 (qR or qRs patterns) suggests RVH (the physician should make sure that there is not a small r in an rsR′ configuration).

6. In the presence of RVH, a wide QRS-T angle with T axis outside the normal range (usually in the 0 degree to -90 degree quadrant) indicates "strain" pattern

Fig. 3-15 is an example of RVH. There is RAD for the patient's age (+150 degrees). The T axis is -10 degrees, and the QRS-T angle is abnormally wide (160 degrees) with the T axis in an abnormal quadrant. The QRS duration is normal. The R waves in III and aVR and the S waves in lead I and V6 are beyond the upper limits of normal, indicating an abnormal rightward force. The R/S ratio in V1 and V2 is larger than the upper limits of normal, and the ratio in V6 is smaller than the lower limits of normal, again indicating RVH. Therefore this tracing shows RVH with "strain."

Right Ventricular Hypertrophy in the Newborn

The diagnosis of RVH in newborns is particularly difficult because of the normal dominance of the RV during that period of life. The following clues, however, are helpful in the diagnosis of RVH in newborns:

1. S waves in lead I, ≥ 12 mm

2. R waves in aVR, ≥ 8 mm

3. Important abnormalities in V1 such as:

   a. Pure R waves (without S) in V1, ≥ 10 mm

   b. R waves V1, ≥ 25 mm

   c. qR pattern in V1 (also seen in 10% of normal newborns)

   d. Upright T waves in V1 in newborns more than 3 days of age (with upright T in V6)

4. QRS axis greater than +180 degrees

Criteria for Left Ventricular Hypertrophy

In LVH some or all of the following abnormalities are present. The greater the number of positive, independent criteria, the greater the probability of an abnormal degree of LVH.

1. LAD for the patient's age (see Table 3-1)

2. QRS voltages in favor of the LV (in the presence of a normal QRS duration)

   a. R in I, II, III, aVL, aVF, V5, or V6 greater than the upper limits of normal for age (see Table 3-4)

   b. S in V1 or V2 greater than the upper limits of normal for age (see Table 3-4)

3. Abnormal R/S ratio in favor of the LV: R/S ratio in V1 and V2 less than the lower limits of normal for the patient's age (see Table 3-5)

4. Q in V5 and V6, 5 mm or more, as well as tall symmetric T waves in the same leads ("LV diastolic overload")

5. In the presence of LVH, a wide QRS-T angle with the T axis outside the normal range indicates "strain" pattern; this is manifested by inverted T waves in lead I or aVF.

Fig. 3-16 is an example of LVH. There is LAD for the patient's age (0 degrees). The R waves in I, aVL, V5, and V6 are beyond the upper limits of normal, indicating abnormal LV force. The QRS duration is normal. The T vector (+55 degrees) remains in the normal quadrant. This tracing shows LVH without "strain."

Criteria for Combined Ventricular Hypertrophy

1. Positive voltage criteria for RVH *and* LVH in the absence of bundle branch block or preexcitation

2. Positive voltage criteria for RVH or LVH and relatively large voltages for the other ventricle

3. Large equiphasic QRS complexes in two or more of the limb leads and in the midprecordial leads (i.e., V2 through V5), called Katz-Wachtel phenomenon

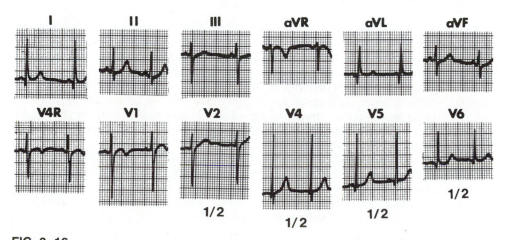

FIG. 3–16.
Tracing from a 4-year-old child with moderate VSD. Note that some precordial leads are in ½ normal standardization.

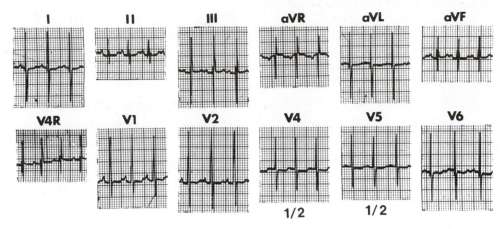

FIG. 3–17.
Tracing from a 2-month-old infant with large-shunt VSD, PDA, and severe pulmonary hypertension.

Fig. 3-17 is an example of combined ventricular hypertrophy (CVH). It is diffi-cult to plot the QRS axis because of large diphasic QRS complexes in limb leads and in the LPLs (i.e., Katz-Wachtel phenomenon). The S waves in I and V6 are abnormally deep (i.e., abnormal rightward force) and the R in V1 (i.e., rightward and anterior force) is also abnormally large, suggesting RVH. The R waves in leads I and aVL (i.e., leftward force) are also abnormally large. Therefore this tracing shows CVH.

VENTRICULAR CONDUCTION DISTURBANCES

Conditions that are grouped together as ventricular conduction disturbances have abnormal prolongation of QRS duration in common. Ventricular conduction distur-bances include the following:

1. RBBB and LBBB

2. Preexcitation (e.g., WPW) syndrome

3. Intraventricular block

In bundle branch blocks and ventricular rhythms, the prolongation is in the terminal portion of the QRS complex (i.e., "terminal slurring"). In the preexcitation, the prolongation is in the initial portion of the QRS complex (i.e., "initial slurring"), producing "delta" waves. In intraventricular block the prolongation is throughout the duration of the QRS complex (Fig. 3-18). The QRS duration varies with age; it is shorter in infants than in older children or adults (see Table 3-3). In adults a QRS duration greater than 0.10 second is required for diagnosis of a bundle branch block or ventricular conduction disturbances. In infants a QRS duration of 0.08 second meets the requirement for a bundle branch block.

By far the most commonly encountered form of ventricular conduction disturbance is RBBB. Although uncommon, the WPW syndrome is a well-defined entity that deserves a brief description. LBBB is extremely rare in children, although common in adults with ischemic and hypertensive heart disease. Intraventricular block is associated with metabolic disorders and diffuse myocardial diseases.

Right Bundle Branch Block

In RBBB delayed conduction through the right bundle branch prolongs the time required for a depolarization of the RV. When the LV is completely depolarized, RV depolarization is still in progress. This produces prolongation of the QRS duration, more specifically, "terminal slurring" (Fig. 3-18, *B*). The terminal slurring of the QRS complex is directed to the *right* and *anteriorly,* since the RV is located rightward and anteriorly in relation to the LV.

Criteria for right bundle branch block

1. RAD, at least for the terminal portion of the QRS complex

2. QRS duration longer than the upper limits of normal for the patient's age (see Table 3-3)

3. Terminal slurring of the QRS complex directed to the right and usually, but not always, anteriorly:

   a. Wide and slurred S in I, V5, and V6

   b. Terminal, slurred R' in aVR and the RPLs (i.e., V4R, V1, V2)

4. ST segment shift and T wave inversion are common in adults, but not in children

Because there is asynchrony of the opposing electromotive forces of each ventricle in RBBB, a greater manifest potential for both ventricles results, making it unsafe to make a diagnosis of ventricular hypertrophy in the presence of RBBB. This also applies to LBBB and the WPW syndrome.

Fig. 3-19 is an example of RBBB. The QRS duration is increased (0.11 second), indicating a ventricular conduction disturbance. There is slurring of the terminal portion of the QRS complex, indicating a bundle branch block, and the slurring is directed to the right (slurred S in I and V6, and slurred R in aVR) and anteriorly (slurred R in V4R and V1), satisfying criteria for RBBB. Although the S waves in I, V5, and V6 are abnormally deep and the R/S ratio in V1 is abnormally large, it cannot be interpreted as RVH in the presence of RBBB.

Two pediatric conditions that are most commonly associated with RBBB are ASD and conduction disturbances after open heart surgery involving right ventriculotomy. Other conditions often associated with RBBB include Ebstein's anomaly, coarctation of the aorta (COA) in infants younger than 6 months of age, ECD, partial anomalous pulmonary venous return (PAPVR), and occasional normal children. The significance of RBBB in children is different from that in adults. In several pediatric examples of RBBB the right bundle is intact. In an ASD the prolonged QRS duration is the result of a longer pathway through a dilated RV, rather than an actual block in the right bundle. Right ventriculotomy for repair of VSD or tetralogy of Fallot (TOF) disrupts the RV subendocardial Purkinje's network and causes prolongation of the QRS duration without necessarily injuring the main right bundle, although the latter may occasionally also be disrupted.

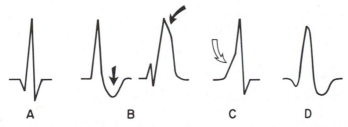

A   B   C   D

FIG. 3–18.
Schematic diagram of three types of ventricular conduction disturbances. **A,** Normal QRS complexes. **B,** QRS complex in RBBB or PVCs with prolongation of the QRS duration in the terminal portion (*black arrows,* terminal slurring). **C,** A preexcitation with delta wave (*open arrow,* initial slurring). **D,** Intraventricular block in which the prolongation of the QRS complex is throughout the duration of the QRS complex.

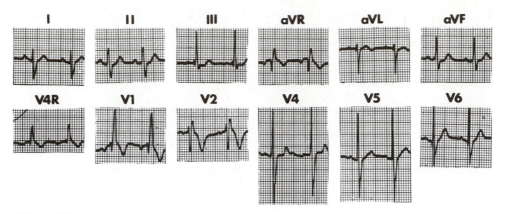

FIG. 3–19.
Tracing from a 6-year-old boy who had corrective surgery for TOF that involved right ventriculotomy for repair of VSD and resection of infundibular narrowing.

Some pediatricians are concerned with the rsR' pattern in V1. Although it is unusual to see this in adults, the rsR' pattern in V1 is *normal* in infants and small children provided that the QRS duration is not prolonged and the voltage of the primary or secondary R waves is not abnormally large. The rsR' pattern may be seen in healthy children because the terminal QRS vector is more rightward and anterior in infants and children than in adults.

Intraventricular Block

In intraventricular block the prolongation is throughout the duration of the QRS complex (see Fig. 3-18, *D*). It is associated with metabolic disorders (e.g., hyperkalemia), myocardial ischemia as seen during cardiopulmonary resuscitation, quinidine or procainamide toxicity, and diffuse myocardial diseases (e.g., myocardial fibrosis, systemic diseases with myocardial involvement).

Wolff-Parkinson-White Syndrome

The WPW syndrome is a form of preexcitation. It results from an anomalous conduction pathway (i.e., bundle of Kent) between the atrium and the ventricle, bypassing the normal delay of conduction in the AV node. The premature depolarization of a ventricle produces a delta wave and results in prolongation of the QRS duration (Fig. 3-18, *C*).

Criteria for Wolff-Parkinson-White syndrome

1. Short PR interval, less than the lower limits of normal for the patient's age

   The lower limits of a normal PR interval are as follows:
   Younger than 3 years old   0.08 seconds
   3 to 16 years old   0.10 seconds
   Older than 16 years old   0.12 seconds

2. Delta wave (initial slurring of the QRS complex)

3. Wide QRS duration beyond the upper limits of normal

Patients with the WPW syndrome are prone to attacks of paroxysmal supraventricular tachycardia (see Chapter 24). The WPW syndrome may mimic other ECG abnormalities such as ventricular hypertrophy, RBBB, or myocardial disorders. In the presence of this syndrome, diagnosis of ventricular hypertrophy cannot be safely made. The often large QRS deflections seen in this condition are usually because of the conduction

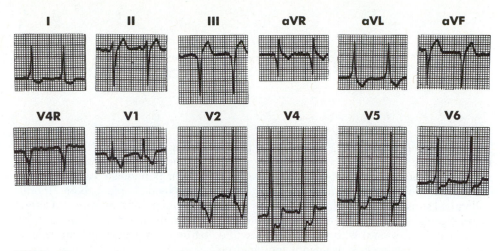

FIG. 3–20.
Tracing from an asymptomatic 2-year-old boy whose VSD underwent spontaneous closure. The tracing shows the WPW syndrome (see text for interpretation).

disturbance, rather than ventricular hypertrophy. The following are two other forms of preexcitation:

1. Lown-Ganong-Levine syndrome is characterized by a short PR interval and normal QRS duration. In this condition James fibers bypass the upper AV node and produce a short PR interval, but the ventricles are depolarized normally through the His-Purkinje system.

2. Mahaim-type preexcitation syndrome is characterized by a normal PR interval and long QRS duration with a "delta wave." There is an abnormal Mahaim fiber that bypasses the bundle of His and "short-circuits" into the RV.

Fig. 3-20 is an example of the WPW syndrome. The most striking abnormalities are a short PR interval (0.08 second) and a wide QRS duration (0.11 second). There are delta waves in most of the leads. Some delta waves are negative, as seen in leads III, aVR, V4R, and V1. The ST segments and T wave are shifted in the opposite direction of the QRS vector, resulting in a wide QRS-T angle. The leftward voltages are abnormally large, but the diagnosis of LVH cannot be safely made in the presence of the WPW syndrome.

4 / Chest Roentgenography

The chest roentgenogram is an essential part of cardiac evaluation. The following information can be gained from x-ray films: heart size and silhouette; enlargement of specific cardiac chambers; pulmonary blood flow (PBF) or pulmonary valve markings (PVM); and other information regarding lung parenchyma, spine, bony thorax, abdominal situs, and so on. Most institutions routinely obtain posteroanterior and lateral views. Special cardiac views (e.g., posteroanterior, lateral, right anterior oblique, and left anterior oblique views) with barium swallow (i.e., barium esophagogram) are seldom used in initial evaluations of infants and children.

HEART SIZE AND SILHOUETTE

Heart Size

Measurement of the cardiothoracic ratio is by far the simplest way to estimate the heart size in older children (Fig. 4-1). The cardiothoracic (CT) ratio is obtained by relating the largest transverse diameter of the heart to the widest internal diameter of the chest:

$$\text{Cardiothoracic ratio} = (A + B) \div C$$

where A and B are maximal cardiac dimensions to the right and to the left of the midline, respectively, and C is the widest internal diameter of the chest. A CT ratio of more than 0.5 indicates cardiomegaly. However, the CT ratio cannot be used with accuracy in newborns and small infants, in whom a good inspiratory chest film is rarely obtained. In this situation the degree of inadequate inspiration should be taken into consideration. Also, an estimation of the cardiac volume should be made by inspecting the posteroanterior and lateral views instead of the CT ratio.

To determine the presence or absence of cardiomegaly, the lateral view of the heart should be taken into consideration. For example, an isolated right ventricular enlargement (RVE) may not be obvious on a posteroanterior film but is obvious on a lateral film. In a patient with a flat chest (or narrow anteroposterior diameter of the chest), a posteroanterior film may erroneously show cardiomegaly.

An enlarged heart on chest x-ray film more reliably reflects a volume overload than a pressure overload. ECGs better represent the pressure overload.

Normal Cardiac Silhouette

The structures that form the cardiac borders in the posteroanterior projection of a chest roentgenogram are as follows (Fig. 4-2). The right cardiac silhouette is formed superiorly by the superior vena cava (SVC) and inferiorly by the right atrium (RA). The left cardiac border is formed from the top to the bottom by the aortic knob, the main pulmonary artery (MPA), and the left ventricle (LV). The left atrial appendage (LAA) is located between the MPA and the LV and is *not* prominent in a normal heart. The right ventricle (RV) does not form the cardiac border in the posteroanterior view. The lateral projection of the cardiac silhouette is formed anteriorly by the RV and posteriorly by the left atrium (LA) above and the LV below. In a normal heart the lower posterior cardiac border (i.e., LV) crosses the inferior vena cava (IVC) line above the diaphragm (Fig. 4-2).

However, in the newborn, a typical, normal cardiac silhouette is rarely seen because of the presence of a large thymus and because the films are often exposed during

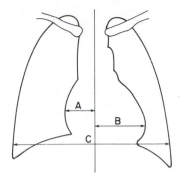

FIG. 4–1.
Diagram showing how to measure the cardiothoracic (CT) ratio from the PA view of a chest x-ray film. The CT ratio is obtained by dividing the largest horizontal diameter of the heart A + B) by the longest internal diameter of the chest (C).

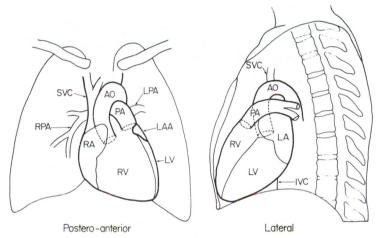

Postero-anterior   Lateral

FIG. 4–2.
PA and lateral projections of normal cardiac silhouette. Note that in the lateral projection, the RV is contiguous with the lower third of the sternum and that the LV normally crosses the posterior margin of the IVC above the diaphragm. *AO,* aorta; *LPA,* left pulmonary artery; *RPA,* right pulmonary artery; *IVC,* inferior vena cava; *LA,* left atrium; *LAA,* left atrial appendage; *LV,* left ventricle; *PA,* pulmonary artery; *RA,* right atrium; *RV,* right ventricle; *SVC,* superior vena cava.

expiration. The thymus is situated in the superoanterior mediastinum. Therefore the base of the heart may be widened with resulting alteration in the normal silhouette in the posteroanterior view. In the lateral view the retrosternal space, which is normally clear in older children, may be obliterated by the large thymus.

Abnormal Cardiac Silhouette

Although discerning individual chamber enlargement often helps determine acyanotic heart defect, the overall shape of the heart sometimes provides important clues to the type of defect, particularly in dealing with cyanotic infants and children. A few examples are presented below with the status of PBF.

1. A "boot-shaped" heart with decreased PBF is a typical shape of the heart in infants with cyanotic tetralogy of Fallot (TOF). This is also seen in some infants with tricuspid atresia. Typical of both conditions is the presence of a hypoplastic MPA segment (Fig. 4-3, *A*). The ECGs are helpful in differentiating these two conditions: the ECG shows right axis deviation (RAD), right ventricular

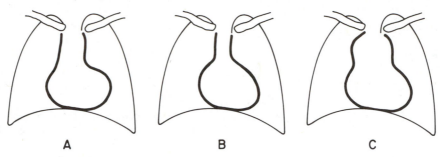

FIG. 4–3.
Abnormal cardiac silhouette. **A,** "Boot-shaped" heart seen in cyanotic TOF or tricuspid atresia. **B,** "Egg-shaped" heart seen in TGA. **C,** "Snowman" sign seen in TAPVR (supracardiac type).

hypertrophy (RVH), and occasional right atrial hypertrophy (RAH) in TOF, while showing a "superior" QRS axis (i.e., left anterior hemiblock), RAH, and left ventricular hypertrophy (LVH) in tricuspid atresia.

2. Narrow waist and "egg-shaped" heart with increased PBF in a cyanotic infant strongly suggests transposition of the great arteries (TGA). The narrow waist results from the absence of a large thymus and the abnormal relationship of the great arteries (Fig. 4-3, *B*).

3. "Snowman" sign with increased PBF is seen in infants with the supracardiac type of total anomalous pulmonary venous return (TAPVR). The left vertical vein, left innominate vein, and dilated SVC make up the "snowman's" head (Fig. 4-3, *C*).

EVALUATION OF CARDIAC CHAMBERS AND GREAT ARTERIES
Individual Chamber Enlargement

Identification of individual chamber enlargement is important in deriving a diagnosis of a specific lesion, particularly in dealing with acyanotic heart defects. Although enlargement of a single chamber is discussed here, more than one chamber is usually involved in a real situation.

Left atrial enlargement. An enlarged LA causes alterations not only of the cardiac silhouette, but also of the various adjacent structures (Fig. 4-4). Mild left atrial enlargement (LAE) is best appreciated in the lateral projection by the posterior protrusion of the LA border. An enlargement of the LA may produce "double density" on the posteroanterior view. With further enlargement, the LAA becomes prominent on the left cardiac border. The left main-stem bronchus is elevated. The barium-filled esophagus is indented to the right.

Left ventricular enlargement. In the posteroanterior view the apex of the heart is not only farther to the left but also downward. In the lateral view of left ventricular enlargement (LVE) the lower posterior cardiac border is displaced further posteriorly and meets the IVC line below the diaphragm level (Fig. 4-5).

Right atrial enlargement. The right atrial enlargement (RAE) is most obvious in the PA projection as an increased prominence of the right lower cardiac silhouette (Fig. 4-6). However, this is not an absolute finding because both false-positive and false-negative results are possible.

Right ventricular enlargement. An isolated right ventrical enlargement (RVE) may not be obvious in the posteroanterior projection, and the normal cardiothoracic ratio may be maintained, since the RV does not make up the cardiac silhouette in the posteroanterior projection. The RVE is best recognized in the lateral view in which it manifests itself by filling of the retrosternal space (Fig. 4-6, *lateral view*).

Size of the Great Arteries

As in the enlargement of specific cardiac chambers, the size of the great arteries often helps make a specific diagnosis.

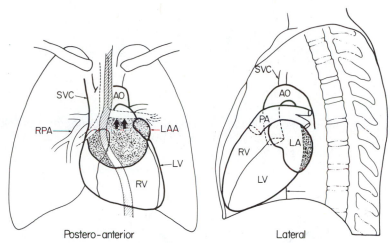

Postero-anterior   Lateral

FIG. 4—4.
Schematic diagram showing roentgenographic findings of LA enlargement in the posteroanterior and lateral projections. *Arrows* show left main-stem bronchus elevation. In the posteroanterior view, "double density" and prominence of the LAA are also illustrated. The barium-filled esophagus (cross-hatched, vertical structure) is indented to the right. In the lateral view, posterior protrusion of the LA border is illustrated. The isolated enlargement of the LA shown here is only hypothetical, since it usually accompanies other changes. Abbreviations are the same as those in Fig. 4-2.

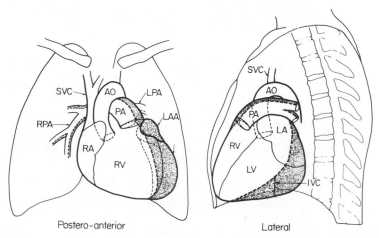

Postero-anterior   Lateral

FIG. 4—5.
Diagrammatic representation of VSD, which demonstrates LV enlargement in addition to the enlargement of the LA and a prominent MPA segment. Abbreviations are the same as those in Fig. 4-2.

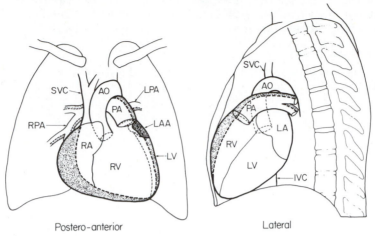

FIG. 4–6.
Schematic diagrams of posteroanterior and lateral chest roentgenograms of ASD. Enlargement of the RA and RV and an increased pulmonary vascularity. Abbreviations are the same as those in Fig. 4-2.

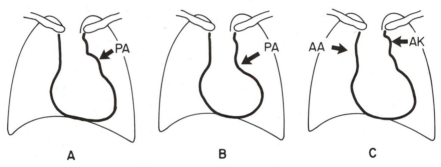

FIG. 4–7.
Abnormalities of the great arteries. **A,** Prominent MPA *(PA)* segment. **B,** Concave PA segment *(PA)* resulting from hypoplasia. **C.** Dilatation of the aorta may be seen as a bulge on the right upper mediastinum by a dilated ascending aorta *(AA)* or as a prominence of the aortic knob *(AK)* on the left upper cardiac border.

Prominent main pulmonary artery segment. The prominence of a normally placed pulmonary artery in the posteroanterior view (Fig 4-7, *A*) results from one of the following:

  a. Poststenotic dilatation (e.g., pulmonary valve stenosis)

  b. Increased blood flow through the pulmonary artery (PA) (e.g., atrial septal defect (ASD), ventricular septal defect (VSD)

  c. Increased pressure in the PA (e.g., pulmonary hypertension)

  d. Occasional normal adolescence, especially in girls

Hypoplasia of the pulmonary artery. A concave MPA segment with resulting "boot-shaped" heart is seen in TOF and tricuspid atresia (Fig. 4-7, *B*); obviously, malposition of the PA must be ruled out

Dilatation of the aorta. An enlarged ascending aorta may be observed in the frontal projection as a rightward bulge of the right upper mediastinum, but a mild degree of enlargement may easily escape detection. Aortic enlargement is seen in TOF and AS (poststenotic dilatation) and less often in patent ductus arteriosus (PDA), coarctation of the aorta (COA), Marfan's syndrome, or systemic hypertension. When the ascending aorta and aortic arch are enlarged, the aortic knob may become prominent on the PA view (Fig. 4-7, C).

PULMONARY VASCULAR MARKINGS

One of the major goals of radiologic examination is the assessment of the pulmonary vasculature. Although many textbooks explain how to detect the increased PBF, this is one of the more difficult aspects in the interpretation of the chest x-ray films of cardiac patients. There is no substitute for the experience gained by looking at many chest x-ray films with normal and abnormal PBF.

Increased Pulmonary Blood Flow

Increased pulmonary vascularity is present when: the right and left pulmonary arteries appear enlarged and extend into the lateral third of the lung field, where they are not usually present; there is an increased vascularity to the lung apices where the vessels are normally collapsed; and the external diameter of the right pulmonary artery (RPA) visible in the right hilus is wider than the internal diameter of the trachea.

An increased PBF in an acyanotic child represents either ASD, VSD, PDA, ECD, partial anomalous pulmonary venous return (PAPVR), or any combination of these. In a cyanotic infant, increased PVMs may indicate TGA, TAPVR, HLHS, persistent truncus arteriosus, or a single ventricle.

Decreased Pulmonary Blood Flow

A decreased PBF is suspected when the hilum appears small, the remaining lung fields appear black, and the vessels appear small and thin. Ischemic lung fields are seen in cyanotic heart diseases with decreased PBF such as critical stenosis or atresia of the pulmonary or tricuspid valves, including TOF.

Pulmonary Venous Congestion

Pulmonary venous congestion is characterized by a hazy and indistinct margin of the pulmonary vasculature. This is caused by pulmonary venous hypertension secondary to left ventricular failure or obstruction to pulmonary venous drainage (e.g., HLHS, MS, TAPVR, cor triatriatum, and so on). Kerley's B lines are short, transverse strips of increased density best seen in the costophrenic sulci. This is caused by engorged lymphatics and interstitial edema of the interlobular septa secondary to pulmonary venous congestion.

Normal Pulmonary Vasculature

Pulmonary vascularity is normal in patients with obstructive lesions such as pulmonary stenosis (PS) or aortic stenosis (AS). Unless the stenosis is extremely severe, pulmonary vascularity remains normal in PS. Patients with small left-to-right shunt lesions also show normal PVMs.

SYSTEMATIC APPROACH

The interpretation of chest x-ray films should include a systematic routine to avoid overlooking important anatomic changes relevant to cardiac diagnosis.

Location of the Liver and Stomach Gas Bubble

The cardiac apex should be on the same side as the stomach or opposite the hepatic shadow. When there is heterotaxia, with the apex on the right and the stomach on the left or vice versa, the likelihood of serious heart defect is great. An even more ominous situation exists with a "midline" liver, associated with asplenia (Ivemark's) syndrome, or polysplenia syndrome (see Fig. 28-1 on p. 373). These infants usually have complex cyanotic heart defects, which are difficult to correct.

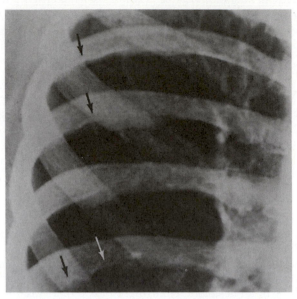

FIG. 4–8.
Rib notching *(arrows)* in an 11-year-old girl with COA. (From Caffey J: *Pediatric x-ray diagnosis,* ed 7, Chicago, 1978, Mosby.)

Skeletal Aspect of Chest X-Ray Film

Pectus excavatum may flatten the heart in the AP dimension and cause a compensatory increase in its transverse diameter, creating the false impression of cardiomegaly. Thoracic scoliosis and vertebral abnormalities are frequent in cardiac patients. Rib notching is a specific finding of COA in the older child (usually older than 5 years) and is usually found between the fourth and eighth ribs (Fig. 4-8).

Identification of the Aorta

Identification of the descending aorta along the left margin of the spine usually indicates a left aortic arch; identification along the right margin of the spine indicates a right aortic arch. When the descending aorta is not directly visible, the position of the trachea and esophagus may help locate the descending aorta. If the trachea and esophagus are located slightly to the right of the midline, the aorta usually descends normally on the left (i.e., left aortic arch). In the right aortic arch, the trachea and esophagus are shifted to the left. Right aortic arch is frequently associated with TOF or persistent truncus arteriosus. In a heavily exposed film, the precoarctation and postcoarctation dilatation of the aorta may be seen as a "figure of 3." This may be confirmed by a barium esophagogram with E-shaped indentation (Fig. 4-9).

Upper Mediastinum

The thymus is prominent in healthy infants and may give a false impression of cardiomegaly. It may give the classic "sail sign" (Fig. 4-10). The thymus often has a wavy border because this structure becomes indented by the ribs. On the lateral view, the thymus occupies the superoanterior mediastinum, obscuring the upper retrosternal space. The thymus shrinks in cyanotic infants or infants under severe stress from congestive heart failure (CHF). In TGA, the mediastinal shadow is narrow ("narrow waist"), partly because of the shrinkage of the thymus gland. Infants with DiGeorge syndrome have an absent thymic shadow and a high incidence of aortic arch anomalies. "Snowman figure" (or figure-of-8 configuration) is seen in infants, who are usually older than 4 months, with anomalous pulmonary venous return draining into the SVC via the left SVC (vertical vein) and the left innominate vein (see Fig. 4-3, *C*).

Pulmonary Parenchyma

Pneumonia is a common complication in patients with high pulmonary venous pressure such as a large PDA or VSD. A long-standing density, particularly in the right lower lung field, suggests bronchopulmonary sequestration in which a segment of the lung is supplied directly by an artery from the descending aorta. A vertical vascular shadow along the right lower cardiac border may suggest PAPVR from the lower lobe and sometimes from the middle lobe of the right lung called *scimitar syndrome*. Bronchopulmonary sequestration is often associated with the scimitar syndrome. In bronchopulmonary sequestration a segment of the lung is supplied by an arterial branch originating from the descending aorta.

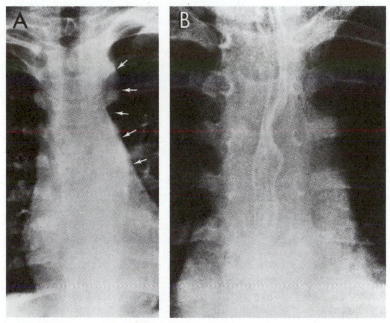

FIG. 4–9.
A, The figure-of-3 configuration indicates the site of coarctation with the large proximal segment of aorta and/or prominent left subclavian artery above and the poststenotic dilatation of the descending aorta below it. **B,** Barium esophagogram reveals the E-shaped indentation or reversed figure-of-3 configuration. (From Caffey J: *Pediatric x-ray diagnosis,* ed 7, Chicago, 1978. Mosby.)

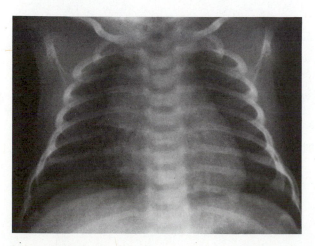

FIG. 4–10.
A roentgenogram showing the typical "sail sign" on the right mediastinal border.

5 / Flow Diagram

A flow diagram that helps arrive at a diagnosis of congenital heart disease (CHD) is shown in Box 5-1. It is based on the presence or absence of cyanosis and on the status of pulmonary blood flow (PBF) whether normal, increased, or decreased. The presence of right ventricular hypertrophy (RVH) or left ventricular hypertrophy (LVH) or both further narrows the possibilities. Only common entities are listed in the flow diagram.

In using this flow diagram certain adjustments are often necessary. For example, in some instances in which pulmonary vascularity on chest x-ray films may be interpreted as normal or at the upper limits of normal, the list may need to be checked under both normal and increased PBF. Likewise, an ECG may show right ventricular (RV) dominance, yet not meet strict criteria for RVH. Such a case may need to be treated as RVH. It should also be remembered that normal ECG and normal pulmonary vascular markings (PVM) on chest x-ray films do not rule out CHD. In fact, many mild, acyanotic heart defects do not show abnormalities on the ECG or chest x-ray films. Diagnosis of these defects rests primarily on findings from the physical examination, particularly on auscultation.

In addition to ventricular hypertrophy seen on ECGs, other ECG findings are occasionally helpful in making the diagnosis. For example, a superiorly oriented QRS axis (i.e., left anterior hemiblock) in an acyanotic infant suggests endocardial cushion defect (ECD), whereas in a cyanotic infant it suggests tricuspid atresia. ECG findings of myocardial infarction may be seen in anomalous origin of the left coronary artery from the pulmonary artery, coronary aneurysms associated with Kawasaki disease, or endocardial fibroelastosis. Common ECG manifestations of some congenital heart diseases are summarized in Table 5-1.

Chest x-ray findings other than PVM also help detect a specific CHD. A few examples follow: (see Chapter 4).

1. Heart size

    a. A large heart indicates large shunt lesions, myocardial failure, or pericardial effusion.

    b. A large heart usually rules out tetralogy of Fallot (TOF).

2. Cardiac silhouette

    a. A "boot-shaped" heart suggests TOF or tricuspid atresia.

    b. An "egg-shaped" heart with increased pulmonary vascularity suggests transposition of the great arteries (TGA).

    c. A "snowman" sign suggests anomalous pulmonary venous return.

3. Right aortic arch is commonly seen in TOF or persistent truncus arteriosus.

4. A midline liver strongly suggests complex cardiac defects associated with asplenia or polysplenia syndrome.

BOX 5–1.
Flow Diagram of CHD

Acyanotic Defects

Increased PBF
  LVH or CVH
    VSD
    PDA
    ECD
  RVH
    ASD (often RBBB)
    PAPVR
    Eisenmenger's physiology secondary to VSD, PDA, and so on
Normal PBF
  LVH
    AS or AR
    COA
    Primary myocardial disease (endocardial fibroelastosis)
    MR
  RVH
    PS
    COA in infants
    MS

Cyanotic Defects

Increased PBF
  LVH or CVH
    Persistent truncus arteriosus
    Single ventricle (common ventricle)
    TGA plus VSD
  RVH
    TGA
    TAPVR
    HLHS
Decreased PBF
  CVH
    TGA plus PS
    Persistent truncus arteriosus with hypoplastic PA
    Single ventricle with PS
  LVH
    Tricuspid atresia
    Pulmonary atresia with hypoplastic RV
  RVH
    TOF
    Eisenmenger's physiology secondary to ASD, VSD, PDA
    Ebstein's anomaly (RBBB)

CHD, congenital heart defect; *PBF*, pulmonary blood flow; *LVH*, left ventricular hypertrophy; *CVH*, combined ventricular hypertrophy; *VSD*, ventricular septal defect; *PDA*, patent ductus arteriosus; *ECD*, endocardial cushion defect; *RVH*, right ventricular hypertrophy; *ASD*, atrial septal defect; *RBBB*, right bundle branch block; *PAPVR*, partial anomalous pulmonary venous return; *AS*, aortic stenosis; *AR*, aortic regurgitation; *COA*, coarctation of the aorta; *MR*, mitral regurgitation; *PS*, pulmonary stenosis; *MS*, mitral stenosis; *TGA*, transposition of the great arteries; *TAPVR*, total anomalous pulmonary venous return; *HLHS*, hypoplastic left heart syndrome; *PA*, pulmonary artery; *RV,* right ventricle; *TOF,* tetralogy of Fallot.

TABLE 5–1.

Common ECG Manifestations of Some CHDs

Congenital Defects	Electrocardiograph Findings
Anomalous origin of the left coronary artery from the PA	Myocardial infarction, anterolateral
Anomalous pulmonary venous return	
Total	RAD, RVH, and RAH
Partial	Mild RVH or RBBB
AS	
Mild to moderate	Normal or LVH
Severe	LVH with or without "strain"
ASD	
Primum type	Left anterior hemiblock (superior QRS axis)
	rsR′ pattern in V1 and aVR (RBBB or RVH)
	First-degree AV block (>50%)
	Counterclockwise QRS loop in the frontal plane of vector cardiogram
Secundum type	RAD, RVH, or RBBB (rsR′ in V1 and aVR)
	First-degree AV block (10%)
COA	
Infants younger than 6 mo	RBBB or RVH
Older children	LVH, normal, or RBBB
Common ventricle or single ventricle	Abnormal Q waves
	Q in V1 and no Q in V6
	No Q in any precordial leads
	Q in all precordial leads
	Stereotype RS complex in most or all precordial leads
	WPW syndrome or SVT
	First-or second-degree AV block
Cor triatriatum	Same as for MS
Ebstein's anomaly	RAH, RBBB
	First-degree AV block
	WPW syndrome
	No RVH
ECD	
Complete	Left anterior hemiblock (superior QRS axis)
	RVH or CVH, RAH
	First-degree AV block, RBBB
Partial	See ASD, primum type
Endocardial fibroelastosis	LVH
	Abnormal T waves
	Myocardial infarction patterns
HLHS (aortic and/or mitral atresia)	RVH
MS, congenital or acquired	RAD, RVH, RAH, LAH (±)
PDA	
Small shunt	Normal
Moderate shunt	LVH, LAH (±)
Large shunt	CVH, LAH
Eisenmenger's syndrome (PVOD)	RVH or CVH
Persistent truncus arteriosus	LVH or CVH
Pulmonary atresia (with hypoplastic RV)	LVH

CHD, congenital heart defect; *PA,* pulmonary artery; *RAD,* right axis deviation; *RVH,* right ventricular hypertrophy; *RAH,* right atrial hypertrophy; *RBBB,* right bundle branch block; *AS,* aortic stenosis; *LVH,* left ventricular hypertrophy; *ASD,* atrial septal defect; *AV,* atrioventricular; *COA,* coarctation of the aorta; *WPW,* Wolff-Parkinson-White; *SVT,* supraventricular tachycardia; *MS,* mitral stenosis; *ECD,* endocardial cushion defect; *CVH,* combined ventricular hypertrophy; *LAH,* left atrial hypertrophy; *PDA,* patent ductus arteriosus; *PVOD,* pulmonary vascular obstructive disease; *RV,* right ventricle.

TABLE 5–1. *Continued*

Congenital Defects	Electrocardiograph Findings
PS	
Mild	Normal or mild RVH
Moderate	RVH
Severe	RVH with "strain," RAH
PVOD (Eisenmenger's syndrome)	RVH or CVH
TOF	RAD
	RVH, moderate or severe
	RAH (±)
D-TGA (complete transposition)	
Intact ventricular septum	RVH, RAH
VSD and/or PS	CVH, RAH, or CAH
L-TGA (congenitally "corrected"	AV block, first- to third-degree
transposition)	Atrial arrhythmias (PAT, atrial fibrillation)
	WPW syndrome
	Absent Q in V5 and V6 and qR pattern in V1
	LAH or CAH
Tricuspid atresia	Left anterior hemiblock (superior QRS axis)
	LVH, RAH
VSD	
Small shunt	Normal
Moderate shunt	LVH, LAH (±)
Large shunt	CVH, LAH
PVOD (Eisenmenger's syndrome)	RVH

PAT, paroxysmal atrial tachycardia; *TGA,* transposition of the great arteries; *CAH,* combined atrial hypertrophy; *VSD,* ventricular septal defect; *PS,* pulmonary stenosis; *TOF,* tetralogy of Fallot.

PART II

Special Tools in Evaluation of Cardiac Patients

Some readers may want to skip this section at this time and come back later as the need arises. Special tools to be discussed in this section may be considered too specialized. Omission of this section does not affect understanding of pathophysiology and most clinical aspects of pediatric cardiac problems.

A number of special tools are available to the cardiologist in the evaluation of cardiac patients. Some tools are readily available and frequently used in tertiary centers, whereas others are more specialized and used less frequently. This section only discusses tests to which noncardiologists are exposed. Echocardiography (echo) (e.g., M-mode, two-dimensional, and Doppler), exercise tolerance test (e.g., stress test), and ambulatory ECG (e.g., Holter monitor) are noninvasive tests; cardiac catheterization and angiocardiography are invasive tests. Although catheter intervention procedures are not diagnostic, this section discusses them because they are usually performed with cardiac catheterization.

Several other tests are not discussed because they are rarely performed or are too specialized. These tests include vectorcardiography, electrophysiologic study, nuclear cardiology (e.g., radionuclide cineangiography, myocardial scintigraphy), and magnetic resonance imaging.

6 / Noninvasive Techniques

ECHOCARDIOGRAPHY

Echo is an extremely useful, safe, and noninvasive method for the diagnosis and management of heart disease. Echo studies, which use ultrasound, provide anatomic diagnosis, as well as functional information. This is especially true with the incorporation of Doppler echo.

The M-mode echo provides an "ice-pick" view of the heart. It has limited capability in demonstrating the spatial relationship of structures but remains an important tool in the evaluation of certain cardiac conditions and functions, particularly for dimensions and timing. The two-dimensional echo provides the enhanced ability to demonstrate the spatial relationship of structures. This capability allows for a more accurate anatomic diagnosis of abnormalities of the heart and great vessels. The Doppler study has added the ability to detect valve regurgitation and cardiac shunts to the echo examination. It also provides some quantitative information such as pressure gradients across a valve, cardiac output, and shunt calculations. Discussion about instruments and techniques is beyond the scope of this book. Normal echo images and their role in the diagnosis of common cardiac problems in pediatric patients are briefly presented.

M-Mode Echocardiography

An M-mode echo is obtained with the ultrasonic transducer placed along the left sternal border and directed toward the part of the heart to be examined. In Fig. 6-1 the ultrasound is shown passing through three important structures of the left side of the heart. Line 1 passes through the aorta and left atrium (LA) where the dimension of these structures is measured. Line 2 traverses the mitral valve. Line 3 goes through the main body of the right ventricle (RV) and left ventricle (LV). Along line 3 the dimensions of the RV and LV and the thickness of the interventricular septum and posterior LV wall are measured. Pericardial effusion is best detected at this level. An M-mode echo of the pulmonary valve is useful in the evaluation of pulmonary hypertension (see Chapter 32).

Although the two-dimensional echo has replaced many roles of the M-mode echo in the diagnosis of cardiac diseases, the M-mode echo still maintains many important applications. The applications include the following:

a. Measurement of the dimensions of cardiac chambers and vessels, thickness of the ventricular septum, and free walls

b. Left ventricular systolic function

c. Study of the motion of the cardiac valves (e.g., mitral valve prolapse (MVP), mitral stenosis (MS), pulmonary hypertension, and so on) and the interventricular septum

d. Detection of pericardial fluid

Normal M-mode echocardiographic values. The dimensions of the cardiac chambers and the aorta increase with increasing age. Table 6-1 shows the mean values and ranges of common M-mode echo measurements according to the patient's weight (see Appendix B, Table B-1 on p. 482). Most dimensions are measured during diastole, coincident with the onset of the QRS complex; the LA dimension and LV systolic dimension are exceptions (Figure 6-1).

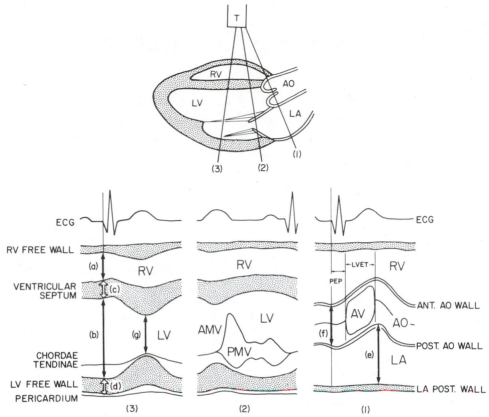

FIG. 6-1.
A cross-sectional view of the left side of the heart along the long axis *(top)* through which "ice-pick" views of the M-mode echo recordings are made *(bottom)*. Many other M-mode views are possible, but only three are shown in this figure. The dimension of the aorta *(AO)* and left atrium is measured along the line *(1)*. Systolic time intervals for the left side are also measured at the level of the aortic valve *(AV)*. The line *(2)* passes through the mitral valve. Measurements made at this level are not useful in pediatric patients. Measurement of chamber dimensions and wall thickness of right and left ventricles is made along the line *(3)*. Normal values of these measurements are shown in Table 6-1. *(a)*, RV dimension; *(b)*, LV diastolic dimension; *(c)*, interventricular septal thickness; *(d)*, LV posterior wall thickness; *(e)*, LA dimension; *(f)*, aortic dimension; *(g)*, LV systolic dimension; *AMV*, anterior mitral valve; *LVET*, left ventricular ejection time; *PEP*, preejection period; *PMV*, posterior mitral valve.

Left ventricular systolic function. LV systolic function is evaluated by the fractional shortening (shortening fraction), ejection fraction, and systolic time intervals. The ejection fraction is a derivative of the fractional shortening and offers no advantages over the fractional shortening. Serial determinations of these measurements are important in conditions in which LV function may change (e.g., in patients with chronic or acute myocardial disease or those with chemotherapy-induced LV dysfunction).

Fractional shortening. Fractional shortening is derived by the following:

$$FS(\%) = Dd - DS/Dd \times 100$$

where FS is fractional shortening, Dd is end-diastolic dimension, and Ds is end-systolic dimension. This is a reliable and reproducible index of LV function, provided there no regional wall-motion abnormality exists and there is concentric contractility of the LV.

TABLE 6–1.

Normal M-Mode Echo Values (mm) by Weight (lb): Mean (Ranges)

	0 to 25 lb	26 to 50 lb	51 to 75 lb	76 to 100 lb	101 to 125 lb	126 to 200 lb
RV dimension	9	10	11	12	13	13
	(3 to 15)	(4 to 15)	(7 to 18)	(7 to 16)	(8 to 17)	(12 to 17)
LV dimension	24	34	38	41	43	49
	(13 to 32)	(24 to 38)	(33 to 45)	(35 to 47)	(37 to 49)	(44 to 52)
LV free wall (or	5	6	7	7	7	8
septum)	(4 to 6)	(5 to 7)	(6 to 7)	(7 to 8)	(7 to 8)	(7 to 8)
LA dimension	17	22	23	24	27	28
	(7 to 23)	(17 to 27)	(19 to 28)	(20 to 30)	(21 to 30)	(21 to 37)
Aortic root	13	17	20	22	23	24
	(7 to 17)	(13 to 22)	(17 to 23)	(19 to 27)	(17 to 27)	(22 to 28)

Modified from Feigenbaum H: *Echocardiography*, ed 4. Philadelphia, 1986, Lea & Febiger.

regional wall-motion abnormality exists and there is concentric contractility of the LV. Mean normal value is 36% with 95% prediction limits of 28% to 44%. The fractional shortening is decreased in a poorly compensated LV regardless of etiology (e.g., pressure overload, volume overload, primary myocardial disorders, doxorubicin cardiotoxicity, and so on). It is increased in compensated LV function such as volume overload (e.g., ventricular septal defect [VSD], patent ductus arteriosus [PDA], aortic regurgitation [AR], mitral regurgitation [MR]) and pressure overload lesions (e.g., moderately severe aortic valve stenosis, hypertrophic obstructive cardiomyopathy [HOCM], and so on).

Ejection fraction. Ejection fraction relates to the change in volume of the LV with cardiac contraction. It is obtained by the following formula:

$$EF(\%) = (Dd)^3 - (Ds)^3/(Dd)^3 \times 100$$

where EF is ejection fraction and Dd and Ds are end-diastolic and end-systolic dimensions respectively. The volume of the LV is derived from a single measurement of the dimension of the minor axis of the LV. In the above formula, the minor axis is assumed to be half of the major axis of the LV; this assumption is incorrect in children. Normal mean ejection fraction is 74% with 95% prediction limits of 64% to 83%.

Systolic time intervals. The systolic time interval of a ventricle includes the preejection period and the ventricular ejection time (see Figure 6-1). The preejection period (from the onset of the Q wave of the ECG to the opening of the semilunar valve) usually reflects the rate of pressure rise in the ventricle during isovolumic systole (i.e., dp/dt). The ventricular ejection time is measured from the cusp opening of the semilunar valve to the cusp closing. Although the preejection period and ventricular ejection time are affected by the heart rate, the ratio of preejection period/ventricular ejection time for both right and left sides is little affected by changes in the heart rate. The method of measuring left preejection period (LPEP) and ventricular ejection time (LVET) is shown in Fig. 6-1 in the right lower panel. Measurement of the right preejection period (RPEP) and ventricular ejection time (RVET) is sometimes difficult, since only the posterior part of the pulmonary valve is normally recorded on the M-mode echo. Normal values and ranges are as follows:

RPEP/RVET = 0.24 (0.16 to 0.30)

LPEP/LVET = 0.35 (0.30 to 0.39)

RPEP/RVET is elevated in a large-shunt VSD and pulmonary hypertension, persistent pulmonary hypertension of the newborn (i.e., PPHN, persistent fetal circulation syndrome), and right bundle branch block (RBBB). In PPHN, the ratio is usually greater than 0.50. LPEP/LVET is elevated in congestive heart failure (CHF) and left bundle branch block (LBBB).

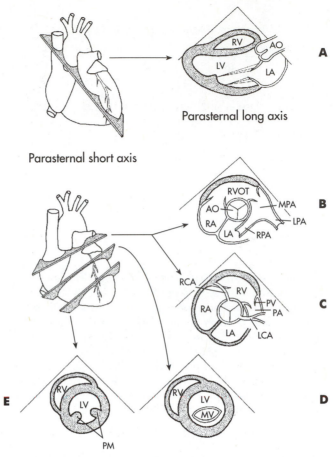

FIG. 6-2.
Diagrammatic illustration of important two-dimensional echo views obtained from the
parasternal transducer position. Parasternal long-axis view **(A)** is shown at the top.
Parasternal short-axis views obtained at various levels: the semilunar valve and great
artery level **(B, C)**, the mitral valve level **(D)**, and the papillary muscle level **(E)**. *AO,*
Aorta; *MV,* mitral valve; *LCA,* left coronary artery; *LPA,* left pulmonary artery; *PM,*
papillary muscle; *RCA,* right coronary artery.

Two-Dimensional Echocardiography

Two-dimensional echo examinations are performed by directing the plane of the
transducer beam along a number of cross-sectional planes through the heart and great
vessels. A routine two-dimensional echo is obtained from four transducer locations—
parasternal, apical, subcostal, and suprasternal notch (SSN) positions. Figs. 6-2 through
6-5 illustrate some standard images of the heart and great vessels. Modified transducer
positions and different angulations make many other views possible. Normal values of
the dimension of the aorta and pulmonary arteries (PAs) are shown in Appendix B (see
Table B-2 on p. 482).

Parasternal views. The parasternal long-axis view is the most basic view and shows
the left ventricular inflow and outflow tracts (Fig. 6-2, *A*). This view is most important
in evaluating the following structures and abnormalities in or near the mitral valve, LA,
LV, LV outflow tract, aortic valve, aortic root, ascending aorta, and ventricular septum.
Pericardial effusion, VSD of tetralogy of Fallot (TOF) and persistent truncus arteriosus,
and overriding of the aorta are best evaluated in this view.

The parasternal short-axis view is the projection that provides cross-sectional images of the heart and the great arteries at different levels. Important views are those taken at the levels of the semilunar valves, mitral valve, and papillary muscles (Fig. 6-2, *B to E*). The parasternal short-axis views are important in the evaluation of the aortic valve (i.e., bicuspid or tricuspid), pulmonary valve, PA and its branches, RV outflow tract, coronary arteries (e.g., absence, aneurysm), LA, LV, ventricular septum, LV outflow tract, the AV valves, and the right side of the heart. PDA is usually visualized in a modified plane similar to Fig. 6-2, *B* (see Fig. 29-5). Doppler interrogation of the ductal shunt is performed in that plane.

Apical views. The apical four-chamber view (Fig. 6-3, *A*) evaluates the atrial and ventricular septa, atrial and ventricular chambers, atrioventricular (AV) valves, pulmonary veins (PVs), identification of anatomic RV and LV, and detection of pericardial effusion. An ECD is well-imaged in this view. The apical four-chamber view that shows LV outflow tract (i.e., apical "five-chamber" view) (Fig. 6-3, *B*) is useful in the visualization of the perimembranous ventricular septum (where the VSD is most often found), LV outflow tract, and ascending aorta, as well as those structures seen in the regular apical four-chamber view. The apical long-axis view (Fig. 6-3, *C*) shows structures similar to those shown in the parasternal long-axis view.

Subcostal views. The subcostal four-chamber view (Fig. 6-4, *A*) demonstrates the atrial and ventricular septa, AV valves, atrial and ventricular chambers, and the drainage of systemic and pulmonary veins. This is the best view for the evaluation of an atrial septal defect (ASD). With further anterior angulation (Fig. 6-4, *B* and *C*), or turning the transducer 90 degrees (Fig. 6-4, *D*), the ventricular outflow tract of both ventricles and the great arteries can be imaged.

Suprasternal notch views. The suprasternal long-axis (Fig. 6-5, *A*) and short-axis (Fig. 6-5, *B*) views are important in the evaluation of anomalies in the ascend-

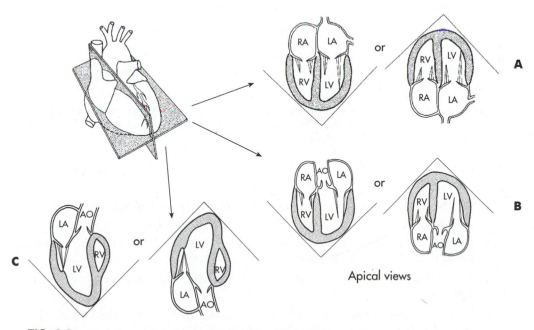

FIG. 6-3.
Diagrammatic illustration of two-dimensional echo views obtained with the transducer at the apical position. Both the apex-down and apex-up images are shown. **A,** Apical four-chamber view. **B,** Apical four-chamber view with LV outflow tract (apical "five-chamber" view). **C,** Apical long-axis view.

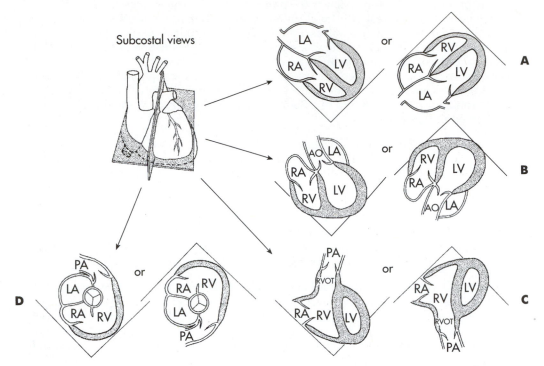

FIG. 6-4.
Diagrammatic illustration of two-dimensional echo views obtained with the transducer at the subcostal position. Both the apex-down and apex-up images are shown. **A,** subcostal four-chamber view. **B,** View showing the LV outflow tract and the proximal aorta (subcostal "five-chamber" view). **C,** View that shows the RV outflow tract and the proximal MPA. **D,** Subcostal short-axis view. LPV, Left pulmonary vein; *RPV,* right pulmonary vein.

ing and descending aortas (e.g., coarctation of the aorta (COA), aortic arch (e.g., interruption), the size of the PAs, and anomalies of systemic veins and pulmonary veins.

Indications. Indications for two-dimensional echo studies are expanding with their increasing diagnostic accuracy. The following are some selected indications for two-dimensional echo examinations.

1. To routinely screen newborns and small infants who appear to have cardiac defects or dysfunction

2. To rule out cyanotic congenital heart disease (CHD) in newborns with clinical findings of PPHN or persistent fetal circulation syndrome.

3. To diagnose PDA, other heart defects, or ventricular dysfunction in a premature infant who is on a ventilator for pulmonary diseases

4. To confirm diagnosis in infants and children with findings atypical of certain defects

5. To rule in or rule out important cardiac conditions that are raised by routine evaluation (e.g., cardiac examination, chest x-ray films, ECG)

6. To follow up on conditions that may change with time and/or treatment (e.g., before and after indomethacin treatment for PDA in premature infants, evaluation of drug therapy for CHF or LV dysfunction, follow-up examination for certain CHD and so on)

7. Before cardiac catheterization and angiocardiography, to have prior knowledge of certain information that can reduce the amount of time spent in the cardiac catheterization laboratory and the amount of the radiopaque dye injected and to supply some information that angiography cannot (Two-dimensional echo is superior to angiocardiography in demonstrating small, thin structures [e.g., subaortic membrane, cor triatriatum, straddling AV valve, Ebstein's anomaly] that may easily be missed by angiocardiography.)

8. To replace cardiac catheterization and angiography in certain situations such as uncomplicated VSD, PDA, or ASD

9. To evaluate the patient after surgery

Doppler Echocardiography

A Doppler echo combines the study of cardiac structure and blood flow profiles. The Doppler effect is a change in the observed frequency of sound that results from motion of the source or target. When the moving object or column of blood moves toward the ultrasonic transducer, the frequency of the reflected sound wave increases (i.e., a positive Doppler shift). Conversely, when blood moves away from the transducer, the frequency decreases (i.e., a negative Doppler shift). Doppler ultrasound equipment detects a frequency shift and determines the direction and velocity of red blood cell flow with respect to the ultrasound beam.

The two commonly used Doppler techniques are continuous wave and pulsed wave. The pulsed wave emits a short burst of ultrasound, and the Doppler echo receiver "listens" for returning information. The continuous wave emits a constant ultrasound beam with one crystal, and another crystal continuously receives returning information. Both techniques have their advantages and disadvantages. The pulsed-wave Doppler can control the site at which the Doppler signals are sampled, but the maximum detectable velocity is limited making it unusable for quantification of severe obstruction. In contrast, continuous-wave Doppler can measure extremely high velocities (e.g., for

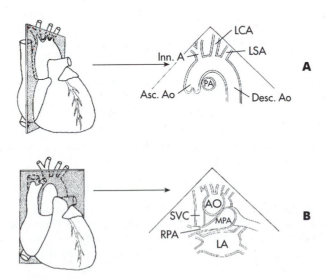

FIG. 6-5.
Diagrammatic drawing of SSN two-dimensional echo views. **A,** Long-axis view. **B,** Short-axis view. *AO,* Aorta; *Asc Ao,* ascending aorta; *Desc Ao,* descending aorta; *Inn A,* innominate artery; *LCA,* left carotid artery; *LSA,* left subclavian artery.

the estimation of severe stenosis), but it cannot localize the site of the sampling; rather, it picks up the signal anywhere along the Doppler beam. When these two techniques are used in combination, clinical application expands.

The Doppler echo determines the direction of flow and flow disturbances. It also quantitates the hemodynamic severity of a cardiac disease noninvasively. Flow disturbances are seen with shunt lesions, stenosis or regurgitation of the cardiac valves, or narrowing of the blood vessels. By convention, velocities of red blood cells moving toward the transducer are displayed above a zero baseline; those moving away from the transducer are displayed below the baseline. The Doppler echo is usually used with color flow mapping to enhance the technique's usefulness. Normal Doppler velocity is less than 1.0 m/sec for the tricuspid and pulmonary valves and may be up to 1.6 m/sec for the ascending and descending aortas.

The Doppler echo technique is useful in studying the direction of blood flow; in detecting the presence and direction of cardiac shunts; in studying stenosis or regurgitation of cardiac valves, including prosthetic valves; in assessing stenosis of blood vessels; in assessing hemodynamic severity of the lesion, including pressures in various compartments of the cardiovascular system; in estimating the cardiac output or blood flow; and in assessing diastolic function of the ventricle (see later discussion).

Measurement of pressure gradients. The simplified Bernoulli equation can be used to estimate the pressure gradient across a stenotic lesion, regurgitant lesion, or shunt lesion. The equation may be one of the following:

$$P_1 - P_2 \text{ (mm Hg)} = 4(V_2{}^2 - V_1{}^2)$$

$$P_1 - P_2 \text{ (mm Hg)} = 4(V \max)^2$$

where $(P_1 - P_2)$ is the pressure difference across an obstruction, V_1 is the velocity (m/sec) proximal to the obstruction, V_2 is the velocity (m/sec) distal to the obstruction in the first equation. When V_1 is less than 1 m/sec it can be ignored, as in the second equation.

To obtain the most accurate prediction of the peak pressure gradient, the Doppler beam should be aligned parallel to the jet flow, and the peak velocity of the jet should be recorded from several different transducer positions. An example of a Doppler study in a patient with a moderate PS is shown in Fig. 6-6. The pressure gradient calculated from the Bernoulli equation is the peak instantaneous pressure gradient *not* the peak-to-peak pressure gradient measured during cardiac catheterization. The peak instantaneous pressure gradient is larger than the peak-to-peak pressure gradient. The difference between the two is more noticeable in patients with mild to moderate obstruction and less apparent in patients with severe obstruction.

Prediction of intracardiac or intravascular pressures. The Doppler echo allows estimation of pressures in the RV, PA, and LV using the flow velocity of certain valvular or shunt jets. Estimation of PA pressure is particularly important in pediatric patients. The following are some examples of such applications:

a. RV (or PA) systolic pressure *(SP)* from tricuspid regurgitation (TR) can be estimated by this equation:

$$\text{RVSP (or PASP)} = 4(V)^2 + \text{RA pressure.}$$

For example, if the TR velocity is 2.5 m/sec, the instantaneous pressure gradient is $4 \times (2.5)^2 = 4 \times 6.25 = 25$ mm Hg. Using an assumed RA pressure of 10 mm Hg, the RV (or PA in the absence of PS) is 35 mm Hg. Similarly, the LV systolic pressure can be estimated from the jet velocity of MR by using an assumed LA pressure of 10 to 15 mm Hg.

b. PA (or RV) systolic pressure *(SP)* can be estimated from VSD jet by this equation:

$$\text{RVSP (or PASP)} = \text{Arm (SP)} - 4(V)^2$$

For example, if the VSD jet flow velocity is 3 m/sec, the instantaneous pressure drop

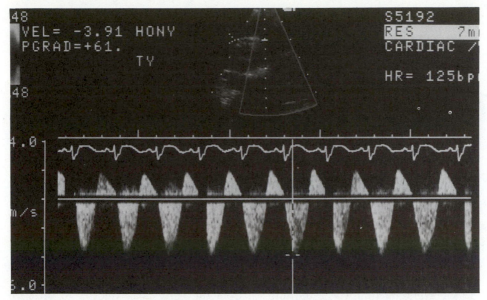

FIG. 6-6.
Doppler echocardiographic study in a child with a moderate pulmonary valve stenosis. The Doppler cursor is placed in the MPA near the pulmonary valve in the parasternal short-axis view. The maximum forward flow velocity (negative flow) is 3.91 m/sec (with an estimated pressure gradient of 61 mm Hg). There is a small regurgitant flow seen during diastole (positive flow).

between the LV and RV is $4 \times 3^2 = 36$ mm Hg. That is, the RV systolic pressure is 36 mm Hg lower than the LV systolic pressure. If the systemic systolic pressure is 90 mm Hg, which is equal to the LV systolic pressure, the RV pressure is estimated to be $90 - 36 = 54$ mm Hg. In the absence of pulmonary stenosis (PS) the PA systolic pressure is also 54 mm Hg.

c. LV systolic pressure *(SP)* from AS jet by this equation:

$$LVSP = 4(V)^2 + \text{Systemic SP}$$

Measurement of cardiac output or blood flow. Both systemic blood flow and pulmonary blood flow (PBF) can be calculated by multiplying the mean velocity of flow and the cross-sectional area as shown in the following equation:

$$\text{Cardiac output (L/min)} = V \times CSA \times 60 \text{ (sec/min)} \div 1000 \text{ cc/L}$$

where V is the mean velocity (cm/sec) obtained either by using a computer program or by manually integrating the area under the curve. CSA is the cross-sectional area of flow (cm^2) measured or computed from the two-dimensional echo. Usually, the PA flow velocity and diameter are used to calculate PBF; the mean velocity and diameter of the ascending aorta are used to calculate systolic blood flow, or cardiac output.

Diastolic function. Signs of diastolic dysfunction may precede those of systolic dysfunction. LV diastolic function can be evaluated by mitral inflow velocities obtained in the apical four-chamber view. The following simple measurements have been useful in evaluating diastolic function of the ventricle (Fig. 6-7):

1. The early (E) and second (A) peak velocities and their ratio: the velocity of an E wave occurring during early diastolic filling and the velocity of an A wave occurring during atrial contraction, as well as the ratio of the two

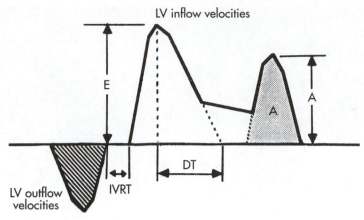

FIG. 6-7.
Selected parameters of diastolic function. See text for discussion.

2. Deceleration time (DT): the interval from the early peak velocity to the zero intercept of the extrapolated deceleration slope

3. Atrial filling fraction: the integral of the A velocity divided by the integral of the total mitral inflow velocities

4. Isovolumic relaxation time (IVRT): the interval between the end of the LV outflow velocity and the onset of mitral inflow; this is easily obtained by pulsed-wave Doppler with the cursor placed in the LV outflow near the anterior leaflet of the mitral valve and is measured from the end of the LV ejection to the onset of the mitral inflow

Abnormalities of diastolic function are easy to find but are usually nonspecific and do not provide independent diagnostic information. In addition, they can be affected by loading conditions (i.e., increase or decrease in preload), heart rate, and the presence of atrial arrhythmias. Two well-known patterns of abnormal diastolic function are a decreased relaxation pattern and a "restrictive" pattern (see Fig. 18-6 on p. 276). The decreased relaxation pattern is seen with hypertrophic and dilated cardiomyopathies, left ventrticular hypertrophy (LVH) of various etiology, ischemic heart disease, other forms of myocardial disease, reduced preload (e.g., dehydration) and increased afterload (e.g., during infusion of arterial vasoconstrictors). The "restrictive" pattern is usually seen in restrictive cardiomyopathy, but is also seen with increased preload (e.g., seen with MR) and a variety of heart diseases with heart failure.

Color Flow Mapping

A color-coded Doppler provides images of the direction and disturbances of blood flow superimposed on the echo structural image. Although systematic Doppler interrogation can obtain similar information, this technique is more accurate and time saving. In general, red is used to indicate flow toward the transducer, and blue is used to indicate flow away from the transducer. Color may not appear when the direction of flow is perpendicular to the ultrasound beam. The turbulent flow is color-coded as either green or yellow.

Contrast Echocardiography

Injection of indocyanine green, dextrose in water, saline, or the patient's blood into a peripheral or central vein produces microcavitations and creates a cloud of echoes on the echocardiogram. Structures of interest are visualized and/or recorded by M-mode or two-dimensional echo at the time of the injection. This technique has successfully detected an intracardiac shunt, validated structures, and identified flow patterns within the heart. For example, an injection of any liquid into an intravenous line may confirm the presence of a right-to-left shunt at the atrial or ventricular level. This technique can be used in the diagnosis of cyanosis resulting from a right-to-left shunt at the atrial level (e.g., PPHN) or in postoperative patients with persistent arterial desaturation. To a large extent, this technique has been replaced by color flow mapping and Doppler studies.

Other Echocardiographic Techniques

Fetal echocardiography. Improvement in image resolution makes visualization of the fetal cardiovascular structure possible, thereby permitting in utero diagnosis of cardiovascular anomalies. Doppler examination and color mapping are also obtained at the same time. To obtain a complete examination, the transducer is placed at various positions on the maternal abdominal wall.

Fetal echo continues to teach physicians more about human fetal cardiac physiology. It also enables physicians to study the effects of cardiovascular abnormalities and abnormal cardiac rhythms in utero, and then assess the need for therapeutic intervention. Indications for fetal echo may include the following:

1. A parent with a history of CHD

2. A history of previous children with CHD

3. The presence of fetal cardiac arrrhythmias

4. The presence of certain maternal diseases (e.g., diabetes mellitus, collagen vascular disease)

5. The presence of chromosomal anomalies

6. The presence of extracardiac anomalies (e.g., diaphragmatic hernia, omphalocele, hydrops)

7. The presence of polyhydramnios or oligohydramnios

8. A history of maternal exposure to certain medications (e.g., lithium, amphetamine, anticonvulsants, addictive drugs, progesterone, and so on)

Transesophageal Echocardiography. By placing a two-dimensional transducer at the end of a flexible endoscope, it is now possible to obtain high-quality, two-dimensional images by way of the esophagus. Color flow mapping and Doppler examination are usually incorporated in this approach. Although multiplane imaging techniques are gaining popularity, physicians commonly use a biplane imaging technique.

If satisfactory images of the heart or blood vessels are not possible from the usual transducer position on the surface of the patient's chest (e.g., patients with obesity or chronic obstructive pulmonary disease), physicians may use a transesophageal echocardiogram (TEE). This approach especially helps assess thrombus in the native or prosthetic valves, endocarditis vegetations, thrombi in the LA chamber and appendage, and aortic dissections. Physicians often use TEE for patients who are undergoing cardiac surgery. The TEE can monitor LV function throughout the surgical procedure, as well as assess cardiac morphology and function before and after surgical repair of valvular heart defects or CHDs. TEE requires general anesthesia or sedation and the presence of an anesthesiologist, since lack of cooperation can result in a serious complication. Pediatric use of this technique is somewhat limited to intraoperative use, some obese adolescents, and adolescents with complicated heart defects for whom the risk of general anesthesia or sedation is worth taking for the expected benefit. Schematic drawing of biplane images of TEE are shown in Appendix B (see Fig. B-1 on p. 484)

Intravascular Echocardiography. To provide an intravascular echo, the ultrasonic transducer can be placed in a small catheter so that vessels can be imaged by means of the lumen. These devices can evaluate atherosclerotic arteries in the adult and coronary artery stenosis or aneurysm in children who had Kawasaki's disease.

EXERCISE TEST

Exercise testing plays an important role in the evaluation of cardiac symptoms by quantifying the severity of the cardiac abnormality, assessing the effectiveness of management, and providing important indications of the need for new or further intervention.

Cardiovascular Response to Exercise

The heart rate, cardiac index, and mean arterial pressure increase during upright exercise. In addition, the systemic vascular resistance (SVR) drops, and the blood flow to the exercising leg muscles greatly increases. Although similar changes occur in pulmonary circulation, the increase in the mean PA pressure (i.e., 100% increase) is twice that of the systemic mean arterial pressure (i.e., 40% increase), and the drop in the PVR is less than that in the SVR (i.e., 17% vs. 49%). This is why children with RV dysfunction (e.g., children who have had a Fontan operation or surgery for TOF or children with pulmonary hypertension) may respond abnormally to exercise and demonstrate a decreased exercise capacity.

A linear relationship exists between the heart rate and progressive workload. The heart rate reaches a maximum plateau just before the level of total exhaustion. People who are the same age tend to have the same maximum heart rate even if their level of conditioning differs.

Indications

Stress testing has been found to be useful in children for following:

1. Aortic stenosis: (AS): Ischemic changes on the ECG during exercise indicate the need for surgical intervention regardless of predicted pressure gradients.

2. AR: Patients who develop ST-segment changes or fail to raise their heart rate with progressive exercise may have LV dysfunction and may need early surgical valve replacement.

3. Evaluation of arrhythmias: Ventricular arrhythmias that increase in frequency with exercise may require initiation of antiarrhythmic therapy. If ventricular arrhythmias are abolished by exercise and not associated with organic cardiac conditions, they can usually be ignored (see Chapter 24). Exercise testing can also evaluate the effectiveness of antiarrhythmic therapy.

4. Evaluation of AV block: AV blocks that worsen with exercise need therapy. Ventricular arrhythmias and symptoms of inadequate cardiac output that appear during exercise testing need further evaluation.

5. Postoperative evaluation of TOF and other cyanotic CHD: A patient who develops multiform premature ventricular contractions (PVCs) or ventricular tachycardia may be a candidate for sudden death. Either antiarrhythmic therapy or surgical intervention should be considered for such patients.

6. Postcoarctectomy patients: Patients who develop an excessive increase in blood pressure with exercise may benefit from antihypertensive measures such as weight reduction, salt restriction, and antihypertensive drug therapy.

7. Adolescents with chest pain: Although cardiac cause of chest pain is rare, testing is occasionally done to rule out cardiac cause.

8. Appropriate exercise prescription for participation in vocational, recreational, and competitive activities.

Types of Exercise Testing

Two types of equipment are used in exercise testing—bicycle ergometers and treadmills. Some exercise laboratories have developed bicycle ergometer protocols, but

TABLE 6–2.
Bruce Treadmill Test Endurance Times (min)

Age Group (yr)	Percentile					Mean	Standard Deviation
	10	25	50	75	90		
Boys							
4 to 5	8.1	9.0	10.0	12.0	13.3	10.4	1.9
6 to 7	9.7	10.0	12.0	12.3	13.5	11.8	1.6
8 to 9	9.6	10.5	12.4	13.7	16.2	12.6	2.3
10 to 12	9.9	12.0	12.5	14.0	15.4	12.7	1.9
13 to 15	11.2	13.0	14.3	16.0	16.1	14.1	1.7
16 to 18	11.3	12.1	13.6	14.5	15.8	13.5	1.4
Girls							
4 to 5	7.0	8.0	9.0	11.2	12.3	9.5	1.8
6 to 7	9.5	9.6	11.4	13.0	13.0	11.2	1.5
8 to 9	9.9	10.5	11.0	13.0	14.2	11.8	1.6
10 to 12	10.5	11.3	12.0	13.0	14.6	12.3	1.4
13 to 15	9.4	10.0	11.5	12.0	13.0	11.1	1.3
16 to 18	8.1	10.0	10.5	12.0	12.4	10.7	1.4

Modified from Cumming GR, Everatt D, Hastman L: Bruce treadmill test in children: normal values in a clinic population, *Am J Cardiol* 41:69, 1978.

this equipment is not standardized and not widely used. On the other hand, the treadmill has become the standard instrument for testing in most hospitals; therefore treadmill protocols are well-standardized and more widely used than bicycle ergometer protocols. The Bruce, both original and modified, and Naughton protocols are popular. In the Bruce protocol, the level of exercise increases by increasing the speed and grade of the treadmill for each 3-minute stage. In the original Bruce protocol, exercise begins at stage 1 (i.e., speed 1.7 mph, 10% grade). After 13 minutes of exercise time with the Bruce protocol, stage IV and 1 minute of stage V have been completed.

Normative Exercise Parameters for the Bruce Protocol

Using the original Bruce protocol, Cumming et al (1978) compiled normative data for endurance time and heart rate, and Klein (1987) compiled data for blood pressure.

1. Endurance time: Endurance times are the best predictors of exercise capacity in children (Table 6-2). The endurance times for boys and girls are close until early adolescence, at which time the endurance of girls diminishes and that of boys increases.

2. Heart rate: A heart rate of 180 to 200 beats/min correlates with maximal oxygen consumption in both girls and boys. Therefore an effort is made to encourage all children to exercise to attain this heart rate range. Patients with increased heart rate response may have diminished cardiac reserve or underlying systemic compromise (e.g., anemia). Trained athletes tend to have lower heart rates at each exercise level.

3. Blood pressure: There is a linear increase in systolic blood pressure with progressive exercise. Systolic pressure in the arm may rise to 180 mm Hg with little change in diastolic pressure (Table 6-3).

Monitoring

During stress testing, the patient is continuously monitored for symptoms such as chest pain or faintness, ischemic changes or arrhythmias on the ECG, and responses in heart rate and blood pressure.

TABLE 6–3.

Maximal Dynamic Systolic Blood Pressure Response (mm Hg) — Bruce Treadmill Protocol
(Mean ± SD)

Age (yrs)	Boys	Girls
10 to 12	151 ± 10	138 ± 14
13 to 15	157 ± 10	157 ± 15
16 to 18	165 ± 17	150 ± 20

Modified from Klein AA: Pediatric exercise testing, *Pediatr Ann* 16:546, 1987. *SD,* Standard deviation.

Heart rate response. Mean maximum exercise heart rate is 180 to 200 beats/min in normal children. Inadequate increments in heart rate may be seen with sinus node dysfunction, in congenital heart block, and after the Fontan operation. An extremely high heart rate at low levels of work may indicate physical deconditioning or marginal circulatory compensation.

Blood pressure response. Failure of arterial blood pressure to rise to the level of 180 mm Hg reflects an inadequate increase in cardiac output. This is commonly seen with cardiomyopathy, LV outflow tract obstruction, coronary artery disease, or the onset of ventricular or atrial arrhythmias. An excessive rise in blood pressure may be seen in patients who have had surgical repair of COA, hypertensive patients, patients with the potential to develop hypertension, and patients with AR.

ECG monitoring. Arrhythmias and ischemic changes are monitored. Arrhythmias, which increase in frequency or begin with exercise, are usually significant and require thorough evaluation. Down-sloping of the ST segment or sustained horizontal depression of the ST segment of 2 mm or greater when measured at 60 to 80 ms or after the J point is considered abnormal (see Fig 27-1 on p. 359).

Safety of Exercise Testing

Physicians should plan and conduct exercise testing with patient safety in mind. The indications and contraindications should be considered, and the physician should know when to terminate the test. Exercise testing should be performed under the supervision of a physician who has been trained to conduct the test.

Contraindications. Good clinical judgment should be foremost in deciding indications and contraindications for exercise testing. Conditions considered to be absolute contraindications for the stress testing include the following:

1. Serious cardiac arrhythmias

2. Acute pericarditis, myocarditis, or myocardial infarction

3. Infective endocarditis

4. Severe AS with symptoms

5. Severe CHF

6. Acute pulmonary embolus or pulmonary infarction

7. Acute or serious noncardiac disorders.

Relative contraindications for exercise testing include the following:

1. Severe systemic or pulmonary hypertension

2. Tachyarrhythmias or bradyarrhythmias

3. Moderate valvular or myocardial disease

4. Hypertrophic cardiomyopathy

5. Psychiatric disorders

In selected cases with relative contraindications even submaximal testing can provide valuable information.

Termination of exercise testing. Absolute indications for terminating exercise testing include the following:

1. A drop in systolic blood pressure despite an increase in workload

2. Onset of anginal chest pain

3. Dizziness or near syncope

4. Signs of poor peripheral perfusion (e.g., cyanosis or pallor)

5. Serious ventricular arrhythmias (e.g., multiform ventricular tachycardia, triplets and runs of PVCs)

6. Patients requesting to stop

Relative indications to stop the test include the following:

1. Excessive ST depression >3 mm

2. Increasing chest pain

3. Fatigue, shortness of breath, wheezing or leg cramps

4. Less serious arrhythmias (e.g., supraventricular tachycardia [SVT]).

AMBULATORY ELECTROCARDIOGRAPHY

Ambulatory ECG monitoring is useful in the diagnosis of arrhythmias that are likely but they are not revealed by a routine ECG. Adhesive ECG electrodes are attached to the chest wall, and an ECG rhythm is continually registered for 24 hours or longer by using a small, battery-driven, cassette tape recorder (i.e., Holter monitor). Two simultaneous channels are usually recorded. This helps distinguish artifacts from arrhythmias. Patients are given a diary so they can record symptoms and activities. The monitor has a built-in timer that is used with the patient's diary to allow subsequent correlation of the symptoms and activities with arrhythmias. The importance of an accurate and complete diary must be impressed on patients and parents. The cassette tape is replayed on a high-speed data analysis system and analyzed by a computerized arrhythmia-detection template. Events of interest can be picked out and printed for review and record. Most analyzers calculate heart rate trends and quantitate supraventricular or ventricular ectopic beats.

Indications

Ambulatory ECG monitoring is obtained for the following reasons:

1. To determine whether symptoms such as chest pain, palpitation, or syncope were caused by cardiac arrhythmias

2. To evaluate the adequacy of medical therapy for an arrhythmia

3. To screen high-risk cardiac patients such as those with hypertrophic cardiomy-opathy or those who had surgical operations known to predispose to arrhythmias (e.g., Mustard, Senning, Fontan-type operation)

4. To evaluate possible intermittent pacemaker failure

5. To determine the effect of sleep on potentially life-threatening arrhythmias.

The Holter recordings should reveal the frequency, duration, and types of arrhythmias, as well as their precipitating or terminating events. Significant arrhythmias rarely cause symptoms such as palpitation, chest pain, and syncope (i.e., fewer than 10% of cases). Marked bradycardia (<50 beats/min in infants, <40 beats/min in older children), SVT with rate >200/min, or ventricular tachycardia are potentially life threatening. These arrhythmias do occur and may worsen during sleep. Ambulatory ECG monitoring is not helpful in the detection of an episode occurring infrequently (i.e., once a week or once a month) and is unnecessary for asymptomatic extrasystoles.

Interpretation

The interpretation of the results usually includes the following:

1. A description of the basic rhythm and the range of the heart rate

2. A description of the characteristics, duration, and frequency of the arrhythmias identified

3. Correlation of the arrhythmias with the patient's activities and symptoms

4. Correlation of ST-segment changes with activities and symptoms if the patient complained of anginal pain.

Findings in Normal Children

Meaningful interpretation of ambulatory ECG recordings performed in patients with organic heart disease or significant systemic illness requires knowledge of the range of heart rate and rhythm variations in normal subjects of comparable age. Ambulatory ECG recordings of healthy pediatric populations have demonstrated that variations in rate and rhythm, which were previously thought to be abnormal, occur quite frequently.

Premature or low-birth-weight infants. The minimum heart rate of premature or low-birth-weight infants can be as low as 73 beats/min, the maximum heart rate can be as high as 211 beats/min. Junctional rhythm was observed in 18% to 70%, premature atrial contractions (PACs) in 2% to 33%, and PVCs in 6% to 17%. First-degree AV block or Wenckebach second-degree AV block occurred in 4% to 6%. Sudden sinus bradycardia and sinus pause occur especially frequently.

Full-term neonates. In full-term neonates, the heart rate can be as low as 75 beats/min and as high as 230 beats/min. Junctional rhythm was present in 28%, PACs in 10% to 35%, and PVCs in 1% to 13%. First-degree AV block or Wenckebach second-degree AV block was recorded in 25% of these neonates. Sinus pause was quite frequent.

Older children between 7 and 16 years of age. During sleep, the heart rate can become as low as 23 beats/min and the maximum rate as high as 110 beats/min in older children. While awake, minimum and maximum heart rates were 45 and 200 beats/min respectively. First-degree AV block and Wenckebach second-degree AV block are also common during sleep (i.e., 3% to 12%). PVCs (i.e., 26% to 57%), which include multiform PVCs; PACs (i.e., 13% to 20%); and junctional rhythm (i.e., 5% to 15%) are also observed.

7 / Invasive Procedures

CARDIAC CATHETERIZATION AND ANGIOCARDIOGRAPHY

Cardiac catheterization and angiocardiography usually constitute the final definitive diagnostic tests for most cardiac patients. They are carried out under general sedation using various sedatives discussed later. For newborns, cyanotic infants, and hemodynamically unstable children, general anesthesia with intubation may be used.

Under local anesthesia and strict aseptic preparation of the skin, catheters are placed in peripheral (most commonly the femoral) vessels and advanced to the heart and central vessels under fluoroscopy with image intensification to reduce radiation exposure. At each location, values of pressure and oxygen saturation of blood are obtained. The oxygen saturation data provide information on the site and magnitude of the left-to-right or right-to-left shunt, if any. The pressure data provide information on the site and severity of obstruction. Cardiac output may be obtained from oxygen saturation data (e.g., the Fick principle), or by indicator dilution (e.g., indocyanine green dye) or thermodilution (e.g., cold saline injection) technique. Selective angiocardiography is usually performed as a part of the catheterization procedure (described later).

Normal Hemodynamic Values

Normal oxygen saturation in the right side of the heart varies between 65% and 80%, depending on cardiac output. Left-sided saturations are usually 95% to 98% in room air. In newborns and heavily sedated children the oxygen saturation may be lower. Pressures are lower in the right side than in the left side of the heart, with systolic pressures in the right ventricle (RV) and pulmonary artery (PA) about 20% to 30% of those in the left side of the heart (Fig. 7-1).

Routine Hemodynamic Calculations

The following calculations are routinely obtained: flow and resistance for systemic and pulmonary circuits and left-to-right or right-to-left shunt.

Flows (cardiac output) and shunts. Flow is calculated by the use of the Fick formula:

$$\text{Pulmonary flow } (\dot{Q}p) = \frac{V_{O_2}}{C_{PV} - C_{PA}}$$

$$\text{Systemic flow } (\dot{Q}s) = \frac{V_{O_2}}{C_{AO} - C_{MV}}$$

where flows are in L/min, V_{O_2} is oxygen consumption (ml/min), C is oxygen content (ml/L) at various positions, PV is pulmonary vein, PA is pulmonary artery, AO is aorta, and MV is mixed systemic venous blood (superior vena cava (SVC) or right atrium). Normal systemic flow or pulmonary flow in the absence of a shunt is 3.1 ± 0.4 L/min/m^2 (i.e., cardiac index).

Oxygen consumption is directly measured during the procedure or is estimated from a table (see Appendix A, Table A-5 on p. 477). *Oxygen capacity* is the maximum quantity of oxygen that can be bound to each gram of hemoglobin (i.e., 1.36 ml × Hb level; each gram of hemoglobin combines maximally with 1.36 ml of oxygen). *Oxygen saturation* is the amount of oxygen bound to hemoglobin compared to the oxygen capacity, and it is expressed as a percentage.

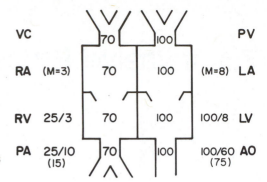

FIG. 7-1.
Pressure and oxygen saturation values in normal children.

When there is a pure left-to-right or right-to-left shunt, the magnitude of the shunt is calculated as follows:

$$\text{Left-to-right shunt} = \dot{Q}p - \dot{Q}s$$

$$\text{Right-to-left shunt} = \dot{Q}s - \dot{Q}p$$

The flow data are subject to much error because of difficulties involved in measuring accurate oxygen consumption or because of the frequent use of assumed oxygen consumption (140 to 160 ml/m²/min) in pediatric patients. Therefore the ratio of pulmonary-to-systemic flow ($\dot{Q}p/\dot{Q}s$) is frequently used, since it does not require an oxygen consumption value. The ratio provides information on the magnitude of the shunt. A $\dot{Q}p/\dot{Q}s$ ratio of 1:1 would indicate no shunting in either direction or bidirectional shunt of equal magnitude. A ratio of 2:1 implies that there is a left-to-right shunt equal to systemic blood flow. A ratio of 0.8:1 signifies that the pulmonary blood flow (PBF) is 20% less than the systemic blood flow (e.g., the flow ratio seen in a cyanotic patient). Patients with a flow ratio greater than 2:1 are usually surgical candidates.

Resistance. Hydraulic resistance *(R)* is defined by analogy to Ohm's law as the ratio of the mean pressure drop (ΔP) to flow (Q) between two points in a liquid flowing in a tube (R = ΔP/Q). Therefore pulmonary vascular resistance (PVR) and systemic vascular resistance (SVR) are calculated using the following formulas:

$$\text{PVR} = \frac{\text{Mean PA pressure} - \text{Mean LA pressure}}{Qp}$$

$$\text{SVR} = \frac{\text{Mean aortic pressure} - \text{Mean RA pressure}}{Qs}$$

The normal SVR varies between 15 and 30 units/m². The normal PVR is high at birth, but reaches values near adult values after 2 to 4 months. Normal values in children and adults are 1 to 3 units/m². Obviously the ratios of PVR/SVR range from 1/10 to 1/20. High values of PVR increase the risk of corrective surgery for many congenital cardiac defects.

Selective Angiocardiography

Information derived from echo and the oxygen saturation and pressure data from catheterization help determine the number and sites of selective angiocardiograms required to delineate cardiovascular structures. A radiopaque dye is rapidly injected into a certain site, and angiograms are recorded on motion picture film at 60 or 90 frames per second, often on biplane views. Depending on the cardiovascular anomaly under study, special views are obtained by moving the fluoroscopic camera (or by positioning the patient at desired angles). Multiple injection sites are often necessary to obtain a complete anatomic diagnosis (Fig. 7-2, *A*).

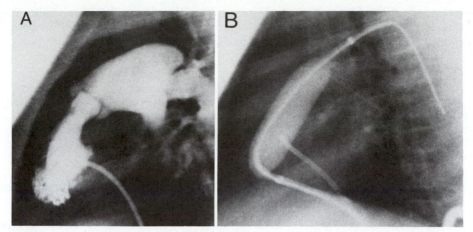

FIG. 7-2.
Angiocardiography and balloon valvuloplasty. **A,** Lateral view of right ventriculogram showing a thick, dome-shaped pulmonary valve and a marked poststenotic dilatation of the PA. **B,** A maximally inflated sausage-shaped valvuloplasty balloon is seen, which suggests that the stenotic pulmonary valve has been widened. The balloon catheter was introduced over a guide wire, which was positioned in the LPA.

Contrast agents used in angiocardiography are water-soluble, complex organic compounds, with three iodine atoms bound to a benzene ring. Old contrast agents (e.g., Renografin 76, Renovist, Hypaque M-75, and Vascoray) are ionic agents with high osmolality (i.e., ionic agents with osmolality of 1690 to 2150 mOsm/kg; much higher than serum osmolality of 275 to 300 mOsm). Nonionic contrast (e.g., Isovue, Omnipaque) are low-osmolality agents (i.e., agents with osmolality of 300 mOsm/kg). After the injection of high-osmolality contrasts, there is a rapid shift of fluid from the interstitial and intracellular spaces into the intravascular space. This causes volume expansion, a slight drop in hematocrit, and a change in electrolyte concentration. These changes adversely affect newborns and infants with congestive heart failure (CHF). Low-osmolality agents cause less volume shift and are safer, but they are considerably more expensive. Other toxic effects of high-osmolality agents include decreased red cell pliability, increased viscosity, osmolar diuresis, proteinuria, hematuria, and renal failure (occasionally).

Risks

Cardiac catheterization and angiocardiography can lead to serious complications and occasionally death. Complications related to catheter insertion and manipulation include serious arrhythmias, heart block, cardiac perforation, hypoxic spells, arterial obstruction, hemorrhage, and infection. Complications related to contrast injection include reactions to the contrast material, intramyocardial injection, and renal complications (e.g., hematuria, proteinuria, oliguria, anuria). Complications related to exposure, sedation, and medications include hypothermia, acidemia, hypoglycemia, convulsions, hypotension, and respiratory depression, which are more likely to occur in newborns.

The risk of cardiac catheterization and angiocardiography varies with the patient's age and illness, the type of lesion, and the experience of the physicians doing the procedure. The reported rate of fatal complications varies from lower than 1% to as high as 5% in the newborn period. In one study the incidence of significant but nonfatal complications requiring treatment (e.g., arrhythmias and arterial complications) was 12% in infants younger than 4 months old. In comparison, the incidence of such complications was 1.5% in the older infants. Major complications (e.g., ventricular arrhythmias, hypotension, arterial complications, perforation of the heart, breakage or knotting of catheters, allergic reactions, hypoxic spells, and so on) occurred 1.4% of the time, and minor complications occurred 6.8% of the time. With better preparation and monitoring, as well as the use of prostaglandin infusion in critically ill newborns, the mortality and morbidity rate can be minimized.

Indications

Indications for these invasive studies vary from institution to institution and from cardiologist to cardiologist. With improved capability of noninvasive techniques (e.g., two-dimensional echo and color flow Doppler studies), many cardiac problems are adequately diagnosed and managed without the invasive studies. The following are considered indications by most cardiologists:

1. Selected newborns with cyanotic congenital heart disease (CHD) who may require palliative surgery or balloon atrial septostomy during the procedure.

2. Selected children with CHD when the lesion is severe enough to require surgical intervention

3. Children who appear to have had unsatisfactory results from cardiac surgery

4. Infants and children with lesions amenable to balloon angioplasty/valvuloplasty

Sedation

A number of sedatives have been used by different institutions with equally good success rates. Smaller doses of sedatives are usually used in cyanotic infants.

1. No sedation is used in the newborn.

2. For small infants weighing less than 10 kg, a combination of chloral hydrate (75 mg/kg, maximum of 2 gm) and diphenhydramine (2 mg/kg, maximum of 100 mg) by mouth has been used with good results.

3. For older children, Demerol compound (i.e., a solution containing 25 mg/ml of meperidine [Demerol], 12.5 mg/ml of promethazine [Phenergan], and 12.5 mg/ml of chloropromazine [Thorazine] is a popular sedative mixture. The dosage of the Demerol compound is 0.11 ml/kg, intramuscularly. Some centers exclude chloropromazine (Thorazine) from the sedative mixture. In cyanotic children the dosage of the Demerol compound is reduced by a third. For children in severe CHF, the dose is reduced by half.

4. Some cardiologists use a combination of meperidine (1 mg/kg) and hydroxyzine (Vistaril) (1 mg/kg) intramuscularly, others use a combination of fentanyl (1.25 μg/kg, maximum of 50 μg) and droperidol (62.5 μg/kg, maximum of 2500 μg) with equal success.

5. Ketamine (3 mg/kg, intramuscularly or 1 to 2 mg/kg, intravenously) may be used, but it can change the hemodynamic data, since it increases the SVR and blood pressure.

6. Morphine (0.1 to 0.2 mg/kg) administered subcutaneously can be used to prevent or treat hypoxic spells.

7. If more sedation is required during the study, intravenous diazepam (Valium) (0.1 mg/kg) or morphine (0.1 mg/kg) is used.

Preparation and Monitoring

Adequate preparation of the patient before the procedure and careful monitoring during the procedure can minimize possible complications and fatality from the invasive studies. The following areas of preparation and monitoring are particularly important:

1. increasing the temperature in the cardiac catheterization laboratory when an infant is being studied

2. using a warming blanket and a rectal thermistor to monitor rectal temperature and avoid hypothermia

3. checking arterial blood gas levels and pH, in addition to correcting acidemia and hypoxemia

4. correcting hypoglycemia or hypocalcemia before the procedure begins, administering glucose during the procedure if hypoglycemia is found

5. monitoring oxygen saturation and administering oxygen (if indicated) during the procedure

6. intubating or readiness for intubating in infants with respiratory difficulties

7. having emergency medications (e.g., atropine, epinephrine, bicarbonate, and so on) drawn up and ready

8. initiating prostaglandin infusion in cyanotic infants who seem to be ductus dependent

9. whenever possible, having another physician (preferably an anesthesiologist) available to monitor the noncardiac aspects of the patient, so that the operator can concentrate on the procedure

CATHETER INTERVENTION PROCEDURES

Recent advances have allowed for the development of a variety of therapeutic procedures using specially modified catheters. These procedures can be performed in the cardiac catheterization laboratory. The lives of critically ill neonates may be saved by these procedures. They may also eliminate or delay elective surgical procedures in children with certain CHD.

Balloon Atrial Septostomy (i.e., Rashkind's Procedure)

Balloon atrial septostomy remains the standard initial palliation of transposition of the great arteries (TGA) and other conditions in which a large atrial communication is desirable. A special balloon-tipped catheter is placed in the left atrium (LA) from the RA through a patent foramen ovale (PFO) or an existing atrial septal defect (ASD). The balloon is inflated with a diluted contrast material, and the catheter is rapidly pulled back to the RA through the interatrial communication, thereby creating a large opening in the atrial septum. This procedure is needed for some infants younger than 4 to 6 weeks of age who have TGA (either with or without associated cardiac anomalies) and total anomalous pulmonary venous return (TAPVR) with restrictive ASD (if surgery is delayed for some reason). The procedure may be appropriate in selected patients with mitral atresia, pulmonary atresia, and tricuspid atresia.

Blade Atrial Septostomy

In infants older than 6 to 8 weeks of age the atrial septum may be too thick to allow an effective balloon septostomy. In such cases the atrial septum can be opened with a blade catheter (i.e., Park blade). The blade catheter uses a small blade that unfolds from the tip of the catheter to actually incise the atrial septum as the catheter tip is withdrawn from the LA to the RA. The opening can be torn further with a balloon catheter. This procedure may eliminate the need for a surgical atrial septectomy (i.e., Blalock-Hanlon operation). Conditions for which the procedure is necessary are the same as those listed for a balloon atrial septostomy.

Balloon Valvuloplasty

Balloon interventional procedures use balloons that are made of special plastic polymers and retain their predetermined diameters. A long guide wire is advanced far beyond the valve of interest, and the balloon catheter is placed over the wire. The middle of the elongated, sausage-shaped balloon is placed in the valve position. The balloon is then inflated with a diluted contrast material to relieve obstruction at the valve.

Pulmonary valve stenosis. This technique is the treatment of choice for valvular pulmonary stenosis (PS) in children and to a large extent, has replaced the surgical pulmonary valvotomy (Fig. 7-2, *B*). The results of this technique are excellent and do not have significant complications. This technique can be used in neonates with critical PS. The effectiveness of a balloon valvuloplasty for a severe dysplastic pulmonary valve is questionable but may be attempted. The procedure is not useful for treatment of infundibular PS that is not associated with valvular PS.

Aortic valve stenosis. This procedure is more difficult and dangerous, especially for infants. The gradient reduction is less effective than for the pulmonary valve. Indications for the balloon valvotomy include peak systolic pressure gradients > 50 to 60 mm Hg without significant aortic regurgitation (AR) in children and adolescents as well as newborns and small infants with critical obstruction regardless of the gradient value. Complications include production or worsening of AR, iliofemoral artery injury and occlusion, ventricular fibrillation, and even death in small infants. Although the effectiveness of the procedure has been questioned, it may be tried in discrete membranous subaortic stenosis, but not in fibromuscular subaortic (or "tunnel") stenosis.

Mitral stenosis. Balloon dilatation valvuloplasty has been effective for rheumatic mitral stenosis (MS) but less effective for congenital MS. Passage of the balloon catheter across the atrial septum is necessary. Complications include perforation of the left ventricle (LV), transient complete atrioventricular (AV) block, tearing of the anterior leaflet of the MV, and severe mitral regurgitation (MR).

Stenosis of prosthetic conduits and valves within conduits. The balloon dilatation procedure may reduce the transconduit gradient across stenotic areas of prosthetic conduits and across valves contained within conduits.

Balloon Angioplasty

Balloon catheters, similar to those used in balloon valvuloplasties, are used for the relief of stenosis of blood vessels. Appropriate guide wires are placed beyond the point of narrowing, and the balloon catheter is placed over the guide wires. The midportion of the balloon is positioned at the point of narrowing, and the balloon is inflated with a diluted contrast media to relieve the narrowing of vascular structures.

Recoarctation of the aorta. This is an extremely useful tool in the management of postoperative residual obstruction of coarctation of the aorta (COA). This procedure has become the procedure of choice for patients with this condition. This is because reoperation carries a significant risk of morbidity and mortality. The procedure's success rate is close to 80%, and late development of an aortic aneurysm rarely occurs.

Native (or unoperated) coarctation of the aorta. The benefit is incomplete and fewer than the benefits resulting from surgery. The complication rate is 17% with an aortic aneurysm formation (both acute and late) in 6% of the patients. The long-term effects of the procedure for native coarctation, which produces tearing of the intima and media of the coarctation segment, are unknown. This is particularly true for the development or worsening of an aortic aneurysm. Surgery may be a better choice than the balloon procedure for native coarctation.

Branch pulmonary artery stenosis. Hypoplastic and stenotic branch PAs are seen with a variety of cardiac malformations, and many of them are seen with postoperative tetralogy of Fallot (TOF). The immediate success rate of the balloon procedure is about 60%, but restenosis occurs in a significant number of patients, and aneurysm formation occurs in approximately 3% of patients. Modification of the balloon technique, using an intravascular stent, may improve the long-term success rate. Because operative treatment of branch PA stenosis is often not possible, attempting the balloon procedure for this condition is justified.

Systemic venous stenosis. For obstructed venous baffles after the Mustard or Senning operation for TGA, the balloon procedure is an attractive alternative. The procedure in stenosis of pulmonary vein (PV) is inappropriate, since stenosis recurs in each case.

Closure Techniques

Various devices have been used to close selected patients with a patent ductus arteriosus (PDA), atrial septal defect (ASD), or muscular ventricular septal defect (VSD)

Closure of patent ductus arteriosus. A double-umbrella plug is used to close the PDA in infants and young children. Now closure is achieved in more than 95% of all cases. Undoubtedly, further experience will continue to improve these results. Recently other devices have successfully been used for this purpose, and the results have been somewhat better than those of the umbrella device. If favorable, late follow-up continues, the transcatheter closure may become the therapy of choice for a PDA.

Catheter closure of a secundum ASD. A double-umbrella device (i.e., Lock Clamshell occluder) has been used to successfully close secundum ASD. The arms of the occluder function like a clamshell, that is, they are hinged and fold back against themselves. This device is delivered through a long sheath that has been placed in the LA. The distal arms of the device are opened in the middle of the left atrium and the distal arms are pulled against the atrial septum. The sheath is then retracted, thereby allowing the proximal arms to open on the right side of the atrial septum. The clamshell devices are not suitable to use for defects that are larger than 25 mm, multiple defects, sinus venosus defects extending into the vena cava, and defects close to the tricuspid valve or right pulmonary veins. A "buttoned," double-disk device has been successfully used in animals to close ASDs through a sheath that is smaller than that used for the clamshell device. This device seems promising.

Transcatheter closure of VSD. Successful closure of a muscular VSD, which is remote from cardiac valves, has been achieved in selected patients by using the double-umbrella, clamshell device.

Embolization of Collaterals and Other Vessels

This technique is used for closing aortopulmonary collaterals (often seen with TOF), Blalock-Taussig shunts, systemic AV fistulas, and pulmonary AV fistulas. Two embolizing devices are available—the Gianturco coil and the White balloons. The Gianturco coils are small, coiled wires, which are coated with thrombogenic Dacron strands that open like a small "pigtail" when placed in the vessel, and then it occludes the vessel by creating a thrombus around the coil. The balloon is placed to a selected spot with an elaborate harpoonlike hydraulic delivery system on a thin catheter. Both devices need a discrete area of stenosis within a tubular vessel for fixation. The vessel should not be more than 6 to 7 mm in diameter. Peripheral embolization of the coil or balloon into the PAs or the aorta is a major risk.

PART III

Pathophysiology

In this section, discussion of fetal and perinatal circulation and the circulatory changes that take place after birth is followed by discussion of pathophysiology of some representative CHDs and acquired heart diseases.

The knowledge of fetal and perinatal circulation is extremely helpful in understanding the clinical manifestations and natural history of CHDs. A few examples of clinical importance in relation to fetal and perinatal circulation are examined. In discussing pathophysiology of CHD and acquired heart disease, attempts were made to explain why particular ECG, chest x-ray, and physical findings are associated with each defect based on hemodynamic abnormalities. In doing so, it was necessary to use a simplistic approach and avoid controversies. Careful study of the pathophysiology section will enable readers to not only explain, but also recall and predict the physical findings and abnormalities of the ECG and chest x-ray films of many cardiac anomalies.

8 / Fetal and Perinatal Circulation

Knowledge of fetal and perinatal circulation is an integral part of understanding the pathophysiology and natural history of congenital heart disease (CHD). Only a brief discussion of clinically important aspects of fetal and perinatal circulation are presented.

FETAL CIRCULATION

Fetal circulation differs from the adult circulation in several ways. Almost all differences are attributable to the fundamental difference in the site of gas exchange. In the adult, gas exchange occurs in the lungs. In the fetus, the placenta provides the exchange of gases and nutrients.

Course of Fetal Circulation

There are four shunts in fetal circulation: placenta, ductus venosus, foramen ovale, and ductus arteriosus (Fig. 8.1). The following summarizes some important aspects of fetal circulation:

1. The placenta receives the largest amount of combined (i.e., right and left) ventricular output (55%) and has the lowest vascular resistance in the fetus.

2. The superior vena cava (SVC) drains the upper part of the body, including the brain (15% of combined ventricular output), whereas the inferior vena cava (IVC) drains the lower part of the body and the placenta (70% of combined ventricular output). Since the blood is oxygenated in the placenta, the oxygen saturation in the IVC (70%) is higher than that in the SVC (40%). The highest Po_2 is found in the umbilical vein (32 mm Hg) (see Fig. 8-1).

3. Most of the SVC blood goes to the right ventricle (RV). About one third of the IVC blood with higher oxygen saturation is directed by the crista dividens to the left atrium (LA) through the foramen ovale, whereas the remaining two thirds enters the RV and main pulmonary artery (MPA). The result is that the brain and coronary circulation receive blood with higher oxygen saturation (Po_2 of 28 mm Hg) than the lower half of the body (Po_2 of 24 mm Hg) (see Fig. 8-1).

4. Less oxygenated blood in the pulmonary artery (PA) flows through the widely open ductus arteriosus to the descending aorta and then to the placenta for oxygenation.

Dimensions of Cardiac Chambers

The proportions of the combined cardiac output traversing the heart chambers and the major blood vessels are reflected in the relative dimensions of these chambers and vessels (see Fig. 8-1).

Since the lungs receive only 15% of combined ventricular output, the branches of the PA are small. This is important in the genesis of the pulmonary flow murmur of the newborn (see Chapters 2 and 28).

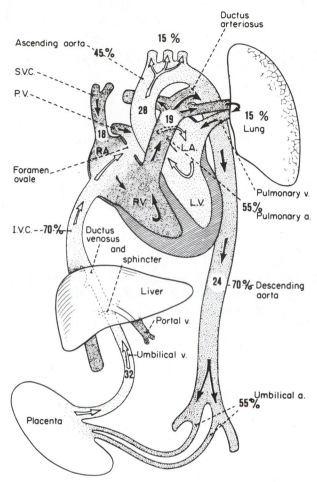

FIG. 8-1.
Diagram of the fetal circulation showing the four sites of shunt: placenta, ductus venosus, foramen ovale, and ductus arteriosus. Intravascular *shading* is in proportion to oxygen saturation, with the lightest shading representing the highest Po_2. The numerical value inside the chamber or vessel is the Po_2 for that site in mm Hg. The percentages outside the vascular structures represent the relative flows in major tributaries and outlets for the two ventricles. The combined output of the two ventricles represents 100%. *a,* artery; *v,* vein; (From Guntheroth WG et al: *Physiology of the circulation: fetus, neonate and child.* In Kelley VC, ed: *Practice of pediatrics,* vol 8, Philadelphia, 1982, 1983, Harper & Row.)

Also, the RV is larger and more dominant than the left ventricle (LV). The RV handles 55% of the combined ventricular output, whereas the LV handles 45% of the combined ventricular output. In addition, the pressure in the RV is identical to that in the LV (unlike in the adult). This fact is reflected in the ECG of the newborn, which shows more RV force than that of the adult.

Fetal Cardiac Output

Unlike the adult heart, which increases its stroke volume when the heart rate decreases, the fetal heart is unable to increase stroke volume when the heart rate falls. Therefore the fetal cardiac output depends on the heart rate; when the heart rate drops, as in fetal distress, a serious fall in cardiac output results.

CHANGES IN CIRCULATION AFTER BIRTH

The primary change in circulation after birth is a shift of blood flow for gas exchange from the placenta to the lungs. The placental circulation disappears, and the pulmonary circulation is established.

1. Interruption of the umbilical cord results in the following:

   a. An increase in systemic vascular resistance (SVR) as a result of the removal of the very-low-resistance placenta

   b. Closure of the ductus venosus as a result of lack of blood return from the placenta

2. Lung expansion results in the following:

   a. A reduction of the pulmonary vascular resistance (PVR), an increase in pulmonary blood flow (PBF), and a fall in PA pressure (Fig. 8-2).

   b. Functional closure of the foramen ovale occurs as a result of increased pressure in the LA in excess of right atrium (RA) pressure. The LA pressure increases as a result of the increased pulmonary venous return to the LA, and the RA pressure falls as a result of closure of the ductus venosus.

   c. Closure of patent ductus arteriosus (PDA) as a result of increased arterial oxygen saturation

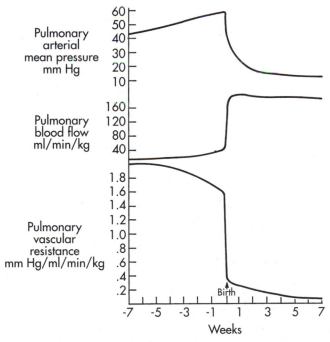

FIG. 8-2.
The changes in PA pressure, PBF, and PVR, during the 7 weeks preceding birth, at birth, and in the 7 weeks after birth. The prenatal data were derived from lambs and the postnatal data from other species. (From Rudolph AM: *Congenital diseases of the heart,* Chicago, 1974, Mosby.)

CHANGES IN PULMONARY VASCULAR RESISTANCE AND CLOSURE OF PATENT DUCTUS ARTERIOSUS

Changes in the PVR and closure of the PDA are so important in understanding many CHDs that further discussion is necessary.

Pulmonary Vascular Resistance

The PVR is as high as the SVR near or at term. The high PVR is maintained by an increased amount of smooth muscle in the walls of the pulmonary arterioles and alveolar hypoxia resulting from collapsed lungs.

With expansion of the lungs and the resulting increase in the alveolar oxygen tension, there is an initial, rapid fall in the PVR. This rapid fall is secondary to the vasodilating effect of oxygen on the pulmonary vasculature (Fig. 8-3). Between 6 and 8 weeks after birth there is a slower fall in the PVR and the PA pressure. This fall is associated with thinning of the medial layer of the pulmonary arterioles. A further decline in the PVR occurs after the first 2 years. This may be related to the increase in the number of alveolar units and their associated vessels.

Many neonatal conditions with inadequate oxygenation may interfere with the normal maturation (i.e., thinning) of the pulmonary arterioles, resulting in persistent pulmonary hypertension or delay in the fall of PVR (Box 8-1). A few examples of clinical importance follow:

1. Infants with a large ventricular septal defect (VSD) may not develop congestive heart failure (CHF) while living at a high altitude, but they may develop CHF if they move to sea level. This is because of the delayed fall in the PVR associated with altitude.

2. Premature infants with severe hyaline membrane disease usually do not develop CHF because of their high PVR, which restricts the left-to-right shunt. Acidosis, which is often present in these infants, may contribute to maintaining a high PVR. CHF may develop as their hyaline membrane disease improves because the resulting increase in arterial Po_2 dilates pulmonary vasculature.

3. In infants with a large VSD, a high PA pressure, resulting from a direct transmission of the LV pressure through the defect, delays the fall in the PVR. As a result, CHF does not develop until 6 to 8 weeks of age or older. In contrast, the PVR falls normally in infants with a small VSD, since direct transmission of the LV pressure to the PA does not occur in this situation.

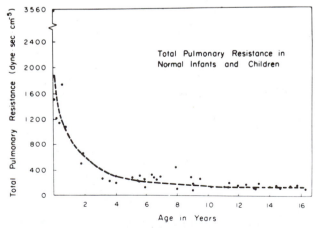

FIG. 8-3.
Postnatal changes in pulmonary vascular resistance. (From Moller JH, et al: *Congenital heart disease,* Kalamazoo, Mich, 1974, Upjohn Company.

BOX 8–1.

Neonatal Conditions That May Interfere With the Normal Maturation of Pulmonary Arterioles

Hypoxia and/or altitude
Lung disease (e.g., hyaline membrane disease)
Acidemia
Increased PA pressure because of large VSD or PDA
Increased pressure in the LA or pulmonary vein

PA, pulmonary artery; *VSD*, ventricular septal defect, *PDA*, patent ductus arteriosus; *LA*, left atrium.

Closure of the Ductus Arteriosus

Functional closure of the ductus arteriosus occurs by constriction of the medial, smooth muscle in the ductus within 10 to 15 hours after birth. Anatomic closure is completed by 2 to 3 weeks of age by permanent changes in the endothelium and subintimal layers of the ductus. Oxygen, prostaglandin E_2 levels, and maturity of the newborn are important factors in the closure of the ductus. Acetylcholine and bradykinin also constrict the ductus.

Oxygen and the ductus. Postnatal increase in oxygen saturation in the systemic circulation is the strongest stimulus for the constriction of the ductal smooth muscle, which leads to the closure of the ductus. The responsiveness of the ductal smooth muscle to oxygen is related to the gestational age of the newborn; the ductal tissue of the premature infant responds less intensely to oxygen than that of the full-term infant. The decreased responsiveness of the immature ductus to oxygen does not result from the lack of smooth muscle development, since the immature ductus constricts well to acetylcholine.

Prostaglandin E and the ductus. A few clinical situations are worth mentioning to show the importance of prostaglandin E series in the maintenance of the patency of the ductus arteriosus in the fetus.

1. A decrease in prostaglandin E_2 levels after birth results in a constriction of the ductus. This decrease results from the removal of the placental source of prostaglandin E_2 production at birth and from the marked increase in PBF, which allows effective removal of circulating prostaglandin E_2 by the lungs.

2. Constricting effects of indomethacin and the dilator effects of prostaglandins E_2 and I_2 are greater in the ductal tissues from an immature fetus than a near-term fetus.

3. Prolonged patency of the ductus can be maintained by intravenous infusion of prostaglandin E_1 in infants such as those with pulmonary atresia, whose survival depends on the patency of the ductus.

4. Indomethacin, a prostaglandin synthetase inhibitor, is used successfully to close a significant PDA in premature infants (see Chapter 29).

5. Maternal ingestion of a large amount of aspirin, an inhibitor of prostaglandin synthetase, may harm the fetus, since the aspirin may constrict the ductus during fetal life, resulting in pulmonary hypertension in the newborn (PPHN). It has been suggested that some cases of PPHN or persistent fetal circulation syndrome may be caused by a premature constriction of the ductus arteriosus.

Reduced arterial Po_2 and increased prostaglandin E_2 concentration. Before true anatomic closure occurs, the functionally closed ductus may be dilated by a reduced arterial Po_2 or an increased prostaglandin E_2 concentration. This may occur in asphyxia and various pulmonary diseases. The ductal closure is delayed at a high altitude. High altitudes have much higher incidence of PDA than areas at sea level.

Responses of Pulmonary Artery and Ductus Arteriosus to Various Stimuli

PA responds to oxygen and acidosis in the opposite manner as the ductus arteriosus. Hypoxia and acidosis relax the ductus arteriosus but constrict the pulmonary arterioles. Oxygen relaxes the pulmonary arterioles but constricts the ductus. The PA are also constricted by sympathetic stimulation and α-adrenergic stimulation (e.g., epinephrine, norepinephrine). Vagal stimulation, β-adrenergic stimulation (e.g., isoproterenol), and bradykinin dilate the PAs.

PREMATURE NEWBORNS

Two important problems that premature infants may face are related to the rate at which PVR falls and the responsiveness of the ductus arteriosus to oxygen (see Chapters 28 and 29).

The ductus arteriosus is more likely to remain open in preterm infants after birth, since the premature infant's ductal smooth muscle does not have a fully developed constrictor response to oxygen. In addition, premature infants have persistently high circulating levels of prostaglandin E_2 (possibly caused by increased production or decreased degradation in the lungs), and the premature ductal tissue exhibits an increased dilatory response to prostaglandin E_2.

In premature infants the pulmonary vascular smooth muscle is not as well developed as that of full-term infants. Therefore the fall in PVR occurs more rapidly than in the mature infant. This accounts for the early onset of a large left-to-right shunt and CHF.

9 / Pathophysiology of Left-to-Right Shunt Lesions

Before discussion of hemodynamic abnormalities of common left-to-right shunt lesions takes place, knowledge of the following model, which is used throughout this section, is helpful. Fig. 9-1 is a block diagram of a normal heart in which one arrow represents a "unit" of normal cardiac output. It is assumed that the cardiac chambers and great arteries and veins, which are indicated with one arrow, are normal in size. If a cardiac chamber or great artery has more than one arrow in it, that chamber or blood vessel will be dilated. A diagram of a normal cardiac roentgenogram was presented in an earlier chapter (see Fig. 4-2 on p. 53). Modification in the appearance of chest roentgenograms because of enlargement or reduction of cardiac chambers or great vessels is presented in diagrammatic drawings to aid in the interpretation of chest x-ray films.

ATRIAL SEPTAL DEFECT

In an atrial septal defect (ASD) the magnitude of the left-to-right shunt is determined by the *size* of the defect and the relative *compliance* of the right ventricle (RV) and left ventricle (LV). Because the compliance of the RV is greater than that of the LV, a left-to-right shunt is present. The magnitude of the shunt is reflected in the degree of cardiac enlargement. Let it be assumed that there is a left-to-right shunt of one arrow at the atrial level. As seen in the block diagram (Fig. 9-2), the right atrium (RA), RV, and main pulmonary artery (MPA) and its branches handle two arrows and therefore are dilated. These findings are translated into the chest x-ray films (Fig. 9-3), which reveal enlargement of the RA, RV, and MPA, as well as an increase in pulmonary vascular markings (PVM). Note that the left atrium (LA) is not enlarged (see Figs. 9-2 and 9-3). This is because the increased pulmonary venous return to the LA does not stay in that chamber; rather it is shunted immediately to the RA. The absence of left atrial enlargement (LAE) is one of the helpful x-ray signs for differentiating an ASD from a ventricular septal defect (VSD).

The dilated RV cavity prolongs the time required for depolarization of the RV because of its longer pathway, producing right bundle branch block (RBBB) pattern (with rsR′ in V1) in the ECG. The RBBB pattern in children with an ASD is not the result of actual block in the right bundle. If the duration of the QRS complex is not abnormally prolonged, the ECG may be read as mild RVH. Therefore either RBBB or mild right ventricular hypertrophy (RVH) is seen on the ECG of children with ASD.

The heart murmur in ASD is not because of the shunt at the atrial level. Since the pressure gradient between the atria is so small and the shunt occurs throughout the cardiac cycle, both in systole and diastole, the left-to-right shunt is silent. The heart murmur in ASD originates from the pulmonary valve because of the increased blood flow (two arrows) through this normal-sized valve (creating relative pulmonary stenosis (PS)) (see Fig. 9-2), therefore, the murmur is systolic in timing. An increased blood flow through the tricuspid valve (two arrows) results in a relative stenosis of this valve and a diastolic rumble at the tricuspid valve area (LLSB). The widely split and fixed S2, which is typical of an ASD, partially results from the RBBB (electric delay in RV depolarization). In addition, the large atrial shunt tends to abolish respiration-related fluctuations in systemic venous return to the right side of the heart. This results in a large venous return to the RA throughout the respiratory cycle, and thereby the fixed S2.

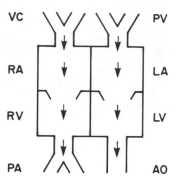

FIG. 9-1.
Diagram of a normal heart. *One arrow* represents a unit of normal cardiac output. *AO,* aorta; *LA,* left atrium; *LV,* left ventricle; *PA,* pulmonary artery; *PV,* pulmonary vein; *RA,* right atrium; *RV,* right ventricle; *VC,* vena cava.

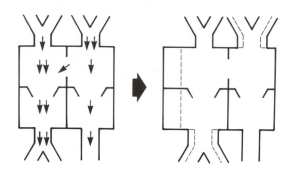

FIG. 9-2.
Block diagram of an ASD. The number of arrows in each chamber represents the amount of blood to be handled by that particular chamber. When one redraws the chambers with two arrows larger than normal, one can predict which chambers will be enlarged.

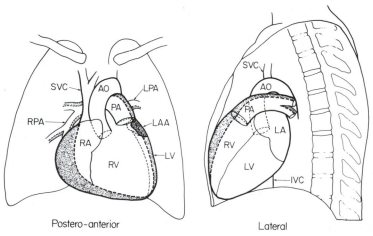

FIG. 9-3.
Posteroanterior and lateral view diagrams of chest roentgenograms. Enlargement of the RA and MPA segment and increased PVMs are present in the posteroanterior view. The RV enlargement is best seen in the lateral view.

Children rarely experience congestive heart failure (CHF). Even in the presence of a large left-to-right shunt, pulmonary artery (PA) pressure remains normal for many years. The PAs handle an increased amount of PBF (without direct transmission of systemic pressure) extremely well for a long time. However, CHF and pulmonary hypertension eventually develop in the third and fourth decade of life.

VENTRICULAR SEPTAL DEFECT

The direction of the shunt in acyanotic VSD is left-to-right. The magnitude of the shunt is determined by the *size*, not the location, of the defect and the level of pulmonary vascular resistance (PVR). With a small defect, a large resistance to the left-to-right shunt is offered at the defect, and the shunt does not depend on the level of PVR. With a large VSD, the resistance offered by the defect is minimal, and the left-to-right shunt depends on the level of PVR. The lower the PVR, the greater the magnitude of the left-to-right shunt. This type of left-to-right shunt is called *dependent shunt.* Even in the presence of a large VSD, the decrease in PVR to a critical level does not occur until the age of 6 to 8 weeks, so the onset of CHF is delayed until that age.

In a VSD of moderate size, the cardiac chambers or vessels with two arrows enlarge, resulting in enlargement of the MPA, LA, and LV, as well as an increase in PVMs (Fig. 9-4). In VSD, it is the LV that does volume overwork, not the RV. This results in LV enlargement; the RV does not enlarge. Since the shunt of VSD mainly occurs during systole when the RV also contracts, the shunted blood goes directly to the PA rather than remain in the RV cavity. Therefore there is no significant volume overload to the RV, and the RV remains relatively normal in size (Figs. 9-4 and 9-5). The difference between VSD and ASD with respect to the presence of LAE should be noted. The similarities between VSD and patent ductus arteriosus (PDA) as to the presence of enlarged LA and LV should also be noted.

Fig. 9-6 summarizes the hemodynamics of VSDs of varying sizes and helps in the understanding of clinical manifestations. The size of a cardiac chamber directly relates

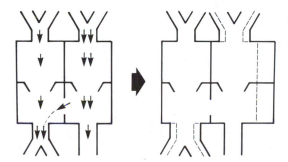

FIG. 9-4.
Block diagram of VSD that shows the chambers and vessels that will be enlarged. There is an enlargement of the LA and LV. The MPA is prominent and the pulmonary vascularity is increased. Note the absence of RV enlargement (see text for explanation).

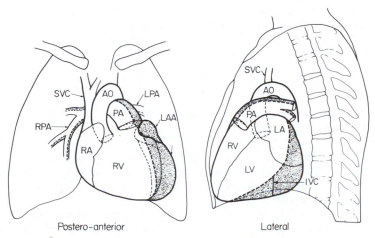

Postero-anterior   Lateral

FIG. 9-5.
Posteroanterior and lateral view diagrams of chest roentgenograms of a moderate VSD. Enlargement of the LA, LV, and MPA and increased PVMs are present. Note the presence of LA enlargement, which is absent in ASD.

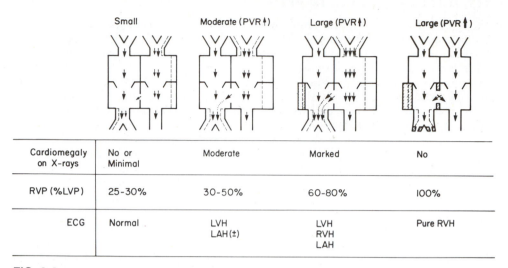

	Small	Moderate (PVR↑)	Large (PVR↑)	Large (PVR↑)
Cardiomegaly on X-rays	No or Minimal	Moderate	Marked	No
RVP (%LVP)	25-30%	30-50%	60-80%	100%
ECG	Normal	LVH LAH(±)	LVH RVH LAH	Pure RVH

FIG. 9-6.
Diagrammatic summary of pathophysiology of VSD. Most of the x-ray and ECG findings can be deduced from this diagram (see text for full description). *LVP*, left ventricular pressure; *RVP*, right ventricular pressure; *PVR*, pulmonary vascular resistance.

to the amount of blood, or the number of arrows, handled by the chamber. The number of arrows in the heart diagram also determine the overall size of the heart.

With a *small* VSD, there is only half of an arrow coming from the LV to the MPA. In addition, the degree of pulmonary vascular congestion and the chamber enlargement is either minimal or too small to result in a significant change of the chest x-ray films (see Fig 9-6). The degree of volume work imposed on the LV is also too small to produce LVH on the ECG. The shunt itself produces a heart murmur (regurgitant systolic), and the intensity of the P2 is normal because the PA pressure is normal.

With a VSD of moderate size (i.e., *moderate VSD*), one arrow shunts from the LV to the RV, and all the chambers that are enlarged handle two arrows. Therefore the cardiomegaly on the x-ray film is of a significant degree. The volume overwork done by the LV is significant so that the ECG produces left ventricular hypertrophy (LVH) of "volume overload" type. Although the shunt is large, the RV is not significantly dilated, and the pressure in this chamber is elevated only slightly (see Fig 9-6). In other words, in a moderate VSD the RV is not under significant volume or pressure overload; therefore ECG signs of RVH are absent. As in a small VSD, a heart murmur (regurgitant systolic type) is produced by the left-to-right shunt. The normal-sized mitral valve handles two arrows. This relative mitral stenosis (MS) produces a middiastolic rumble at the apex. The PA pressure is mildly elevated; therefore the intensity of the P2 may increase slightly.

With a *large* VSD, the overall heart size is larger than that seen with a moderate VSD because there is a much greater shunt. Since there is direct transmission of the LV pressure through the large defect to the RV, in addition to a much greater shunt, the RV becomes enlarged and hypertrophied. Therefore the x-ray film shows biventricular enlargement, LAE, and greatly increased pulmonary vascularity (see Fig 9-6). The ECG shows combined ventricular hypertrophy (CVH) and sometimes left atrial hypertrophy (LAH). A large VSD usually results in CHF.

When a large VSD is left untreated, irreversible changes take place in the pulmonary arterioles. With gradual development of the *pulmonary vascular obstructive disease* (*PVOD* or *Eisenmenger's syndrome*), which may take years to develop, striking changes occur in the heart size, ECG, and clinical findings. Since the PVR is notably elevated at this stage, approaching the systemic level, the magnitude of the left-to-right shunt decreases. This results in the removal of a volume overload placed on the LV. Therefore the size of the LV and the overall heart size decreases, and the ECG evidence of LVH disappears, leaving RVH because of the persistence of pulmonary hypertension. Although the heart size becomes small, the MPA segment remains enlarged because of persistent pulmonary hypertension. In other words, with development of PVOD, the heart size returns to normal except for a prominent MPA segment, and a pure RVH on the ECG results. A bidirectional shunt causes cyanosis. Since the shunt is small, the loudness of the murmur decreases or may even disappear. The S2 is loud and single because of pulmonary hypertension.

PATENT DUCTUS ARTERIOSUS

The hemodynamics of PDA are similar to those of VSD. The magnitude of the left-to-right shunt is determined by the *resistance* offered by the ductus (i.e., diameter, length, and tortuosity) when the ductus is small, and by the level of *PVR* when the ductus is large (i.e., dependent shunt). Therefore the onset of CHF with a PDA is similar to that with a VSD.

The chambers and vessels that enlarge are the same as those in a VSD, except for an enlarged aorta to the level of the PDA (i.e., enlarged ascending aorta) (Fig. 9-7). Therefore in PDA, chest x-ray films show enlargement of the LA and LV, large ascending aorta and MPA, and an increase in PVMs (Fig. 9-8). Although the aorta is enlarged, it usually does not produce an abnormal cardiac silhouette, since the aorta does not form the cardiac silhouette. Therefore chest x-ray films of PDA are indistinguishable from those of VSD.

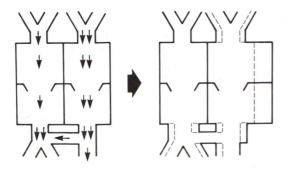

FIG. 9-7.
Block diagram of the heart in PDA. Note the similarities between PDA and VSD as to the chamber enlargement. There is an enlargement of the aorta to the level of the ductus arteriosus.

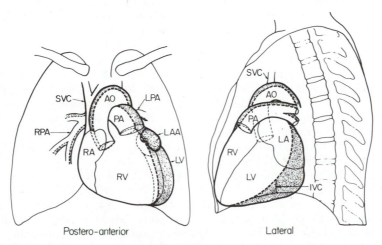

Postero-anterior   Lateral

FIG. 9-8.
Diagrammatic drawing of the posteroanterior and lateral chest x-ray films of PDA. Note the similarities in chest x-ray films between PDA and VSD.

Hemodynamic consequences of PDA are similar to those of VSD. In PDA with a small shunt the LVE is minimal; therefore the ECG and chest x-ray findings are close to normal. Since there is a significant pressure gradient between the aorta and the PA in both systole and diastole, the left-to-right shunt occurs throughout the cardiac cycle, thereby producing the characteristic continuous murmur of this condition. With a small shunt, the intensity of the P2 is normal because the PA pressure is normal.

In PDA with a moderately large shunt the heart size is moderately enlarged with increased pulmonary blood flow (PBF). The chambers enlarged are the LA, LV, and the MPA segment. The ECG shows LVH as in moderate VSD. In addition to the characteristic continuous murmur, there may be an apical diastolic flow rumble as a result of relative MS. The P2 slightly increases in intensity if it can be separated from the loud heart murmur.

In a large PDA, marked cardiomegaly and increased PVMs are present. The volume overload is on the LV and LA, which produces LVH and occasional LAH on the ECG. The free transmission of the aortic pressure to the PA produces pulmonary hypertension and RV hypertension with resulting RVH on the ECG. Therefore the ECG shows CVH and LAH, as in a large VSD. The continuous murmur is present with a loud apical diastolic rumble because of a relative MS. The P2 is accentuated in intensity because of pulmonary hypertension.

An untreated large PDA can also produce PVOD, with a resulting bidirectional (i.e., right-to-left and left-to-right) shunt at the ductus level. The bidirectional shunt may produce cyanosis only in the lower half of the body (i.e., differential cyanosis). As in VSD with Eisenmenger's syndrome, the heart size returns to normal because of the reduced magnitude of the shunt. The peripheral pulmonary vascularity decreases, but the central hilar vessels and the MPA segment are greatly dilated because of severe pulmonary hypertension. The ECG shows pure RVH because the LV is no longer under volume overload. Auscultation no longer reveals the continuous murmur or the apical rumble because of the reduced shunt. The S2 is single and loud because of pulmonary hypertension.

ENDOCARDIAL CUSHION DEFECT

During fetal life the endocardial cushion tissue contributes to the closure of both the lower part of the atrial septum (i.e., ostium primum) and the upper part of the ventricular septum, in addition to the formation of the mitral and tricuspid valves. The failure of this tissue to develop may be complete or partial. A simple way of understanding the complete form of ECD is that the tissue in the center of the heart is missing, with resulting VSD, primum type of ASD, and clefts in the mitral and tricuspid valves. In the partial form of the defect, only an ASD is present in the ostium primum septum (primum-type ASD), often associated with a cleft in the mitral valve.

Hemodynamic abnormalities of primum type of ASD are similar to those of secundum-type ASD, in which the RA and RV are dilated with increased PBF (Fig 9-9). These changes are expressed in the chest x-ray films (see Fig. 9-3). The cleft mitral valve is usually insignificant from a hemodynamic point of view, since blood regurgitated into the LA is immediately shunted to the RA, thereby decompressing the LA. The physical findings are also similar to those of secundum ASD—a widely split and fixed S2, a systolic ejection murmur at the upper left sternal border (ULSB), and a middiastolic rumble of relative tricuspid stenosis (TS), at the LLSB. In addition, a systolic murmur of MR is occasionally present. The ECG findings are also similar—RBBB (with rsR' in V1) or mild RVH. One exception, which is important in differentiating between the two types of ASDs, is the presence of a "superior" QRS axis or left anterior hemiblock (in the range of −20 degrees to −150 degrees) in the primum type of ASD. The abnormal QRS axis seen in ECD (both partial and complete forms) is not the result of axis deviation or any of the hemodynamic abnormalities mentioned; rather the abnormal QRS occurs because of a primary abnormality in the development of the His bundle and the bundle branches.

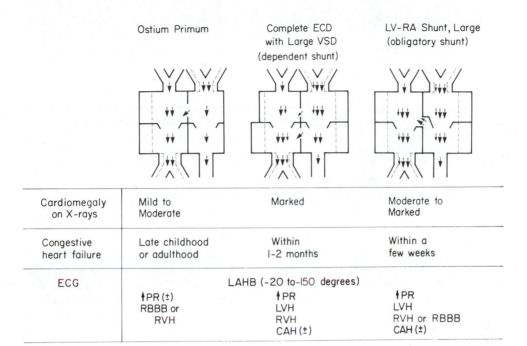

	Ostium Primum	Complete ECD with Large VSD (dependent shunt)	LV-RA Shunt, Large (obligatory shunt)
Cardiomegaly on X-rays	Mild to Moderate	Marked	Moderate to Marked
Congestive heart failure	Late childhood or adulthood	Within 1-2 months	Within a few weeks
ECG	LAHB (−20 to −150 degrees)		
	↕PR (±) RBBB or RVH	↕PR LVH RVH CAH (±)	↕PR LVH RVH or RBBB CAH (±)

FIG. 9-9.
Hemodynamic changes in different types of ECD. Hemodynamics of the ostium primum type of ASD are identical to those of the secundum type of ASD. The cleft mitral valve is usually not significant from a hemodynamic point of view. In complete ECD, the hemodynamic changes are the sum of those of VSD and ASD, resulting in enlargement of all four cardiac chambers and increased PBF. Again, the cleft mitral valve is not significant, and its effect is not shown here. The shunt depends on the level of the PVR tance (dependent shunt). In the LV-RA shunt, the shunt depends not on the level of PVR but on the size of the defect (obligatory shunt). Therefore CHF may occur within the first weeks of life. *LAHB,* Left anterior hemiblock.

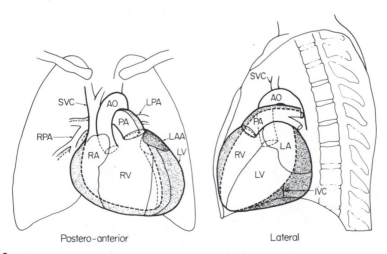

Postero-anterior   Lateral

FIG. 9-10.
Diagrammatic drawing of chest roentgenograms in the complete form of ECD. All four cardiac chambers are enlarged with increased PVMs.

Hemodynamic changes seen with complete ECD are the sum of the changes of ASD and VSD. The magnitude of the left-to-right shunt in both ASD and VSD is determined by the level of PVR (i.e., dependent shunt). It has volume overload on the LA and LV as in a VSD and partially because of mitral regurgitation (MR). In addition, it has volume overload of the RA and RV as in an ASD (see Fig. 9-9). This is translated to the chest x-ray films as biatrial and biventricular enlargement (Fig. 9-10). The ECG also reflects these changes as CVH and occasional combined atrial hypertrophy (CAH). Left anterior hemiblock is also characteristic of ECD. Physical examination is characterized by a hyperactive precordium and regurgitant systolic murmurs of VSD and MR, loud and narrowly split S2 (because of pulmonary hypertension), apical and/or tricuspid diastolic rumble, and signs of CHF. Those who survive infancy may develop PVOD, as already discussed for a large VSD or large PDA.

A direct communication between the LV and RA may occur as part of ECD or as an isolated defect unrelated to ECD. The direction of the shunt is from the high-pressure LV to the low-pressure RA. The magnitude of the shunt is determined by the *size* of the defect, regardless of the state of PVR; blood shunted to the RA must go forward through the lungs even if the PVR is high. This type of shunt, which is independent of the status of PVR, is called an *obligatory shunt* (see Fig. 9-9). CHF occurs within a few weeks, which is much earlier than in the usual VSD. The enlarged chambers are identical to those of the complete form of ECD. Therefore the chest x-ray films and ECG findings are similar to those seen in complete ECD. Physical findings also resemble those of complete ECD, although the holosystolic murmur may be more prominent at the mid-right sternal border (MRSB).

10 / Pathophysiology of Obstructive and Valvular Regurgitant Lesions

This chapter discusses hemodynamic abnormalities of obstructive and valvular regurgitant lesions of congenital and acquired etiologies. For convenience, they are divided into the following three groups based on their hemodynamic similarities:

1. Ventricular outflow obstructive lesions (e.g., aortic stenosis (AS), pulmonary stenosis (PS), coarctation of the aorta (COA))

2. Stenosis of atrioventricular (AV) valves (e.g., mitral stenosis (MS), tricuspid stenosis (TS))

3. Valvular regurgitant lesions (e.g., mitral regurgitation (MR), tricuspid regurgitation (TR), aortic regurgitation (AR), pulmonary regurgitation (PR))

OBSTRUCTION TO VENTRICULAR OUTPUT

Common congenital obstructive lesions to ventricular output are AS, PS, and COA. All of these obstructive lesions produce the following three pathophysiologic changes (Fig. 10-1):

1. An ejection systolic murmur (as seen in auscultation)

2. Hypertrophy of the respective ventricle (as seen in ECG)

3. Poststenotic dilatation (as seen in chest-x ray films); (This is not seen with subvalvar stenosis or isolated infundibular stenosis.)

Aortic and Pulmonary Valve Stenoses

An ejection type of systolic murmur can best be heard when the stethoscope is placed over the area distal to the obstruction. Therefore the murmur of AS is usually loudest over the ascending aorta (i.e., upper right sternal border (URSB) or aortic valve area), and the murmur of PS is loudest over the main pulmonary artery (MPA) (i.e., ULSB or pulmonary valve area). However, the actual location of the aortic valve is under the sternum at the level of third left intercostal space (3LICS); therefore the murmur of AS may be quite loud at 3LICS.

In isolated stenosis of the pulmonary or aortic valve the intensity and duration of the ejection type of systolic murmur are directly proportional to the severity of the stenosis. In mild stenosis of a semilunar valve the murmur is of low intensity (grade 1 to 2/6) and occurs early in systole with the apex of the "diamond" in the first half of the systole. With increasing severity of the stenosis, the murmur becomes louder (often with a thrill), and the apex of the murmur moves toward the S2. With mild pulmonary valve stenosis, the S2 is normal or split widely because of prolonged "hangout time" (see Chapter 2). With severe PS, the murmur is long and may continue beyond the A2, the S2 splits widely, and the intensity of the P2 decreases (Fig. 10-2, A). With severe AS, the S2 becomes single or splits paradoxically because of the delayed A2 in relation to the P2 (Fig. 10-2, B). In semilunar valve stenosis an ejection click may be audible. The click is produced

FIG. 10-1.
Three secondary changes in ventricular
outflow obstructive lesions that are typically
seen in aortic valve stenosis and pulmonary
valve stenosis. They are a systolic ejection
murmur, hypertrophy of the responsible
ventricle, and poststenotic dilatation. A normal-
sized ventricle and a great artery are shown in
broken lines. A similar change occurs with
coarctation of the aorta.

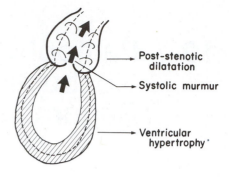

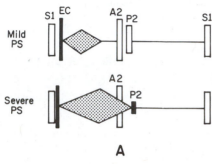

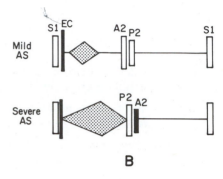

A   **B**

FIG. 10-2.
Systolic murmurs of pulmonary valve stenosis **(A)** and aortic valve stenosis **(B).** The
duration and intensity of the murmur increase with increasing severity of the stenosis.
Note the changes in the splitting of S2 (see text). An ejection click *(EC)* is present in
both conditions. Abnormal heart sounds are shown as *black bars.*

by a sudden checking of the valve motion or possibly by the sudden distention of the
dilated great arteries.

If the obstruction is severe, the ventricle that has to pump blood against the obstruction will hypertrophy. The left ventricle (LV) will hypertrophy in AS and the right ventricle (RV) in PS, which results in left ventricular hypertrophy (LVH) and right ventricular hypertrophy (RVH) respectively on the ECG. Cardiac output is maintained unless
myocardial failure occurs in severe cases; therefore, the heart size remains normal.

Poststenotic dilatation is the hallmark of an obstruction at the valvular level. It is not
seen with subvalvular stenosis; it is seen only mildly or not at all with supravalvular
stenosis. It is believed that the fatigue of collagen fibers, resulting from sustained
vibration of the vessel distal to the narrowing, causes the poststenotic dilatation. In
pulmonary valve stenosis a prominent MPA segment is visible on chest x-ray film (see
Fig. 4-7, A on p. 56). In aortic valve stenosis, a dilated aorta may look like a bulge on
the right upper mediastinum or as a prominence of the aortic knob on the left upper
mediastinum (see Fig. 4-7, C on p. 56). Mild dilatation of the ascending aorta secondary
to aortic valve stenosis is usually not visible on the plain chest x-ray films, since the
ascending aorta does not form the cardiac border.

Coarctation of the Aorta

In older children with COA a systolic ejection murmur (SEM) is present over the
descending aorta, but distal to the site of coarctation (i.e., in the left interscapular area).
Since many of these patients also have an abnormal aortic valve (most commonly a
bicuspid aortic valve), a soft AS murmur and an occasional AR murmur may be heard.
Depending on the obstruction's severity, the femoral pulses in the lower extremities are
either weak and delayed or absent. The weak pulse primarily results from a slow

upstroke of the arterial pulse in the lower extremity sites. On chest x-ray films, poststenotic dilatation of the descending aorta (distal to the coarctation) often produces the figure-of-3 sign on the plain film or an E-shaped indentation on the barium esophagogram (see Fig. 4-9 on p. 59). The ECG shows LVH because of a pressure overload placed on the LV. In newborns and small infants RVH or right bundle branch block (RBBB) is commonly seen, but LVH is not.

Previously, physicians used terms such as *preductal* and *infantile coarctation* to describe symptomatic infants. Terms such as *postductal* and *adult type coarctation* described asymptomatic children. Neither terminology is correct (see Chapter 13). The coarctation is almost always juxtaductal (i.e., located opposite the entry of the ductus arteriosus). Major differences in pathology between symptomatic infants and asymptomatic children often occur and contribute significantly to hemodynamic abnormalities (Fig. 10-3).

1. Many patients who become symptomatic early in life have an associated ventricular septal defect (VSD) and/or left-sided obstructive lesions, which tend to decrease blood flow to the ascending aorta and through the aortic isthmus (i.e., the segment between the left subclavian artery and the ductus arteriosus) during fetal life. The obstructive lesions may be in the LV outflow tract, the aortic valve, or the proximal aorta (see Fig. 10-3, *A*).

2. The associated anomalies result in more volume work delegated to the RV, which supplies blood to the descending aorta through a large ductus arteriosus. The RV becomes more dilated and hypertrophied, and the LV becomes smaller than normal. Even in the absence of associated lesions, the RV handles more volume work than the LV, and the LV is relatively small. A relatively small amount of blood goes to the ascending aorta. The aorta becomes somewhat hypoplastic.

During fetal life there is no need for a forward flow from the ascending to the descending aorta. This absence does not stimulate the development of collateral circulation between the ascending and descending aortas. When the ductus closes after birth, a sudden increase in the pressure work imposed on the relatively small LV occurs. This results in a noticeable decrease in the perfusion of the descending aorta (with resulting circulatory shock), renal failure, and signs of left heart failure (i.e., dyspnea and

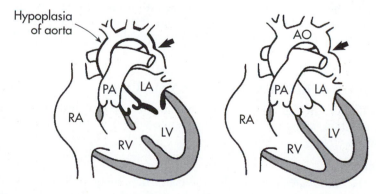

FIG. 10-3.
Diagrammatic comparison of the heart and aorta in symptomatic infants and asymptomatic children with coarctation of the aorta. **A,** In symptomatic infants, associated defects are frequently found, which include VSD, aortic and mitral valve diseases, and hypoplasia of the ascending and transverse aortas. These abnormalities are shown in heavy lines. **B,** In asymptomatic children, the coarctation is usually an isolated lesion, except for bicuspid aortic valve (not shown).

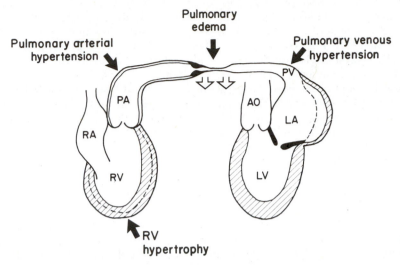

FIG. 10-4.
Hemodynamic changes in severe MS. LAE and LAH, pulmonary venous hypertension, and possible pulmonary edema result. Reflex vasoconstriction of pulmonary arterioles leads to pulmonary arterial hypertension and RVH.

pulmonary venous congestion). Even in the absence of associated lesions, some infants develop LV failure. The presence of the pressure gradient between the proximal and distal aortas gradually stimulates the development of collateral circulation between them. Most of these infants, who do not have associated defects, tolerate the postnatal closure of the ductus well and remain asymptomatic (see Fig. 10-3, *B*).

The previously described changes in fetal circulation account for the presence of RVH or RBBB on the ECG. During fetal life the RV normally performs 55% of the combined ventricular volume work, and the LV performs 45%. This combined ventricular volume work has an RV:LV volume work ratio of 55:45. This is the reason why normal newborn infants have RV dominance on the ECG. An associated VSD and/or obstructive lesions delegate more volume work to the RV; for example, if the RV:LV volume work ratio is 70:30, the RV dominance is greater than normal with resulting RVH on the ECG. Thus RVH seen in symptomatic infants usually results from an increased volume overload placed on the RV during fetal life. The RVH is gradually replaced by LVH by 2 years of age.

STENOSIS OF ATRIOVENTRICULAR VALVES

Stenosis of the AV valves produces obstruction to pulmonary or systemic venous return. Passive congestion in the pulmonary or systemic venous system result in the clinical manifestations.

Mitral Stenosis

Stenosis of the mitral valve is more often rheumatic than congenital in origin. It produces diastolic murmurs because of pressure gradients that develop in diastole between the left atrium (LA) and LV, in addition to a series of changes in the LA, pulmonary veins, pulmonary arteries (PAs), and the RV, which are structures proximal to the point of obstruction.

When significant MS is present, the LA becomes dilated and hypertrophied (Fig. 10-4). The pressure in the LA is raised with a pressure gradient between the LA and LV during diastole. The elevated LA pressure then raises PV and capillary pressures. Pulmonary edema may result if the hydrostatic pressure in the capillaries exceeds the osmotic pressure of the blood. Therefore chest x-ray films may reveal pulmonary vein congestion or pulmonary edema and LA enlargement. This produces dyspnea, with or without exertion, and orthopnea. The high pulmonary capillary pressure results in reflex arteriolar constriction. The pulmonary arteriolar constriction may help prevent pulmonary edema but causes pulmonary artery hypertension and hypertrophy of the RV (reflected as RVH on the ECG and as a prominent MPA segment on chest x-ray films) and ultimate right heart failure (reflected as cardiomegaly on x-ray films).

The pressure gradient during diastole produces a middiastolic rumble that is best heard at the apex on auscultation. When the mitral valve is mobile (not severely stenotic), an opening snap precedes the murmur (see Fig. 21-1 on p. 311). During the last part of diastole, the pressure gradient persists and the LA contracts, producing a presystolic murmur. At the time of the onset of ventricular contraction, the mitral valve leaflets are relatively wide apart because of a prolonged atrial contraction, thereby producing a loud S1. If cardiac output reduces significantly, thready pulses result. The dilated LA contributes to the frequent occurrence of atrial fibrillation in adults, which would result in the loss of the presystolic murmur.

The following conditions, which are characterized by an elevated pulmonary vein pressure, have similar pathophysiology and require differentiation from MS:

1. Total anomalous pulmonary venous return (TAPVR) with obstruction (see Chapter 14)

2. Cor triatriatum (see Chapter 17)

3. Stenosis of individual pulmonary vein

4. Hypoplastic left heart syndrome (HLHS) (see Chapter 29)

5. Left atrial myxoma (see Chapter 22)

Tricuspid Stenosis

Stenosis of the tricuspid valve is rare and usually congenital. It produces dilatation and hypertrophy of the right atrium (RA) for obvious reasons. Therefore chest x-ray films reveal right atrial enlargement (RAE), and the ECG shows right atrial hypertrophy (RAH).

Increased pressure in the systemic veins produces hepatomegaly, distended neck veins, and rarely splenomegaly. A pressure gradient across this valve during diastole produces a middiastolic murmur. A prolonged contraction of the RA to push blood through the narrow valve may produce a presystolic murmur. It is occasionally associated with congenital hypoplasia of the RV, which exaggerates the obstruction to the blood flow into the RV.

VALVULAR REGURGITANT LESIONS

Important valvular regurgitant lesions are AR and MR. Severe pulmonary valve regurgitation is relatively rare, except in a postoperative state. Tricuspid valve regurgitation is also rare.

In general, when regurgitation is severe, the chambers both proximal *and* distal to a regurgitant valve become dilated with volume overload of these chambers. With MR, both the LV and LA dilate, whereas with AR, the LV enlarges and the aorta enlarges or increases its pulsation. If the regurgitation is minimal, only auscultatory abnormalities indicate its presence.

Mitral Regurgitation

The major problem in MR is a volume overload of both the LA and LV with resulting enlargement of these chambers (Fig. 10-5). Therefore chest x-ray films reveal enlargement of the LA and LV, and the ECG may show LVH and left atrial hypertrophy (LAH).

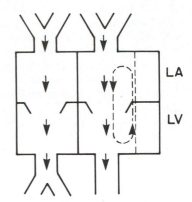

FIG. 10-5.
Diagrammatic representation of hemodynamic changes in MR. Note that the chambers with *two arrows* (LA and LV) are enlarged.

Regurgitation of blood from the LV to the LA produces a regurgitant systolic murmur that is best heard near the apex. Because of an abnormal increase in the flow across the mitral orifice during the rapid filling phase, the S3 is usually loud. When the regurgitation is severe, a middiastolic rumble may be present because of "relative" MS that results from handling an excessive amount of left atrial blood through the normal-sized mitral orifice. The dilated LA chamber tends to dampen the transmission of the pressure from the LV, and the pressure in the LA is usually not notably elevated. Therefore marked pulmonary hypertension only occurs occasionally.

Tricuspid Regurgitation

Hemodynamic changes similar to those described for MS result. The RA and RV enlarge for obvious reasons. The ECG may show RAH and RVH (or RBBB).

A systolic regurgitant murmur, a loud S3, and a diastolic rumble develop as in MR, but they are audible at the tricuspid area (both sides of the lower sternal border) rather than at the apex. With severe regurgitation, pulsation of the liver and neck veins may occur.

Aortic Regurgitation

There is volume overload of the LV, since this chamber must handle normal cardiac output in addition to the amount that leaks back to the LV (Fig. 10-6). This is represented as LV enlargement on x-ray films and LVH on the ECG. Because of the increase in stroke volume received by the aorta, the aorta pulsates more than normal and becomes somewhat dilated, although the aorta does not retain all of the increased stroke volume.

An increase in systolic pressure results from an increase in stroke volume. The diastolic pressure is lower because of a continuous leak back to the LV during diastole. This results in a wide pulse pressure and bounding peripheral pulse. The regurgitation during diastole produces a high-pitched decrescendo diastolic murmur immediately after the S2 (see Fig. 21-4 on p. 315). The regurgitant flow is directed toward the apex; therefore the diastolic decrescendo murmur is well audible at the apex and in the 3LICS. The AR flow, which coincides with the forward flow of left atrial blood, produces a flutter motion of the MV. This produces an Austin-Flint murmur in diastole. With severe AR, a high LV end-diastolic pressure approximates the mitral valve leaflets at the onset of the ventricular systole, resulting in a reduced intensity of the S1.

Pulmonary Regurgitation

Pathophysiology of PR is similar to that of AR. The RV dilates, and the PA may enlarge. This is represented in x-ray films as RV enlargement and a prominence of the MPA segment. The ECG may show RVH or RBBB.

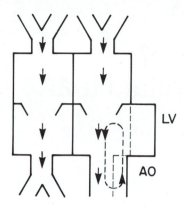

FIG. 10-6.
Diagrammatic representation of hemodynamic changes in AR. Note that the LV and aorta, with *two arrows,* are enlarged.

Because of the low diastolic pressure of the PA, the murmur of PR is low pitched, and the gap between the S2 and the onset of the decrescendo diastolic murmur is wider than that seen in AR. In the presence of pulmonary hypertension; however, the murmur of PR resembles that of AR. The direction of the regurgitation is to the body of the RV; therefore the PR murmur is audible along the left sternal border rather than at the apex, as in AR. This auscultatory finding is helpful in differentiating between PR and AR.

11 / Pathophysiology of Cyanotic Congenital Heart Defects

PATHOPHYSIOLOGY OF CYANOSIS

Clinical Cyanosis

Cyanosis is a bluish discoloration of the skin and mucous membrane resulting from an increased concentration of reduced hemoglobin. Clinical cyanosis occurs when the amount of reduced hemoglobin in the cutaneous veins reaches a critical level, about 5 g/100 ml. The critical level of the reduced hemoglobin in the cutaneous vein may result from either desaturation of arterial blood or an increased extraction of oxygen by peripheral tissue. The latter occurs in the presence of normal arterial saturation that results from a sluggish flow of blood (e.g., circulatory shock, hypovolemia, vasoconstriction from cold). Cyanosis secondary to desaturation of arterial blood is called *central cyanosis;* cyanosis with normal arterial oxygen saturation is called *peripheral cyanosis.*

The level of hemoglobin greatly influences the occurrence of cyanosis. Normally about 2 g/100 ml of reduced hemoglobin is present in the venules, so an additional 3 g/100 ml of reduced hemoglobin in arterial blood produces clinical cyanosis. Cyanosis is recognized at a higher level of oxygen saturation in patients with polycythemia and at a lower level of oxygen saturation in patients with anemia (Fig. 11-1). For a normal person with hemoglobin of 15 g/100 ml, 3 g of reduced hemoglobin is 20% desaturation. When the oxygen saturation reaches about 80%, cyanosis occurs. In a patient with polycythemia with hemoglobin of 20 g/100 ml, 3 g of reduced hemoglobin with 15% desaturation (or 84% arterial saturation) is needed when cyanosis is recognized. On the other hand, in a patient with a marked anemia (i.e., hemoglobin 6 g/100 ml), 3 g of reduced hemoglogin is a 50% desaturation when cyanosis occurs. Cyanosis may result from a number of causes (see box on p. 115).

Early detection. Cyanosis of cardiac origin must be diagnosed early for proper management, but the detection of mild cyanosis is difficult. In a newborn, acrocyanosis, which is a normal finding in this age group, may cause confusion. In addition, some newborns are polycythemic, which contributes to the appearance of cyanosis. Cyanosis is more difficult to detect in children with dark pigmentation and is better perceived in natural light than in artificial light. In older infants and children, chronic cyanosis of a mild degree, which may be difficult to detect, produces clubbing.

When in doubt, arterial oxygen saturation can be obtained by a pulse oximeter or arterial Po_2 by blood gas determination. When cyanosis occurs because of lung diseases or disorders of the central nervous system, crying may improve the cyanosis; however, crying usually worsens cyanosis in children with cyanotic heart defects. When cyanosis results from noncardiac causes, inhalation of 100% oxygen usually increases the arterial Po_2 to 300 to 400 mm Hg or greater and at least to 100 mm Hg (see Chapter 29).

Circumoral cyanosis. *Circumoral cyanosis* refers to a bluish color of skin around the mouth. Isolated circumoral cyanosis is of no concern unless it occurs because of a low cardiac output. In this situation the arterial oxygen saturation is normal. This reflects a sluggish capillary blood flow in a child with fair skin, and it may be seen in healthy children with vasoconstriction from the cold.

114

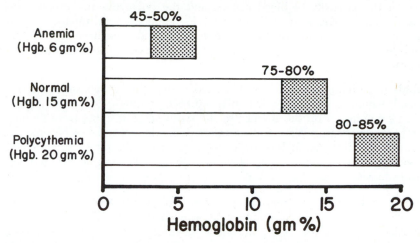

FIG. 11–1.
Influence of hemoglobin levels on clinical recognition of cyanosis. Cyanosis is recognizable at a higher arterial oxygen saturation in patients with polycythemia and at a lower arterial oxygen saturation in patients with anemia. See text for explanation.

BOX 11–1

Causes of Cyanosis

Reduced arterial oxygen saturation (i.e., central cyanosis)
　Inadequate alveolar ventilation
　　Central nervous system depression
　　Inadequate ventilatory drive (e.g., obesity, pickwickian syndrome)
　　Obstruction of the airway, congenital or acquired
　　Structural changes in the lungs and/or ventilation-perfusion mismatch (e.g., pneumonia, cystic fibrosis, hyaline membrane disease, pulmonary edema, CHF, and so on)
　　Weakness of the respiratory muscles
　Desaturated blood bypassing effective alveolar units
　　Intracardiac right-to-left shunt (i.e., cyanotic CHD)
　　Intrapulmonary shunt (e.g., pulmonary atrioventicular (AV) fistula, chronic hepatic disease resulting in multiple micro-AV fistulas in the lungs)
　　Pulmonary hypertension with the resulting right-to-left shunt at the atrial, ventricular, or ductal levels (e.g., Eisenmenger's syndrome, persistant pulmonary hypertension of the newborn [PPHN])
Increased deoxygenation in the capillaries (i.e., peripheral cyanosis)
　Circulatory shock
　CHF
　Acrocyanosis of newborns
Abnormal hemoglobin (unrelated to the degree of oxygenation)
　Methemoglobinemia (e.g., well water ingestion, aniline dye, congenital methemeglobinemia)
　Carbon monoxide poisoning

Consequences and Complications

Polycythemia. Low arterial oxygen content stimulates bone marrow through erythropoietin release from the kidneys and produces an increased number of red blood cells. Polycythemia, with a resulting increase in the oxygen-carrying capacity, benefits cyanotic children. However, when the hematocrit reaches 65% or higher, a sharp increase in the viscosity of blood occurs, and the polycythemic response becomes disadvantageous, particularly if there is CHF. Some cyanotic infants have relative anemia with normal or lower than normal hematocrit and hypochromia on blood smear. Although less cyanotic, these infants are usually more symptomatic and improve when iron therapy raises the hematocrit.

Clubbing. Clubbing is a hypertrophic osteoarthropathy as a consequence of central cyanosis. It usually does not appear until a child is 6 months or older, and it is seen first and most pronounced on the thumb. In the early stage it appears as shininess and redness of the finger tips. When fully developed, the fingers and toes become thick and wide and have convex nail beds (see Fig. 2-1 on p. 13). Clubbing is also seen in patients with liver disease, subacute bacterial endocarditis (SBE), and on a hereditary basis without cyanosis.

Hypoxic spells and squatting. Although most frequently seen in infants with TOF, the hypoxic spell may occur in infants with other forms of CHD. The hypoxic spell is characterized by a period of uncontrollable crying, rapid and deep breathing (i.e., hyperpnea), deepening of cyanosis, limpness or convulsions, and occasionally death. A special posture, called *squatting*, is commonly seen in children with a right-to-left shunt. This posture increases arterial oxygen saturation, probably by a temporary trapping desaturated blood in the lower extremities.

Central nervous system complications. Cyanotic infants, particularly those with severe hypoxia, are prone to develop disorders of the central nervous system, such as brain abscess or cerebrovascular accident. Cyanotic CHDs account for 5% to 10% of all cases of brain abscesses. The predisposition for brain abscesses may partially result from the fact that right-to-left intracardiac shunts may bypass the normally effective phagocytic filtering actions of the pulmonary capillary bed. This predisposition may also result from the fact that polycythemia and the consequent high viscosity of blood lead to tissue hypoxia and microinfarction of the brain, which are later complicated by bacterial colonization. However, SBE is rarely associated with a brain abscess. The triad of symptoms of brain abscesses are fever, headaches, and focal neurologic deficit.

Cerebrovascular accident caused by embolization arising from thrombus in the cardiac chamber or in the systemic veins may be associated with surgery or cardiac catheterization. Cerebral venous thrombosis may occur, often in infants younger than 2 years of age who have cyanosis and relative iron-deficiency anemia. A possible explanation for these findings is that microcytosis further aggravates hyperviscosity resulting from polycythemia.

Bleeding disorders. Disturbances of hemostasis are frequently present in children with severe cyanosis and polycythemia. Most frequently noted are thrombocytopenia and a defective platelet aggregation. Other abnormalities include prolonged prothrombin time and partial thromboplastin time and lower levels of fibrinogen and factors V and VIII. Clinical manifestations may include easy bruising, petechiae of the skin and mucous membranes, epistaxis, and gingival bleeding. Red cell withdrawal and replacement with an equal volume of plasma tends to correct the hemorrhagic tendency and lower blood viscosity.

Depressed intelligent quotient. Children with chronic hypoxia and cyanosis have a lower-than-expected intelligence quotient, as well as a poorer perceptual and gross motor function than children with acyanotic CHDs, even after surgical repair of cyanotic heart defects.

Scoliosis. Children with chronic cyanosis, particularly girls and patients with TOF, often have scoliosis.

Hyperuricemia and gouts. Hyperuricemia and gouts tend to occur in older patients with uncorrected or inadequately repaired cyanotic heart defects.

COMMON CYANOTIC HEART DEFECTS

D-Transposition of the Great Arteries

D-Transposition of the great arteries (D-TGA), commonly called complete TGA, is the most common cyanotic CHD in newborns. In this condition the aorta arises from the RV, and the PA arises from the LV. Therefore the normal anteroposterior relationship of the great arteries is reversed so that the aorta is anterior to the PA (transposition), but the aorta remains to the right of the PA; therefore the prefix D is used for dextroposition. In levo-transposition of the great arteries (L-TGA or congenitally corrected TGA), the aorta is anterior to and to the left of the PA; therefore the prefix L is used (see Chapter 14). The atria and ventricles are in normal relationship. The coronary arteries arise from the aorta, as in a normal heart. Desaturated blood returning from the body to the RA flows out of the aorta without being oxygenated in the lungs and then returns to the RA. Therefore tissues, including vital organs such as the brain and heart, are perfused by blood with a low oxygen saturation. On the other hand, well-oxygenated blood returning to the LA flows out of the PA and returns to the LA. This results in a complete separation of the two circuits. The two circuits are said to be *in parallel* rather than *in series*, as in normal circulation (Fig. 11-2). This defect is incompatible with life unless communication between the two circuits occurs to provide the necessary oxygen to the body. This communication can occur at the atrial, ventricular, or ductal level or at any combination of these levels.

In the most frequently encountered form of D-TGA only a small communication exists between the atria, usually a patent foramen ovale (PFO) (Fig. 11-3, *A*). The newborn is notably cyanotic from birth and has an arterial oxygen saturation of 30% to 50%. The low arterial Po_2 which ranges from 20 to 30 mm Hg, causes an anaerobic glycolysis with resulting metabolic acidosis. The hypoxia and acidosis are detrimental to myocardial function. Normal postnatal decrease in PVR results in increased PBF and volume overload to the LA and LV. The severe hypoxia and acidosis with a resulting decrease in myocardial function and the volume overload to the left side of the heart cause CHF during the first week of life. Therefore chest x-ray films show cardiomegaly and increased pulmonary vascularity. Unless hypoxia and acidosis are eliminated, the condition of these infants deteriorates rapidly. Hypoxia and acidosis stimulate the carotid and cerebral chemoreceptors, causing hyperventilation and a low Pco_2 in the pulmonary circulation. Other metabolic problems encountered are hypoglycemia, which is probably secondary to pancreatic islet hypertrophy and hyperinsulinism, and a tendency toward hypothermia. The ECG shows RVH, but RVH may be difficult to diagnose in the first days of life because of the normal dominance of the RV at this age. Usually no heart murmur is noted in a neonate with D-TGA, although a murmur is

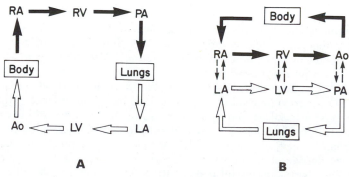

A   **B**

FIG. 11–2.

Circulation pathways of normal *in series* circulation (**A**) and the *in parallel* circulation of transposition of the great arteries (**B**). *Open arrows,* Oxygenated blood; *closed arrows,* desaturated blood.

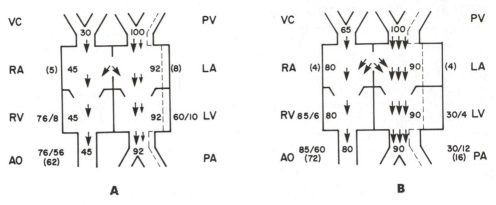

FIG. 11–3.
Diagrammatic representation of hemodynamics of TGA with inadequate mixing **(A)** and with a good mixing at the atrial level **(B).** Numbers within the diagram denote oxygen saturation values, and those outside the diagram denote pressure values. *VC,* Vena cava; *AO,* aorta; *PV,* pulmonary veins.

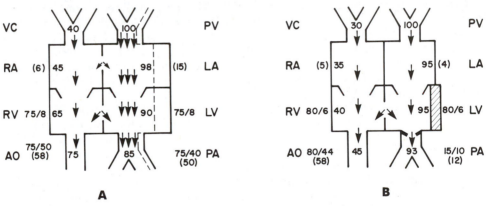

FIG. 11–4.
Diagrammatic representation of hemodynamic abnormalities in TGA with a large VSD **(A)** and with VSD and PS **(B).** Numbers within the diagram denote oxygen saturation values, and those outside the diagram denote pressure values.

commonly found in other forms of cyanotic heart defects. The S2 is single, mainly because the pulmonary valve is farther from the chest wall, causing the P2 to be inaudible. A deeply cyanotic newborn with increased PVMs and cardiomegaly without heart murmur can be considered to have TGA until proved otherwise.

The presence of a large ASD is most desirable in infants with TGA. The frequency of a large ASD occurring naturally in TGA is low, but when a large ASD is present, infants have good arterial oxygen saturation (as high as 80% to 90%) because of good mixing (Fig. 11-3, *B*). Therefore hypoxia and metabolic acidosis are not the problems in these children. In fact, the idea of the balloon atrial septostomy (i.e., Rashkind procedure) was derived from the natural history of infants with TGA and a large ASD. Infants who have had a successful balloon atrial septostomy behave like those with a naturally occurring ASD. As the PVR falls after birth, PBF increases with an increase in the size of the LA and LV. Although these infants are not hypoxic or acidotic, CHF develops because of volume overload to the left side of the heart. Since the RV is the systemic ventricle, RVH becomes evident on the ECG.

When associated with a large VSD, only minimal arterial desaturation is present, and cyanosis may be missed (Fig 11-4, A). Therefore metabolic acidosis does not develop, but left-sided heart failure results within the first few weeks of life as the PBF increases with decreasing PVR. Chest x-ray films reflect this, showing cardiomegaly with increased PVMs. The ECG may show combined venticular hypertrophy (CVH) when the VSD is large: RVH because of the systemic RV and LVH because of volume overload of the left side of the heart (see Fig. 11-4, A). A heart murmur of VSD is present, and the S2 is single because the P2 is inaudible or pulmonary hypertension is present.

Although the VSD helps good mixing the volume of fully saturated blood, which is returning from the lungs to be shunted to the systemic circulation, is inadequate because of PS (Fig. 11-4, B). Likewise, even after a well-performed Rashkind procedure, the arterial oxygen saturation does not increase because of the decreased PBF. These infants have severe hypoxia and acidosis and may succumb early in life. This is a good illustration of how the magnitude of PBF affects the arterial oxygen saturation in a given cyanotic CHD. Since PBF is not increased, the left cardiac chambers are not under increased volume work; therefore cardiac enlargement and CHF do not develop. X-ray films reflect this as a normal heart size and normal or decreased pulmonary vascularity. The ECG shows evidence of CVH; the LVH component is present because of PS, and RVH is present because of the nature of TGA. Physical examination reveals a PS murmur and a single S2, in addition to cyanosis.

Persistent Truncus Arteriosus and Single Ventricle

In persistent truncus arteriosus (Fig. 11-5, A), a single arterial blood vessel (truncus arteriosus) arises from the heart. The PA or its branches arise from the truncus arteriosus, and the truncus continues as the aorta. A large VSD is always present in this condition. In single (or common) ventricle (Fig. 11-5, B), two AV valves empty into a single ventricular chamber from which a great artery (either the aorta or PA) arises. The other great artery arises from a rudimentary ventricular chamber attached to the main ventricle. No ventricular septum of significance is present (see Fig. 14-51 on p. 231).

The following similarities exist between persistent truncus arteriosus and single ventricle from the hemodynamic point of view:

1. There is almost complete mixing of systemic venous and pulmonary venous blood in the ventricle, and the oxygen saturation of blood in the two great arteries is similar.

2. Pressures in both ventricles are identical.

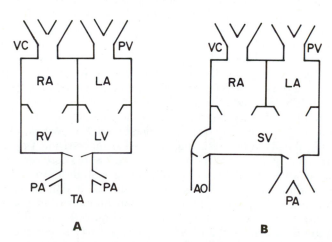

FIG. 11–5.
Diagrammatic representation of persistent truncus arteriosus **(A)** and a common form of single ventricle **(B)**. *VC,* Vena cava; *TA,* truncus arteriosus; *SV,* single ventricle.

3. The level of oxygen saturation in the systemic circulation is proportional to the magnitude of PBF.

In addition to the level of PVR, the magnitude of PBF is determined by the caliber of the PA in the case of persistent truncus arteriosus and by the presence or absence of PS in the case of single ventricle. When the PBF is large, the patient is minimally cyanotic but may develop CHF because of an excessive volume overload placed on the ventricle. In contrast, when the PBF is small, the patient is severely cyanotic and does not develop CHF, since there is no volume overload. This latter group and TOF share similarities.

Physical examination reveals varying degrees of cyanosis depending on the magnitude of PBF. A heart murmur of the VSD is rarely audible because a huge defect is present. There may be an SEM caused by the stenosis of the pulmonary valve or the PA. An early diastolic murmur of truncal valve regurgitation may be heard. The ECG usually shows CVH in both conditions. In persistent truncus arteriosus, the ECG is similar to that of the large VSD that produces CVH. In single ventricle the QRS complexes of all precordial leads (i.e., V1 through V6) are recorded over *one* ventricle, unopposed by the other ventricle. Therefore QRS complexes over the entire precordial leads are similar (poor R/S progression), suggesting CVH. Chest x-ray findings are determined by the magnitude of PBF — if the magnitude is large, the heart size is large and the pulmonary vascularity increases. If the magnitude is small, the heart size is small and the pulmonary vascularity decreases. With increased PBF and resulting pulmonary hypertension, CHF and later PVOD (i.e., Eisenmenger's syndrome) may develop.

Tetralogy of Fallot

The classic description of TOF includes the following four abnormalities: VSD, PS, RVH, and overriding of the aorta. From a physiologic point of view, TOF requires only two abnormalities — a VSD large enough to equalize systolic pressures in both ventricles, as well as in the aorta, and a stenosis of the RV outflow tract in the form of infundibular stenosis, valvular stenosis, or both. RVH is secondary to PS, and the overriding of the aorta is not always present. Depending on the severity of the RV outflow tract obstruction, the direction and the magnitude of the shunt through the VSD vary. With mild stenosis, the shunt is left-to-right, and the clinical pictures resemble those of a VSD. This is called *acyanotic* or *pink TOF* (Fig. 11-6, *A*). With a more severe stenosis, the shunt is right-to-left and results in "cyanotic" TOF (Fig 11-6, *B*). In the extreme form of TOF the pulmonary valve is atretic with right-to-left shunting of the entire systemic venous return through the VSD. PBF is provided through a PDA. In TOF, regardless of the ventricular shunt's direction, the systolic pressure in the RV equals that of the LV and the aorta (Fig. 11-6). The mere combination of a small VSD and a PS is not TOF; the size of the VSD must be nearly as large as the anulus of the aortic valve to equalize the pressure in the RV and LV.

In *acyanotic TOF* a small-to-moderate, left-to-right ventricular shunt is present, and the systolic pressures are equal in the RV, LV, and aorta (Fig. 11-6, *A*). The PA pressure is slightly elevated and has a moderate pressure gradient between the PA and RV. Since the presence of the PS minimizes the magnitude of the left-to-right shunt, the heart size and the pulmonary vascularity increase slightly to moderately. These increases are indistinguishable from those of a small-to-moderate VSD. However, the ECG always shows RVH, since the RV pressure is high, as well as an occasional presence of LVH. The heart murmurs originate from the PS and in the VSD. Therefore the murmur is a superimposition of an SEM of PS and a regurgitant systolic murmur of a VSD. The murmur is best audible along the LLSB and MLSB, and it sometimes extends to the ULSB. Therefore in a child who has physical and x-ray findings similar to those of a small VSD, the presence of RVH or CVH on ECG should raise the possibility of acyanotic TOF. (Small VSD is associated with LVH or normal ECG rather than with RVH or CVH.) Right aortic arch, if present, confirms the diagnosis. Infants with acyanotic TOF become cyanotic with time, usually by 1 or 2 years of age, and have clinical pictures of cyanotic TOF, including exertional dyspnea and squatting.

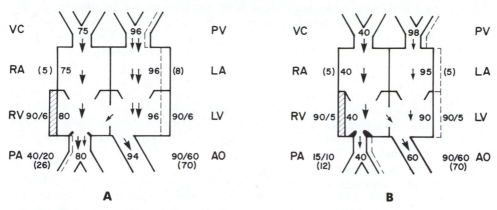

FIG. 11–6.
Hemodynamics of acyanotic **(A)** and cyanotic **(B)** TOF. Numbers within the diagram denote oxygen saturation values, and those outside the diagram denote pressure values. In both conditions, the systolic pressure in the RV is identical to that in the LV and the aorta, and there is a significant pressure gradient between the RV and the PA. In acyanotic form **(A)**, PBF is slightly to moderately increased, whereas in cyanotic form **(B)**, PBF is decreased.

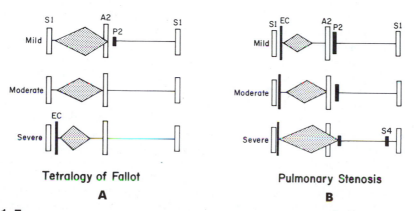

FIG. 11–7.
Comparison of SEMs in TOF **(A)** and isolated pulmonary valve stenosis **(B)** (see text), *EC,* ejection click.

In infants with classic, *cyanotic TOF* the presence of a severe PS produces a right-to-left shunt at the ventricular level (i.e., cyanosis) and a decrease in PBF (Fig. 11-6, *B*). The PAs are small, and the LA and LV may be slightly smaller than normal because of a reduction in the pulmonary venous return to the left side of the heart. Therefore chest x-ray films show a normal heart size with decreased pulmonary vascularity. The systolic pressures are identical in the RV, LV, and aorta. The ECG demonstrates RVH because of the pressure overload on the RV. The right-to-left ventricular shunt is silent, and that the heart murmur originates from the PS (ejection type). The ejection murmur is best audible at the MLSB (over the infundibular stenosis) or occasionally at the ULSB (in cases with pulmonary valve stenosis). The intensity and the duration of the heart murmur are proportional to the amount of blood flow through the stenotic valve. When the PS is mild, a relatively large amount of blood goes through the stenotic valve with a relatively small right-to-left ventricular shunt, thereby producing a loud, long systolic murmur. However, with severe PS, there is a relatively large right-to-left ventricular shunt that is silent, and only a small amount of blood goes through the PS, thereby producing a short, faint systolic murmur. In other words, the intensity and duration of the systolic murmur are *inversely* proportional to the severity of the PS. These findings are in contrast to those seen in isolated PS (Fig. 11-7). Because of low pressure in the PA, the P2 is soft and often inaudible, resulting in a single S2. The heart size on x-ray films is normal in TOF. If a cyanotic infant has a large heart on the chest x-ray examination, especially with an increase in pulmonary vascularity, TOF is extremely unlikely unless the child has undergone a large systemic-PA shunt operation. Another important point is that the infant with TOF does not develop CHF. This is because no cardiac chamber is under volume overload and the pressure overwork placed on the RV is tolerated well, since the RV pressure does not exceed that of the aorta, which is under the baroreceptor control.

The extreme form of TOF is that associated with *pulmonary atresia,* in which the only source of PBF is through a constricting PDA. All systemic venous return is shunted right-to-left at the ventricular level, resulting in a marked systemic arterial desaturation. Probably the more important reason for such severe cyanosis is the markedly reduced pulmonary venous return to the left side of the heart, since the PBF is severely reduced in this condition. Unless the patency of the ductus is maintained, the infant will die. Infusion of prostaglandin E_1 has been successful in this and other forms of cyanotic CHDs that rely on the patency of the ductus arteriosus for PBF. Heart murmur is absent, or a faint murmur of PDA is present. RVH is present on the ECG as in other forms of TOF. Chest x-ray films show a small heart because of markedly reduced PBF.

It is important to understand what controls the degree of cyanosis and the amount of PBF, since this concept applies to understanding the mechanism and treatment of the "hypoxic" spell of TOF. Since the VSD of TOF is large enough to equalize systolic pressures in both ventricles, the RV and LV may be treated as a single chamber that ejects blood to the systemic and pulmonary circuits (Fig. 11-8). The ratio of flows to the pulmonary and systemic circuits ($\dot{Q}p/\dot{Q}s$) is related to the ratio of resistance offered by the RV outflow obstruction (see *PR*, pulmonary resistance, found in Fig. 11-8) and SVR. Either an increase in pulmonary resistance or a decrease in SVR increases the degree of the right-to-left shunt. Likewise, more blood passes through the RV outflow obstruction when the SVR increases or the pulmonary resistance decreases. Although controversies exist, pulmonary resistance is considered fairly constant. This is because pulmonary valve stenosis has a fixed resistance and the infundibular stenosis, which consists of disorganized muscle fibers intermingled with fibrous tissue, is relatively nonreactive. Therefore the degree of the right-to-left shunt or the amount of PBF is primarily controlled by changes in the SVR. A decrease in the SVR increases the right-to-left shunt and decreases the PBF with a resulting increase in cyanosis. On the other hand, an increase in the SVR decreases the right-to-left shunt and forces more blood through the stenotic RV outflow tract. This results in an improvement in the arterial oxygen saturation.

Also, excessive tachycardia or hypovolemia can increase the right-to-left shunt through the VSD, resulting in a fall in the systemic arterial oxygen saturation. The resulting hypoxia can initiate the hypoxic spell. Further narrowing of the RV outflow tract obstruction, as in HOCM for the LV, or a reduction of the SVR have been proposed

FIG. 11–8.
Simplified concept of TOF that demonstrates how a change in the SVR or RV outflow obstruction (pulmonary resistance, *PR*) affects the direction and the magnitude of the ventricular shunt.

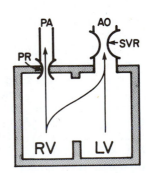

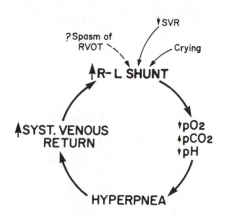

FIG. 11–9.
Mechanism of hypoxic spell. A decrease in the arterial Po_2 stimulates the respiratory center, and hyperventilation results. Hyperpnea increases systemic venous return. In the presence of a fixed RV outflow tract *(RVOT)*, the increased systemic venous return results in increased right-to-left shunt, worsening cyanosis. A vicious cycle is established.

as possible mechanisms for the tachycardia- or hypovolemia-induced hypoxic spell. Slowing of the heart rate, widening of the RV outflow tract by β-adrenergic blockers or volume expansion, or interventions that increase the SVR may all be used to terminate the hypoxic spell. The mechanisms of hypoxic spells discussed so far is used in the treatment of hypoxic spells.

The *hypoxic spell,* also called *cyanotic spell* or *tet spell,* occurs in young infants with TOF. It consists of hyperpnea (i.e., *rapid* and *deep* respiration), worsening cyanosis, and the disappearance of the heart murmur. This occasionally results in complications of the central nervous system and even death. Any event such as crying, defecation, or increased physical activity that suddenly lowers the SVR or produces a large right-to-left ventricular shunt may initiate the spell by establishing a vicious cycle of hypoxic spells (Fig. 11-9). The sudden onset of tachycardia or hypovolemia can also cause the spell. The resulting fall in arterial Po_2, in addition to an increase in Pco_2 and a fall in pH, stimulates the respiratory center and produces hyperpnea. In turn, this makes the negative thoracic pump more efficient and results in an increase in the systemic venous return. In the presence of a fixed opening or fixed resistance at the RV outflow tract (i.e., pulmonary resistance) the increased systemic venous return to the RV must go out the aorta. This leads to a further decrease in the arterial oxygen saturation, which establishes a vicious cycle of hypoxic spells (Fig. 11-9).

Treatment of hypoxic spells are aimed at breaking this cycle by using one or more of the following maneuvers:

1. Using the knee-chest position and holding the baby traps systemic venous blood in the legs, thereby decreasing the systemic venous return and helping to calm the baby. The knee-chest position may also increase SVR by reducing arterial blood flow through the femoral arteries.

2. Morphine sulfate suppresses the respiratory center and abolishes hyperpnea.

3. Sodium bicarbonate ($NaHCO_3$) corrects acidosis and eliminates the respiratory center-stimulating effect of acidosis.

4. Administration of oxygen may improve arterial oxygen saturation a little.

5. Vasoconstrictors such as phenylephrine raise SVR.

6. Ketamine is a good drug to use, since it simultaneously increases the SVR and sedates the patient. Both effects are known to terminate the spell.

7. Propranolol has been used successfully in some cases, both acute or chronic. Its mechanism of action is not entirely clear. When administered for acute cases, propranolol may reduce the spasm of the RV outflow tract and slow the heart rate. The successful use of propranolol in the prevention of hypoxic spells is more likely the result of the drug's peripheral action. It may stabilize vascular

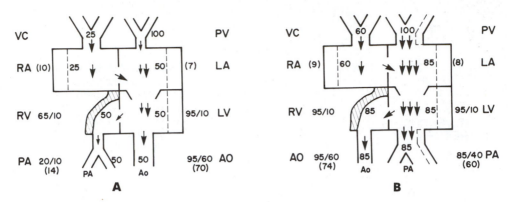

FIG. 11–10.
Hemodynamics of tricuspid atresia with normally related **(A)** and transposed **(B)** great arteries. Numbers within the diagram denote oxygen saturations, and those outside the diagram denote pressure values.

reactivity of the systemic arteries, thereby preventing a sudden decrease in the SVR (see Chapter 14).

Tricuspid Atresia

In tricuspid atresia the tricuspid valve and a portion of the RV do not exist (Fig. 11-10, A and B). Since no direct communication exists between the RA and RV, systemic venous return to the RA must be shunted to the LA through an ASD or a PFO. The pressure in the RA is elevated in excess of that in the LA, and the RA chamber enlarges (i.e., RAH on the ECG and RAE on x-ray films). The LA and LV receive both the systemic venous and pulmonary venous returns and therefore dilate (i.e., LAE and LVE on x-ray films). The volume overload placed on the LV is unopposed by the hypoplastic RV, resulting in LVH on the ECG. Therefore the ECG shows RAH and LVH, and the x-ray films show RAE, LAE, and LVE. In addition, left anterior hemiblock (or superior QRS axis) is a characteristic ECG finding in tricuspid atresia as in ECD. Embryologically there is a similarity between these two defects; tricuspid atresia results from an abnormal development of the endocardial cushion tissue, that is, an incomplete shift of the common AV canal to the right. This abnormal shift may explain the similar QRS axis in both conditions.

Oxygen saturation values are equal in the aorta and the PA, since there is a complete mixing of systemic and pulmonary venous blood in the LV from which both the systemic and pulmonary circuits receive blood. The level of arterial saturation directly relates to the magnitude of PBF. Anatomically the great arteries are normally related in about 70% of cases and transposed in about 30% of cases. In patients with normally related great arteries (Fig. 11-10, A) the PBF is generally reduced, since it comes through a small VSD, hypoplastic RV, and/or small PAs. Therefore arterial oxygen saturation is low, and the infant is notably cyanotic. In infants with TGA (Fig. 11-10, B) the PBF is usually greatly increased. Therefore these infants are only mildly cyanotic; their heart size is large, and their PVMs are increased. However, because of an interplay of other factors such as the size of VSD, the presence or absence of PS or pulmonary atresia, as well as the patency of the ductus arteriosus, some infants with normally related great arteries may have increased PBF, and some infants with TGA may have decreased PBF. In tricuspid atresia the magnitude of PBF determines not only the level of arterial oxygen saturation, but also the degree of enlargement of the cardiac chambers.

No physical findings are characteristic of tricuspid atresia. These infants have varying degrees of cyanosis, and most have a heart murmur of VSD. A PS murmur, if present, is characteristic. In patients with increased PBF, an increased amount of blood passing through the mitral valve may produce an apical diastolic rumble. The liver may be enlarged because of increased pressures in the RA, which may result from an inadequate interatrial communication or heart failure.

In summary, tricuspid atresia is the most likely diagnosis if a cyanotic infant shows a superiorly oriented QRS axis (i.e., left anterior hemiblock), RAH and LVH on the ECG, as well as RAE with or without the LAE and LVE, a concave MPA segment as the result of hypoplasia of the PA, and decreased PVMs on chest x-ray examinations.

Pulmonary Atresia

In pulmonary atresia direct communication between the RV cavity and the PA does not exist; the PDA is the major source of blood flow to the lungs. The systemic venous return to the RA must go to the LA through an ASD or a PFO. The RA enlarges and hypertrophies to maintain a right-to-left atrial shunt (e.g., RAE on x-ray film and RAH on the ECG). The RV is usually hypoplastic with a thick ventricular wall, but occasionally the RV is normal in size, and TR is usually present. Systemic venous and pulmonary venous returns mix in the LA and go to the LV to supply the body and lungs (Fig. 11-11). The volume load placed on the left side of the heart (i.e., LA and LV) is proportionally related to the magnitude of PBF. Since the PDA is the major source of PBF and it may close after birth, the PBF is usually decreased. Therefore the infant is severely cyanotic, and the overall heart size is normal or only slightly increased. The hypoplasia of the RV and possible volume overload to the LV produces LVH on the ECG.

The infant is usually notably cyanotic, and the S2 is single because there is only one semilunar valve to close. A faint, continuous murmur of PDA may be present. Closure of the ductus results in a rapid deterioration of these infants' conditions. Reopening or maintaining the patency of the ductus arteriosus with infusion of prostaglandin E_1 increases PBF, improves cyanosis, and stabilizes the infant's condition.

In summary, a severely cyanotic newborn with decreased pulmonary vascularity and normal or slightly enlarged heart size on chest x-ray films, and RAH or CAH and LVH on the ECG may have pulmonary atresia. The QRS axis is usually normal, a finding in contrast to the superior QRS axis seen in tricuspid atresia. Either a faint, continuous murmur of a PDA or a soft regurgitant systolic murmur of TR may be present.

Total Anomalous Pulmonary Venous Return

In TAPVR the pulmonary veins drain abnormally to the RA, either directly or indirectly, through its venous tributaries. An ASD is usually present to send blood from the RA to the LA and LV. Depending on the drainage site, TAPVR may be divided into the following three types (see Fig. 14-27 on p. 205):

1. Supracardiac: The common pulmonary vein drains to the SVC through the vertical vein and the left innominate vein.

2. Cardiac: The pulmonary veins empty into the RA directly or indirectly through the coronary sinus.

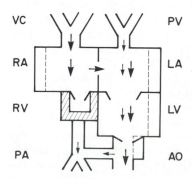

FIG. 11-11.
Hemodynamics of pulmonary atresia. The chambers that enlarge are similar to those in tricuspid atresia; therefore x-ray findings are similar in tricuspid atresia and pulmonary atresia. The ECG also shows LVH but without the characteristic left anterior hemiblock of tricuspid atresia. Because of the decreased PBF, the aortic saturation is low, and the infant is notably cyanotic.

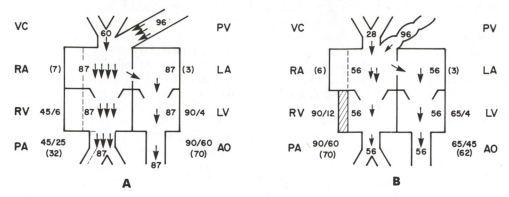

FIG. 11–12.
Hemodynamics of TAPVR without **(A)** and with **(B)** obstruction to the pulmonary venous return. In the nonobstructive type **(A),** the hemodynamics are similar to those of a large ASD, with the exception of a mild systemic arterial desaturation. In the obstructive type **(B),** the hemodynamics are characterized by pulmonary venous hypertension, pulmonary edema, pulmonary arterial hypertension, and a marked arterial desaturation. The heart size is not enlarged on chest x-ray films. Severe RVH is present on the ECG.

3. Infracardiac (or subdiaphragmatic): The common pulmonary vein traverses the diaphragm and drains into the portal or hepatic vein or the IVC.

Physiologically, however, TAPVR may be divided into two types—obstructive and nonobstructive—depending on the presence or absence of obstruction to the pulmonary venous return. The infracardiac type is usually obstructive, and the majority of the cardiac and supracardiac types are nonobstructive.

The hemodynamics of the nonobstructive types of TAPVR are similar to those of a large ASD. The amount of blood that goes to the LA through the ASD, rather than to the RV, is determined by the size of the interatrial communication and the relative compliance of the ventricles. Since the RV compliance normally increases after birth with a rapid fall in the PVR and the ASD may be of inadequate size, more blood enters the RV than the LA. This results in volume overload of the right side of the heart and the pulmonary circulation. This causes the RA, RV, PA, and pulmonary veins to enlarge (Fig. 11-12, A). Chest x-ray films show this as RAE and RVE, a prominent MPA segment, and increased pulmonary vascularity. The pressures in the RV and PA are slightly elevated. The ECG shows RBBB or RVH, as in secundum ASD, and occasional RAH. Since there is a complete mixing of systemic and pulmonary venous return in the RA, oxygen saturation values are almost identical in the aorta and the PA. Physical examination reveals an ejection systolic murmur at the ULSB because of the increased flow through the pulmonary valve and a diastolic flow rumble of relative TS, since these valves handle three arrows (Fig. 11-12, A). The S2 splits widely for the same reasons as it does for ASD. This contributes to the characteristic "quadruple" rhythm of TAPVR, which consists of an S1, a widely split S2, and an S3 or S4. Children with a large PBF are only minimally desaturated, and cyanosis is often missed because the arterial oxygen saturation ranges from 85% to 90% (Fig. 11-12, A).

If there is an obstruction to the pulmonary venous return, the hemodynamic consequences are notably different from those without pulmonary venous obstruction. The obstruction to the pulmonary venous return is usually present in the infracardiac type and sometimes in cases of supracardiac and cardiac types of TAPVR. The obstruction to the pulmonary venous return causes pulmonary venous hypertension and secondary PA and RV hypertension (Fig. 11-12, B) a situation similar to that seen in MS (see Chapter 10). Pulmonary edema results when the hydrostatic pressure in the capillaries exceeds the osmotic pressure of the blood. As long as a large ASD permits a right-to-left shunt, the RV cavity remains relatively small (i.e., smaller than one arrow). This is because the RV hypertension prevents the RV compliance from increasing and the PVR remains elevated. Therefore chest x-ray films show a relatively small heart and characteristic patterns of pulmonary venous congestion or pulmonary edema (i.e., "ground-glass" appearance). The ECG reflects the high pressure in the RV (i.e., RVH). The oxygen saturation values are equal in the aorta and the PA because of the complete mixing of systemic and pulmonary venous return at the RA level, and the arterial saturation becomes much lower than that found in patients without obstruction. The degree of arterial desaturation or cyanosis inversely relates to the amount of PBF. Since this is an extremely important concept, it is further discussed in the two extreme examples of TAPVR discussed later in the chapter. Infants with obstruction have severe cyanosis and respiratory distress. The latter results from pulmonary edema and may cause pulmonary rales on auscultation. The pulmonary valve closure sound (P2) is loud because of pulmonary hypertension, which results in a single, loud S2. The heart murmur may be absent because of the lack of increased flow through the pulmonary or tricuspid valve (i.e., smaller than one arrow) (Fig. 11-12, *B*).

Full comprehension of the relationship between the magnitude of PBF and the systemic arterial oxygen saturation helps in understanding and managing most cyanotic CHDs. The two extreme examples of TAPVR shown in Fig. 11-12 discuss this relationship.

If the PBF is 3 times as great as the systemic blood flow (i.e., $\dot{Q}p/\dot{Q}s = 3:1$), as in most nonobstructive cases, the arterial oxygen saturation is close to 90%, and cyanosis does not become obvious. This figure is derived as follows: an assumed pulmonary vein saturation of 96% and a vena caval saturation of 60% results in an average mixed venous saturation of 87%:

$$\frac{(96 \times 3) + (60 \times 1)}{4} = 87(\%)$$

The difference in the arterial and venous oxygen saturation is kept at 27% to indicate the absence of heart failure (Fig. 11-12, *A*)

If an obstruction to the pulmonary venous return exists and the PBF is small, a marked arterial desaturation results based on the following calculation. It assumed that the PBF is 70% of the systemic flow (i.e., $\dot{Q}p/\dot{Q}s = 0.7:1$) and the pulmonary vein saturation 96%:

$$\frac{(96 \times 0.7) + (28 \times 1)}{1.7} = 56(\%)$$

It is also assumed that the infant is not experiencing heart failure (i.e., the systemic AV difference is 28%) (Fig. 11-12, *B*).

This relationship holds true for other forms of cyanotic CHD. For a given defect, an *increase* in the magnitude of the PBF results in a rise in the systemic arterial oxygen saturation, and a *decrease* in the PBF results in a decrease in the arterial oxygen saturation. An improvement in cyanosis after a systemic-PA shunt operation in an infant with decreased PBF is an example of this relationship. On the other hand, an infant with CHF from a single ventricle in which a large PBF and pulmonary hypertension are present may improve after a PA banding (the procedure that decreases the PBF and lowers PA pressure), but the arterial oxygen saturation usually decreases, and cyanosis worsens.

PART IV

Specific Congenital Heart Defects

The following three chapters discuss common left-to-right shunt lesions, obstructive lesions, and cyanotic cardiac defects. Other chapters in this part discuss aortic arch anomalies, primarily "vascular ring" and cardiac malposition. Miscellaneous, rare anomalies that do not belong to these categories are grouped and briefly discussed in yet another chapter. These chapters are intended to be used as a quick reference; therefore, descriptions are brief.

12 / Left-to-Right Shunt Lesions

This chapter discusses common left-to-right shunt lesions such as ASD, VSD, PDA, ECD, and PAPVR.

ATRIAL SEPTAL DEFECT

Prevalence

ASD (ostium secundum defect) occurs as an isolated anomaly in 5% to 10% of all CHDs. It is more common in females than in males (i.e., M:F = 1:2). About 30% to 50% of children with CHDs have an ASD as part of their cardiac defects.

Pathology

1. Three types of ASDs exist—secundum defect, primum defect, and sinus venosus defect. PFO does not ordinarily produce intracardiac shunts (see Chapter 17).

2. Ostium secundum defect is the most common type of ASD, making up 50% to 70% of all ASDs. This defect is present at the site of fossa ovalis, allowing left-to-right shunting of blood from the LA to the RA (Fig. 12-1). Anomalous pulmonary venous return is present in about 10% of cases.

3. Ostium primum defects occur in about 30% of all ASDs, if including those that occur as part of a complete ECD (Fig. 12-1). Isolated ostium primum ASD occurs in about 15% of all ASDs. This is discussed in greater detail in the section on partial ECD.

4. Sinus venosus defect, which occurs in about 10% of all ASDs, is most commonly located at the entry of the SVC into the RA (i.e., superior vena caval type) and rarely at the entry of the IVC into the RA (i.e., inferior vena caval type). The right PVs may drain anomalously into the RA. More commonly, the right PVs may enter normally into the LA at the point near the ASD and give an appearance of an anomalous entry of these veins into the RA. True anomalous PV return of the right PVs into the IVC occurs in the scimitar syndrome. (see Chapter 17).

5. An unroofed coronary sinus is a rare communication between the coronary sinus and the LA, which produces clinical pictures similar to other types of ASD.

6. Mitral valve prolapse (MVP) occurs in 20% of patients with either ostium secundum or sinus venosus defects.

Clinical Manifestations

History. Infants and children with ASDs are usually asymptomatic.

Physical examination (Fig. 12-2).

1. A relatively slender body build is typical. (The body weight of many is less than the 10th percentile.)

2. A widely split and fixed S2 and a grade 2-3/6 systolic ejection murmur are characteristic findings of the ASD in older infants and children. With a large left-to-right shunt, a middiastolic rumble resulting from relative TS may be audible at the LLSB.

3. The typical auscultatory findings may be absent in infants, even infants who have a large defect.

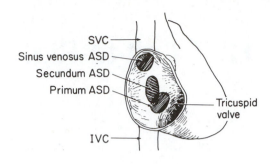

FIG. 12–1.
Anatomic types of ASDs, viewed with
the RA wall removed.

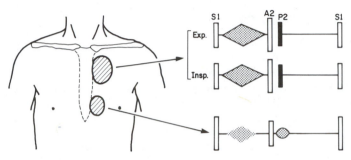

FIG. 12–2.
Cardiac findings of ASD. Throughout this book, heart murmurs *with solid borders* are
the primary murmurs, and those *without solid borders* are transmitted murmurs or those
occurring occasionally. Abnormalities in heart sounds are shown in *black. Exp,*
Expiration; *Insp.,* inspiration.

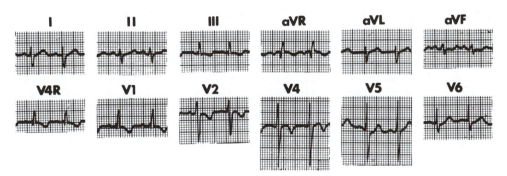

FIG. 12–3.
Tracing from a 5-year-old girl with secundum-type ASD.

Electrocardiography (Fig. 12-3). RAD of $+90$ to $+180$ degrees and mid-RVH or
RBBB with an rsR' pattern in V1 are typical findings.

X-ray studies (Fig. 12-4).

1. Cardiomegaly with RAE and RVE are visible.

2. A prominent MPA segment and increased PVMs can be seen.

Echocardiography.

1. A two-dimensional echo study is diagnostic. The study shows the position as well as
   the size of the defect, which can best be seen in the subcostal four-chamber view (Fig.

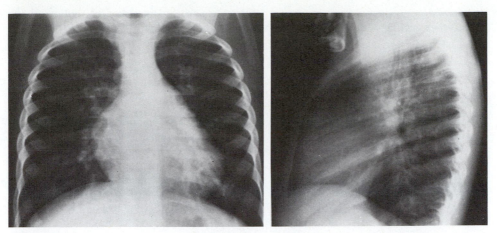

FIG. 12–4.
PA and lateral views of chest roentgenogram from a 10-year-old child with ASD. The heart is mildly enlarged with involvement of the RA (best seen in PA view) and the RV (best seen in the lateral view with obliteration of the retrosternal space). Pulmonary vascularity is increased, and the MPA segment is slightly prominent.

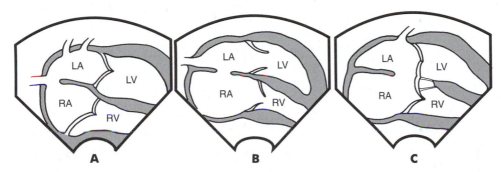

FIG. 12–5.
Diagram of two-dimensional echo of the three types of ASD. The subcostal transducer position provides the most diagnostic view. **A,** Sinus venosus defect. Defect is located in the posterosuperior atrial septum, usually just beneath the orifice of the SVC. This defect is often associated with partial anomalous return of the right upper pulmonary vein. **B,** Secundum ASD. Defect is located in the middle portion of the atrial septum. **C,** Primum ASD. Defect is located in the anteroinferior atrial septum, just over the inflow portion of each AV valve.

12-5). In the secundum ASD a dropout can be seen in the midatrial septum. The primum type shows a defect in the lower atrial septum; the SVC type of sinus venous defect shows a defect in the posterosuperior atrial septum.

2. Indirect signs of a left-to-right shunt are always present. These include RVE and RAE, as well as a dilated PA, which often accompanies an increase in the flow velocity. These findings provide the functional significance of the defect.

3. Pulsed-Doppler examination reveals a characteristic flow pattern with the maximum left-to-right shunt occurring in diastole. Color-flow mapping enhances the evaluation of the hemodynamic status of the ASD. Doppler examination can estimate pressures in the RV and PA.

4. M-mode echo may show increased RV dimension and paradoxical motion of the interventricular septum, which signals RV volume overload.

5. In older children and adolescents adequate imaging of the atrial septum may not always be possible by the ordinary echo study. Transesophageal echo (TEE) may be used as an alternative.

Natural History

1. Earlier reports indicated that spontaneous closure of the secundum defect occurred in about 40% of patients in the first 4 years of life (actually between 14% and 55% of patients). The defect may decrease in size in some patients. However, a recent report indicates an overall rate of spontaneous closure to be 87%. In patients with an ASD diagnosed before 3 months of age spontaneous closure occurs in 100% of patients with a defect <3 mm at 1½ years of age. Spontaneous closure occurs more than 80% of the time for patients with defects between 3 and 8 mm before 1 ½ years of age. An ASD with a diameter >8 mm rarely closes spontaneously.

2. Most children with an ASD remain active and asymptomatic, although CHF develops in infancy. This rarely occurs.

3. If untreated, CHF and pulmonary hypertension develop in adults who are in their 20s and 30s.

4. With or without surgery, atrial arrhythmias (flutter/fibrillation) may occur as an adult.

5. Infective endocarditis does not occur in patients with isolated ASDs. Therefore SBE prophylaxis is unnecessary for these patients unless their condition is associated with other defects.

6. Cerebrovascular accident, resulting from paradoxical embolization through an ASD, is a rare complication.

Management
Medical.

1. Exercise restriction is unnecessary.

2. Prophylaxis for infective endocarditis is not indicated unless the patient has associated MVP.

3. In infants with CHF medical management is recommended because of its high success rate and the possibility of spontaneous closure of the defect.

4. Nonsurgical closure of the secundum ASD by the use of either the "clamshell" device or the "buttoned" device is still undergoing investigation.

Surgical.

Indications. A left-to-right shunt with a a $\dot{Q}p/\dot{Q}s$ of ≥1.5:1 indicates the need for surgical closure. Some physicians consider a smaller shunt to be a surgical indication because of the risk of paradoxical embolization and cerebrovascular accident. High PVR (i.e., ≥10 units/m², >7 units/m² with vasodilators) is a contraindication for surgery.

Timing. Surgery is usually delayed until 3 to 4 years of age because the possibility of spontaneous closure exists. However, surgery is performed during infancy if CHF does not respond to medical management or if oxygen and other medical therapy are needed for infants with associated bronchopulmonary dysplasia.

Procedure. The defect is repaired under cardiopulmonary bypass with either a simple suture or a pericardial or Teflon patch.

Mortality. Fewer than 1% of patients die; however, there is a greater risk for small infants and those with increased PVR.

Complications. Cerebrovascular accident and postoperative arrhythmias may develop in the immediate postoperative period.

Postoperative Follow-Up

1. Cardiomegaly on x-ray film and enlarged RV dimension on echo, in addition to a wide splitting of the S2, may persist for 1 or 2 postoperative years.

2. Atrial or nodal arrhythmias occur in between 7% and 20% of postoperative patients. Occasionally, sick sinus syndrome, which occurs especially after the repair of sinus venosus defect, may require antiarrhythmic drugs and/or pacemaker therapy.

3. Some patients may show symptoms of associated MVP.

VENTRICULAR SEPTAL DEFECT

Prevalence

VSD is the most common form of CHD and accounts for 15% to 20% of all CHDs, not including those occurring as part of cyanotic CHDs.

Pathology

1. The ventricular septum may be divided into a small membranous portion and a large muscular portion (Fig. 12-6, *A*). The muscular septum has three components — the inlet, the trabecular septum, and the outlet (infundibular) septum. The trabecular septum is further divided into central, marginal, and apical portions. A VSD may be classified into perimembranous, inlet, outlet (infundibular), central muscular, marginal muscular, and apical muscular defects (Fig. 12-6, *B*).

    a. The membranous septum is a relatively small area immediately beneath the aortic

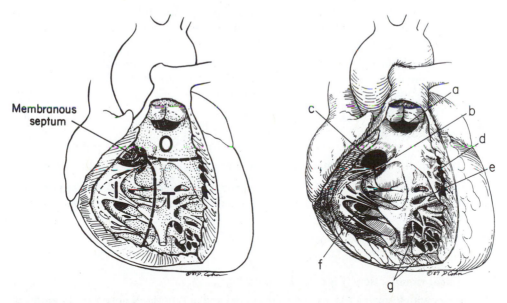

FIG. 12–6.
Anatomy of ventricular septum and VSD. **A,** Ventricular septum viewed from the RV side. The membranous septum is small. The large muscular septum has three components: the inlet, the trabecular septum, and the outlet (or infundibular septum). **B,** Anatomic locations of various VSDs and landmarks, viewed with the RV free wall removed. *I,* Inlet septum; *T,* trabecular septum; *O,* outlet (or infundibular) septum; *a,* outlet (infundibular)defect; *b,* papillary muscle of the conus; *c,* perimembranous defect; *d,* marginal muscular defect; *e,* central muscular defect; *f,* inlet defect; *g,* apical muscular defect.
(From Graham TP Jr et al: *Moss's heart disease in infants, children, adolescents,* 1989, Williams & Wilkins.)

valve. The membranous defect involves varying amounts of muscular tissue adjacent to the membranous septum (perimembranous VSD). According to the accompanying defect in the adjacent muscular septum, perimembranous VSDs have been called *perimembranous inlet (i.e., AV canal type), perimembranous trabecular,* or *perimembranous outlet (i.e., tetralogy type) defect.* Perimembranous defect occurs most commonly (i.e., 70%).

   b. Outlet defects account for 5% to 7% of all VSDs in the Western world and about 30% in Far Eastern countries. It is located in the outlet septum, and part of its rims is formed by the aortic and pulmonary annulus. It has been called *supracristal, conal, subpulmonary,* or *subarterial defect.*

   c. Inlet defects account for 5% to 8% of all VSDs. It is located posterior and inferior to the perimembranous defect, beneath the septal leaflet of the tricuspid valve, and inferior to the papillary muscle of the conus when seen from the RV (see Fig. 12-6, *B*).

   d. Trabecular (muscular) defects account for 5% to 20% of all VSDs. They frequently appear to be multiple when viewed from the right side. Central muscular defect is posterior to the septal band. Apical muscular defect is near the cardiac apex and is difficult to visualize and repair. The marginal defects are usually multiple, small, and tortuous. The "Swiss cheese" type of multiple muscular defects is extremely difficult to close surgically.

2. The defects vary in size, ranging from a tiny defect without hemodynamic significance to a large defect with accompanying CHF and pulmonary hypertension.

3. The bundle of His is related to the posteroinferior quadrant of perimembranous defects and the superoanterior quadrant of the inlet muscular defect. Defects in other parts of the septum are usually unrelated to the conduction tissue.

4. In an infundibular defect the right coronary cusp of the aortic valve may herniate through the defect. This results in AR and an obstruction in the RV outflow tract. A similar herniation of the right and/or noncoronary cusp may occasionally occur through perimembranous defects.

Clinical Manifestations
   History.
1. With a small VSD, the patient is asymptomatic with normal growth and development.

2. With a moderate to large VSD, delayed growth and development, decreased exercise tolerance, repeated pulmonary infections, and CHF are relatively common during infancy.

3. With long-standing pulmonary hypertension, a history of cyanosis and a decreased level of activity may be present.

   Physical examination (Figs. 12-7 and 12-8).
1. Infants with a small VSD are well-developed and acyanotic. Before 2 or 3 months of age, infants with a large VSD may have poor weight gain or show signs of CHF. Cyanosis and clubbing may be present in patients with PVOD (Eisenmenger's syndrome).

2. A systolic thrill may be present at the LLSB. Precordial bulge and hyperactivity are present with a large-shunt VSD.

3. The intensity of the P2 is normal with a small shunt and moderately increased with a large shunt. The S2 is loud and single in patients with PVOD. A grade 2-5/6 regurgitant systolic murmur is present at the LLSB (see Figs. 12-7 and 12-8). It may be holosystolic or early systolic. An apical diastolic rumble is present with a moderate to large shunt.

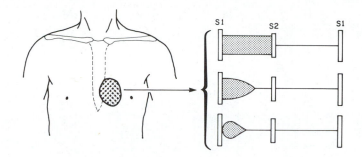

FIG. 12–7.
Cardiac findings of a small VSD. A regurgitant systolic murmur is best audible at the LLSB; it may be holosystolic or less than holosystolic. Occasionally, the heart murmur is in early systole. A systolic thrill *(dots)* may be palpable at the LLSB. The S2 splits normally, and the P2 is of normal intensity.

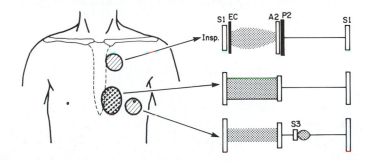

FIG. 12–8.
Cardiac findings of a large VSD. A classic holosystolic regurgitant murmur is audible at the LLSB. A systolic thrill is also palpable at the same area *(dots)*. There is usually a middiastolic rumble resulting from relative MS, at the apex. The S2 is narrowly split, and the P2 is accentuated in intensity. Occasionally an ejection click *(EC)* may be audible in the ULSB when associated with pulmonary hypertension. The heart murmurs shown without solid borders are transmitted from other areas and are not characteristic of the defect. Abnormal sounds are shown in *black*.

4. With infundibular VSD, a grade 1-3/6 early diastolic decrescendo murmur of AR may be audible. This murmur occurs because of herniation of an aortic cusp.

Electrocardiography.

1. With a small VSD, the ECG is normal.

2. With a moderate VSD, LVH and occasional LAH may be seen.

3. With a large defect, the ECG shows combined verticle hypertrophy (CVH) with or without LAH (Fig. 12-9).

4. If PVOD develops, the ECG shows RVH only.

X-ray studies (Fig. 12-10).

1. Cardiomegaly of varying degrees is present and involves the LA, LV, and RV (sometimes). PVMs increase. The degree of cardiomegaly and the increase in PVMs directly relate to the magnitude of the left-to-right shunt.

2. In PVOD the MPA and the hilar PAs enlarge noticeably, but the peripheral lung fields are ischemic. The heart size usually remains normal.

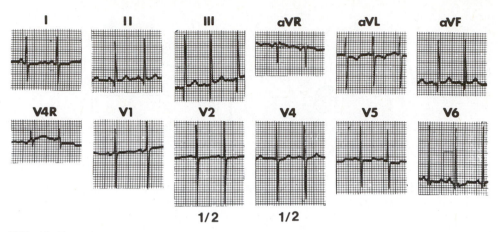

FIG. 12–9.
Tracing from a 3-month-old infant with large VSD, PDA, and pulmonary hypertension. The tracing shows CVH with left dominance. Note that V2 and V4 are in ½ standardization.

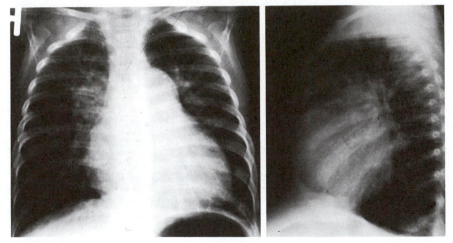

FIG. 12–10.
PA and lateral views of chest roentgenogram in VSD with large shunt and pulmonary hypertension. The heart size is moderately increased, with enlargement on both sides. PVMs are increased, with a prominent MPA segment.

Echocardiography. Two-dimensional and Doppler echo can identify the number, size, and exact location of the defect, estimate PA pressure by using the modified Bernuoulli equation; identify other associated defects; and estimate the magnitude of the shunt.

To identify the precise location of a VSD by two-dimensional echo, the way in which the planes of the ultrasound beam of various echo views traverse the ventricular septum must be known. The lines drawn in Fig. 12-11 represent ultrasound planes seen with various transducer positions.

1. Line *1* (see Fig. 12-11, *A* and *B*) corresponds to the ultrasound plane seen with the apical and subcostal four-chamber views. It cuts through the inlet septum and the trabecular septum.

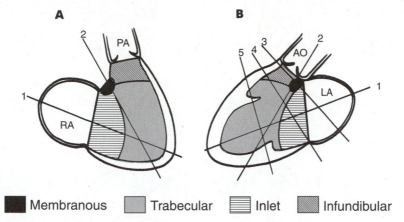

Membranous ▪ Trabecular ▪ Inlet ▪ Infundibular

FIG. 12–11.
Components of the ventricular septum and various echo planes. The membranous, inlet, trabecular, and infundibular septa are shown in different shades. **A,** The ventricular septum is viewed with the free wall of the RVs removed. Line *1* corresponds with the four-chamber views, and line *2* with the five-chamber views. **B,** The septum is viewed with the LV posterior wall removed. Three lines, marked *3* through *5,* represent the echo planes of the parasternal short-axis view. Lines *1* and *2* are the same as in **A.**

2. Line *2* (see Fig. 12-11, *A* and *B*) corresponds to the ultrasound plane seen with the apical and subcostal *five-chamber* views. This line cuts through the membranous septum, located just under the aortic valve, and the trabecular septum including the apex.

3. Lines *3* through *5* (see Fig. 12-11, *B*) correspond to different levels of the parasternal short-axis view. Line *3* cuts through the membranous septum and the infundibular septum. Line *4* corresponds to the short-axis view at the mitral valve level, and it cuts through the infundibular or trabecular septum anteriorly and the inlet septum posteriorly. Line *5* corresponds to the short-axis view at the papillary muscle level, and it cuts through the midportion of the trabecular septum.

VSDs are imaged in two-dimensional echo as areas of echo dropout in the ventricular septum. Examination for a VSD in the ventricular septum, which is a large structure, should be carried out in a systematic manner. When possible, more than one view should be obtained. Preferably, these views should combine the long- and short-axis planes.

1. Membranous VSD is best imaged in the apical or subcostal five-chamber views (Fig. 12-12, *G* and *H*), located just under the aortic valve and in the parasternal short-axis view at the level of aortic valve adjacent to the tricuspid valve (Fig. 12-12, *B*). Fig. 12-13 shows a perimembranous VSD imaged in the apical five-chamber view.

2. Inlet VSD, as either an isolated defect or a perimembranous inlet VSD seen in ECD, is best imaged in the apical or subcostal four-chamber views beneath the AV valves (Fig. 12-12, *E* and *F*). It can also be seen equally well in the parasternal short-axis view in the posterior interventricular septum at the levels between the mitral valve and the papillary muscle (Fig. 12-12, *C*).

3. Trabecular VSD is imaged in the midportion to apical portion of the septum in the parasternal long-axis view (Fig. 12-12, *A*) and in the four- or five-chamber views (Fig. 12-12, *E, F, G,* or *H*). In the parasternal short-axis view it is imaged in either the anterior septum at the mitral valve level (Fig. 12-12, *C*) or the entire septum at the level of the papillary muscle (Fig. 12-12, *D*). For imaging of an apical

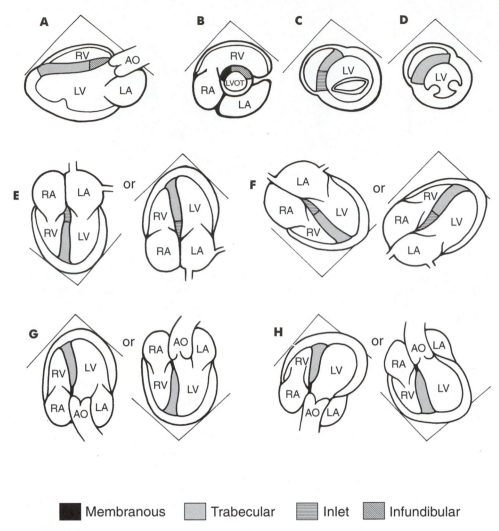

FIG. 12–12.
Diagrammatic representation of different parts of the ventricular septum seen in various two-dimensional echo views. **A,** Parasternal long-axis view. **B** through **D,** Different levels of the parasternal short-axis view. **E** and **F,** Apical and subcostal four-chamber views, respectively. **G** and **H,** Apical and subcostal five-chamber views, respectively.

muscular VSD, the transducer must be maximally angled toward the cardiac apex. The marginal muscular VSD is seen in the anterior part of the trabecular septum (Fig. 12-12, *C* or *D*).

4. Infundibular VSD is easily imaged in the parasternal long-axis view as a defect immediately beneath the aortic valve (Fig. 12-12, *A*). This is usually associated with the overriding of the VSD by the aorta as seen in TOF. In the parasternal short-axis view, it is imaged as a defect in the 12 o'clock to 2 o'clock position at the level of or slightly below the aortic valve (Fig. 12-12, *B*).

Natural History

1. Spontaneous closure occurs in 30% to 40% of patients with membranous VSDs and muscular VSDs during the first 6 months of life. It occurs more frequently in small

defects. These VSDs do not become bigger with age; rather, they decrease in size. Inlet defects and infundibular defects do not become smaller or close spontaneously.

2. CHF develops in infants with large VSDs but usually not until 6 to 8 weeks of age.

3. PVOD may begin to develop as early as 6 to 12 months of age in patients with large VSDs, but the resulting right-to-left shunt usually does not develop until the teenage years.

4. Infundibular stenosis may develop in some infants with large defects and result in a decrease in the magnitude of the left-to-right shunt (i.e., acyanotic TOF) with an occasional production of a right-to-left shunt.

5. Infective endocarditis rarely occurs.

Management.

Understanding the natural history of a VSD is important when planning its management.

Medical.

1. Treatment of CHF, if developed, is indicated with digoxin and diuretics (see Chapter 30) for 2 to 4 months to see if growth failure could be improved. Frequent feedings of high-calorie formulas, either by nasogastric tube or oral feeding, may help. Anemia, if present, should be corrected by oral iron therapy.

2. No exercise restriction is required in the absence of pulmonary hypertension.

3. Maintenance of good dental hygiene and antibiotic prophylaxis against infective endocarditis are important (see Chapter 19).

4. "Umbrella" closure of selected muscular defects is possible but is still in the experimental stage.

Surgical.

Indications and timing. Small infants who have large VSDs and develop CHF and growth retardation are managed first with digoxin and diuretics. If growth failure cannot be improved by medical therapy, the VSD should be operated on within the first 6 months of age. Surgery should be delayed for infants who respond to medical therapy.

After 1 year of age, a significant left-to-right shunt with Qp/Qs of at least 2:1 indicates surgical closure is needed regardless of the PA pressure.

Infants with evidence of pulmonary hypertension but no CHF or growth failure should have a cardiac catheterization at 6 to 12 months of age. Surgery should follow soon after cardiac catheterization. Older infants with large VSDs and evidence of elevated PVR should be operated on as soon as possible.

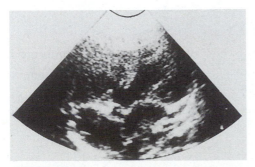
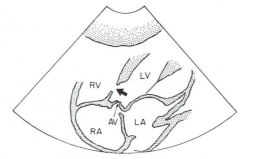

FIG. 12–13.
Apical four-chamber view with LV outflow tract (apical five-chamber view) in a patient with perimembranous VSD *(arrow)*. *AV,* Aortic valve.

Infants who have small VSDs and have reached the age of 6 months without CHF and evidence of pulmonary hypertension are usually not candidates for surgery. Surgery is not indicated for a small VSD with $\dot{Q}p/\dot{Q}s < 1.5:1$.

Surgery is contraindicated in patients with PVR/SVR of ≥ 0.5 or PVOD with a predominant right-to-left shunt.

Procedure. PA banding as a palliative procedure is no longer performed unless additional lesions make complete repair difficult. Direct closure of the defect under cardiopulmonary bypass and/or deep hypothermia is preferably carried out through an atrial approach rather than right ventriculotomy.

Mortality. Surgical mortality is 2% to 5% after the age of 6 months. Mortality is higher for small infants younger than 2 months of age, in infants with associated defects, or infants with multiple VSDs.

Complications. RBBB is common in patients repaired via right ventriculotomy.

RBBB and left anterior hemiblock, which occurs in fewer than 10% of patients, is a controversial cause of sudden death.

Complete heart block occurs in fewer than 5% of patients.

Residual shunts remain in about 20% of patients, and cerebrovascular accident is extremely rare.

Surgical approaches for special situations.

vsd + pda. If the PDA is large, the ductus alone may be closed in the first 6 to 8 weeks in the hope that the VSD is restrictive. If the VSD is not restrictive, it may be closed at an appropriate time after trying medical management.

vsd + coa. Controversies exist. A recommended approach is to initially repair the COA alone either with or without PA banding. The VSD is closed later, if indicated.

vsd + ar syndrome. The prolapsed aortic cusp, with resulting AR, is usually associated with infundibular VSD and occasionally with perimembranous VSD. It occurs in about 5% of patients with VSD. In Far Eastern countries it occurs in 15% to 20% of children. The adjacent (i.e., right and/or noncoronary) aortic valve cusps prolapse through the defect into the RV outflow tract. Once AR appears it gradually worsens. An operation is usually performed promptly when AR is present, even if the $\dot{Q}p/\dot{Q}s$ is $< 2:1$, so that progression of AR is either aborted or abolished. When AR is trivial or mild, the VSD alone is closed. When AR is moderate or severe, the aortic valve is repaired or replaced. Not every case of VSD + AR results from the prolapsed aortic cusps; it may be the result of a VSD and bicuspid aortic valve.

Development of subaortic stenosis. A discrete fibrous or fibromuscular subaortic stenosis is occasionally associated with perimembranous VSD. It is also seen in patients with COA and VSD, after PA banding or repair of a VSD. The mechanism for the development is unclear. Because of its progressive nature and potential damage to the aortic valve, surgical resection is usually undertaken relatively early if a gradient more than 30 mm Hg is present. Long-term follow-up of these stenoses is mandatory because they tend to recur.

Postoperative Follow-Up

1. An office examination should be scheduled every 1 to 2 years.

2. Activity should not be restricted unless complications have resulted from surgery.

3. SBE prophylaxis may be discontinued 6 months after surgery. If a residual shunt is present, SBE prophylaxis should be continued indefinitely on indications.

4. The patient's postoperative history of transient heart block with or without pacemaker therapy requires long-term follow-up.

PATENT DUCTUS ARTERIOSUS

Prevalence

PDA occurs in 5% to 10% of all CHDs, excluding premature infants. It is more common in females then in males (i.e., M:F = 1:3). PDA is a common problem in premature infants (see Chapter 29).

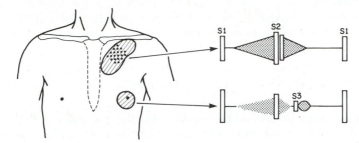

FIG. 12–14.
Cardiac findings of PDA. A systolic thrill may be present in the area shown by *dots*.

Pathology

1. There is a persistent patency of a normal fetal structure between the left PA and the descending aorta, that is, about 5 to 10 mm distal to the origin of the left subclavian artery.

2. The ductus is usually cone-shaped with a small orifice to the PA, which is restrictive to blood flow. The ductus may be short or long, straight or tortuous.

Clinical Manifestations
History.

1. Patients are usually asymptomatic when the ductus is small.

2. A large-shunt PDA may cause a lower respiratory tract infection, atelectasis, and CHF (accompanied by tachypnea and poor weight gain).

Physical examination (Fig. 12-14).

1. Tachycardia and exertional dyspnea may be present in infants with a large-shunt PDA. With PVOD, a right-to-left ductal shunt results in cyanosis only in the lower half of the body (i.e., differential cyanosis).

2. The precordium is hyperactive. A systolic thrill may be present at the ULSB. Bounding peripheral pulses with wide pulse pressure, with elevated systolic pressure and lower diastolic pressure, are characteristic findings.

3. The P2 is usually normal, but its intensity may be accentuated if pulmonary hypertension is present. A grade 1-4/6 continuous ("machinery") murmur is best audible at the left infraclavicular area or ULSB. The heart murmur may be crescendo systolic at the ULSB in small infants or infants with pulmonary hypertension. An apical diastolic rumble may be heard when the PDA shunt is large.

Electrocardiography. The ECG findings for PDA are similar to those of VSD. Normal or LVH may be seen with small to moderate PDA. CVH is seen with large PDA. If PVOD develops, RVH may be seen.

X-ray studies. X-ray findings are also similar to those of VSD.

1. Chest x-ray films may be normal with a small-shunt PDA.

2. Cardiomegaly of varying degrees occurs with enlargement of the LA, LV, and the ascending aorta. PVMs are increased.

3. With PVOD, the heart size is normal with a marked prominence of the MPA segment and hilar vessels.

Echocardiography.

1. The PDA can be imaged in most of the patients. Its size can be assessed by two-dimensional echo in a high parasternal view or in a suprasternal notch view (see Fig. 29-5 on p.390).

2. Doppler studies that are performed with the sample volume in the PA immediately proximal to the ductal opening provide important functional information (see Chapter 29).

3. The dimensions of the LA and LV provide an indirect assessment of the magnitude of the left-to-right ductal shunt. The larger the shunt, the greater the dilatation of these chambers.

Natural History

1. Unlike PDAs in premature infants, spontaneous closure of a PDA does not usually occur. This is because the PDA in term infants results from a structural abnormality of the ductal smooth muscle rather than a decreased responsiveness of the premature ductus to oxygen.

2. CHF and/or recurrent pneumonia develop if the shunt is large.

3. PVOD may develop if a large PDA with pulmonary hypertension remains untreated.

4. SBE, which may be more frequent with small PDAs than with large ones, may occur.

5. Although rare, an aneurysm of PDA may develop and possibly rupture.

Differential Diagnosis

The following conditions occur with a continuous murmur and/or bounding pulses, and they require differentiation from PDA:

1. *Coronary AV fistula:* A continuous murmur is usually maximally audible along the right sternal border, not at the left infraclavicular area or ULSB.

2. *Systemic AV fistula:* A bounding pulse with a wide pulse pressure and signs of CHF may develop without continuous murmur over the precordium. A continuous murmur is present over the fistula (i.e., head or liver).

3. *Pulmonary AV fistula:* A continuous murmur is audible over the back. Cyanosis and clubbing are present in the absence of cardiomegaly.

4. *Venous hum:* A venous hum is maximally audible in the right and/or left infraclavicular and supraclavicular areas when the patient is sitting. It usually disappears when the patient lies in a supine position.

5. *Collaterals in COA or TOF:* A continuous murmur is audible in the intercostal spaces, usually bilaterally.

6. *VSD with AR:* A to-and-fro murmur, rather than a continuous murmur, is audible at the MLSB or LLSB.

7. *Absence of the pulmonary valve:* A to-and-fro murmur ("sawing wood" sound) is audible at the ULSB. Large hilar PAs on x-ray films and RVH on the ECG are characteristic. These patients are frequently cyanotic, since this is usually associated with TOF.

8. *Persistent truncus arteriosus:* A continuous murmur is occasionally audible at 2RICS or at the back in a cyanotic infant, rather than in the ULSB. The ECG may show CVH, and chest x-ray films show varying degrees of cardiomegaly and increased pulmonary vascularity. A right aortic arch is frequently found.

9. *Aortopulmonary septal defect (AP window):* A bounding pulse is present, but the murmur resembles that of a VSD. CHF develops in early infancy.

10. *Peripheral PA stenosis:* A continuous murmur is audible all over the thorax. The

ECG may show RVH if the stenosis is severe. This often accompanies rubella syndrome or Williams syndrome.

11. *Ruptured sinus of Valsalva aneurysm:* The sudden onset of chest pain and signs of severe heart failure with dyspnea develop. A continuous murmur or a to-and-fro murmur is present at the base. This condition is more commonly seen in patients with Marfan's syndrome.

12. *TAPVR draining into the RA:* A murmur that sounds similar to a venous hum may be heard along the right sternal border in a child with mild cyanosis. The ECG shows RVH in the presence of cardiomegaly and increased PVMs on chest x-ray films.

13. When obstruction to pulmonary venous return occurs after the *Mustard operation* for TGA, a soft, continuous murmur may be audible along the MRSB or LRSB.

Management
Medical.

1. Indomethacin is ineffective in term infants with PDA. Therefore it should not be used.

2. No exercise restriction is needed in the absence of pulmonary hypertension.

3. Prophylaxis for SBE is indicated when indications arise.

4. Catheter closure of the ductus using several different devices (e.g., double-umbrella device, adjustable buttoned device, Gianturco coils) has been reported with varying success but it is in the experimental stage. A recent comparison between the surgical and catheter closure of the ductus shows that the catheter closure carries a lower success rate with residual shunt in 20% to 30%, a higher complication rate, and a higher cost. Although catheter closure techniques may continue to improve with further modification and experience, surgical closure appears to be preferable at this time.

Surgical.

Indications. Anatomic existence of a PDA, regardless of size, is an indication for surgery. The presence of PVOD is a contraindication to surgery.

Timing. The surgical procedure is performed at any time between 6 months and 2 years of age or when the diagnosis is made in an older child. In infants with CHF, pulmonary hypertension, or recurrent pneumonia, surgery is performed on an urgent basis.

Procedures. Ligation and division through left posterolateral thoracotomy without cardiopulmonary bypass.

Mortality. Death occurs in fewer than 1% of patients.

Complications. Complications are rare. Injury to the recurrent laryngeal nerve (i.e., hoarseness), the left phrenic nerve (i.e., paralysis of the left hemidiaphragm), or the thoracic duct (i.e., chylothorax) is possible. Recanalization (reopening) of the ductus is possible, although rare, occurring after ligation alone and without division.

Postoperative Follow-Up

1. Regular follow-up is unnecessary after PDA ligation unless surgical complications are present.

2. Unless pulmonary hypertension persists, activity does not need to be restricted.

3. SBE prophylaxis is not needed beyond 6 months after surgery.

COMPLETE ENDOCARDIAL CUSHION DEFECT
Prevalence

ECD (complete AV canal defect or AV communis) occurs in 2% of all CHDs. Of patients with ECD, 30% are children with Down syndrome. Of children with Down syndrome,

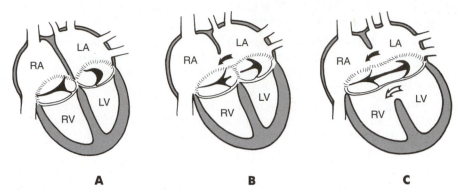

FIG. 12–15.
Diagrammatic illustration of the AV valve and cardiac septa in partial and complete ECDs. **A,** Normal AV valve anatomy with no septal defects. **B,** Partial ECD with clefts in the mitral and tricuspid valves and an ostium primum ASD *(solid arrow).* **C,** Complete ECD. There is a common AV valve with large anterior and posterior bridging leaflets. An ostium primum ASD *(solid arrow)* and an inlet VSD are present.

40% have CHDs, and 40% of the defects are ECD. ECD is a component of heart defects in asplenia or polysplenia syndrome (see Chapter 14).

Pathology

1. Structural abnormalities that are seen in complete ECD are usually the structures normally derived from the endocardial cushion tissue. Ostium primum ASD, VSD in the inlet ventricular septum, and clefts in the anterior mitral valve and the septal leaflet of the tricuspid valve (forming the common AV valve) are all present in the complete form of ECD (Fig. 12-15). The combination of these defects may result in interatrial and/or interventricular shunts, LV-to-RA shunt, and/or AV valve regurgitation. Although rare, the entire atrial septum and/or a large portion of the ventricular septum may be absent. When two AV valve orifices are present without an interventricular shunt, the defect is called *partial ECD* or *ostium primum ASD*.

2. Both complete and partial forms of ECD are characterized by a deficiency of the inlet portion of the ventricular septum with a "scooped-out" appearance of the muscular septum and an excessively long infundibular septum, as well as by an abnormal position of the aortic valve (i.e., anterosuperior to, rather than wedged between, the right and left AV valves) (Fig. 12-16). The latter results in the lengthening and narrowing of the LV outflow tract, thereby producing the characteristic "goose neck deformity" on angiocardiogram.

3. In complete ECD a single valve orifice connects the atrial and the ventricular chambers, whereas in the partial form, there are separate mitral and tricuspid orifices. The common AV valve usually has five leaflets—the anterior bridging leaflet, the posterior bridging leaflet, the right and left mural leaflets, and the right anterosuperior leaflet (see Fig. 12-16). The arrangement of the LV papillary muscles may be abnormal, in that either they are closer together or only one papillary muscle is present in the LV, which makes surgical repair difficult.

4. In the majority of complete ECD cases the AV orifices are equally committed to the RV and LV. In some patients, however, the orifices are committed primarily to one ventricle with hypoplasia of the other ventricle (i.e., RV or LV "dominance."). Occasionally, an ipsilateral atrium is also hypoplastic. Hypoplasia of one ventricle may create problems for surgical repair.

5. A universally accepted classification for complete ECD does not exist. Anderson and

his co-workers provide a new interpretation to the Rastelli classification (1967) (Fig. 12-17). According to this new interpretation, the anterior bridging leaflet is undivided in all three types. The Rastelli classification was based on the relationships of only the anterior bridging leaflets to the crest of the ventricular septum or RV papillary muscles, but did not consider equal variability in the arrangement of the posterior bridging leaflet. In type A the anterior bridging leaflet is mostly contained in the LV and usually tightly tethered to the crest of the ventricular septum. This type is

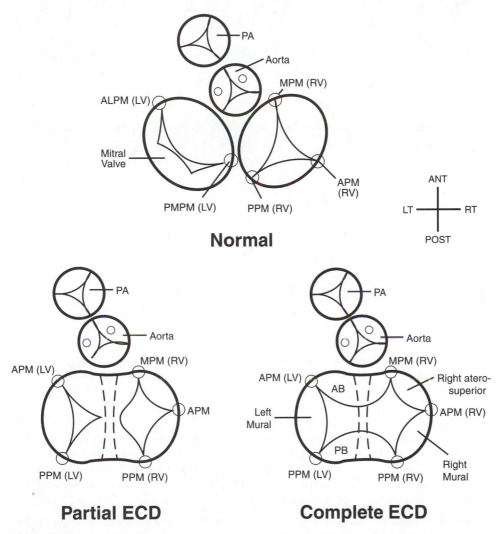

FIG. 12–16.
Anatomy of the AV valve and papillary muscle positions in the normal heart and partial and complete ECDs as viewed from above. There are five leaflets in complete ECD. In partial ECD, the connection of the anterior and posterior bridging leaflets (connecting tongue) produces the partitioning of the AV valve orifice. The aortic valve in a normal heart is deeply wedged between the mitral and tricuspid annuli, whereas the aortic valve is unwedged in ECDs. The names of the leaflets in partial ECD are the same as those in complete ECD. *AB,* Anterior bridging leaflet; *ALPM,* anterolateral papillary muscle; *APM,* anterior papillary muscle; *MPM,* medial papillary muscle; *PB,* posterior bridging leaflet; *PMPM,* posteromedial papillary muscle; *PPM,* posterior papillary muscle. (Modified from Yoo S-J, Choi Y-H: *Angiocardiograms in congenital heart disease,* Seoul, 1989, Korea Publishing Co.)

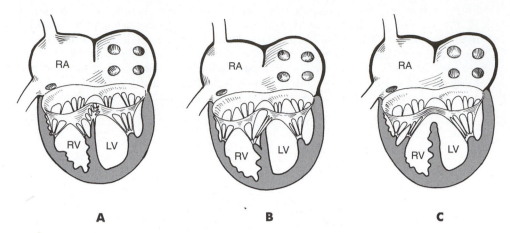

FIG. 12–17.
Rastelli's classification of complete ECD. **A,** Type A. **B,** Type B. **C,** Type C (see text for description).

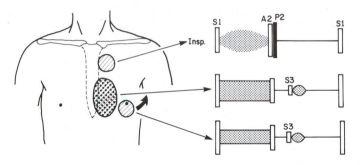

FIG. 12–18.
Cardiac findings of complete ECD, which resemble those of large VSD. A systolic thrill may be present at the LLSB *(dotted area),* where the systolic murmur is loudest. *Insp.,* Inspiration.

commonly associated with Down syndrome. In type B the anterior bridging leaflet extends into the RV and is not attached to the ventricular septum; rather it is attached to an anomalous RV papillary muscle. In type C a free-floating, anterior leaflet extends further into the RV and is attached to the anterior papillary muscle. This type is often seen in the asplenia syndrome.

6. Additional cardiac anomalies such as PDA and TOF, both of which occur in 10% of all ECD cases, may be present in children without Down syndrome. Associated defects are rare in children with Down syndrome.

Clinical Manifestation

History. Failure to thrive, repeated respiratory infections, and signs of CHF are common.

Physical examination (Fig. 12-18).

1. Infants with ECD are usually undernourished and have tachycardia and tachypnea. This defect is common in infants with Down syndrome.

2. Hyperactive precordium with a systolic thrill at the LLSB is common (shown as the area with dots in Fig. 12-18).

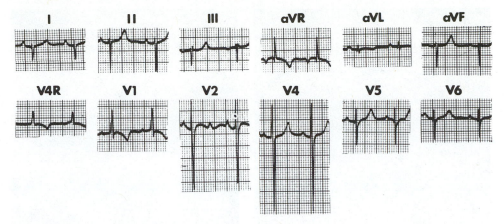

FIG. 12–19.
Tracing from a 5-year-old boy with Down syndrome and complete AV canal. Note the superior QRS axis (-110 degrees) and RVH.

3. The S1 is accentuated. The S2 narrowly splits, and the P2 increases in intensity. A grade 3-4/6 holosystolic regurgitant murmur may be heard along the LLSB. The systolic murmur may transmit well to the left back and be heard well at the apex because of MR. A middiastolic rumble may be present at the LLSB or at the apex as a result of relative stenosis of the tricuspid or mitral valve.

4. Signs of CHF (e.g., hepatomegaly, gallop rhythm) may be present.

Electrocardiography.

1. Left anterior hemiblock (i.e., "superior" QRS axis) with the QRS axis between -40 and -150 degrees is characteristic of the defect (Fig. 12-19).

2. Most patients have a prolonged PR interval (i.e., first-degree AV block).

3. RVH or RBBB is present in all cases, and many patients have LVH, too.

X-Ray Studies. Cardiomegaly is always present and involves all four cardiac chambers. PVMs are increased, and the MPA segment is prominent.

Echocardiography. Two-dimensional and Doppler echo studies allow imaging of all components of ECD, in addition to an assessment of the severity of these components. The following surgically important information can be gained: the size of the ASD and VSD, the size of the AV valve orifices, the anatomy of leaflets, chordal attachment, relative and absolute size of the RV and LV, and the left papillary muscle architecture.

1. The apical and subcostal four-chamber views are most useful in evaluating the anatomy and the functional significance of the defect. These views show both an ostium primum ASD and an inlet muscular VSD (Fig. 12-20). Either the anterior bridging leaflet crosses the ventricular septum, or the right and left AV valve leaflets can be seen at the same level from the crest of the ventricular septum. The full extent of the ASD and VSD can be imaged during systole when the common anterior leaflet is closed.

2. A combined use of the subcostal transducer position (i.e., about 45 degrees clockwise from a standard four-chamber view) and the parasternal short-axis examination may show a cleft in the mitral valve, the presence of bridging leaflets, the number of AV valve orifices, and the AV valve leaflets. These views may also image the abnormal position of the anterolateral papillary muscle, which is

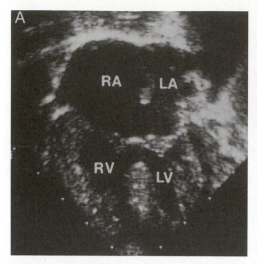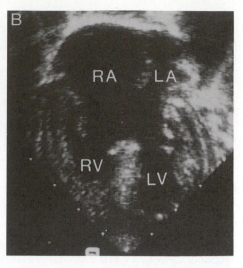

FIG. 12–20.
Apical four-chamber views in systole **(A)** and diastole **(B)** from a patient with a complete ECD. In systole, an ostium primum defect and an inlet VSD are imaged. The AV valve appears to be attached to the crest of the ventricular septum by chordae (type A). When the AV valve opens in diastole, a large deficiency in the center of the heart is visible. Note that there is a common AV valve, instead of two separate AV valves. (From Snider AR, Serwer GA: *Echocardiography in pediatric heart disease,* Chicago, 1990, Mosby.)

displaced posteriorly from its normal position, and the number (i.e., single or triple) of papillary muscles.

3. The subcostal five-chamber study may image a goose-neck deformity, which is characteristic of an angiocardiographic finding (Fig. 12-21).

4. In real time the subcostal and apical four-chamber views can image the chordal attachment of the anterior bridging leaflet either to the crest of the ventricular septum (i.e., type A), to the right side of the septum (i.e., type B), or to a papillary muscle at the apex of the RV or on its free wall (i.e., type C). A similar analysis of the posterior bridging leaflet can be made from the subcostal transducer position.

Natural History

1. For patients with ECD, heart failure occurs 1 to 2 months after birth, and recurrent peumonia is common.

2. Without surgical intervention, most patients die by the age of 2 to 3 years.

3. In the latter half of the first year of life the survivors begin to develop PVOD. These survivors usually die in late childhood or as young adults. Infants with Down syndrome are particularly prone to the early development of PVOD during infancy. As a result, surgery should be performed during infancy.

Management
   Medical.

1. In small infants with CHF anticongestive management, using digoxin, diuretics, captopril, and so on, should be started.

2. Antibiotics and other supportive measures are indicated for pneumonia and other infections.

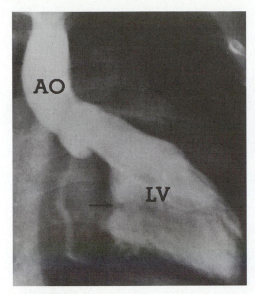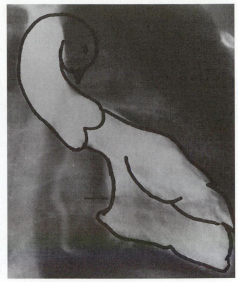

FIG. 12–21.
Frontal view of a left ventriculogram of a patient with partial ECD showing goose-neck deformity. The LV outflow tract is elongated and narrowed. The arrow points to the mitral cleft.

3. Antibiotic prophylaxis against SBE is recommended on indications.

Surgical.

Indications. The presence of complete ECD indicates the need for surgery, since an important hemodynamic derangement is usually present. Most of these infants have CHF that is unresponsive to medical therapy, and some have elevated PVR.

Timing. Although timing varies with institutions and with the hemodynamics of the defects, most centers perform the repair at 3 to 8 months of age. Early surgical repair is especially important for infants with Down syndrome and complete ECD because of their known tendency to develop early PVOD.

Procedures.

PALLIATIVE. A banding in early infancy is no longer recommended unless other associated abnormalities make complete repair a high-risk procedure. The mortality rate for PA banding may be as high as 15%.

CORRECTIVE. Given two ventricles of suitable size and no additional defects, closure of the primum ASD and inlet VSD and reconstruction of the left AV valves as a "trileaflet" valve are carried out under cardiopulmonary bypass and/or deep hypothermia (Fig. 12-22). The repair of complete ECD is technically more difficult than repairs of a secundum ASD and a perimembranous VSD. Mitral valve replacement may become necessary in only a few patients.

Mortality. The mortality rate has decreased to 5% to 10% in recent years. The survival rate is the same for patients with and without Down syndrome. Factors that increase the surgical risk are young age, severe AV valve regurgitation, hypoplasia of the LV, increased and fixed PVR, and severe preoperative symptoms. Other defects (e.g., double-orifice mitral valve, single left-sided papillary muscle, additional muscular VSD) increase the surgical risk.

Special situations.

1. Because of the early development of PVOD in patients with Down syndrome and complete ECD, a cardiac catheterization should be performed before 3 months of age,

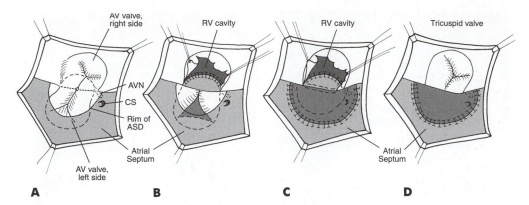

FIG. 12–22.
Surgery for AV canal. **A,** Complete ECD is viewed from the RA side. Part of the left side of the common AV valve is visible through the ostium primum ASD. The inlet VSD is shown by a broken line. **B,** The right-sided AV valve is retracted, the VSD is repaired by a patch, and the cleft in the left-sided AV valve is sutured. **C,** The ASD is closed with an oversized patch to include the AV node and the coronary sinus. **D,** The repair is complete.

and elective surgery should follow shortly thereafter. Down syndrome itself is not a risk factor.

2. Patients with severe hypoplasia of the LV and low PA pressure may receive a combination of Fontan-type operation and the Damus Kaye-Stansel operation (see Fig. 14-9 on p. 184). The proximal MPA is anastomosed end-to-side to the ascending aorta, and the venae cavae are anastomosed to the RPA.

3. TOF and complete ECD (i.e., "canal tet"): If severely cyanotic, a systemic-to-PA shunt is carried out during infancy. A complete repair is done between 2 and 4 years of age.

Complications.

1. MR becomes persistent or worsens 10% of the time.

2. Although complete heart block occurs rarely (in fewer than 5% of patients), it occurs more frequently when mitral valve replacement is required (as many as 20% of patients).

3. Postoperative arrhythmias occur and are usually supraventricular.

Postoperative Follow-Up.

1. An office evaluation should be given every 6 months to 1 year.

2. SBE prophylaxis on indications should be continued even after surgery.

3. Medications (e.g., digitalis, diuretics, captopril, and so on) may be required if residual hemodynamic abnormalities are present.

4. Some restriction of activities may be necessary if significant MR or other complications exist.

PARTIAL ENDOCARDIAL CUSHION DEFECT
Prevalence
Partial ECD (partial AV canal defect or ostium primum ASD) occurs in 1% to 2% of all CHDs, which is considerably less than a secundum ASD.

Pathology

1. In partial ECD there is a deficiency of the atrioventricular septum, as in complete ECD. A defect is present in the lower part of the atrial septum near the AV valves without an interventricular communication (see Fig. 12-1). The anterior and posterior bridging leaflets are fused by a connecting tongue to form separate right and left AV orifices (see Figs. 12-15 and 12-16). There are "clefts" in the septal leaflets of the mitral and tricuspid valves. The conjoined leaflets are displaced into the ventricle and are usually firmly attached to the crest of the ventricular septum. The aortic valve and AV valves are distanced from one another, which accounts for the characteristic "goose-neck" deformity in angiocardiograms (see Fig. 12-21).

2. Less common forms of partial ECD include common atrium, VSD of the inlet septum (i.e., AV canal type VSD), and isolated cleft of the mitral valve. A common atrium, in which the atrial septum is virtually absent, is either a characteristic lesion in patients with the Ellis van Creveld syndrome or a component of complex cyanotic heart defects such as those associated with asplenia or polysplenia syndrome.

Clinical Manifestations

History.

1. Patients with ostium primum ASD are usually asymptomatic during childhood.

2. History of symptoms such as dyspnea, fatigability, recurrent respiratory infections, and growth retardation may be present early in life if associated with major MR or common atrium.

Physical examination.

1. Cardiac findings are the same as those of a secundum ASD (see Fig. 12-2) with the exception of a regurgitant systolic murmur of MR, which may be present at the apex.

2. Mild cyanosis and clubbing may be present in patients with a common atrium.

Electrocardiography.

1. Left anterior hemiblock (i.e., "superior" QRS axis) with the QRS axis ranging from -30 to -150 degrees is characteristic of the condition (see Fig. 12-19).

2. RVH or RBBB (with rsR' pattern in V1) is present as in a secundum ASD.

3. First-degree AV block (i.e., prolonged PR interval) is present in 50% of cases.

X-ray studies. The x-ray films are the same as those of a secundum ASD (see Fig. 12-4) except for LAE and LVE when MR is significant. A characteristic "goose-neck deformity" is seen on a left ventriculogram (see Fig. 12-21).

Echocardiography.

1. Two-dimensional and Doppler echo allows accurate diagnosis of a primum ASD. A defect is in the lower atrial septum (see Fig. 12-5). No visible or Doppler-detectable VSD is present. The septal portions of the AV valves insert at the same level on the crest of the ventricular septum.

2. A cleft in the anterior leaflet of the mitral valve is commonly imaged. Less common abnormalities of the mitral valve include double-orifice mitral valve and parachute mitral valve.

3. The atrial septum is completely absent in a patient with a common atrium.

4. Color-flow and Doppler studies are useful in the detection of stenosis or regurgitation of the AV valve and in the assessment of the RV and PA pressures.

Natural History

1. CHF may develop in childhood earlier than secundum ASD. CHF is related to major MR or other associated defects.

2. Pulmonary hypertension (i.e., PVOD) develops in adulthood.

3. SBE, usually of the AV valves, is a rare complication.

4. Arrhythmias occur in 20% of patients.

Management
Medical.

1. No exercise restriction is indicated.

2. Precaution against SBE should be observed.

3. Anticongestive measures with digoxin and diuretics may be indicated for some patients.

Surgical.
Indications. The presence of a partial AV canal or primum ASD is an indication for surgical repair. Spontaneous closure of primum ASD does not occur.

Timing. Elective surgery can be performed in children who are between the ages of 1 and 2 years old and who have no symptoms. Surgery can be performed earlier in infants with CHF, failure to thrive, MR or a common atrium.

Procedures. The ASD is closed, and the cleft mitral and tricuspid valves are reconstructed under cardiopulmonary bypass.

Mortality. The surgical mortality rate is approximately 3%. Risk factors include the presence of CHF or cyanosis, failure to thrive, and the presence of moderate to severe MR.

Complications. Reoperation is needed in about 15% of the patients who have residual or worsening MR.

Atrial or nodal arrhythmias occasionally occur.

Complete heart block rarely results and requires a permanent pacemaker.

Although rare, subaortic stenosis is either missed preoperatively or develops after surgery.

Postoperative Follow-Up

1. Usually no restriction in activity is indicated.

2. Unlike secundum ASD, continued SBE prophylaxis is indicated even after completing surgery.

3. Sinus node dysfunction may require permanent pacemaker therapy.

4. Periodic evaluation for the development of subaortic stenosis and for worsening of MR should be performed.

PARTIAL ANOMALOUS PULMONARY VENOUS RETURN
Prevalence

PAPVR occurs in fewer than 1% of all CHDs.

Pathology

1. One or more (but not all) pulmonary veins drain into the RA or its venous tributaries such as the SVC, IVC, coronary sinus, and left innominate vein. The right pulmonary veins are involved twice as often as the left pulmonary veins.

2. The right pulmonary veins may drain into the SVC, which is often associated with sinus venosus defect (Fig. 12-23, *A*), or drain into the IVC (Fig. 12-23, *B*) in association with the atrial septum intact and bronchopulmonary sequestration (see Chapter 17).

3. The left pulmonary veins either drain into the left innominate vein (Fig. 12-23, *C*) or drain into the coronary sinus (Fig. 12-23, *D*). ASD is usually present with anomalous drainage of the left pulmonary veins.

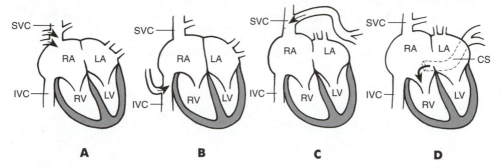

FIG. 12–23.
Common types of PAPVR. **A,** The right pulmonary veins drain anomalously to the SVC. Sinus venosus ASD is usually present. **B,** The right lower pulmonary vein drains anomalously into the IVC, usually without an associated ASD. **C,** The left pulmonary veins drain into the left innominate vein. **D,** The left pulmonary veins drain into the coronary sinus.

Pathophysiology

1. Hemodynamic alterations are similar to those in ASD. PBF increases as a result of recirculation through the lungs.

2. The magnitude of the pulmonary recirculation is determined by the number of anomalous pulmonary veins, the presence and size of ASD, and the PVR.

Clinical Manifestations

History. Children with PAPVR are usually asymptomatic.

Physical examination.

1. Cardiac findings are similar to those of ASD (see Fig. 12-2).

2. When associated with ASD, the S2 is split widely and fixed. When the atrial septum is intact, the S2 is normal. A grade 2-3/6 SEM is present at the ULSB. A middiastolic rumble, resulting from relative TS, may be present.

Electrocardiography. RVH, RBBB, or a normal ECG may be seen.

X-ray studies. The findings are similar to those of secundum ASD (see Fig. 12-4).

1. Cardiomegaly involving the RA, and RV, enlargement of the MPA segment, and increased pulmonary vascularity are all present.

2. Occasionally a dilated SVC, a crescent-shaped vertical shadow in the right lower lung (i.e., scimitar syndrome), or a distended vertical vein may suggest the site of anomalous drainage.

Echocardiography. The diagnosis of PAPVR requires a high index of suspicion. A systematic attempt to visualize each pulmonary vein should be made during any routine echo studies.

1. The inability to visualize all four pulmonary veins in the presence of a mild dilatation of the RA and RV strongly suggests the diagnosis of PAPVR, especially in the presence of demonstrable ASD.

2. PAPVR is frequently found in patients with ASD of any type and in those with persistent left SVC.

3. In sinus venosus defect the chance of anomalous drainage of the right upper pulmonary vein is high.

Natural History

1. Cyanosis and exertional dyspnea may develop during the patient's 20s and 30s. This results from pulmonary hypertension and PVOD.

2. Pulmonary infections are common in patients with anomalous drainage of the right PVs to the IVC (see Chapter 17).

Management
Medical.

1. Exercise restriction is not required.

2. SBE prophylaxis is probably not indicated.

Surgical.
Procedures. Surgical correction is carried out under cardiopulmonary bypass. The procedure to be performed depends on the site of the anomalous drainage.

TO THE RA. The ASD is widened, and a patch is sewn in such a way that the anomalous PVs drain into the LA (similar to that shown in Fig. 14-30, *B* on p. 209).

TO THE SVC. A tunnel is created between the anomalous vein and the ASD through the SVC and the RA by using a Teflon or pericardial patch. A plastic or pericardial gusset is placed in the SVC to prevent obstruction to the SVC.

TO THE IVC. In scimitar syndrome the resection of the involved lobe(s) may be indicated without connecting the anomalous vein to the heart. When the anomalous venous drainage is an isolated lesion, the vein is reimplanted to the RA, and an intraatrial tunnel is created to drain into the LA.

TO THE CORONARY SINUS. It is repaired in the same manner as for TAPVR to the coronary sinus (see Fig. 14-30, *C* on p. 209).

Indications. Indications for surgery are a significant left-to-right shunt with a $\dot{Q}p/\dot{Q}s$ > 2:1, and if the anatomy is uncomplicated, a ratio is > 1.5:1. Surgery is indicated in patients with scimitar syndrome with severe hypoplasia of the right lung even with a $\dot{Q}p/\dot{Q}s$ <2:1. Isolated single lobe anomaly without an ASD is usually not corrected.

Timing and mortality. Surgery is carried out between the age of 2 and 5 years. Surgical mortality occurs less than 1% of the time.

Complications.

1. SVC obstruction for those patients with the anomalous drainage into the SVC.

2. Postoperative arrhythmias (usually supraventricular) occurs.

Postoperative Follow-Up

1. An examination should be done every 1 to 2 years, or at a longer interval.

2. No restriction in activities is indicated.

3. SBE prophylaxis is not indicated beyond 6 months after surgery.

13 / Obstructive Lesions

Lesions that produce obstruction to ventricular outflow such as PS, AS, and COA are summarized throughout this chapter.

PULMONARY STENOSIS

Prevalence

PS occurs in 8% to 12% of all CHDs.

Pathology

1. PS may be valvular, subvalvular (infundibular), or supravalvular. An obstruction may occur within the RV cavity by an abnormal muscle bundle (i.e., "double-chambered RV").

2. In **valvular PS,** the pulmonary valve is thickened, with fused or absent commissures and, a small orifice. (Fig. 13-1, *A*). Although the RV is usually normal in size, it is hypoplastic in infants with critical PS (with nearly atretic valve). Dysplastic valves (consisting of thickened irregular, immobile tissue and a variably small pulmonary valve annulus) are frequently seen with Noonan's syndrome.

3. Isolated **infundibular PS** is rare; it is usually associated with a large VSD (TOF) (Fig. 13-1, *B*).

4. Aberrant hypertrophied muscular bands (running between the ventricular septum and the anterior wall) divide the RV cavity into a proximal high-pressure chamber and a distal low-pressure chamber (i.e., double chambered RV). A "dimple" in the ordinarily smooth RV surface is found at surgery (see Chapter 17).

5. **Supravalvar PS,** also called *stenosis of the main PA,* is occasionally seen with rubella syndrome and Williams syndrome (Fig. 13-1, *C*).

Clinical Manifestations

History.

1. Children with mild PS are completely asymptomatic.

2. Exertional dyspnea and fatigability may be present in patients with moderately severe cases.

3. Heart failure or exertional chest pain may develop in severe cases.

Physical examination (Fig. 13-2).

1. Most patients are acyanotic and well developed. Newborns with critical PS are cyanotic and tachypneic.

2. A right ventricular tap and a systolic thrill may be present at the ULSB (and occasionally in the SSN).

3. A systolic ejection click is present with valvular stenosis at the ULSB. The S2 may split widely, and the P2 may diminish in intensity. A SEM (grade 2-5/6) is best audible at the ULSB, and it transmits well to the back, too. The louder and longer the murmur, the more severe the stenosis (see Fig. 13-2).

4. Hepatomegaly may be present if CHF develops.

157

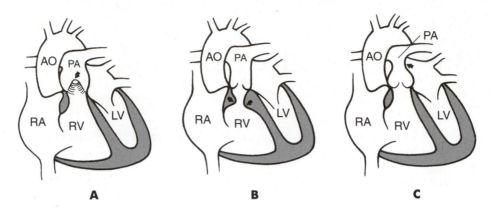

FIG. 13-1.
Anatomic types of PS. **A,** Valvular stenosis. **B,** Infundibular stenosis. **C,** Supravalvar PS (or stenosis of the MPA). Abnormalities are indicated by arrows.

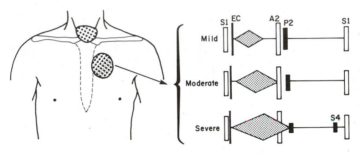

FIG. 13-2.
Cardiac findings of pulmonary valve stenosis. Abnormal sounds are shown in *black.* *Dots* represent areas with systolic thrill. *EC,* Ejection click.

Electrocardiography.

1. The ECG is normal in mild cases.

2. RAD and RVH are present in moderate PS. The degree of RVH on the ECG correlates with the severity of PS (i.e., the R wave in V1 > 20 mm is usually associated with systemic pressure in the RV).

3. RAH and RVH with strain may be seen in severe PS.

4. Neonates with critical PS may show LVH because of hypoplastic RV and relatively large LV.

X-ray study.

1. Heart size is usually normal, but the MPA segment is prominent (i.e., poststenotic dilatation) (Fig. 13-3). Cardiomegaly is present if CHF develops.

2. PVMs are usually normal but may decrease with severe PS.

Echocardiography.

1. Two-dimensional echo in the parasternal short-axis view shows thick pulmonary valve cusps with restricted systolic motion (doming). The size of the pulmonary valve annulus can be estimated. The MPA is often dilated (poststenotic dilatation).

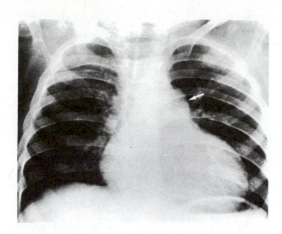

FIG. 13-3.
A PA view of chest film in pulmonary valve stenosis. Note a marked poststenotic dilatation *(arrow)* and normal pulmonary vascularity. (Courtesy Dr. Ewell Clarke, San Antonio, Texas).

2. Dysplastic valves are characterized by noticeably thickened and immobile leaflet and hypoplasia of the pulmonary valve annulus.

3. The Doppler study can estimate the pressure gradient (see Fig. 6-6 on p. 75). Multiple transducer locations should be used to obtain the maximum flow velocity. The instantaneous pressure gradient estimated by Doppler echo is slightly greater than the peak-to-peak systolic pressure gradient obtained by cardiac catheterization (i.e., about 10% greater).

Natural History

1. The severity of stenosis is usually not progressive in mild PS, but it does tend to progress with age in moderate or severe PS.

2. CHF may develop in patients with severe stenosis.

3. SBE occasionally occurs.

4. Sudden death is possible in patients with severe stenosis during heavy physical activities.

Management
  Medical.

1. Restriction of activity is not necessary, except in cases of severe PS.

2. Antiobiotic prophylaxis against SBE should be observed when indications arise.

3. Balloon valvuloplasty, which is performed at the time of cardiac catheterization, is preferable to surgical repair for significant pulmonary valve stenosis (i.e., RV systolic pressure of ≥50 mm Hg). This procedure is useful even for dysplastic pulmonary valves, and it has been successfully applied in neonates with severe PS.

4. Newborns with critical PS and cyanosis may improve by prostaglandin E_1 infusion, which reopens the ductus, and other supportive measures. Percutaneous balloon valvotomy may be performed; if unsuccessful, surgery is usually needed.

  Surgical.
Indications and timing.

1. Children with valvular PS and a RV pressure ≥80 mm Hg and in whom balloon valvuloplasty is unsuccessful (e.g., dysplastic pulmonary valve) require surgery on an elective basis.

2. Other types of obstruction (e.g., infundibular stenosis, anomalous RV muscle bundle) with significant pressure gradients also require surgery on an elective basis.

3. Infants with critical PS and CHF require surgery or balloon valvotomy on an urgent basis.

Procedures.

1. Pulmonary valvotomy is performed for pulmonary valve stenosis under cardiopulmonary bypass and/or deep hypothermia. Neonates with critical PS may require a transventricular valvotomy and/or the insertion of a transannular patch while receiving prostaglandin E_1 infusion. If severe infundibular hypoplasia is present, a left Gore-Tex shunt is also performed.

2. Dysplastic valves often require complete excision of the valves.

3. Anomalous muscle bundles require surgical resection.

4. Stenosis at the PA level requires patch widening of the narrow portion.

5. Infundibular stenosis requires resection of the infundibular muscle and patch widening of the RV outflow tract.

Mortality.

   Surgical mortality occurs in fewer than 1% of older children. This rate is about 10% in critically ill infants.

Postoperative follow-up.

1. SBE prophylaxis is needed even after relief of stenosis.

2. Periodic echo and Doppler studies are needed to estimate the pressure gradient.

AORTIC STENOSIS

Prevalence

AS represents 3% to 6% of all patients with CHDs, and it occurs more often in males (M:F = 4:1).

Pathology

1. Stenosis may be at the valvular, subvalvular, or supravalvular level (Fig. 13-4).

2. Valvular AS may be because of a bicuspid aortic valve, an unicuspid aortic valve, or stenosis of the tricuspid aortic valve (Fig. 13-4 *B*). A bicuspid aortic valve with a fused commissure and an eccentric orifice accounts for the most common form of aortic valve stenosis (Fig. 13-5, *B*). Less common is the unicuspid valve with one lateral attachment (Fig. 13-5, *A*). A valve that has three unseparated cusps with a stenotic central orifice is the least common form (Fig. 13-5, *C*).

3. Supravalvular AS is an annular constriction above the aortic valve at the upper margin of the sinus of Valsalva (Fig. 13-4, *C*). Occasionally, the ascending aorta is diffusely hypoplastic. This is often associated with Williams syndrome, which includes mental retardation, characteristic facies, and PA stenosis.

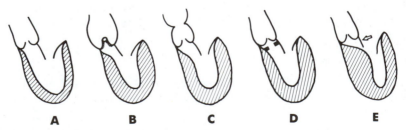

FIG. 13-4.
Anatomic types of AS. **A,** Normal. **B,** Valvular stenosis. **C,** Supravalvular stenosis. **D,** Discrete subaortic stenosis. **E,** IHSS. IHSS is discussed in Chapter 18.

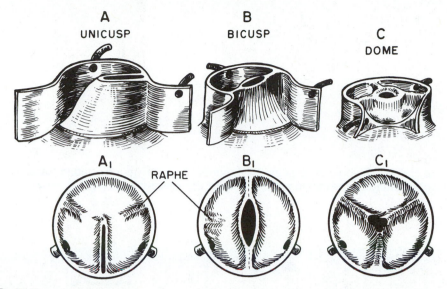

FIG. 13-5.
Anatomic types of aortic valve stenosis. Top row is side view, and bottom row is the view as seen in surgery during aortotomy. **A,** Unicuspid aortic valve. **B,** Bicuspid aortic valve. **C,** Stenosis of a tricuspid aortic valve. (From Goor DA, Lillehei CW: *Congenital malformations of the heart,* New York, 1975, Grune & Stratton.

4. Subvalvular (subaortic) stenosis may result from a simple diaphragm (discrete) (Fig. 13-4, *D*) or from a long, tunnel-like fibromuscular narrowing (tunnel stenosis) of the LV outflow tract.

   a. Discrete subaortic stenosis accounts for about 10% of all AS cases, and it occurs more often than tunnel stenosis. It is common among patients with COA and VSD. For some reason, discrete subaortic stenosis develops after PA banding or repair of a VSD.

   b. A tunnel-like subaortic stenosis is often associated with hypoplasia of the ascending aorta and aortic valve ring, as well as with thickened aortic valve leaflets.

   c. Another type of subvalvular stenosis is IHSS (Fig. 13-4, *E*), a primary disorder of the heart muscle (see Chapter 18).

Clinical Manifestations
  History.

1. Most children with mild to moderate AS are asymptomatic. Occasionally, exercise intolerance may be present.

2. Exertional chest pain, fatigability, or syncope may occur with a severe degree of obstruction.

3. Infants with critical stenosis of the aortic valve may develop CHF within the first few months of life.

  Physical examination (Fig. 13-6).

1. Patients are acyanotic and have developed normally.

2. Blood pressure is normal in most patients, but a narrow pulse pressure is present in severe AS. Patients with supravalvular AS may show a higher systolic pressure in the right arm than in the left.

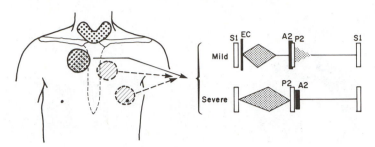

FIG. 13-6.
Cardiac findings of aortic valve stenosis. Abnormal sounds are indicated in *black*.
Systolic thrill may be present in areas with *dots*. *EC,* Ejection click.

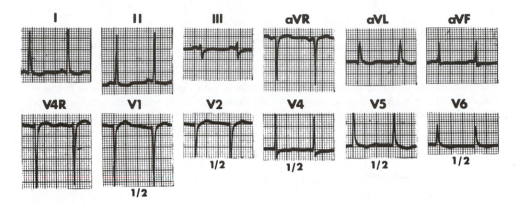

FIG. 13-7.
Tracing from a 7-year-old boy with severe AS. It shows LVH with probable "strain"
pattern.

3. A systolic thrill may be palpable at the URSB, in the SSN, or over the carotid arteries.

4. An ejection click may be heard with valvular AS. The S2 splits either normally or a bit narrowly. The S2 may split paradoxically in severe AS (see Fig. 13-6). A harsh, grade 2-4/6, SEM may best be heard at the 2RICS or 3LICS with good transmission to the neck and apex. A high-pitched, early diastolic decrescendo murmur, which results from AR, may be audible in patients with bicuspid aortic valve and in those with discrete subvalvular stenosis.

5. Peculiar "elfin facies" and mental retardation may be associated with supravalvular AS (e.g., Williams syndrome).

6. Newborns with critical AS may develop CHF. The heart murmur may be absent or faint, and the peripheral pulses are weak and thready. The heart murmur becomes louder when CHF improves.

Electrocardiography. In mild cases the ECG is normal. LVH with strain pattern may be present in severe cases (Fig. 13-7). Correlation of the severity of AS and the ECG abnormalities is relatively poor.

X-ray studies.
1. The heart size is usually normal in children, but a dilated ascending aorta or a prominent aortic knob may be seen occasionally in valvular AS, resulting from poststenotic dilatation.

2. Significant cardiomegaly does not develop unless CHF occurs later in life or if AR becomes substantial.

3. Newborns with critical AS show generalized cardiomegaly with pulmonary venous congestion.

Echocardiography.

1. Valvular AS:

   a. The coaptation line is seen in the center of the aortic root in an M-mode echo of a normal aortic valve (Fig. 13-8, *A*). In M-mode echo of a bicuspid valve, an eccentric closure line or multiple closure lines of the aortic valve may be present during diastole (Fig. 13-8, *B* and *C*).

   b. In the parasternal short-axis view of two-dimensional echo, normal aortic valves are tricuspid with three cusps of approximately equal size. In diastole the normal aortic cusp margins form a Y pattern (see Fig. 13-9). A bicuspid aortic valve appears as a noncircular (i.e., football-shaped) orifice in systole (Fig. 13-10). Stenosis of the tricuspid aortic valve appears as a heavy Y pattern in diastole and as a small, centrally located orifice in systole with three thickened commissures distinctly visible. A unicommissural aortic valve, which may usually be seen in infants with critical AS, is seen as a circular orifice positioned eccentrically within the aortic root and without visible distinct cusps.

   c. In the parasternal long-axis view of two-dimensional echo, doming of the thick aortic valve with restriction to the opening is seen in systole. Reverse doming during diastole commonly occurs in the unicuspid valve, occurs less frequently in the bicuspid valve, and does not occur with the tricuspid aortic valve.

2. The parasternal long-axis view, apical long-axis view, and/or apical five-chamber view show the discrete subaortic membrane as a thin echo stretching across the LV outflow tract just beneath the aortic valve. The fibromuscular type (i.e., tunnel stenosis) involves a more extensive area of the LV outflow tract as seen in the parasternal long-axis view or apical long-axis view.

3. Supravalvar AS is seen as a narrowing that results from a discrete membrane in the parasternal long-axis view and apical long-axis view. The suprasternal view best shows diffuse hypoplasia of the ascending aorta.

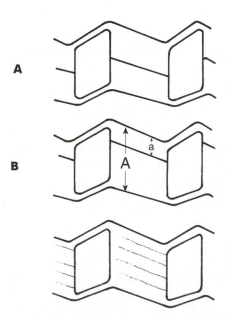

FIG. 13-8.
Diagram demonstrating M-mode echo of normal aortic valve **(A)** and various patterns seen with bicuspid aortic valves **(B,C).** In bicuspid aortic valve, the eccentricity index (0.5 × A/a) is usually greater than 1.5, where A is the aortic root diameter and a is the distance from the diastolic closure line to the nearest aortic wall. The normal eccentricity index is 1.0 to 1.2.

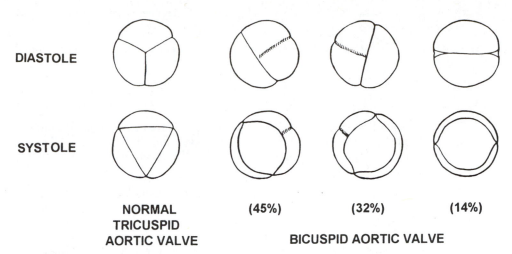

| | DIASTOLE | | | |
| SYSTOLE | | | | |

DIASTOLE

SYSTOLE

NORMAL
TRICUSPID
AORTIC VALVE   (45%)   (32%)   (14%)

BICUSPID AORTIC VALVE

FIG. 13-9.
Diagram of parasternal short-axis scan shows normal tricuspid (left column) and
bicuspid aortic valves (three right columns) during diastole and systole. Three nearly
equal-sized aortic cusps are imaged in a normal aortic valve, which opens widely during
systole. Systolic opening pattern distinguishes a raphe from a commissure. With a
bicuspid aortic valve, various commissural orientations are imaged. The most common
pattern demonstrates commissures at the 4 or 5 o'clock and the 9 or 10 o'clock
positions, with raphe at the 1 or 2 o'clock position (46%). Less common patterns are
those with commissures at the 7 and 1 o'clock positions and those with commissures at
the 3 and 9 o'clock positions. (Modified from Brandenburg RO Jr, Tajik AJ, Edwards
WD, et al: Accuracy of 2-dimensional echocardiographic diagnosis of congenitally
bicuspid aortic valve: echocardiographic-anatomic correlation in 115 patients, *Am J
Cardiol* 51:1469-1473, 1983.)

4. Doppler studies can estimate the severity of the stenosis by using the simplified
   Bernoulli equation (see Chapter 6). The Doppler-derived gradient (i.e., instantaneous
   gradient) is as much as 30 mm Hg higher than the peak-to-peak systolic pressure
   gradient for mild to moderate stenosis.

Natural History

1. Chest pain, syncope, and even sudden death (1% to 2% of cases) may occur in children
   with severe AS.

2. Heart failure occurs with severe AS during the newborn period or later in adult life.

3. A significant increase in the pressure gradient frequently occurs with growth, since
   cardiac output increases with growth.

4. The stenosis may worsen with aging as the result of calcification of the valve cusps.
   This worsening condition requires valve replacement in many adult patients.

5. Progressive worsening of AR is possible in discrete subaortic stenosis.

6. SBE occurs in approximately 4% of patients with valvar AS.

Management
   Medical.

1. Maintenance of good oral hygiene and antibiotic prophylaxis against bacterial
   endocarditis are especially important for patients with AS regardless of the type or
   severity of the stenosis (see Chapter 19).

2. Children with moderate to severe AS should not perform sustained, strenuous activities.

3. To prepare for surgery, anticongestive measures with inotropic agents and diuretics, prostaglandin E_1 infusion, and oxygen administration are necessary for critically ill newborns with CHF.

4. Percutaneous balloon valvuloplasty to relieve the stenosis may be tried at the time of cardiac catheterization on selected patients, including newborns. Although the results are promising, they are not as good as those for PS.

5. Serial echo-Doppler ultrasound evaluation is needed every 2 years in asymptomatic children with mild to moderate stenosis and more often in children with severe stenosis.

Surgical.
Procedures.

1. Closed aortic valvotomy, using calibrated dilators or balloon catheters without cardiopulmonary bypass, may be performed in sick infants. This procedure has a low surgical mortality.

2. Other procedures are performed under cardiopulmonary bypass or total circulatory arrest and deep hypothermia.

   a. In aortic valve commissurotomy, fused commissures are divided with a knife to within 1 mm of the aortic wall. Only commissures with adequate leaflet attachments to the aortic wall are opened, since division of rudimentary commissures produces AR.

   b. Aortic valve replacement may be required for a unicuspid or a severely dysplastic bicuspid aortic valve. These situations usually found in extremely sick neonates. Older children and adolescents who have already had aortic valvotomies may also need valve replacement. Valve replacement is done by using either a prosthetic valve, a porcine bioprosthesis, an aortic valve allograft, or a pulmonary valve autograft. The prosthetic valve requires anticoagulation. A porcine valve or aortic allografts do not necessitate anticoagulation and have limited durability.

   c. In pulmonary-root autografts (i.e., Ross procedure) the autologous pulmonary valve replaces the aortic valve, and an aortic or a pulmonary allograft replaces the pulmonary valve. Although the Ross procedure is more complex than simple aortic-aortic valve replacement because the procedure requires coronary artery implantation, it can be carried out with a low mortality rate in selected patients (Fig. 13-10). The pulmonary valve autograft has the advantage of documented, long-term durability, that does not require anticoagulation and remains uncompromised by host reactions. There is evidence of the autograft's growth, making it an attractive option for aortic valve replacement in infants and children. Mild regurgitation of the neoaortic valve occurs frequently, which may result from a preexisting pulmonary valve regurgitation.

   d. Patients with severe annular narrowing or tunnel-like narrowing may need aortic root enlargement (i.e., Konno operation) before valve replacement.

   e. Excision of the membrane is done for discrete subvalvular AS. Myectomy or myotomy of the septal muscle tends to improve the result.

   f. Widening of the stenotic area by using a diamond-shaped fabric patch is performed for discrete supravalvar AS.

Indications and timing.

1. Neonates and young infants with CHF from critical AS require urgent surgery.

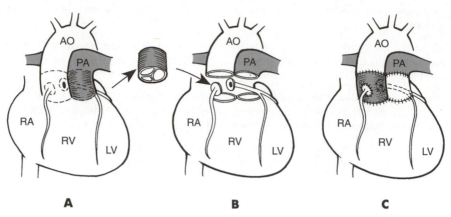

FIG. 13-10.
Ross procedure (pulmonary root autograft). **A,** Two horizontal lines on the aorta and PA and two broken circles around the coronary artery ostia are lines of proposed incision. The pulmonary valve with a small rim of RV muscle, and the adjacent PA are removed. **B,** The aortic valve and the adjacent aorta have been removed, leaving buttons of aortic tissue around the coronary arteries. **C,** The pulmonary autograft is sutured to the aortic annulus and to the distal aorta, and the coronary arteries are sutured to openings made in the PA. The pulmonary valve is replaced with either an aortic or pulmonary allograft.

2. Children with severe AS with a peak systolic pressure gradient of 75 mm Hg or a calculated effective orifice area <0.5 cm^2/m^2 receive surgery on an elective basis.

3. Children with a peak systolic pressure gradient of 50 to 75 mm Hg are a controversial group. They may be closely watched and have their activity limited until a more opportune time, or they may be operated on if their pressure gradients increase. Valve replacement surgery should be delayed, if possible, until an adult-sized valve can be used.

4. Asymptomatic children with a systolic pressure gradient <50 mm Hg do not usually require surgery.

5. Symptoms related to AS (e.g., anginal chest pain, syncope) with strain pattern on the ECG or abnormal exercise test are indications for surgery even if the systolic gradient is 50 mm Hg.

6. An earlier elective operation may be considered for discrete subvalvular AS of moderate degree (i.e., gradient >50 mm Hg) because of the progressive nature of AR.

7. Surgery is advisable for patients with supravalvar AS when the peak pressure gradient across the stenosis is ≥ 50 mm Hg. The operation is performed whenever the patient meets the criteria for surgery.

Mortality. The overall mortality rate for infants and small children with aortic valvular stenosis ranges from 15% to 20%. Sick neonates and those with poor preoperative functional status have a mortality rate as high as 40%. The hospital mortality in older children is 1% to 2%. Death occurs for discrete subvalvular and supravalvular stenosis in fewer than 1% of cases.

Complications. Significant AR may develop after aortic valvotomy.

Postoperative follow-up.

1. Annual examination with an ECG and chest x-ray is necessary for all patients who had aortic valve surgery in order to detect further degenerative changes. A pressure

gradient may develop again 5 to 10 years after a valvotomy, especially in children requiring the valvotomy during the neonatal period or in infancy. Approximately 25% of patients require valve replacement 15 to 20 years after the original surgery for valvar AS. Recurrence of discrete subaortic stenosis often occurs after surgical resection of the membrane and requires periodic follow-up.

2. Restriction from competitive, strenuous sports may be necessary for children with moderate residual AS and/or AR.

3. SBE prophylaxis should be used on indications after surgery for all types of aortic valve surgery. The incidence of SBE does not decrease with valve surgery, rather it may increase.

4. Anticoagulation is needed after a prosthetic mechanical valve replacement, but not after tissue valve replacement.

COARCTATION OF THE AORTA

Prevalence

COA occurs in 8% to 10% of all CHDs cases. It is more common in males than in females (M:F = 2:1). Of patients with Turner's syndrome, 30% have COA.

Pathology

1. The terms *preductal* and *postductal*, as well as *infantile* or *adult type COA* are misleading. COA is almost always in a juxtaductal position (i.e., neither preductal nor postductal).

2. In *symptomatic infants* with COA the descending aorta is supplied by right heart blood via the ductus arteriosus during fetal life and at birth. Other cardiac defects such as aortic hypoplasia, abnormal aortic valve, VSD (50%), PDA (60%), and mitral valve anomalies are often present. All of these cardiac defects tend to decrease antegrade aortic blood flow in utero (see Fig. 10-3 on p. 109). Occasionally, infants without associated defects may become symptomatic because of LV failure, which results from a sudden increase in pressure work in early postnatal life. COA also occurs as part of TGA and DORV (e.g., Taussig-Bing abnormality). With ductal closure, these infants become symptomatic early in life. Good collateral circulation has not developed in these infants (see Chapter 10).

3. In *asymptomatic children* with COA the descending aorta is supplied by LV blood via the ascending aorta and the aortic isthmus during fetal life. Associated cardiac defects, except for bicuspid aortic valve, are rare in these children. Good collateral circulation gradually develops between the proximal aorta and the distal aorta (Fig. 13-11).

4. As many as 85% of patients with COA have a bicuspid aortic valve.

Symptomatic Infants

Clinical manifestations.

History. Poor feeding, dyspnea, and poor weight gain or signs of acute circulatory shock may develop in the first 6 weeks of life. Fig. 13-12 provides an explanation for hemodynamic deterioration in the newborn period. Newborn discharge examination may have been normal as a result of incomplete obliteration of the aortic end of the ductus that would permit blood flow to the descending aorta.

Physical examination.

1. Infants with COA are pale and experience varying degrees of respiratory distress. Oliguria or anuria, general circulatory shock, and severe acidemia are common. Differential cyanosis may be present; for example, only the lower half of the body is cyanotic because of a right-to-left ductal shunt.

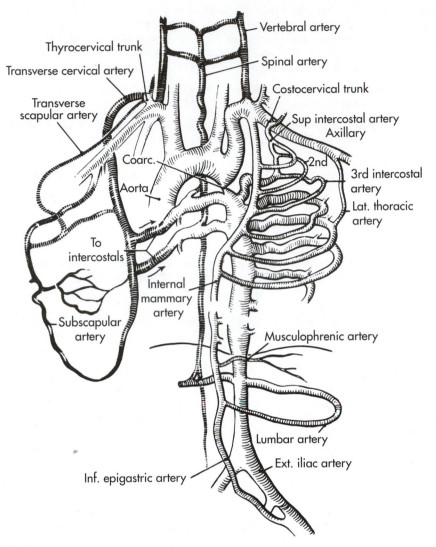

FIG. 13-11.
Collateral circulation in COA. Anteriorly, the internal mammary artery leads to the epigastric arteries for the supply to the lower extremity. The arteries arising from the subclavian artery and supplying the scapula communicate, by way of intercostal arteries, with the descending aorta thereby supplying blood to the abdominal organs. The anterior spinal artery is also enlarged. (From Moller JH, Amplatz K, Edwards JE: *Congenital heart disease,* Kalamazoo, Michigan, 1971, Upjohn Co.)

2. Peripheral pulses may be weak and thready as a result of CHF. A blood pressure differential may become apparent only after improvement with administration of inotropic agents.

3. The S2 is single and loud; a loud S3 gallop is usually present. No heart murmur is present in 50% of sick infants. A nonspecific systolic ejection murmur is audible over the precordium. The heart murmur may become louder after treatment.

Electrocardiography. Normal or rightward QRS axis and RVH or RBBB are present in most infants with COA, rather than LVH, which is seen in older children (see Chapter 10) (Fig. 13-13).

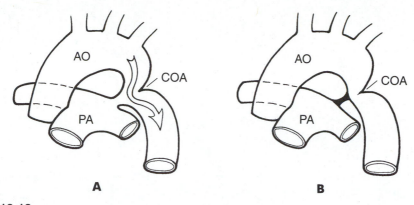

FIG. 13-12.
Explanation for hemodynamic deterioration seen in some infants with COA in the first days of life. **A,** Coarctation is at the juxtaductal position, so that space is added to the narrowed aorta by ductus. **B,** After ductal obliteration, the added lumen is lost, and the aorta becomes severely obstructed, although the severity of the coarctation is unchanged.

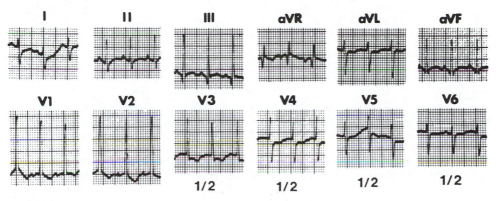

FIG. 13-13.
Tracing from a 3-week-old infant with COA. Note a marked RVH.

X-ray studies. Marked cardiomegaly and pulmonary edema or pulmonary venous congestion are usually present.

Echocardiography. Two-dimensional echo and color-flow Doppler studies usually show the site and the extent of the coarctation.

1. In the superasternal notch view, a wedge-shaped "shelf" of tissue is imaged in the posterior and lateral aspects of the upper descending aorta, which is distal to the left subclavian artery. Other associated defects such as VSD can be imaged. Cardiac catheterization is usually unnecessary.

2. Doppler studies above and below the coarctation site, in conjunction with two-dimensional echo, are useful in assessing the severity of the narrowing.

Natural history.

1. About 20% to 30% of all patients with COA develop CHF by 3 months of age.

2. If undetected and/or untreated, early death may result from CHF and renal shutdown in symptomatic infants with COA.

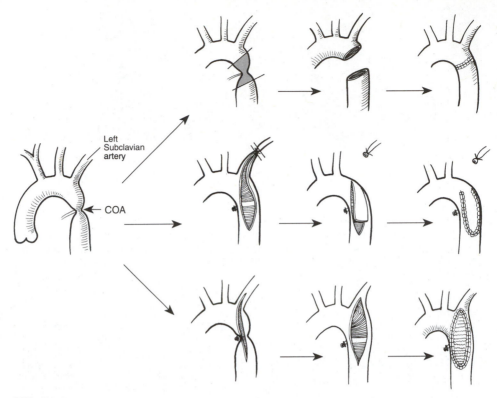

FIG. 13-14.
Surgical techniques for repair of COA. *Top,* End-to-end anastomosis. A segment of coarctation is resected, and the proximal and distal aortas are anastomosed end-to-end. *Middle,* Subclavian flap procedure. The distal subclavian artery is divided, and the flap of the proximal portion of this vessel is used to widen the coarcted segment. *Bottom,* Patch aortoplasty. An elliptical woven Dacron patch is inserted to expand the diameter of the lumen. Regardless of the type of operative procedure, the ductus arteriosus is always ligated and divided.

Management.
Medical.

1. Prostaglandin E$_1$ infusion should be started to reopen the ductus arteriosus and establish flow to the descending aorta and the kidneys during the first weeks of life.

2. Intensive anticongestive measures with short-acting inotropic agents (e.g., dopamine, dobutamine), diuretics, and oxygen should be started.

3. Balloon angioplasty can be a useful procedure for sick infants in whom standard surgical management carries a high risk. This is controversial, however.

Surgical.
PROCEDURES. Surgical procedures vary greatly from institution to institution, but the following procedures are popular (Fig. 13-14).

1. Resection and end-to-end anastomosis consists of resecting the coarctation segment and anastomosing the proximal and distal aortas (Fig. 13-14, *top*).

2. Subclavian flap aortoplasty consists of dividing the distal subclavian artery and inserting a flap of the proximal portion of this vessel between the two sides of the longitudinally split aorta throughout the coarctation segment (Fig. 13-14, *middle*).

3. With patch aortoplasty, the aorta is opened longitudinally through the coarctation segment and extending to the left subclavian artery, and the fibrous shelf and any existing membrane are excised. An eliptical, woven Dacron patch is inserted to expand the diameter of the lumen (Fig. 13-14, *bottom*).

4. A conduit insertion between the ascending and descending aorta may be performed for severe, long-segment COA (not shown in Fig. 13-14).

INDICATIONS AND TIMING.

1. If CHF or circulatory shock develops early in life, surgery should be performed on an urgent basis. A short period of medical treatment, as described earlier, improves the patient's condition before surgery; prolonged medical treatment is not recommended.

2. If there is a large associated VSD, one of the following procedures may be performed:

   a. Only coarctation repair is performed without PA banding. If CHF cannot be managed medically, VSD is surgically closed within days or weeks.

   b. If the PA pressure remains high after completing COA surgery, PA banding is performed. This approach is necessary only for infants with multiple VSDs, large apical VSD, single ventricle, or other complex lesions. Later VSD is closed, and the PA band is removed between 6 and 24 months of age.

MORTALITY. The mortality rate for COA patients is less than 5%.

COMPLICATIONS.

1. Postoperative renal failure is the most common cause of death.

2. Residual obstruction and/or recoarctation occurs in 6% to 33% of all cases.

Postoperative follow-up.

1. An examination every 6 to 12 months to check for the recurrence of COA is necessary, since recoarctation is possible. This is especially important if surgery is performed in the first year of life.

2. SBE prophylaxis should be continued on indications because of the frequently associated bicuspid aortic valve and residual coarctation.

3. Balloon angioplasty may be performed if a significant recoarctation develops.

4. Physicians should watch for and treat systemic hypertension.

Asymptomatic Children
Clinical manifestations.
History. Most children are asymptomatic. Occasionally, a child complains of weakness and/or pain in the legs after exercise.

Physical examination (Fig. 13-15).

1. Patients grow and develop normally.

2. Arterial pulses in the leg are either absent or weak and delayed. There is hypertension in the arm, or blood pressure readings in the arm are higher than those found in the leg. In normal children the oscillometric systolic pressure in the thigh or calf is 5 to 10 mm Hg higher than that in the arm. With the use of the auscultatory method, the leg systolic pressure may be as much as 20 mm Hg higher than in the arm (see Chapter 2).

3. A systolic thrill may be present in the SSN. The S2 splits normally, and the A2 is accentuated. An ejection click is frequently audible at the apex and/or at the base, which results from the associated bicuspid aortic valve or systemic hypertension. A systolic ejection murmur (SEM), grade 2-4/6 can be heard at the URSB, MLSB, or LLSB. A well-localized systolic murmur is also audible in the left interscapular area in the back. Occasionally, an early diastolic decrescendo murmur of AR from the bicuspid aortic valve may be audible in 3LICS (Fig. 13-15).

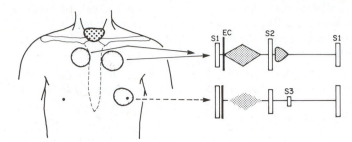

FIG. 13-15.
Cardiac findings of COA. A systolic thrill may be present in the SSN (area shown by *dots*). *EC,* Ejection click.

Electrocardiography. Leftward QRS axis and LVH are commonly found. The ECG appears normal in 20% of patients.

X-ray study.

1. The heart size may be normal or slightly enlarged.

2. Dilatation of the ascending aorta may be seen.

3. An E-shaped indentation on the barium-filled esophagus, or a "3 sign" on overpenetrated films, suggests COA (see Fig. 4-9 on p. 59).

4. Rib notching between the fourth and eighth ribs may be seen in older children but rarely in children younger than 5 years of age (see Fig. 4-8 on p. 58).

Echocardiography.

1. A discrete shelf-like membrane is imaged in the posterolateral aspect of the descending aorta by two-dimensional echo, usually in SSN view. Cardiac catheterization is usually unnecessary in children with clinically uncomplicated COA.

2. Bicuspid aortic valve is frequently present.

3. Doppler examination reveals disturbed flow distal to the coarctation, and it can estimate the severity of the obstruction by the Bernoulli equation. A more accurate estimation of the gradient is obtained by the expanded Bernoulli equation in which the peak velocities obtained from the segments proximal and distal to the coarctation site are used. In severe COA with extensive collaterals the Doppler-estimated gradient may underestimate the severity of the coarctation because the blood flow decreases through the obstruction.

Natural history.

1. A bicuspid aortic valve may cause stenosis and/or regurgitation with age.

2. SBE can occur on either the aortic valve or the coarctation.

3. LV failure, rupture of the aorta, intracranial hemorrhage (i.e., rupture of a berry aneurysm of the arterial circle of Willis), hypertensive encephalopathy, and hypertensive cardiovascular disease may develop during adulthood.

Management.
Medical.

1. Good dental hygiene and precaution against SBE are important.

2. Children with mild COA should be watched closely for hypertension in the arm or for increasing pressure differences between the arm and leg.

3. Hypertensive crisis, if it develops, should be diagnosed and treated appropriately (see Chapter 31).

4. Balloon angioplasty for native (unoperated) coarctation is controversial; however, it may produce aortic aneurysm with the possibility of serious late complications.

Surgical.
INDICATIONS AND TIMING.

1. COA with hypertension in the upper extremities or with a large systolic pressure gradient of 20 mm Hg or greater between the arms and the legs indicates that elective surgical correction is necessary between the ages of 2 and 4. In older children it is operated on soon after the diagnosis is made. To produce this much pressure gradient, the diameter of the descending aorta needs to be reduced to less than one third of normal, resulting in the appearance of severe coarctation. Late complications (e.g., hypertension, endocarditis, central nervous system bleeding) rarely occur if surgery is performed earlier; however, early surgery (i.e., before 1 year of age) increases the chance of recoarctation.

2. If severe hypertension, CHF, or cardiomegaly is present, surgery is performed at an earlier age.

3. Children with mild COA (i.e., < 20 mm Hg gradient) may be considered for surgery if a prominent gradient develops with exercise.

PROCEDURES.

1. Resection of the coarctation segment and end-to-end anastomosis is the procedure of choice for discrete COA in children (see Fig. 13-14).

2. Occasionally, subclavian artery aortoplasty or circular or patch grafts may be performed.

MORTALITY. The mortality rate is less than 1% in older children.
COMPLICATIONS.

1. Spinal cord ischemia producing paraplegia may develop after cross-clamping of the aorta during surgery, which is probably related to limited collateral circulation. This develops in 0.4% of cases.

2. Postoperative rebound hypertension or postcoarctectomy syndrome may occur (see Chapter 36).

Postoperative follow-up.

1. Annual examinations should pay attention to the following:

   a. Persistence or resurgence of hypertension in the arm and legs of some patients (The cause of the hypertension is not clearly understood.)

   b. Blood pressure differences in the arm and leg, which suggests recoarctation

   c. Associated abnormalities such as bicuspid aortic valve or mitral valve disease

   d. Persistent myocardial dysfunction that was present before surgery

   e. Subaortic AS evolving years after the initial surgery in some patients

2. The physician should emphasize the need to continue SBE prophylaxis on indications.

3. If recurrence of COA occurs, balloon dilatation of the COA should be considered. Balloon angioplasty of recoarctation is considered safe.

INTERRUPTED AORTIC ARCH
Prevalence
Interrupted aortic arch accounts for about 1% of all critically ill infants who have CHDs.

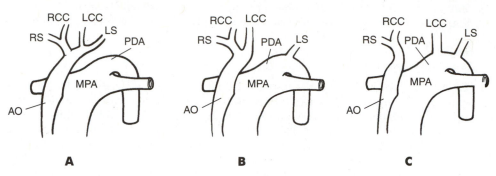

FIG. 13-16.
Three types of aortic arch interruption. **A,** Type A. **B,** Type B. **C,** Type C (see text).

Pathology

1. This is an extreme form of coarctation of the aorta in which the aortic arch is atretic or a segment of the arch is absent.

2. Depending on the location of the interruption, the defect is divided into the following three types (Fig. 13-16):

    a. Type A: The interruption is distal to the left subclavian artery (occurs in 30% of cases).

    b. Type B: The interruption is between the left carotid and left subclavian arteries (occurs in 43% of cases). An aberrant right subclavian artery is common. Di George syndrome is reported in about 50% of patients.

    c. Type C: The interruption is between the innominate and left carotid arteries (occurs in 17% of cases).

3. Interrupted aortic arch is usually associated with PDA and VSD. A bicuspid aortic valve occurs in 60% of all cases. Often there is mitral valve deformity (occurs in 10% of cases), persistent truncus arteriosus (occurs in 10% of cases), or subaortic stenosis (occurs in 20% of cases).

Clinical Manifestations

1. Respiratory distress, variable degrees of cyanosis, poor peripheral pulses, and signs of CHF or circulatory shock develop during the first days of life. Differential cyanosis is uncommon because of the frequent association of VSD.

2. Chest x-ray films show cardiomegaly, increased PVMs, and pulmonary venous congestion or pulmonary edema. The upper mediastinum may be narrow because of the absence of the thymus, as commonly found with Di George syndrome. The ECG may show RVH in uncomplicated cases.

3. Echo is useful in the diagnosis of the interruption and associated defects. Angiocardiography is usually indicated for accurate diagnosis of the anatomy.

Management

1. Medical treatment consists of prostaglandin E_1 infusion (preferably before 4 days of age) with intubation and oxygen administration. Workup for Di George syndrome (i.e., serum calcium) should be done. Hyperventilation that causes respiratory alkalosis and tetany should be avoided, and citrated blood (which causes hypocalcemia by chelation) should not be transfused in patients with Di George syndrome. Blood should be irradiated before the transfusion.

2. Primary complete repair of the interruption and the VSD is recommended if the interruption is associated with a simple VSD. If associated with complex anomalies, the initial procedures should be banding the PA and repairing the interruption. Debanding and repair of the VSD and other cardiac anomalies should be done at a later date. A primary anastomosis, Dacron vascular graft, or venous homograft may be used to repair the interruption. Surgical mortality can be as low as 10% for initial surgery.

14 / Cyanotic Congenital Heart Defects

This chapter discusses well-known CHDs that produce cyanosis. Some of these defects increase PBF, whereas others decrease PBF. Defects discussed in this chapter include complete TGA (D-TGA), TOF, TAPVR, tricuspid atresia, pulmonary atresia with an intact ventricular septum, Ebstein's anomaly, persistent truncus arteriosus, single ventricle, DORV and splenic syndromes. Although uncomplicated cases of congenitally corrected TGA (L-TGA) do not produce cyanosis, they are included in this chapter, since the majority of cases are associated with other cardiac defects resulting in cyanosis.

COMPLETE TRANSPOSITION OF THE GREAT ARTERIES

Prevalence

D-TGA occurs in about 5% of all CHDs. It is more common in males than in females (M:F = 3:1).

Pathology

1. In D-TGA the aorta arises anteriorly from the RV carrying desaturated blood to the body, and the PA arises posteriorly from the LV carrying oxygenated blood to the lungs. There is a fibrous continuity between the pulmonary and mitral valves, and subaortic conus is present. (In normal hearts the aorta arises from the LV and lies posterior to and right of the pulmonary valve, and there are aortic-mitral fibrous continuity and subpulmonary conus). The result of D-TGA is complete separation of the pulmonary and systemic circulations. This results in hypoxemic blood circulating throughout the body and hyperoxemic blood circulating in the pulmonary circuit (see Fig. 11-2 on p. 117). Defects that permit mixing of the two circulations (e.g., ASD, VSD, and PDA) are necessary for survival.

2. About half of these infants do not have associated defects other than PFO or a small PDA (i.e., simple TGA). Dynamic obstruction of the LV outflow tract (i.e., subpulmonary obstruction), which results from bowing of the ventricular septum to the left because of a greater RV pressure, occurs in about 20% of the patients. Anatomic subpulmonary stenosis or abnormal mitral chordal attachment rarely cause obstruction of the LV outflow tract.

3. VSD is present in 30% to 40% of the patients with D-TGA and may be located anywhere in the ventricular septum. A combination of VSD and significant obstruction of the LV outflow tract occurs in about 10% of all patients with D-TGA. The LV outflow trait obstruction occurs in about 30% of patients with both D-TGA and VSD. Other associated defects are more common in infants with associated VSD than in those without. Such associated defects include COA, interrupted aortic arch, pulmonary atresia and an overriding or straddling of the AV valve.*

---

* Overriding is an abnormal relationship between the AV valve annulus and the ventricular septum. The AV valve annulus commits to both ventricular chambers, and it is the result of malalignment of the atrial and ventricular septa. Straddling is present when the chordae tendinea insert into the contralateral ventricle through a septal defect. Type A straddling is a mild form in which chordae insert near the crest of the ventricular septum. In type B the insertion is along the ventricular septum. In type C straddling chordae insert onto the free wall of the contralateral ventricle. Overriding and straddling may occur independently or coexist in the same valve.

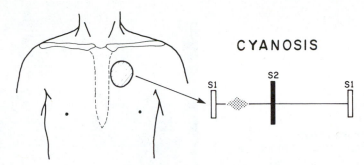

FIG. 14–1
Cardiac findings of TGA. Heart murmur is usually absent, and the S_2 is single in the majority of patients.

4. The classic complete TGA is called *D-transposition in* which the aorta is located anteriorly and to the right of the PA. This is why the prefix *D* is used. When the transposed aorta is located to the left of the PA, it is called *L-transposition* (see Fig. 16-4 on p. 254).

Clinical Manifestations
History.

1. History of cyanosis from birth is always present.

2. Signs of CHF with dyspnea and feeding difficulties develop during the newborn period.

Physical examination (Fig. 14-1).

1. Moderate to severe cyanosis is present, especially in large, male newborns. Such an infant is tachypneic but without retraction unless CHF supervenes.

2. The S2 is single and loud. No heart murmur is heard in infants with an intact ventricular septum. A systolic (regurgitant) murmur of VSD may be audible in less cyanotic infants with associated VSD. A soft systolic ejection murmur (SEM) of PS may be audible.

3. If CHF supervenes, hepatomegaly and dyspnea develop.

Laboratory studies.

1. Severe arterial hypoxemia with or without acidosis is present. Hypoxemia does not respond to oxygen inhalation.

2. Hypoglycemia and hypocalcemia are occasionally present.

Electrocardiography.

1. There is a rightward QRS axis (i.e., +90 to +200 degrees).

2. RVH is usually present after the first few days of life. After 3 days of life, an upright T wave in V1 may be the only abnormality suggestive of RVH.

3. CVH may be present in infants with large VSD, PDA, or PVOD because all of these conditions produce an additional LVH.

4. Occasionally RAH may be present.

X-ray studies.

1. Cardiomegaly with increased pulmonary vascularity is usually present.

2. An egg-shaped cardiac silhouette with a narrow, superior mediastinum is characteristic (Fig. 14-2).

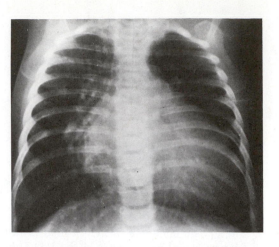

FIG. 14–2
A PA view of the chest roentgenogram from a 2-month-old infant with D-TGA. Note cardiomegaly (cardiothoracic ratio of 0.7), "egg-shaped" heart with narrow waist, and increased pulmonary vascular markings, which are characteristic of this condition.

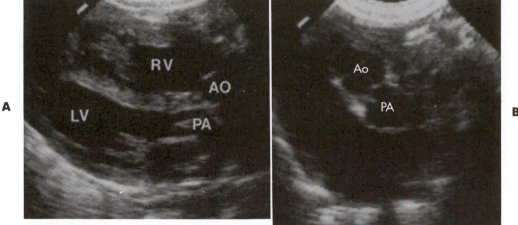

FIG. 14–3
Parasternal echo views in D-TGA. **A,** In this parasternal long-axis view, the great arteries are seen in parallel alignment. The posterior artery is directed posteriorly, bifurcates into two branches, and is therefore a PA. **B,** In the parasternal short-axis view, the aorta (AO) and the PA are seen in cross section as double circles. (From Snider AR, Serwer GA: *Echocardiography in pediatric heart disease,* St Louis, 1990 Mosby.)

Echocardiography. Two-dimensional echo and color-flow Doppler studies usually provide all the anatomic and functional information needed for the management of infants with D-TGA.

1. In the parasternal long-axis view, the posterior great artery has a sharp posterior angulation toward the lungs, which suggests that this artery is the PA (Fig. 14-3, *A*). In contrast to the normal intertwining of the great arteries, the proximal portion of the great arteries runs parallel.

2. In the parasternal short-axis view, the "circle and sausage" appearance of the normal great arteries is not visible. Instead, the great arteries appear as "double circles" (Fig. 14-3, *B*). The PA is in the center of the heart, and the coronary arteries do not arise from this great artery. The aorta is usually anterior and slightly to the right of the PA.

3. In the apical and subcostal five-chamber views the PA (i.e., the artery that bifurcates) arises from the LV, and the aorta arises from the RV.

4. The status of atrial communication, both before and after the balloon septostomy, is best evaluated in the subcostal view. Doppler examination and color-flow mapping should aid in the functional evaluation of the atrial shunt.

5. Frequently, associated defects such as VSD, LV outflow tract obstruction (dynamic or fixed), or pulmonary valve stenosis can be evaluated. Subaortic stenosis or COA rarely occurs.

6. The coronary arteries can be imaged in most patients by using parasternal and apical views (Fig. 14-4).

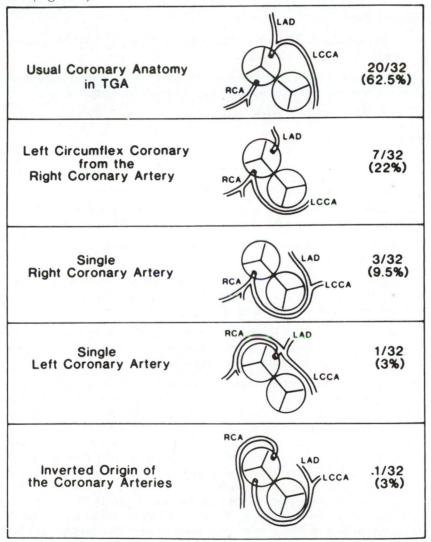

FIG. 14—4
Diagram of the coronary artery anatomy in 32 patients with TGA. The orientation of the figures is that of a parasternal short-axis echo view. *LAD,* Left anterior descending artery; *LCCA,* left circumflex coronary artery; *RCA,* right coronary artery. (From Pasquini L, Sanders SP, Parness IA et al: Diagnosis of coronary artery anatomy by two-dimensional echocardiography in patients with transposition of the great arteries, *Circulation* 75:557-564, 1987).

Natural History

1. Progressive hypoxia and acidosis result in death unless the mixing of the systemic and pulmonary blood improves. CHF develops in the first weeks of life. Without surgical intervention, death occurs in 90% of patients before they reach 6 months of age.

2. Infants with intact ventricular septum are the sickest group, but demonstrate the most dramatic improvement after the Rashkind balloon atrial septostomy. These infants have a tendency to develop PVOD at an earlier age than those with other forms of CHD, making surgical repair necessary during early infancy.

3. Infants with VSD are the least cyanotic group but the most likely to develop CHF and PVOD. Many infants with TGA + large VSD develop moderate PVOD by 3 to 4 months of age. Thus surgical procedures are recommended before reaching that age.

4. Infants with a significant PDA are similar to those with a large VSD, in terms of their development of CHF and PVOD.

5. The combination of VSD and PS allows considerably longer survival without surgery, but this combination carries a high surgical risk for correction.

6. Cerebrovascular accident is rarely a complication.

Management
  Medical.

1. The following measures should be carried out before an emergency cardiac catheterization (if performed) or a surgical procedure:

   a. Arterial blood gases and pH should be obtained, and a hyperoxitest should be carried out (see Chapter 29) to confirm the presence of a cyanotic CHD.

   b. Metabolic acidosis should be corrected, and hypoglycemia and/or hypocalcemia should be treated.

   c. Prostaglandin E_1 infusion should be started to improve arterial oxygen saturation by reopening the ductus. This should be continued throughout the cardiac catheterization and until the time of surgery.

   d. Oxygen should be administered for severe hypoxia. Oxygen may help lower pulmonary vascular resistance (PVR) and increase PBF, as well as result in the increase of systemic arterial oxygen saturation.

2. Before surgery, cardiac catheterization and a balloon atrial septostomy (i.e., the Rashkind procedure) are often carried out to have some flexibility in planning surgery. If adequate interatrial communication exists and the anatomic diagnosis of TGA is clear by echo examination, the patient may go to surgery without cardiac catheterization or the balloon atrial septostomy. In the balloon atrial septostomy a balloon-tipped catheter is advanced into the LA through the patent foramen ovale. The balloon is inflated with diluted radiopaque dye and abruptly withdrawn to the RA under fluoroscopic or echo monitoring. This procedure creates a large defect in the atrial septum through which the intracardiac mixing occurs. It carries a minimal complication rate and often improves the arterial oxygen saturation. An increase in the oxygen saturation of 10% or more and a minimal interatrial pressure gradient are considered satisfactory results of the procedure.

3. For older infants and those for whom the initial balloon atrial septostomy was only temporarily successful, blade atrial septostomy may be performed. This procedure widens the interatrial communication by cutting it with a surgical blade built in a catheter and then repeating the balloon procedure.

4. CHF may be treated with digoxin and diuretics.

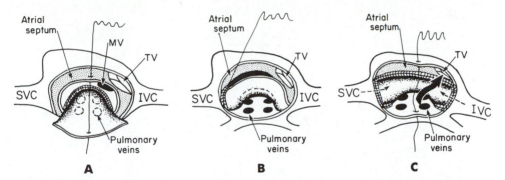

FIG. 14–5
The Mustard operation viewed through an incision made on the RA free wall. **A,** Atrial septum *(dotted area)* has been excised at the site of ASD. A pericardial patch is placed in the LA in such a way to redirect pulmonary venous blood to the right atrium. The pulmonary veins *(four broken circles)* are seen under the baffle. The mitral valve *(MV)* and tricuspid valve *(TV)* are seen. *SVC,* Superior vena cava; *IVC,* inferior vena cava. **B,** The remaining edge of the pericardial baffle is reflected and sewn along the right margin of the openings of the SVC and IVC and to the anterior edge of the ASD. **C,** Atrial incision is closed. When completed, systemic venous blood from the SVC and IVC goes to the anatomical left atrium and the MV. Pulmonary venous blood *(heavy arrow)* goes to the TV.

Surgical.

Palliative procedure. The Blalock-Hanlon operation, involving a surgical excision of the posterior aspect of the atrial septum without cardiopulmonary bypass, is now only rarely performed. It used to be performed when the Rashkind procedure and blade atrial septostomy failed to increase arterial oxygen saturation. The mortality rate of this procedure is too high (i.e., 10% to 25%) to justify routine use.

Definitive repairs. Definitive surgeries performed for TGA are procedures that switch right- and left-sided blood at three levels. These levels included the following: the atrial level (the intraatrial repair surgeries such as the Senning or Mustard operations), the ventricular level (the Rastelli operation), and the great artery level (arterial switch operation or the Jatene operation). The Damus-Kaye-Stansel operation in conjunction with the Rastelli operation can be used in patients with VSD and subaortic stenosis.

Procedures and their complications.

1. The following are intraatrial repair operations:

    a. The Mustard operation: This oldest form of surgical technique redirects the pulmonary and systemic venous return at the atrial level by using either a pericardial or prosthetic baffle (Fig. 14-5).

    b. The Senning operation: This is a modification of the Mustard operation. It uses the atrial septal flap and the RA free wall to redirect the pulmonary and systemic venous return (Fig. 14-6).

    c. Complications of intraatrial repair surgeries: Numerous early and late complications may arise especially after the Mustard operation. Such complications include the following:
       (1) Obstruction to the pulmonary venous return (<5% of all cases)
       (2) Obstruction to the systemic venous return (<5% of all cases)
       (3) Residual intraatrial baffle shunt (≤20% of all cases)
       (4) Tricuspid valve regurgitation (rarely occurs)
       (5) Absence of sinus rhythm (>50% of all cases) and frequent supraventricular arrhythmias

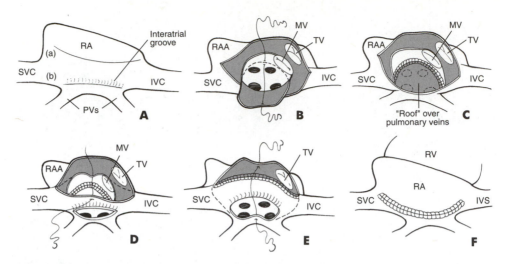

FIG. 14–6
The Senning operation. **A,** This procedure requires two incisions, *(a)* and *(b)*. The incision *(b)* is made along the left side of the interatrial groove. **B,** The initial procedure is performed through the opening created by incision *(a)*. An atrial septal flap is made. A patch closure of the ASD or alternative measures to augment the atrial septal flap is sometimes required. **C,** The atrial septal flap is sewn in the left atrium in such a way to direct pulmonary venous blood to the RA through an opening created by incision *(b)*. **D,** The posterior right atrial flap is then sewn to the atrial septum *(dotted lines)* and the anterior margin of the ASD in such a way to direct blood from the superior and inferior venae cavae to the anatomic LA. **E and F,** The anterior atrial flap is sewn to the RA free wall *(dotted lines)* and to the left atrial flap created by incision *(b)*. Patch augmentation may become necessary between the anterior atrial flap and the left atrial flap to provide enough room to the pulmonary venous blood pathway.

    (6) Depressed RV (i.e., systemic ventricular) function during exercise
    (7) Sudden death attributable to arrhythmias (3% of survivors)
    (8) PVOD

2. The Rastelli operation: In patients with VSD and severe PS, the redirection of the pulmonary and systemic venous blood is carried out at the ventricular level. The LV is directed to the aorta by creating an intraventricular tunnel between the VSD and the aortic valve. A conduit is placed between the RV and the PA (Fig. 14-7). Complications after the Rastelli operation include conduit obstruction (especially with those containing porcine heterograft valves) and complete heart block (rarely occurs).

3. Arterial switch operation (or the Jatene operation): The coronary arteries are transplanted to the PA, and the proximal great arteries are connected to the distal end of the other great artery, resulting in an anatomic correction (Fig. 14-8). This procedure has advantages over the intraatrial repair surgeries because it is a physiologic correction and results in fewer long-term complications such as arrhythmias, RV dysfunction, baffle stenosis, and TR. For patients with simple TGA, normal sinus rhythm is usually present, arrhythmias are extremely rare, and LV function is normal. However, PA stenosis at the site of reconstruction occurs in 5% to 10% of cases; complete heart block occurs in 5% to 10%. AR is a late complication occurring in more than 20% of patients, especially in patients who already had PA banding. An important cause of AR may be an unequal size of the pulmonary cusps that lead to eccentric coaptation. This is present in most patients. Another early or late complication is coronary artery obstruction, which may lead to myocardial ischemia, infarction, and even death (see Chapter 27, Appendix A, and Fig. AA-3).

The following factors are important for a successful arterial switch operation and should be carefully evaluated when selecting cases.

a. LV that can support the systemic circulation after surgery must exist. The LV pressure should be near systemic levels at the time of surgery, or the switch should be performed shortly after birth (i.e., before 2 weeks of age). In patients whose LV pressure is low, LV pressure can be raised by a PA banding either with or without a shunt, for 7 to 10 days (in cases of rapid, two-stage switch operation) or for 5 to 9 months before undertaking the switch operation. LV pressure greater than 85% and LV posterior wall thickness greater than 4.5 mm appear to be satisfactory.

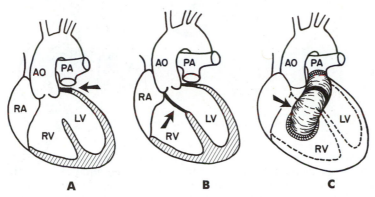

FIG. 14–7
The Rastelli operation. **A,** The PA is divided from the LV, and the cardiac end is oversewn *(arrow).* **B,** An intracardiac tunnel *(arrow)* is placed between the large VSD and the aorta so that the LV communicates with the aorta. **C,** The RV is connected to the divided PA by an aortic homograft or a valve-bearing prosthetic conduit. *RA,* Right atrium; *AO,* aorta.

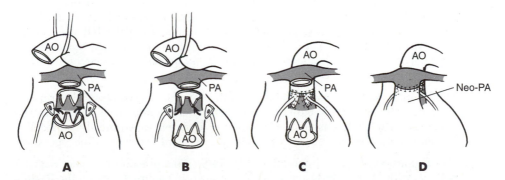

FIG. 14–8
Arterial switch operation. **A,** The aorta is transected slightly above the coronary ostia, and the PA is also transected at about the same level. The ascending aorta is lifted, and both coronary arteries are removed from the aorta with triangular buttons **B,** Triangular buttons of similar size are made at the proper position in the PA trunk. **C,** The coronary arteries are transplanted to the PA. The ascending aorta is brought behind the PA and is connected to the proximal PA, to form a neoaorta. **D,** The triangular defects in the proximal aorta are repaired, and the proximal aorta is connected to the PA. Note that the neo-PA is in front of the neoaorta.

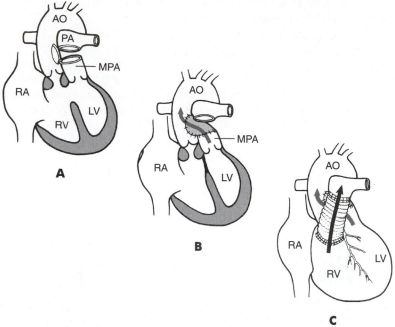

FIG. 14–9
Damus-Kaye-Stansel operation for D-TGA + VSD + subaortic stenosis. **A,** D-TGA with VSD and subaortic stenosis are illustrated. The main pulmonary artery is transected near its bifurcation. An appropriately positioned and sized incision is made in the ascending aorta. **B,** The proximal main pulmonary artery is anastomosed end-to-side to the ascending aorta using either a Dacron tube or Gore-Tex. This channel will direct LV blood to the aorta. The aortic valve is either closed or left unclosed. **C,** Through a right ventriculotomy, the VSD is closed, and a valved conduit is placed between the RV and the distal PA. This channel will carry RV blood to the PA.

   b. There must be a coronary artery pattern amenable to transfer to the neoaorta without distortion or kinking. Most coronary artery patterns in TGA are amenable to the arterial switch operation, but the risk is high when the left main or left anterior descending coronary artery passes anteriorly between the aorta and the PA. Such a situation is usually accompanied by an intramural course of the artery in the aortic wall.

   c. The LV inflow and outflow tracts must be free of significant structural abnormality. Patients with severe LV outflow tract obstruction should have a Rastelli-type operation. Mild pulmonary valve stenosis or dynamic or surgically remediable subpulmonary stenosis do not preclude a successful arterial switch operation.

   d. The Damus-Kaye-Stansel operation (Fig. 14-9): This procedure is necessary for patients with TGA + VSD and subaortic stenosis in conjunction with the Rastelli procedure. In this procedure, the subaortic stenosis is bypassed by connecting the proximal PA trunk to the ascending aorta. The VSD is closed and a conduit is placed between the RV and the distal PA. The Damus-Kaye-Stansel operation is also applicable in patients with single ventricle + TGA with an obstructive bulboventricular foramen or DORV with a subaortic stenosis (see Fig. 14-52). A procedure that supplies blood flow to the lungs is necessary (e.g., a bidirectional cavopulmonary shunt, a systemic-PA shunt, a Fontan-type operation).

Surgical Procedures for Transposition of the Great Arteries

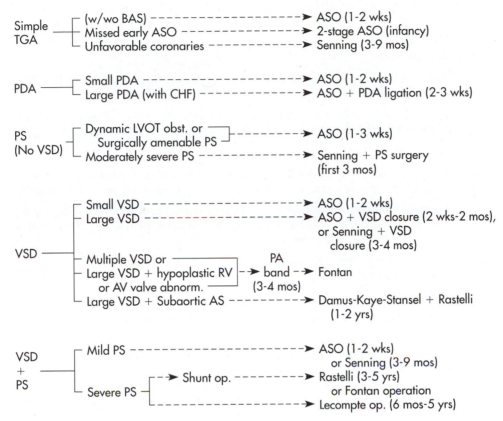

FIG. 14–10
Management flow diagram for TGA (see text for discussion). *ASO,* Arterial switch operation (Jatene operation); *BAS,* balloon atrial septostomy; *LVOT,* left ventricular outflow tract; *PS,* pulmonary stenosis.

PREFERRED PROCEDURE, TIMING, AND MORTALITY. Preferred procedure, timing, and mortality vary greatly from institution to institution and are subject to change with the development of new information and new procedures. The intraatrial repair surgeries have had extensive experiences and carry a high incidence of early and late complications. The arterial switch operation is considered the procedure of choice by most centers. The following is a partial list of popular approaches according to the anatomic complexity (Fig. 14-10).

1. Infants with simple TGA (i.e., with intact ventricular septum):

   a. The arterial switch operation is the procedure of choice in most centers and is preferably performed in the first 2 weeks of life and definitely before 4 weeks of age. Early surgical mortality occurs about 2% to 5% of the time. The overall 5-year survival after the arterial switch operation occurs 82% of the time.

b. If the opportunity for an early arterial switch is missed (i.e., after 1 month of age), a two-stage procedure can be performed. This procedure involves PA banding, with or without a shunt, followed by the switch operation.

c. Between 3 and 9 months of age, infants who have an unfavorable coronary anatomy may receive an intraatrial repair by means of either the Senning or Mustard procedure.

2. Infants with PDA:

a. Infants with a small PDA are handled in the same way as infants with intact ventricular septum.

b. Infants with a large PDA and CHF require the arterial switch operation and PDA ligation within the first 2 to 3 weeks. The mortality rate is less than 5%.

3. Infants with PS:

a. Infants with dynamic LV outflow tract obstruction should receive the arterial switch operation. This type of obstruction resolves itself after the switch surgery.

b. Infants with mild structural narrowing at the pulmonary valve or subvalvar region, which is surgically remediable, can have the arterial switch operation with a surgical risk similar to that for simple TGA.

c. Infants with more severe PS may receive the Senning operation and surgical relief of PS by 3 months of age.

4. Infants with VSD:

a. Infants with a small VSD may be handled in the same way as infants with simple TGA.

b. For infants with a large VSD, many centers prefer the arterial switch operation and VSD closure without PA banding between 2 weeks and 2 months of age. The mortality rate for this procedure is about 5%. As an alternative, the Senning operation + VSD closure can be carried out without PA banding at 3 to 4 months of age, but this approach is less desirable.

c. Infants with multiple VSDs, however, may receive a PA banding by 3 to 4 months of age. A Fontan-type operation is then performed at a later date.

d. For infants with large VSD and associated subaortic stenosis, the Damus-Kaye-Stansel operation and the Rastelli operation can be performed at 1 to 2 years of age. The mortality rate has been considerable, ranging from 15% to 30%.

e. Infants with large VSD and hypoplastic RV or straddling AV valve cannot be candidates for the arterial switch operation or the Senning operation. They can have a PA banding initially and a Fontan-type operation later.

5. Infants with VSD + PS:

a. Infants with a VSD and mild PS that may be fixed surgically can be treated like infants with a large VSD, or they may receive the Senning operation between 3 and 9 months of age.

b. Infants with a large VSD and severe PS may need a systemic-PA shunt surgery during infancy (see Fig. 14-20). The Rastelli operation can be performed at 3 to 5 years of age. The recent mortality rate is less than 5% for the Rastelli operation. Alternatively, a Fontan-type operation can be performed between 2 and 4 years of age.

c. For infants with a large VSD and severe PS, the Lecompte intraventricular repair can be performed between the ages of 6 months and 5 years. The mortality rate is less than 5%. In this operation the LV is connected to the aorta, and the RV is connected to the PA by a technique that does not require an extracardiac conduit (Fig. 14-11).

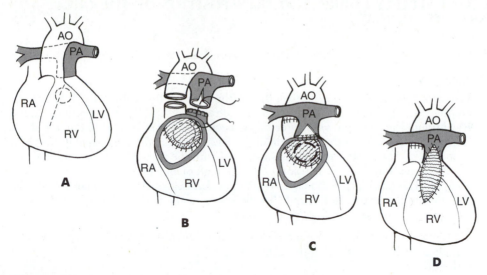

FIG. 14–11
The Lecompte operation. **A,** Anatomy of D-TGA is shown. A right ventriculotomy is made along the vertical heavy, broken line. Note that the VSD is shown as a broken circle. **B,** Through the right ventriculotomy, the VSD has been enlarged, and the resection of the infundibular septum has been accomplished *(broken circle).* A Dacron patch is sewn into place in such a way to connect the LV and the aorta (to create an LV-Aorta pathway). The aorta *(AO)* and PA trunk *(PA)* are transected. The proximal segment of the pulmonary trunk is sutured. The distal pulmonary trunk is enlarged by an anterior vertical incision. **C,** The aorta is repositioned behind the PA bifurcation and reconstructed. The posterior lip of the distal segment of the PA is anastomosed to the superior end of the right ventriculotomy. This forms the floor of the RV-PA pathway. **D,** A Dacron patch is placed over the right ventriculotomy and the anterior aspect of the distal segment of the pulmonary trunk, as a roof over the RV-PA pathway. A monocusp valve is placed beneath the patch.

Postoperative follow-up

POSTOPERATIVE SENNING/MUSTARD OPERATION. Follow-up every 6 to 12 months is recommended in order to detect arrhythmias, sick sinus syndrome, TR, or depressed RV function.

1. Atrial arrhythmias are quite common (occurring in more than 50% of all cases) and rarely causes late, sudden death (occurring in 3 to 5% of all cases). Arrhythmias include ectopic atrial tachycardia, sick sinus syndrome with a slow nodal rate, and AV conduction disturbances. Permanent pacemaker implantation and antiarrhythmic agents may be needed to treat bradytachyarrhythmias.

2. TR may worsen with time, and afterload reducing agents may be needed.

3. Depressed RV (i.e., systemic ventricle) function during exercise often begins years after surgery and may require restriction of activities. Some of these patients require diuretics, anticongestive medications, and antiarrhythmic agents years after surgery.

POSTSWITCH PATIENTS. Although the complication rate is much lower than with intraatrial repair, a regular follow-up is needed to detect stenosis of the PA or aorta in the supravalvar regions; coronary artery obstruction with myocardial ischemia or infarction, ventricular dysfunction, and/or arrhythmias; and semilunar valve regurgitation. These complications are, for the most part, hemodynamically insignificant or infrequent.

CONGENITALLY CORRECTED TRANSPOSITION OF THE GREAT ARTERIES (L-TGA)

Prevalence

L-TGA (or ventricular inversion) occurs in fewer than 1% of all patients with CHDs.

Pathology

1. Visceroatrial relationship is normal; that is, the RA is to the right of the LA. The RA empties into the anatomic LV through the mitral valve, and the LA empties into the RV through the tricuspid valve. For this to occur, the RV is located to the left of the LV, and the LV is located to the right of the RV, which is called *ventricular inversion* (Fig. 14-12). The great arteries are transposed with the aorta rising from the RV and the PA rising from the LV. The aorta is located left of and anterior to the PA (see Fig 16-4, *D*). The result is functional correction, in that oxygenated blood comes into the LA, goes to the anatomic RV, and then flows out of the aorta. This is why the term *corrected* is used to describe this condition.

2. Theoretically, no functional abnormalities exist, but unfortunately, most cases are complicated by associated intracardiac defects, AV conduction disturbances, and arrhythmias.

   a. VSD occurs in 80% of all cases.

   b. PS, both valvar and subvalvar, occurs in 50% of patients and is usually associated with VSD.

   c. Systemic AV valve (tricuspid) regurgitation occurs in 30% of patients.

   d. Both varying and progressive degrees of AV block and paroxysmal supraventricular tachycardia are frequently found.

3. The cardiac apex is in the right chest (dextrocardia) in about 50% of cases.

4. The coronary arteries show a mirror-image distribution. The right coronary artery supplies the anterior descending branch and gives rise to a circumflex; the left coronary artery resembles a right coronary artery.

Clinical Manifestations

History.

1. Patients are asymptomatic when L-TGA is not associated with other defects.

2. During the first months of life, most patients with associated defects become symptomatic with cyanosis resulting from VSD + PS, or CHF, resulting from large VSD.

FIG. 14–12
Diagram of congenitally corrected TGA (L-TGA). There is an inversion of ventricular chambers with their corresponding atrioventricular valves. The great arteries are transposed, but functional *correction* results, with oxygenated blood going to the aorta. Unfortunately, a high percentage of the patients with L-TGA have associated defects with resulting cyanosis.

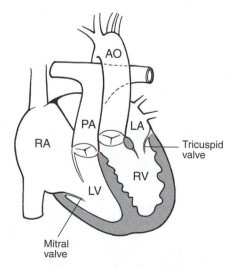

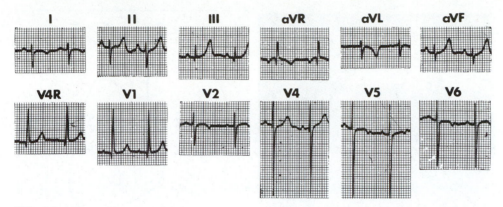

FIG. 14–13

Tracing from an 8-year-old girl with L-TGA, VSD, and PS. Note that no Q waves are seen in leads I, V5, and V6. Instead, the Q waves are seen in V4R and V1. This suggests ventricular inversion. The electrocardiogram also suggests hypertrophy of the right ventricle (anatomic LV).

3. Exertional dyspnea and easy fatigability may develop with systemic AV valve regurgitation.

Physical examination.

1. The patient is cyanotic if PS and VSD are present.

2. Hyperactive precordium occurs in the presence of a large VSD. Systolic thrill occurs in the presence of PS, with and without VSD.

3. The S2 is loud and single at the ULSB or URSB. A grade 2-4/6 harsh, regurgitant holosystolic murmur along the LLSB indicates the presence of VSD or systemic AV valve (tricuspid valve) regurgitation. A grade 2-3/6 ejection systolic murmur is present at the ULSB or URSB if PS is present. An apical diastolic rumble may be present because of large VSD or significant TR.

Electrocardiography.

1. The absence of Q waves in I, V5, and V6 and/or the presence of Q waves in V4R or V1 is characteristic of the condition (Fig. 14-13). This is because the direction of ventricular septal depolarization is from the embryonic LV to RV.

2. Varying degrees of AV block are common. First-degree AV block is present in 50% of patients. Second-degree AV block may progress to become complete heart block.

3. Atrial arrhythmias and WPW syndrome are occasionally present.

4. Atrial and/or ventricular hypertrophy may be present in complicated cases (see Fig. 14-13).

X-ray study.

1. Straight, left upper cardiac border, formed by the ascending aorta, is a characteristic finding (Fig. 14-14).

2. Cardiomegaly and increased PVMs are present when the condition is associated with VSD.

3. Pulmonary venous congestion and LAE may be seen with severe AV valve regurgitation.

4. Positional abnormalities (e.g., dextrocardia, mesocardia, and so on) may be present.

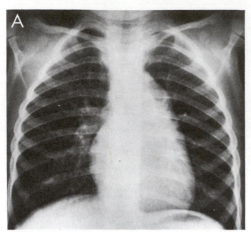
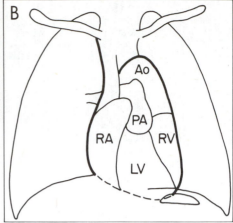

FIG. 14–14
A posteroanterior view of actual **(A)** and a diagram **(B)** of chest roentgenogram from a
10-year-old child with L-TGA. Note the straight left cardiac border formed by the
ascending aorta.

Echocardiography. By the use of the segmental approach (see Chapter 16), diagnosis
of L-TGA can be made easily, and associated anomalies can be detected and quantitated.

1. The parasternal long-axis view is obtained from a more vertical and leftward scan
   than with a normal heart. The aorta, which arises from the posterior ventricle, is
   not in fibrous continuity with the AV valve.

2. In the parasternal short-axis scanning, a "double circle" is imaged instead of the
   normal "circle and sausage" pattern. The posterior circle is the PA without
   demonstrable coronary arteries. The aorta is usually anterior to and left of the PA.
   The LV, which has two well-defined papillary muscles, is seen anteriorly and on
   the right and is connected to the characteristic "fish mouth" appearance of the
   mitral valve.

3. In the apical and subcostal four-chamber views the LA is connected to the tricuspid
   valve with a more apical attachment to the ventricular septum, and the RA is
   connected to the mitral valve. The anterior artery (aorta) arises from the left-sided
   morphologic RV, and the posterior artery with bifurcation (PA) arises from the
   right-sided morphologic LV.

4. The situs solitus of the atria is confirmed by the drainage of systemic veins (i.e.,
   IVC, SVC) into the right-sided atrium and the drainage of pulmonary veins into
   the left-sided atrium.

5. The following associated abnormalities should be looked for and their functional
   significance should be assessed by the Doppler technique and color-flow mapping:
   type and severity of PS, size and location of VSD, straddling of the AV valve.

Natural History

The clinical course is determined by the presence or absence of associated defects and
complications.

1. Some palliative surgeries are usually needed in infancy when L-TGA is associated
   with other defects, for example, PA banding for large VSD or a systemic-PA shunt
   for PS. Without these procedures 20% to 30% of patients die in the first year. CHF
   is the most common cause of death.

2. Regurgitation of the systemic AV valve (i.e., tricuspid valve) develops in about 30% of patients. This often happens as a result of dysplastic or Ebstein-like valves.

3. Progressive AV conduction disturbances may occur, including complete heart block in up to 30%. These disturbances occur more often in patients without VSD than in those with VSD. Sudden death rarely occurs.

4. Occasionally adult patients without major associated defects are asymptomatic.

Management
Medical.

1. Treatment with anticongestive agents is necessary if CHF develops.

2. Antiarrhythmic agents are used for arrhythmias.

3. Prophylaxis against SBE should be observed when indications arise.

Surgical.
Palliative procedures

1. A PA banding may be needed for uncontrollable CHF.

2. Systemic-PA shunt is necessary for patients with severe PS (usually associated with VSD).

Definitive procedures

1. Closure of VSD is indicated when the defect is associated with VSD. Complete heart block is a complication of the surgery occurring in 10% to 20% of the time. The mortality rate is 5% to 10%, which is higher than that for a simple VSD.

2. Corrective surgery for VSD + PS is more difficult, with a higher mortality rate (i.e., 10% to 15%) than closure of VSD alone. A conduit between the LV and the MPA is often necessary to repair PS.

3. Valve replacement for significant TR is required in about 15% of patients.

4. Pacemaker implantation is required for either spontaneous or postoperative complete heart block.

Postoperative follow-up.

1. Follow-up every 6 to 12 months is required for a possible progression of AV conduction disturbances or worsening of anatomic tricuspid valve regurgitation.

2. Antibiotic prophylaxis against SBE should be reminded.

3. Routine pacemaker care, if a pacemaker is implanted, should be conducted.

4. Activity restriction is indicated if significant hemodynamic abnormalities persist.

TETRALOGY OF FALLOT
Prevalence

TOF occurs in 10% of all CHDs. This is the most common cyanotic heart defect seen in children beyond infancy.

Pathology

1. The original description of TOF included the following four abnormalities: a large VSD, RV outflow tract obstruction, RVH, and an overriding of the aorta. In actuality only two abnormalities are required—a VSD large enough to equalize pressures in both ventricles and an RV outflow tract obstruction. The RV hypertrophy is secondary to the RV outflow tract obstruction and to VSD. The overriding of the aorta varies (Fig. 14-15).

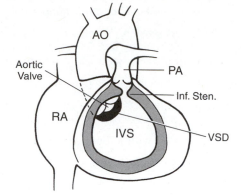

FIG. 14–15
Diagram of TOF. A large subaortic VSD is present through which aortic cusps are visualized. There is PS, which is either infundibular, valvular, or a combination. The RV muscle is hypertrophied. *IVS*, interventricular septum.

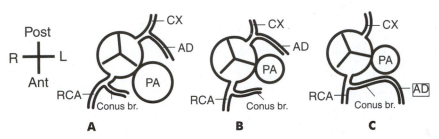

FIG. 14–16
Schema of coronary arteries in TOF. **A,** Normal. **B,** TOF with normal coronary arteries. **C,** Tetralogy with anterior descending *(AD)* from right coronary artery *(RCA)*. *CX*, Circumflex artery.

2. The VSD in TOF is a perimembranous defect with extention into the subpulmonary region.

3. The RV outflow tract obstruction is most frequently in the form of infundibular stenosis (45%). The obstruction is rarely at the pulmonary valve level (10%). A combination of the two may also occur (30%). The pulmonary valve is atretic in the most severe form of the anomaly (15%). In some children, pulmonary atresia develops with time.

4. The pulmonary annulus and MPA are hypolastic in most patients. The PA branches are usually small with variable peripheral stenosis. Obstruction at the origin of the left PA is particularly common. Systemic collateral arteries feeding into the lungs are occasionally present, especially more often seen with severe cases of TOF.

5. Right aortic arch is present in 25% of the cases.

6. In about 5% of TOF patients, abnormal coronary arteries are present. The most common abnormality is when the anterior descending branch arises from the right coronary artery and passes over the RV outflow tract, which prohibits a surgical incision in the region (Fig. 14-16).

Clinical Manifestations
  History.
1. A heart murmur is audible at birth.

2. Most patients are symptomatic with cyanosis at birth. Dyspnea on exertion, squatting, or hypoxic spells develop later in mildly cyanotic infants.

3. Infants with *acyanotic* TOF may be asymptomatic or may show signs of CHF from a large left-to-right ventricular shunt.

4. Immediately after birth severe cyanosis is seen in patients with TOF and pulmonary atresia.

Physical examination (Fig. 14-17).

1. Varying degrees of cyanosis, tachypnea, and clubbing are present.

2. RV tap along the left sternal border and a systolic thrill at the upper and middle LSBs are commonly present (50%).

3. An ejection click that originates in the aorta may be audible. The S2 is usually single, since only the aortic component may be heard. A long, loud (i.e., grade 3-5/6) systolic ejection murmur is heard at the middle and upper LSBs. This murmur may be easily confused with the holosystolic regurgitant murmur of a VSD. The more severe the obstruction of the RV outflow tract, the shorter and softer the systolic murmur. Occasionally, a continuous murmur representing a PDA shunt may be audible in a deeply cyanotic neonate (with TOF with pulmonary atresia).

4. In the acyanotic form a long systolic murmur, resulting from VSD and infundibular stenosis, is audible along the entire LSB, and cyanosis is absent. Thus auscultatory findings resemble those of a small-shunt VSD, but the ECG shows RVH or CVH.

Electrocardiography.

1. RAD (+120 to +150 degrees) is present in cyanotic TOF. In the acyanotic form the QRS axis is normal.

2. RVH is usually present, but the strain pattern is unusual. CVH may be seen in the acyanotic form. RAH is occasionally present.

X-ray study.
Cyanotic TOF.

1. The heart size is normal or smaller than normal, and PVMs are decreased. "Black" lung fields are seen in TOF with pulmonary atresia.

2. A concave MPA segment with an upturned apex (i.e., "boot-shaped" heart or coeur en sabot) is characteristic (Fig. 14-18).

3. RAE (25%) and right aortic arch (25%) may be present.

Acyanotic TOF. X-ray findings of acyanotic TOF are indistinguishable from those of a small to moderate VSD, but patients with TOF have RVH rather than LVH on the ECG.

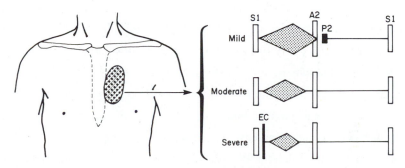

FIG. 14–17
Cardiac findings in cyanotic TOF. A long SEM at the MLSB and ULSB, and a loud, single S2 are characteristic auscultatory findings of TOF.

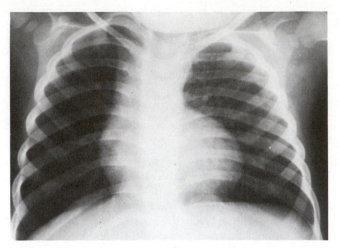

FIG. 14–18
A posteroanterior view of chest roentgenogram in TOF. The heart size is normal, and
pulmonary vascular markings are decreased. A hypoplastic MPA segment contributes to
the formation of the "boot-shaped" heart.

Echocardiography. Two-dimensional echo and Doppler studies can make the
diagnosis and quantitate the severity of TOF.

1. A large, perimembranous infundibular VSD and overriding of the aorta are imaged
   in the parasternal long-axis view (Fig. 14-19).

2. Anatomy of the RV outflow tract, the pulmonary valve, the pulmonary annulus, the
   MPA, and its branches are imaged in the parasternal short-axis view.

3. Doppler studies estimate the pressure gradient across the obstruction.

4. With pulmonary atresia, a *vertical* ductus can be imaged showing the direction of flow
   from the aorta to the PA (see Fig. 14-22).

5. Anomalous coronary artery distribution can be imaged or suspected (see Fig. 14-16).

6. Associated anomalies such as ASD and persistence of the left SVC can be imaged.

Natural History

1. Infants with acyanotic TOF gradually become cyanotic. Patients who are already
   cyanotic become more cyanotic as a result of the worsening condition of the
   infundibular stenosis and polycythemia.

2. Hypoxic spells may develop in infants (see Chapter 11).

3. Some patients, particularly those with severe TOF, develop AR.

4. Growth retardation may be present if cyanosis is severe.*

5. Brain abscess and cerebrovascular accident rarely occur (see Chapter 11).*

6. SBE is occasionally a complication.*

7. Polycythemia develops secondary to cyanosis.*

8. Physicians need to watch for the development of relative iron-deficiency (i.e.,
   hypochromic) anemia (see Chapter 11).*

---

* This occurs in all types of cyanotic CHD.

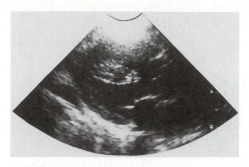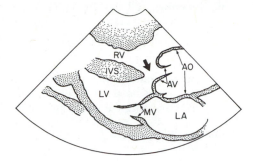

FIG. 14–19
Parasternal long-axis view in a patient with TOF. Note a large subaortic VSD *(arrow)* and a relatively large aorta *(AO)* overriding the interventricular septum *(IVS)*. *AV,* Aortic valve; *MV,* mitral valve.

9. Coagulopathy is a late complication of a long-standing cyanosis.

Hypoxic Spell

Hypoxic spell (i.e., cyanotic spell, "tet" spell) of TOF requires immediate recognition and appropriate treatment, since it can lead to serious complications of the central nervous system.

Hypoxic spells are characterized by a paroxysm of hyperpnea (i.e., *rapid* and *deep* respiration), irritability and prolonged crying, increasing cyanosis, and decreasing intensity of the heart murmur. The hypoxic spells occur in infants. The peak incidence of hypoxic spells is found between 2 and 4 months of age. These spells usually occur in the morning after crying, feeding, or defecation. A severe spell may lead to limpness, convulsion, cerebrovascular accident, or even death. There appears to be no relationship between the degree of cyanosis at rest and the likelihood of having hypoxic spells (see Chapter 11).

Treatment of the hypoxic spell strives to break the vicious cycle of the spell (see Fig. 11-9). Physicians may use one or more of the following to treat the spell:*

1. The infant should be picked up and held over the shoulder, or the infant should be held in a knee-chest position with or without a forearm behind the knees.

2. Morphine sulfate, at 0.2 mg/kg administered subcutaneously or intramuscularly, suppresses the respiratory center and abolishes hyperpnea.

3. Oxygen is usually administered, but it has little demonstrable effect on arterial oxygen saturation.

4. Acidosis should be treated with sodium bicarbonate ($NaHCO_3$), at 1 mEq/kg administered intravenously. The same dose may be repeated in 10 to 15 minutes. $NaHCO_3$ reduces the respiratory center–stimulating effect of acidosis. With the previous treatments, the infant usually becomes less cyanotic, and the heart murmur becomes louder, which indicates increased PBF through the stenotic RV outflow tract.

If the hypoxic spells do not fully respond to these measures, the following medications may be tried:*

5. Vasoconstrictors such as phenylephrine (Neo-Synephrine), at 0.02 mg/kg administered intravenously, may be effective.

---

* Treatments are listed in decreasing order of preference.

6. Ketamine, at 1 to 3 mg/kg (average of 2 mg/kg) administered intravenously over 60 seconds, works well. It increases the SVR and sedates the infant.

7. Propranolol, at 0.01 to 0.25 mg/kg (average 0.05 mg/kg) administered by slow intravenous push, reduces the heart rate and may reverse the spell.

8. Oral propranolol therapy, at 2 to 6 mg/kg/day administered in three to four divided doses, may be used to prevent the recurrence of hypoxic spells and to delay corrective surgical procedures in high-risk patients.

Management
Medical.

1. Physicians should recognize and treat hypoxic spells (see Chapter 11). It is important to educate parents to recognize the spell and what to do.

2. Oral propranolol therapy, at 0.5 to 1.5 mg/kg every 6 hours, is occasionally used to prevent hypoxic spells while waiting for an optimal time for corrective surgery.

3. Balloon dilatation of the RV outflow tract and pulmonary valve, though not widely practiced, has been attempted to delay repair for several months.

4. Maintenance of good dental hygiene and practice of antibiotic prophylaxis against SBE on indications are important (see Chapter 19).

5. Relative iron-deficiency anemia should be detected and treated. Anemic children are more susceptible to cerebrovascular accident. Normal hemoglobin or hematrocrit values or decreased red blood indices indicates iron-deficiency anemia in cyanotic patients.

Surgical.
Palliative shunt procedures.

INDICATIONS. Shunt procedures are performed to increase PBF. Indications vary from institution to institution. Indications may include the following, but many institutions prefer primary repair without a shunt operation regardless of the patient's age:

1. neonates with TOF and pulmonary atresia

2. infants with hypoplastic pulmonary annulus, which requires transanular patch for complete repair

3. children with hypoplastic PAs

4. severely cyanotic infants younger than 3 months of age

5. infants younger than 3 to 4 months old, who have medically unmanageable hypoxic spells

PROCEDURES, COMPLICATIONS, AND MORTALITY. Only Blalock-Taussig shunt and Gore-Tex interposition shunt (i.e., modified Blalock-Taussig) are performed at this time and have a surgical mortality rate of 1% or less.

1. Classic Blalock-Taussig shunt, anastomosed between the subclavian artery and the ipsilateral PA, may be the procedure of choice for infants older than 3 months (Fig. 14-20). A right-sided shunt is performed in patients with left aortic arch; a left-sided shunt is performed for right aortic arch.

2. Gore-Tex interposition shunt, placed between the subclavian artery and the ipsilateral PA, is the procedure of choice for small infants younger than 3 months and sometimes for older infants (see Fig. 14-20). A left-sided shunt is preferred for patients with left aortic arch, whereas a right-sided shunt is preferred for patients with right-sided aortic arch.

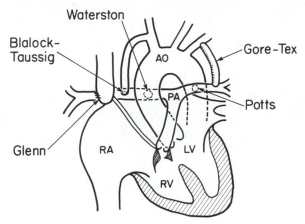

FIG. 14–20
Palliative procedures that can be used in patients with cyanotic cardiac defects with decreased PBF. The Glenn procedure (anastomosis between the superior vena cava and right PA) may be performed in older infants with hypoplastic RV, such as is seen with tricuspid atresia.

3. The Waterston shunt, anastomosed between the ascending aorta and the right PA, is no longer performed because of a high incidence of surgical complications (see Fig. 14-20). Complications resulting from this procedure include too large a shunt leading to CHF and/or pulmonary hypertension, and narrowing and kinking of the right PA at the site of the anastomosis. The latter creates difficult problems in closing the shunt and reconstructing the right PA at the time of corrective surgery.

4. The Potts operation, anastomosed between the descending aorta and the left PA, is no longer performed either (see Fig. 14-20). It may result in heart failure or pulmonary hypertension, as in the Waterston operation. A separate incision (i.e., left thoracotomy) is required to close the shunt during corrective surgery, which is performed through a midsternal incision.

Conventional repair surgery. Timing of this operation varies from institution to institution, but an early surgery is generally preferred.

Indications and timing.

1. Symptomatic infants who have favorable anatomy of the RV outflow tract and PAs may have primary repair at any time after 3 to 4 months of age. Some centers perform primary repair even in younger infants and newborns. Advantages cited for early primary repair include diminution of hypertrophy and fibrosis of the RV, the normal growth of PAs and alveolar units, and reduced incidence of postoperative ventricular ectopic beats and sudden death.

2. Asymptomatic and minimally cyanotic children may have repair between 3 and 24 months of age, depending on the degree of the annular and PA hypoplasia.

3. Mildly cyanotic infants who have had previous shunt surgery may have total repair 1 to 2 years after the shunt operation.

4. Asymptomatic and acyanotic children (i.e., "pink tet") have the operation at 1 to 2 years of age.

5. Asymptomatic children with coronary artery anomalies may have repair at 3 to 4 years of age, since a conduit may be required between the RV and the PA.

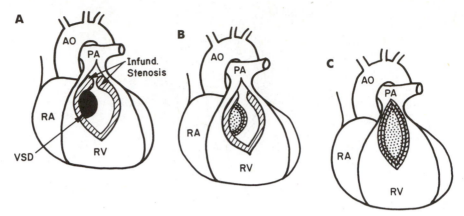

FIG. 14–21
Total correction of TOF. **A,** Anatomy of TOF showing a large VSD, infundibular stenosis, and hypoplasia of the pulmonary valve anulus. **B,** Patch closure of the VSD and resection of the infundibular stenosis. **C,** Placement of a fabric patch on the outflow tract of the RV.

PROCEDURE. Total repair of the defect is carried out under cardiopulmonary bypass and circulatory arrest. The procedure includes patch closure of the VSD and a widening of the RV outflow tract by resection of the infundibular tissue and placement of a fabric patch (Fig. 14-21).

MORTALITY. For patients with uncomplicated TOF, the mortality rate is 2% to 5% during the first 2 years. Patients at risk are those younger than 3 months and older than 4 years, as well as those with severe hypoplasia of the pulmonary annulus and trunk. Other risk factors include multiple VSDs, large aortopulmonary collateral arteries, and Down syndrome. For TOF with pulmonary atresia or other complicated anatomies, the mortality rate is higher (i.e., 5% to 20%).

COMPLICATIONS.

1. Bleeding problems that occur during the postoperative period, especially in older polycythemic patients.

2. Pulmonary valve regurgitation that is well-tolerated.

3. CHF, although usually transient, that may require anticongestive measures.

4. RBBB on the ECG, caused by right ventriculotomy, which occurs in over 90% of patients and is well tolerated.

5. Complete heart block (i.e., <1%) or ventricular arrhythmia are both rare

Rastelli operation.
PROCEDURE. Fig. 14-7 shows a schematic drawing of the procedure.

INDICATIONS, TIMING, AND MORTALITY. Patients with severe hypoplasia or atresia of the RV outflow tract and those with coronary artery anomalies may have the procedure performed at about 5 years of age at which time adult-sized homograft-valved conduits can be used. The mortality rate for this procedure is 10% or less.

Postoperative follow-up

1. A long-term follow-up with office examinations every 6 to 12 months is recommended, especially for patients with residual VSD shunt, residual obstruction of the RV outflow tract, residual PA obstruction, or arrhythmias or conduction disturbances.

2. Some children develop late arrhythmias, particularly ventricular tachycardia, which may result in sudden death. Arrhythmias are primarily related to persistent RVH as the result of unsatisfactory repair. Complaints of dizziness, syncope, or palpitation may suggest arrhythmias. A 24-hour Holter monitoring or exercise test may be needed.

3. Varying levels of activity limitation may be necessary.

4. For a patient who had TOF repair, SBE prophylaxis should be observed throughout life.

5. Children with sinus node dysfunction may require pacemaker therapy.

6. Pacemaker follow-up care is required for patients with implanted pacemakers secondary to surgically induced complete heart block or sinus node dysfunction.

TETRALOGY OF FALLOT WITH PULMONARY ATRESIA

Prevalence

Pulmonary atresia occurs in about 15% to 20% of patients with TOF.

Pathology

1. The intracardiac pathology resembles that of TOF in all respects except the presence of pulmonary atresia, the extreme form of RV outflow tract obstruction. The atresia may be at the infundibular or valvar level.

2. The PBF is most commonly mediated through PDA (70%) and less commonly through multiple systemic collaterals (30%). The ductus is small and long and arises from the left aortic arch at an acute angle (instead of the normal oblique junction) and the courses downward ("vertical" ductus) (Fig. 14-22).

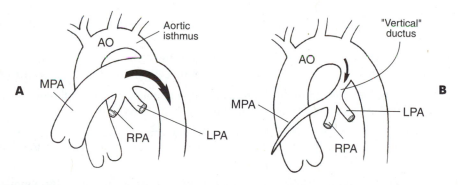

FIG. 14–22
Anatomy of the ductus arteriosus in pulmonary atresia. The size and the direction of the ductus arteriosus are different between a normal fetus and a fetus with pulmonary atresia. **A,** In a normal fetus, the ductus is large, since it transmits about 60% of combined ventricular output. It joins the aorta at an obtuse angle because flow is directed downward to the descending aorta. The aortic isthmus (the portion of the aorta between the left subclavian artery and the ductus) is narrower than the descending aorta. **B,** In pulmonary atresia, the ductus is small because flow to the descending aorta does not go through the ductus and because the lungs receive only about 15% of combined ventricular output. Furthermore, since flow is from the aorta to the PA, the connection of the ductus with the aorta has an acute inferior angle (sometimes called *vertical ductus*). The aortic isthmus has the same diameter as the descending aorta. This type of ductus arteriosus is also found in some patients with tricuspid atresia.

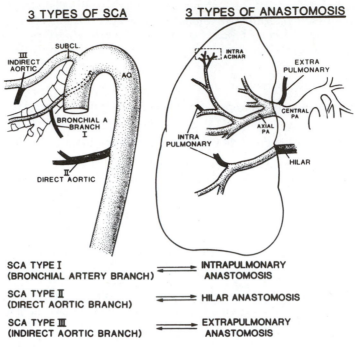

FIG. 14–23
The three types of systemic collateral artery *(SCA)* and three types of anastomosis with the PA. The characteristic pattern of anastomosis for each type of SCA is given. *SUBCL,* Subclavian; *AO,* aorta (From Rabinovitch M, Herzera-deLeon V, Castaneda AR et al: Growth and development of the pulmonary vascular bed in patients with tetralogy of Fallot with or without pulmonary atresia, *Circulation* 64:1234-1249, 1981.

3. PA anomalies are common in the form of hypoplasia, nonconfluence, and abnormal distribution.

   a. The central PA is hypoplastic in most patients with TOF + pulmonary atresia but more frequently in patients with only systemic collaterals than those with PDA.

   b. The central PAs are confluent in 85% of patients; they are nonconfluent in 15%. Confluent PAs are usually found in patients with PDAs (70%).

   c. Among patients with confluent PAs, 50% have incomplete arborization (distribution) of one or both PAs. About 80% of the patients with nonconfluent PAs have incomplete arborization.

4. Three types of systemic collaterals and their patterns of anastomosis with pulmonary circulation have been identified (Fig. 14-23). Some of these collateral circulations communicate with the central PA (i.e., dual blood supply). Others do not communicate with the central PA and are the sole supplier of the target pulmonary segments.

   a. *Bronchial artery branches* (type I) arise from one of the normal bronchial arteries, which originates in the ascending aorta, and makes an intrapulmonary anastomosis.

   b. *Direct aortic branches* (type II) may number 1 to 6 and are found in about two thirds of patients. They arise from the descending thoracic aorta and feed the pulmonary circulation through the hilar PAs. These collaterals occasionally take a tortuous course, but invariably have an obstruction within the collateral vessels

(Fig. 14-24). The central PA is smaller than found with the other types of systemic collaterals.

    c. *Indirect aortic branches* (type III) arise from branches of the aorta other than bronchial arteries such as subclavian, internal mammary, and intercostal arteries. They usually anastomose with the central PA.

Clinical Manifestations

1. These patients are cyanotic at birth. The degree of cyanosis depends on whether the ductus is patent and how extensive the systemic collateral arteries are.

2. Usually a heart murmur cannot be heard. However, a faint, continuous murmur may be audible from the PDA or collaterals. The S2 is loud and single. A systolic click is occasionally present.

3. The ECG shows RAD and RVH.

4. Chest x-ray images show a normal heart size, the heart often appears as a boot-shaped silhouette (see Fig. 14-18) and the pulmonary vascularity is markedly decreased (i.e., "black" lung field).

5. Echo studies show all anatomic findings of TOF plus absence of a direct connection between the RV and the PA. The branch PAs and the vertical ductus are well-imaged from a high-parasternal or suprasternal position (see Fig. 14-22).

Natural History

1. Without immediate attention to the establishment of PBF during the newborn period, most neonates who have this condition die during the first 2 years of life; however, infants with extensive collateral may survive for a long time, perhaps for more than 15 years.

2. Occasionally, patients with excessive collateral circulation develop hemoptysis during late childhood.

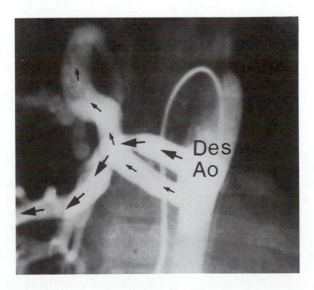

FIG. 14–24
A descending aortogram in a 6-year old child with TOF and pulmonary atresia. Two large collateral arteries (type II, direct aortic branch) arise from the descending aorta *(Des Ao)* to supply the right lung. The collateral arteries make hilar anastomoses. One of the collaterals *(thin arrows)* follows a tortuous course before making the anastomosis. Collateral arteries are not seen to the left lung, and there was no identifiable LPA.

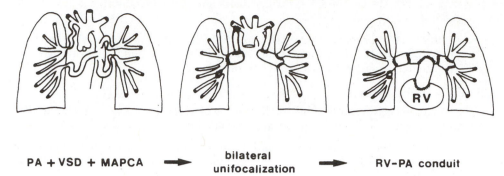

PA + VSD + MAPCA ➡ **bilateral unifocalization** ➡ **RV-PA conduit**

FIG. 14–25
Schematic drawing of the staged operation. *Left,* Typical systemic collateral arteries in TOF + pulmonary atresia *(PA)* with multiple aortopulmonary collateral arteries *(MAPCA).* *Middle,* Complete unifocalization in the first-stage surgery. *Right,* Second-stage repair in which a conduit is placed between a newly created central PA and the RV (Sawatari K et al: Staged operation for pulmonary atresia and ventricular septal defect with major aortopulmonary collateral arteries, *J Thorac Cardiovasc Surg* 98:738-750, 1989).

Management
Medical.

1. Prostaglandin E_1 infusion should be started as soon as the diagnosis is made or suspected to keep the ductus open for cardiac catheterization and to prepare for surgery. The starting dose of Prostin VR Pediatric solution is 0.05 to 0.1 µg/kg/min. When the desired effect is obtained, the dosage should be gradually reduced to 0.01 µg/kg/min.

2. Emergency cardiac catheterization is usually performed to delineate anatomy of the PAs and systemic arterial collaterals.

Surgical.

Single-stage repair. Complete, primary surgical repair in patients with TOF + pulmonary atresia is only possible when central PAs of adequate size exist (i.e., 50% of normal PA dimension) and the central PA connects without obstruction to sufficient regions of the lungs (i.e., at least enough regions to equal one whole lung). Primary repair of this condition consists of closing the VSD, establishing a continuity between the RV and the central PA (this may be done by using a pericardial or Dacron patch or a conduit with a tissue valve), and interrupting collateral circulations. The mortality rate varies between 5% and 20%.

Staged repair. When the requirements for single stage repair are not met, palliative procedures aimed at inducing the growth of the central PA are initially performed. Complete surgery occurs later. To achieve a good result, the surgery should be performed early in the patient's life; a first-stage repair should be performed before 1 or 2 years of age, and complete repair should be done before age 3 or 4.

Most infants with a small, confluent, central PA require a systemic-PA shunt to promote growth of the central PA. Sometimes a transannular patch or a conduit between the RV and the PA can be placed in infants with a reasonably sized, confluent, central PA as a temporary procedure. The VSD may be left open or closed with a fenestrated patch to increase the PBF.

For patients with multiple systemic collateral arteries supplying different regions of the lungs (i.e., nonconfluent, central PA), a surgical connection between or among the isolated regions of the lungs may be made so they might be perfused from a single source, called *unifocalization* of PBF (Fig. 14-25). These procedures can improve the PA arborization pattern. The mortality rate of unifocalization ranges from 5% to 15%, and the patency rate of the shunt noticeably varies. A conduit between the RV and a newly created central PA can be made later. About half to a quarter of the original patients can undergo the final procedure.

Occlusion of collateral arteries by coil embolization. Occlusion of collateral arteries by coil embolization should be performed preoperatively if adequate, alternative flow to that area of the lung can be identified. When it is evident or demonstrated by testing that too much hypoxia would result from preoperative closure, closure is done in the operating room.

Postoperative follow-up

1. Frequent follow-up is needed to assess the palliative surgery and decide appropriate times for further surgeries.

2. Some patients develop AR. This occurs more often in patients with TOF + pulmonary atresia than those without pulmonary atresia.

3. Patients with conduit may require conduit replacement at a later time.

4. Antibiotic prophylaxis for SBE should be observed for an indefinite amount of time.

5. A certain level of activity restriction is needed, since many of these children have exercise intolerance.

6. If hemoptysis develops as a late complication, conservative management is recommended.

TETRALOGY OF FALLOT WITH ABSENT PULMONARY VALVE

Prevalence

TOF with absent pulmonary valve occurs in approximately 2% of patients with TOF.

Pathology and Pathophysiology

1. The pulmonary valve leaflets are either completely absent or have an uneven rim of rudimentary valve tissue present. The annulus of the valve is stenotic and displaced distally. A massive aneurysmal dilatation of the PAs exists. This anomaly is usually associated with a large VSD, similar to that seen in TOF. It rarely occurs with intact ventricular septum.

2. The massive PA aneurysm (Fig 14-26) and large RV stroke output, which results from

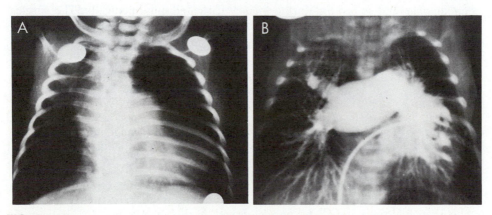

FIG. 14–26
A posteroanterior view of plain chest film **(A)** showing hyperinflated areas in the left upper lobe and right lower portion of the chest in a 1-month-old infant with absence of the pulmonary valve. An anteroposterior view of pulmonary arteriogram **(B)** showing massive aneurysmal dilatation of both the RPA and LPA.

PR, compress anteriorly the lower end of the developing trachea and bronchi throughout the fetal life. This produces signs of airway obstruction and respiratory distress during infancy. Pulmonary complications (e.g., atelectasis, pneumonia, and so on) are the usual causes of death, rather than the intracardiac defect. The ductus arteriosus is absent in some patients with a more severe aneurysmal dilatation of the PAs.

3. Since the stenosis at the pulmonary valve ring is only of moderate degree, an initial bidirectional shunt becomes predominantly a left-to-right shunt after the newborn period.

4. In some infants, tufts of PAs entwine and compress the intrapulmonary bronchi, resulting in reduced numbers of alveolar units. This may preclude successful surgical correction.

Clinical Manifestations

1. A mild cyanosis may be present as a result of a bidirectional shunt during the newborn period when the PVR is relatively high. Cyanosis disappears, and signs of CHF may develop after the newborn period.

2. A to-and-fro murmur (with "sawing-wood" sound) at the upper and middle LSBs is a characteristic auscultatory finding of the condition. This murmur occurs because of mild PS and free PR. The S2 is loud and single. The RV hyperactivity is palpable.

3. The ECG shows RAD and RVH.

4. Chest x-ray images reveal a noticeably dilated MPA and hilar PAs. The heart size is either normal or mildly enlarged, and PVMs may be slightly increased. The lung fields may show hyperinflated areas, representing partial airway obstruction (see Fig. 14-26, A).

5. Echo reveals a large, subaortic VSD with overriding of the aorta, distally displaced pulmonary annulus (with thick ridges present instead of fully developed pulmonary valve leaflets), and gigantic aneurysm of the MPA and branch PAs. Doppler studies reveal evidence of stenosis at the annulus and PR. Cardiac catherization and angiocardiography (see Fig. 14-26, B) are usually unnecessary for accurate diagnosis.

Natural History

1. More than 75% of infants with severe pulmonary complications (e.g., atelectasis, pneumonia, and so on) die during infancy if treated only medically. The surgical mortality of infants with pulmonary complication is as high as 40%.

2. Infants who survive infancy without serious pulmonary problems do well for 5 to 20 years and have fewer respiratory symptoms during childhood. They become symptomatic later and die from intractable right-sided heart failure.

Management

Medical. In the past, medial management was preferred because of poor surgical results in newborns; however, the mortality rate of medical management is extremely high. Once the pulmonary symptoms appear, neither surgical nor medical management have good results.

Surgical. Early surgical treatment is advocated before respiratory symptoms develop. Doing so reduces the effect of the compression by the pulmonary aneurysms on the tracheobronchial trees and allows normal growth of the airways.

Two-stage operation. Initially, ligation or tight banding of the MPA is performed to eliminate PR, excessive RV stroke output, and secondary PA dilatation and airway obstruction along with a systemic-PA Gore-Tex shunt. Between 2 and 4 years of age, closure of the VSD, reconstruction of the PA with reduction of the size of the PA aneurysm, and occlusion of the shunt are completed. Some surgeons use a homograft valve at the pulmonary valve position and others do not.

Primary repair. With recent advances in infant cardiac surgery, complete primary repair of the defect may be the procedure of choice before respiratory symptoms develop.

TOTAL ANOMALOUS PULMONARY VENOUS RETURN

Prevalence

TAPVR accounts for 1% of all CHDs. There is a marked male preponderance for the infracardiac type (i.e., M:F = 4:1).

Pathology

1. No direct communication exists between the pulmonary veins and the LA. Instead, they drain anomalously into the systemic venous tributaries or into the right atrium. Depending on the drainage site of the pulmonary veins, the defect may be divided into the following four types (Fig. 14-27):

    a. Supracardiac: This accounts for 50% of TAPVR patients. The common pulmonary venous sinus drains into the right SVC through the left vertical vein and the left innominate vein (see Fig. 14-27, *A*).

    b. Cardiac: The accounts for 20% of TAPVR patients. The common pulmonary venous sinus drains into the coronary sinus (see Fig. 14-27, *C*), or the pulmonary veins enter the RA separately through four openings (only two openings are illustrated in Fig. 14-27, *B*).

    c. Infracardiac (subdiaphragmatic): This accounts for 20% of TAPVR patients. The common pulmonary venous sinus drains to the portal vein, ductus venosus, hepatic vein, or IVC. The common pulmonary vein penetrates the diaphragm through the esophageal hiatus (see Fig. 14-27, *D*).

    d. Mixed type: This accounts for 10% of TAPVR patients. This type is a combination of the other types.

2. An interatrial communication, either as an ASD or PFO, is necessary for survival.

3. The left side of the heart is relatively small.

4. Many patients with supracardiac and cardiac types of TAPVR and most patients with the infracardiac type have pulmonary hypertension secondary to obstruction of the pulmonary venous return.

Clinical Manifestations

Clinical manifestations differ depending on whether there is obstruction to the pulmonary venous return. They will be presented separately.

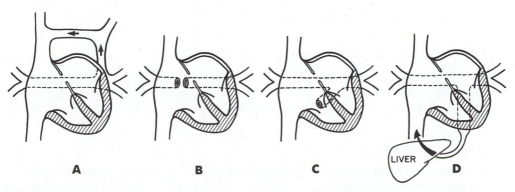

FIG. 14–27
Anatomic classification of TAPVR. **A,** Supracardiac. **B** and **C,** Cardiac. **D,** Infracardiac.

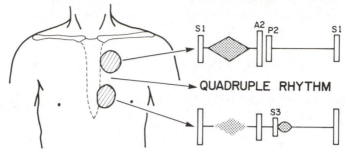

FIG. 14–28
Cardiac findings of TAPVR without obstruction to pulmonary venous return.

Without pulmonary venous obstruction
History.

1. CHF with growth retardation and frequent pulmonary infection are common in infancy.

2. A history of mild cyanosis from birth is present.

Physical examination.

1. The infant is undernourished and mildly cyanotic. Signs of CHF (e.g., tachypnea, dyspnea, tachycardia, and hepatomegaly) are present.

2. Precordial bulge with hyperactive RV impulse is present. Cardiac impulse is maximal at the xyphoid process and the LLSB.

3. Characteristic quadruple or quintuple rhythm is present. The S2 is widely split and fixed, and the P2 may be accentuated. A grade 2-3/6 ejection systolic murmur is usually audible at the ULSB. A middiastolic rumble is always present at the LLSB (Fig 14-28).

Electrocardiography. RVH of the so called volume overload type (i.e., rsR′ in V1) and occasional RAH are present.

X-ray study.

1. Moderate to marked cardiomegaly involving the RA and RV is present with increased PVMs.

2. "Snowman" sign or figure-of-8 configuration may be seen in the supracardiac type, but rarely before 4 months of age (Fig. 14-29).

With pulmonary venous obstruction
History.

1. Marked cyanosis and respiratory distress develop in the neonatal period with failure to thrive.

2. Worsening of cyanosis with feeding, especially in infants with infracardiac type resulting from compression of the common pulmonary vein by the food-filled esophagus.

Physical examination.

1. Moderate to marked cyanosis and tachypnea with retraction are present in newborns or undernourished infants.

2. Cardiac findings may be minimal. A loud, single S2 and gallop rhythm are present. Heart murmur is usually absent. If present, however, it is usually a faint SEM at the ULSB.

3. Pulmonary rales and hepatomegaly are usually present.

Electrocardiography. Invariably RVH in the form of tall R waves in the right precordial leads is present. RAH is occasionally present.

X-ray study. The heart size is normal or slightly enlarged. The lung fields reveal findings of pulmonary edema (i.e., diffuse reticular pattern and Kerley's B lines). These findings may be confused with pneumonia or hyaline membrane disease.

Echocardiography.

COMMON FEATURES.

1. Large RV with compressed LV (i.e., relative hypoplasia of the LV) is the most striking initial finding. Large RA and small LA, with deviation of the atrial septum to the left and dilated PAs, are also present.

2. An interatrial communication is usually present. PFO occurs in 70% of patients, and secundum ASD occurs in 30%.

3. A large, common chamber (i.e., common pulmonary venous sinus) may be imaged posterior to the LA in the parasternal long-axis view.

4. An M-mode echo may show signs of RV volume overload, which includes abnormal motion of the interventricular septum.

5. Doppler studies reveal an increased flow velocity in the MPA, an increased flow velocity or continuous flow at the site of the pulmonary venous drainage, and findings suggestive of pulmonary hypertension.

FEATURES OF THE SUPRACARDIAC TYPE. The most common site of connection is the left SVC (i.e., left vertical vein) with subsequent drainage to the dilated left innominate vein and right SVC. These abnormal pathways can be imaged in the SSN short-axis view. Color-flow mapping and Doppler ultrasound are helpful in defining the direction of the flow in the left SVC.

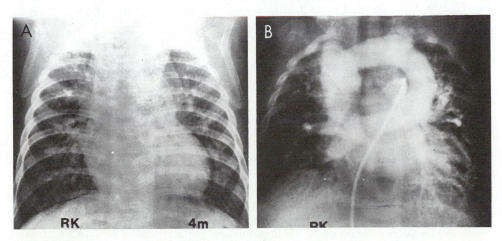

FIG. 14–29
A posteroanterior view of plain chest film demonstrating "snowman" sign **(A)** and an angiocardiogram demonstrating anatomic structures that participate in the formation of the "snowman" sign **(B)**; the vertical vein (left superior vena cava), the left innominate vein, and the right superior vena cava.

FEATURES OF THE CARDIAC TYPE. The most common site of entry is to the coronary sinus, occurring in 15% of cases. A dilated coronary sinus, best imaged in the parasternal long-axis view and the apical four-chamber view, may be the first clue to this condition. The confluence of each pulmonary vein can be imaged.

FEATURES OF THE INFRACARDIAC TYPE. A dilated vein descending to the abdominal cavity through the diaphragm is imaged using the subcostal sagittal and transverse scans. All four pulmonary veins that connect to the confluence must be imaged. They are best imaged on the subcostal coronal scan or the SSN short-axis view.

POSSIBILITY OF THE MIXED TYPE. Unless all four pulmonary veins are imaged to connect to the confluence, the possibility of the mixed type of TAPVR is not eliminated. In the most common mixed type the left lung, usually the upper lobe, drains to the left SVC, and the remaining pulmonary veins in both lungs drains to the coronary sinus.

Natural History

1. CHF occurs in both types of TAPVR and involves growth retardation and repeated pneumonias.

2. Without surgical repair, two thirds of the infants without obstruction die before reaching 1 year of age. They usually die from superimposed pneumonia.

3. Patients with infracardiac type rarely survive for longer than a few weeks without surgery. Most die before 2 months of age.

Management
Medical.

1. Intensive anticongestive measures with digitalis and diuretics should be provided for infants without pulmonary venous obstruction.

2. Patients should receive oxygen, diuretics for pulmonary edema, and correction of metabolic acidosis, if present.

3. Infants with severe pulmonary edema resulting from infracardiac type and other types with obstruction, should be intubated and receive ventilator therapy with oxygen and positive end-expiratory pressure if necessary, before cardiac catheterization and surgery.

4. If the size of the interatrial communication appears to be obstructive and immediate surgery is not indicated, balloon atrial septostomy or blade atrial septostomy may be performed to enlarge the communication.

Surgical.
Indications and timing. Corrective surgery is necessary for all patients with this condition. No palliative procedure exists.

1. All infants with pulmonary venous obstruction should be operated on soon after diagnosis, even in the newborn period.

2. Infants who do not have pulmonary venous obstruction but do have heart failure that is difficult to control are usually operated on between 4 and 6 months of age.

Procedures. Although procedures vary with the site of the anomalous drainage, all procedures intend to redirect the pulmonary venous return to the LA (Fig. 14-30). Surgery may be performed under cardiopulmonary bypass, profound hypothermia, and total circulatory arrest.

SUPRACARDIAC TYPE. A large, side-to-side anastomosis is made between the common pulmonary venous sinus and the LA. The vertical vein is ligated. The ASD is closed with a cloth patch (see Fig. 14-30, *A*).

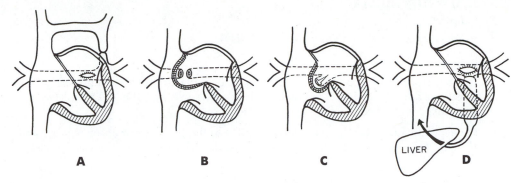

FIG. 14–30
Surgical approaches to various types of TAPVR (see text).

TAPVR TO THE RA. The atrial septum is excised and a patch is sewn in such a way that the pulmonary venous return is diverted to the LA (see Fig. 14-30, *B*).

TAPVR TO THE CORONARY SINUS. An incision is made in the anterior wall of the coronary sinus to make a communication between the coronary sinus and the LA. A single patch closes the original ASD and the ostium of the coronary sinus. This results in the drainage of coronary sinus blood with low oxygen saturation into the LA (see Fig. 14-30, *C*).

INFRACARDIAC TYPE. A large anastomosis is made between the common pulmonary venous sinus and the LA. The common pulmonary vein, which descends vertically to the abdominal cavity, is ligated at the upper end (see Fig. 14-30, *D*).

Mortality. Surgical management is superior to medical management. The mortality rate is between 5% and 10% for infants with the unobstructed type. This rate can be as high as 20% for infants with the infracardiac type. Two common causes of death are postoperative paroxysms of pulmonary hypertension and the development of pulmonary vein stenosis.

COMPLICATIONS.

1. Paroxysms of pulmonary hypertension, which relate to a small and poorly compliant left heart with resulting cardiac failure and pulmonary edema, may require a prolonged respiratory support postoperatively.

2. Postoperative arrhythmias are usually atrial.

3. Obstruction at the site of anastomosis or pulmonary vein stenosis rarely occurs.

Postoperative follow-up

1. An office evaluation every 6 to 12 months is recommended for such possible late complications as pulmonary vein obstruction and atrial arrhythmias.

2. Pulmonary vein obstruction at the anastomosis site or delayed development of pulmonary vein stenosis may develop in about 10% of the patients and requires reoperation. These complications are usually evident within the first 6 to 12 months of the repair. The possibility of pulmonary vein stenosis requires cardiac catheterization and angiocardiography. If present, it is nearly impossible to correct.

3. Some patients develop atrial arrhythmias, including sick sinus syndrome that requires medical treatment and/or pacemaker therapy.

4. Activity restriction is usually unnecessary unless pulmonary venous obstruction occurs.

5. SBE prophylaxis is usually not needed unless an obstruction is present.

TRICUSPID ATRESIA

Prevalence

Tricuspid atresia accounts for 1% to 3% of CHDs.

Pathology

1. The tricuspid valve is absent, and the RV is hypoplastic, with the absence of the inflow portion of the RV. The associated defects such as ASD, VSD, or PDA are necessary for survival.

2. Tricuspid atresia is usually classified according to the presence or absence of PS and of TGA. The great arteries are normally related in about 70% of the cases and are

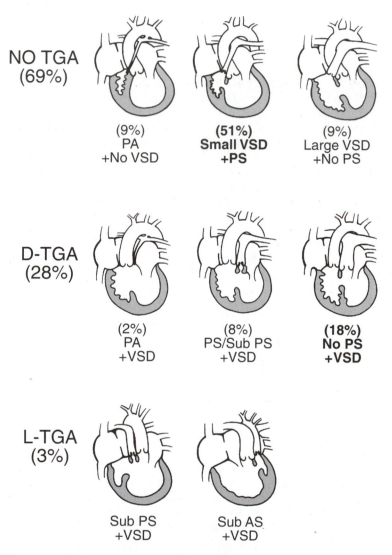

NO TGA (69%)

| (9%) PA +No VSD | **(51%) Small VSD +PS** | (9%) Large VSD +No PS |

D-TGA (28%)

| (2%) PA +VSD | (8%) PS/Sub PS +VSD | **(18%) No PS +VSD** |

L-TGA (3%)

| Sub PS +VSD | Sub AS +VSD |

FIG. 14–31
Anatomic classification of tricuspid atresia. In about 50% of cases the great arteries are normally related, and there is a small VSD with associated hypoplasia of the PAs. When the great arteries are transposed, the VSD is usually large, and the PAs are large with increased PBF. (Data from Keith JD, Rowe RD, Vlad P: *Heart disease in infancy and childhood,* ed 3, New York, 1978, Macmillan.)

transposed in 30%. They usually appear in D-form. In 3% of cases the L-form occurs. (Fig. 14-31).

3. In patients with normally related great arteries the VSD is usually small, and PS is present with resulting hypoplasia of the PAs. This is the most common type, occurring in about 50% of all patients with tricuspid atresia. Occasionally, the VSD is large with normal-sized PAs, or the ventricular septum is intact with pulmonary atresia.

4. When TGA is present, the pulmonary valve is normal with increased PBF in two thirds of cases. In one third of cases, it is either stenotic or atretic with decreased PBF. Patients with TGA need a fairly large VSD to maintain normal systemic cardiac output. Less than adequate size or spontaneous reduction of the VSD creates problems with a decreased systemic cardiac output. Such a situation is similar to single ventricle with obstructed bulboventricular foramen and has an unfavorable surgical outlook.

5. COA or interrupted aortic arch is a frequently associated anomaly that is more commonly seen in patients with TGA.

Clinical Manifestations
History.

1. Cyanosis is usually severe from birth. Tachypnea and poor feeding usually manifest.

2. History of hypoxic spells may be present in infants with this condition.

Physical examination (Fig. 14-32).

1. Cyanosis, either with or without clubbing, is always present.

2. A systolic thrill is rarely palpable when associated with PS.

3. The S2 is single. A grade 2-3/6 systolic regurgitant murmur of VSD is usually present at the LLSB. A continuous murmur of PDA is occasionally present. An apical diastolic rumble is rarely audible with large PBF.

4. Hepatomegaly may indicate an inadequate interatrial communication or CHF.

Electrocardiography.

1. Superior QRS axis or left anterior hemiblock (with the QRS axis between 0 and -90 degrees) is characteristic. It appears in most patients without TGA (Fig. 14-33). The superior QRS axis is present in only 50% of patients with TGA.

2. LVH is usually present; RAH or CAH is common.

X-ray study. The heart size is normal or slightly increased, with enlargement of the

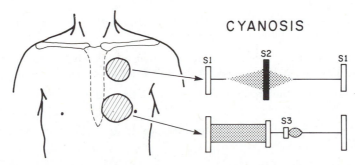

FIG. 14–32
Cardiac findings of tricuspid atresia associated with PDA and VSD. Left anterior hemiblock and cyanosis are characteristic of the defect.

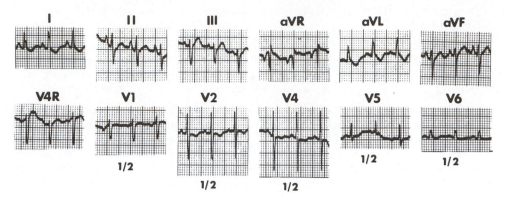

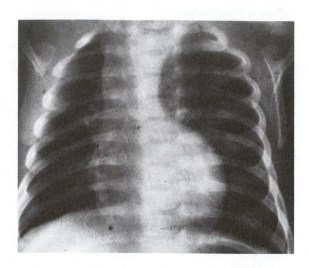

FIG. 14–33
Tracing from a 6-month-old girl with tricuspid atresia showing left anterior hemiblock (−30 degrees), RAH, and LVH.

FIG. 14–34
A posteroanterior view of chest roentgenogram in an infant with tricuspid atresia with normally related great arteries. The heart is minimally enlarged. The PVMs are decreased, and the MPA segment is somewhat concave.

RA and LV. Pulmonary vascularity decreases in most patients (Fig. 14-34), although it may increase in infants with TGA. Occasionally, the concave MPA segment may produce a boot-shaped heart, like the x-ray findings of TOF.

Echocardiography. Two-dimensional echo readily establishes the diagnosis of tricuspid atresia.

1. Absence of the tricuspid orifice, marked hypoplasia of the RV, and a large LV can be imaged in the apical four-chamber view.

2. The bulging of the atrial septum toward the left, in addition to the size of an interatrial communication, are easily imaged in the subcostal four-chamber view.

3. The size of the VSD, the presence and severity of PS, and the presence of TGA should all be investigated.

4. Patients with TGA should be examined for possible subaortic stenosis and aortic arch anomalies.

Natural History

1. Few infants with tricuspid atresia and normally related great arteries survive beyond 6 months of age without surgical palliation.

2. Occasionally, patients with increased PBF develop CHF.

3. For patients who survive into their second decade of life, the chronic volume overload of the LV usually produces secondary cardiomyopathy and reduced contractility of that ventricle.

Management
Medical.

1. Prostaglandin E$_1$ should be started in neonates with severe cyanosis to maintain the patency of the ductus before planned cardiac catheterization or cardiac surgery.

2. The Rashkind procedure (i.e., balloon atrial septostomy) may be performed as part of the initial catheterization to improve the RA-to-LA shunt, especially when the interatrial communication is considered inadequate by echo studies.

3. Treatment of CHF is rarely needed in infants with TGA without PS.

4. Infants with normally related great arteries and adequate PBF through a VSD do not need any of these other procedures; rather, they need to be closely watched for decreasing oxygen saturation resulting from spontaneous reduction of the VSD.

Surgical.
Palliative surgery. Most infants with tricuspid atresia require a palliative procedure before a Fontan-type operation can be performed.

SHUNT OPERATIONS. Most patients who have tricuspid atresia with decreased PBF need either a systemic-PA shunt or a cavopulmonary shunt to increase PBF and arterial oxygen saturations.

1. The Blalock-Taussig shunt or Gore-Tex shunt (see Fig. 14-20) can be performed at any age. The mortality rate of this shunt operation is about 1% for infants and slightly higher for newborns.

2. An end-to-side SVC to RPA shunt (i.e., bidirectional superior cavopulmonary shunt, or bidirectional Glenn procedure) can be performed in older infants (Fig. 14-35, A). The IVC blood still bypasses the lungs. This is a widely accepted palliative procedure that satisfactorily increases oxygen saturation, which averages 85%, without adding volume work to the LV. This is the first of the two-stage Fontan-type operation. The mortality rate for this procedure is between 5% and 10%. This option should be considered for children with PVR between 2 and 4 U/m^2 or other borderline risk factors. For these children a complete Fontan operation may carry a high rate of mortality.

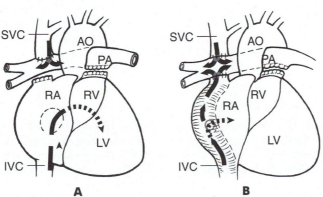

FIG. 14–35
Currently popular modified Fontan operation. **A,** Bidirectional Glenn operation or SVC-to-RPA anastomosis. **B,** Cavocaval baffle-to-PA connection, with or without fenestration. See text for description of these procedures.

PULMONARY ARTERY BANDING. PA banding is very rarely necessary for infants with CHF resulting from increased PBF. PA banding may be performed at any age with a mortality rate of less than 5%.

DAMUS-KAYE-STANSEL + SHUNT OPERATION. For infants with TGA and restrictive VSD, PA banding has a high mortality rate for the same reason as that for single ventricle with obstructed bulboventricular foramen and transposed aorta. The Damus-Kaye-Stansel procedure, in addition to systemic-PA shunt, may be preferred for infants with TGA and restrictive VSD. In the Damus-Kaye-Stansel operation the MPA is transected, the distal PA is sewn over, and the proximal PA is connected end-to-side to the ascending aorta (see Fig. 14-9). A Fontan-type operation can be performed at a later time.

Definitive surgery (e.g., Fontan-type operation).

PROCEDURE (FIG. 14-35, B). A modified Fontan operation is the definitive procedure for patients with tricuspid atresia. At the present time, the procedure of choice is a cavocaval baffle-to-PA connection with or without fenestration. Fontan-type operations can also be performed in patients with single ventricle, complicated DORV, HLHS, and heterotoxia.

1. The cavocaval baffle-to-PA anastomosis consists of an end-to-side anastomosis of the cephalic end of the SVC to the RPA (i.e., bidirectional Glenn operation); an end-to-side anastomosis of the cardiac end of the SVC to the undersurface of the RPA; and the construction of an intraatrial cavocaval baffle, which is a tubular pathway created from the orifice of the IVC to the orifice of the SVC (see Fig. 14-35, B).

2. "Fenestrated Fontan" procedure has been advocated as an alternative to the cavocaval baffle-to-PA anastomosis, especially in high-risk patients. A fenestration of 4 to 6 mm is made in the intraatrial baffle, which can later be closed in the cardiac catheterization laboratory using a clamshell device* (Fig. 14-35, B).

INDICATIONS AND TIMING. Cavocaval baffle-to-PA anastomosis can be performed in most patients with tricuspid atresia and patients with a functional single ventricle. The following are risk factors: high PVR (> 2 U/m^2) or high mean PA pressure (> 18 mm Hg); distorted PAs secondary to previous shunt operations; poor systolic or diastolic ventricular function, with LV-end diastolic pressure greater than 12 mm Hg or an ejection fraction less than 60%; and functional AV valve regurgitation. The presence of two or more of these risk factors constitutes a high-risk situation.

Younger than 4 years of age is no longer considered a risk factor. This procedure can even be performed on infants. The age should be balanced against the potential adverse effects of the additional shunt operation that may produce PA distortion or depressed LV function by volume overload. Children older than 10 years may be a risk factor, since some of these children already have LV dysfunction. PA size is not considered a surgical risk factor, however, a recent report indicates that the small PA size is a risk factor. The mortality rate for this procedure has been reduced to about 5%.

COMPLICATIONS.

1. Low cardiac output, heart failure, or both are early postoperative complications.

2. Persistent pleural effusion occurs more often on the right. The following treatments may be used for this complication: prolonged chest tube drainage, a low-fat diet with a medium-chain triglyceride oil supplement or total parenteral nutrition, chemical or talc pleurodesis, a pleuroperitoneal shunt, and thoracic duct ligation, which is a major surgery.

3. Thrombus formation in the systemic venous pathways is suspected if cyanosis and inadequate perfusion develop. Transesophageal echocardiography may be better

---

* The clamshell device has been taken off of the market for safety reasons.

than surface echo in the detection of the thrombus for older children. Treatment consists of warfarin, streptokinase thrombolysis, or surgical removal.

4. Reoperation is often necessary for the revision of conduits and for pacemaker implantation.

5. Although rare, acute liver dysfunction with SGPT greater than 1000 U/L can occur during the first week after surgery from possible hepatic hypoperfusion, (which is caused by low cardiac output).

6. Complete heart block rarely occurs.

Postoperative follow-up.

Of patients with tricuspid atresia, 70% are still living 5 years after surgery, and 65% survive 10 years. During years 11 to 16 after surgery, follow-up shows acceptable results with the majority of patients. Of these patients, 48% are classified in New York Heart Association as class I, and 16% as class II (see Appendix A, Table A-4).

1. Long-term follow-up on a regular basis is necessary to detect the following late complications:

   a. Prolonged hepatomegaly and ascites require treatment with digitalis, diuretics, and afterload-reducing agents.

   b. Supraventricular arrhythmia is one of the most troublesome late complications and occurs in 12% to 20% of patients. Supraventricular arrhythmia may result in CHF, fluid retention, and even death. Antiarrhythmic agents and pacemaker implantation may be required.

   c. A progressive decrease in arterial oxygen saturation may result from an obstruction of the venous pathways, leakage in the intraatrial baffle, or the development of pulmonary arteriovenous fistula. A decreased ratio of upper/lower lobe perfusion may be a factor in the development of the pulmonary arteriovenous fistula.

   d. Protein-losing enteropathy with hypoproteinemia or hypoalbuminemia occurs in 10% to 15% of patients 5 to 10 years after surgery. This is more common in patients with heterotaxia than those patients with tricuspid atresia.

   e. Patients who received an older modification of the Fontan-type operation may develop stenosis and fibrosis of the conduit valve (porcine heterograft) or obstruction of the Dacron conduit. As a result, they may require reoperation.

2. Patients should maintain a low-salt diet.

3. Patients should not participate in competitive, strenuous sports.

4. Antibiotic prophylaxis against SBE should be observed when indications arise.

Evolution of the Fontan-type operation. The Fontan-type operation applies to many complex CHDs of which most are otherwise uncorrectable. Therefore this procedure can be considered a major advancement in the pediatric cardiac surgery during the last 2 decades. Many modifications have been made since the original Fontan operation (1971). An overview of these modifications has recently been discussed by Aldo Castaneda (from Glenn to Fontan, Circulation, 86[suppl II]:II-80. 1992). In the 1940s and 1950s, systemic-to-PA shunts (such as Blalock-Taussig) were applied to children with tricuspid atersia to increase PBF. During this time, animal studies were being performed, leading to the present-day Fontan-type operation.

The results of animal experiments conducted in the 1940s and 1950s suggested that the RV could be successfully bypassed. Dogs survived for as long as 2 months after the bypass of the RV by anastomosis of the RA appendage to the MPA and ligation of the proximal MPA. Experiments also showed that when the tricuspid valve was obliterated in steps, dogs could survive the anastomosis of the RA appendage to the MPA. Robicsek and associates (1966) were able to completely bypass both the RA and RV in dogs by using a four-step process over a period of 8 or 9 months. The eventual bypass procedures developed combine the Glenn operation and transplantation of the IVC to the LA. Carlon and associates (1951) experimented with dogs and successfully connected end-to-end between the azygous vein and the distal end of the RPA with ligation of the caudal end of the SVC. This anastomosis is the forerunner of the Glenn shunt, which is an end-to-end anastomosis of the SVC to the distal end of the RPA (see Fig. 14-20). This anastomosis was considered to be more effective than the Blalock-Taussig shunt because it increased PBF with venous blood instead of the mixture of arterial and venous blood.

The original Fontan operation (1971) consisted of a Glenn shunt, connection of the RA and the RPA with insertion of an aortic homograft, insertion of another allograft valve in the IVC-RA junction, and closure of the ASD (see Fig. 14-36 A). At that time, RA contractions were thought to be important in pulsatile assistance to the pulmonary circulation. It became evident later that inlet and outlet valves were more problematic than beneficial.

Kreutzer and associates (1973) made a direct anastomosis between the RA appendage and the PA trunk using either a homograft or the patient's own pulmonary valve. The ASD was closed (see Fig. 14-36, B). Subsequently, modifications of the connection were made between the RA and RV (see Fig. 14-36, C), as well as between the RA and the MPA or RPA (see Fig. 14-35, D), by direct anastomosis of the two structures or by using patches or conduits with or without an interposed valve. It became evident later that a direct connection between the RA appendage and the RPA without an interposed valve provided equally good hemodynamic results, and that the incorporation of a portion of the RV was not beneficial.

Kawashima and associates (1984) reported a new operation. In this operation the systemic venous return completely bypassed the RA and RV in patients with an interrupted IVC with azygous or hemiazygos continuation and other complex intracardiac anomalies. The right and/or left SVC(s), which receives blood from the entire systemic venous system, were connected end-to-side to the ipsilteral PAs. This procedure proved that the RA and RV can be completely bypassed in people.

In cavocaval baffle-to-PA connection, the latest modification of the Fontan operation, the RA and RV are both completely bypassed in patients with normal IVCs (see Fig. 14-35, E) (de Leval et al, 1988, Jonas et al, 1988). The following are advantages of this procedure: a lower risk of damage to the AV node; less of the atrial wall exposed to high pressure, thereby possibly decreasing the risk of early or late atrial arrhythmias; a reduced risk of atrial thrombosis, and hemodynamic superiority to the RA-PA connection. As shown by de Leval and associates, the interposition of a compliant RA chamber between the systemic vein and the PA is a major cause of energy loss in the RA, and cavocaval baffle-PA anastomosis presents significant hydrodynamic advantages.

Two-stage Fontan operation was recommended for high-risk patients (see Fig. 14-35 A). Initially, a bidirectional cavopulmonary anastomosis (i.e., an end-to-side SVC to RPA anastomosis, a bidirectional Glenn shunt) was performed. This was later followed by the completion of the cavocaval baffle-to-RPA anastomosis. After the first procedure there was often a noticeable improvement in oxygen saturation and symptoms which raised questions about the necessity of the second procedure.

Fenestrated Fontan has been recommended for high-risk patients (see Fig. 14-36, F). Reported advantages of the fenestration include the following: lower early surgical mortality, reduced incidence and/or duration of postoperative pleural effusion, shorter hospital stay, and the right-to-left shunt through the fenestration that may help maintain cardiac output if blood flow through the lungs decreases. The following are possible disadvantages: paradoxical embolization and stroke, lower arterial oxygen saturation, and the need to close the fenestration.

Extracardiac right heart bypass with an IVC-to-RPA Dacron conduit and SVC-to-PA anastomosis has also been performed (see Fig. 14-36, G). This procedure may reduce the incidence of late atrial arrhythmia.

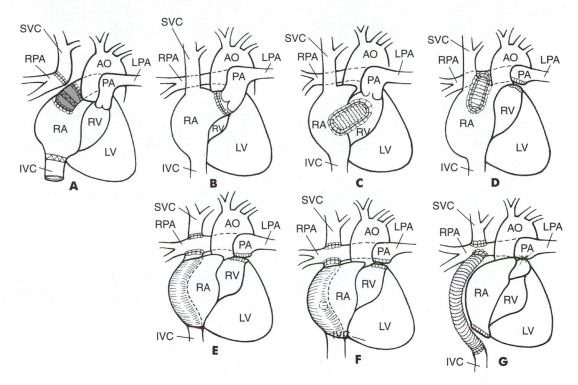

FIG. 14–36

Modifications of the Fontan operation. **A,** The original Fontan operation (Fontan and Baudet, 1971) consisted of an end-to-end anastomosis of the RPA to SVC, an end-to-end anastomosis of right atrial appendage to proximal end of the right PA by means of an aortic valve homograft, closure of ASD, insertion of a pulmonary valve homograft into the IVC, and ligation of the MPA. **B,** Modification by Kreutzer et al (1973) consisted of an anastomosis of the right atrial appendage and the MPA with its intact pulmonary valve (which was excised from the RV) after closure of the ASD and VSD. A Glenn operation was not performed, and no IVC valve was used. **C,** A later modification by Bjork et al (1979) which consisted of a direct anastomosis between the right atrial appendage and the RV outflow tract in patients with a normal pulmonary valve, using a roof of pericardium to avoid a synthetic tube graft. **D,** The direct anastomosis of the RA to the RPA. **E** and **F,** Separate anastomosis of the two ends of the divided SVC to the RPA and insertion of IVC to SVC intraatrial baffle (total cavopulmonary connection) with **(F)** and without **(E)** fenestration. **G,** Extracardiac conduit between the IVC and the RPA and a bidirectional Glenn operation.

PULMONARY ATRESIA WITH INTACT VENTRICULAR SEPTUM

Prevalence

Pulmonary atresia with intact ventricular septum accounts for fewer than 1% of all CHDs. It comprises 2.5% of the critically ill infants with CHDs.

Pathology

1. In 80% of these patients the pulmonary valve is atretic with a diaphragm-like membrane. The infundibulum is atretic in 20% of these patients. The valve ring and the MPA are hypoplastic. The PA trunk is rarely atretic. The ventricular septum remains intact.

2. RV size varies and relates to survival. In 1982, Bull and associates classified this

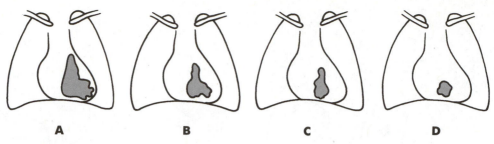

FIG. 14–37
Schematic diagram of right ventriculograms which illustrate three types of pulmonary atresia with intact ventricular septum. **A,** Normal right ventricle. **B,** Tripartite type which shows all three portions (inlet, trabecular, and infundibular portions) of the RV.
C, Bipartite type in which only the inlet and infundibular portions are present.
D, Monopartite type in which only the inlet portion of the RV is present.

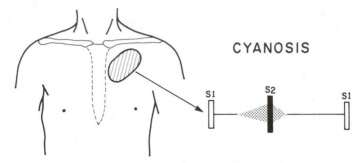

FIG. 14–38
Cardiac findings of pulmonary atresia. These are nonspecific for the defect and may be found in TOF with pulmonary atresia as well.

condition into three types based on the presence or absence of the three portions of the RV—inlet, trabecular, and infundibular portions (Fig. 14-37). All three of these portions are present and the RV is almost normal in size in the *triparite type* of pulmonary atresia. In the *bipartite type* the inlet and infundibular portions are present, but the trabecular portion is obliterated. The inlet is the only portion present, and the RV size is diminutive in the *monopartite type*.

3. The high pressure in the RV is decompressed through dilated coronary microcirculation (i.e., coronary sinusoids) into the left or right coronary artery (see Fig. 14-39). Often the proximal coronary arteries are obstructed. Sinusoid channels are demonstrable by a right ventriculogram in 30% to 50% of cases. If proximal coronary artery obstruction is present, coronary circulation is perfused by desaturated RV blood. Tricuspid valve regurgitation often occurs. The prevalence of the sinusoids directly relates to the RV pressure and inversely relates to the amount of TR.

4. An interatrial communication (i.e., either ASD or PFO) and PDA are necessary for the patient to survive.

Clinical Manifestations

   History. A history of severe cyanosis since birth is present.

   Physical examination (Fig. 14-38).

1. Severe cyanosis and tachypnea are seen in distressed neonates.

2. The S2 is single. A heart murmur is usually absent, but a soft murmur of either TR or a soft continuous murmur of PDA may be audible.

3. Inadequate interatrial communication causes the presence of hepatomegaly.

Electrocardiography.

1. The QRS axis is normal (i.e., +60 to +140 degrees), in contrast to a superiorly oriented QRS axis of tricuspid atresia. This distinction between the two conditions is important.

2. LVH is usually present. Occasionally RVH is seen in infants with a relatively large RV cavity. RAH is common, occurring in 70% of cases.

X-ray study. The heart size may be normal or large, resulting from RA enlargement. PVMs are decreased with clear lung fields. The MPA segment is concave.

Echocardiography. Diagnostic features include thickened, immobile, atretic pulmonary valve with no Doppler evidence of blood flow through it; hypertrophied RV wall with a small cavity; patent, but small, tricuspid valve; a right-to-left atrial shunt through an ASD demonstrated by color-flow and Doppler studies; and a ductus arteriosus running vertically from the aortic arch to the PA (i.e., vertical ductus) (see Fig. 14-22). The RPA and LPA branches are usually well developed but are sometimes variably hypoplastic. Multiple sinusoids may be imaged.

Natural History

Without appropriate medical management, including prostaglandin E_1 infusion and surgery, prognosis is exceedingly poor. About 50% of these patients die by the end of the first month if not managed properly; about 85% die by 6 months of age. Death usually coincides with the spontaneous closure of the ductus arteriosus.

Management
  Medical.

1. Prostaglandin E_1 (Prostin VR Pediatric solution) infusion should begin as soon as the diagnosis is suspected or confirmed, so that the patency of the ductus arteriosus is maintained. Infusion is continued during cardiac catheterization and surgery. The starting dose of Prostin is 0.05 to 0.1 µg/kg/min. When the desired effect is achieved, the dosage is gradually reduced to 0.01 µg/kg/min.

2. Cardiac catheterization and angiocardiography are recommended for most patients with pulmonary atresia. A right ventriculogram demonstrates sinusoids (Fig. 14-39), and an ascending aortogram identifies stenosis or interruption of the coronary arteries. Both are important in surgical decision-making. A balloon atrial septostomy may be performed as part of the cardiac catheterization to improve the right-to-left atrial shunt, but it is recommended only if RV sinusoids are identified.

3. For survivors, prophylaxis against SBE required when indications arise.

  Surgical.
  Urgent procedures. Three categories of surgical decision for infants with pulmonary atresia with intact ventricular septum exist. These categories depend on the size of the RV and the presence or absence of coronary sinusoids or coronary artery anomalies.

1. When the RV appears to be an adequate size for future growth, a connection is established between the RV and the MPA to prepare for a two-ventricular repair. A systemic-PA shunt is performed at the same time.

   a. Placement of a transannular RV outflow patch and a systemic-PA shunt seems most promising for a two-ventricular repair at a later date (Fig. 14-40). The mortality rate is about 20%. An equally good result has been reported with 2 to 3 weeks of prostaglandin E_1 infusion to maintain ductal patency, which is used

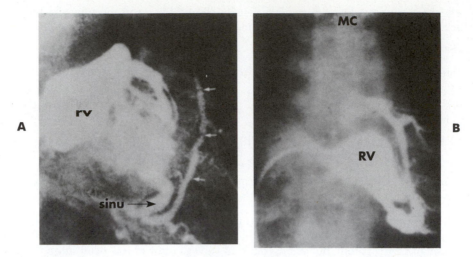

FIG. 14–39
Right ventriculograms in a patient with pulmonary atresia. **A,** Contrast medium filling the
right ventricle *(rv)* passes into the ventricle-coronary fistula *(sinu)* and left anterior
descending *(LAD)* coronary artery. Small white arrows point to multiple stenotic areas in
the LAD. **B,** Massive filling of a dilated and irregular LAD coronary artery from the right
ventriculare injection *(RV)*. (From Williams WG, Burrows P, Freedom RM et al:
Thromboexclusion of the right ventricle in children with pulmonary atresia and intact
ventricular septum, *J Thorac Cardiovasc Surg* 101:222-229, 1991.)

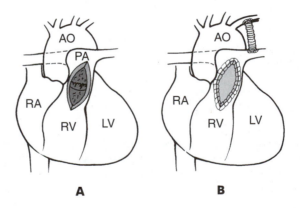

FIG. 14–40
Initial surgery for tripartite or bipartite type of pulmonary atresia. **A,** A longitudinal
incision is made across the pulmonary annulus. The pulmonary valve is incised, and the
RV outflow tract is carefully widened. **B,** A piece of pericardium is used for the
transannular patch. A left-sided Gore-Tex shunt is made between the left subclavian
artery and the LPA.

instead of the shunt. The one year survival rate is 80%. Balloon atrial septostomy
is not recommended with this approach so that a high RA pressure is maintained
to maximize the forward RV output.

b. A popular approach combines closed transpulmonary valvotomy without cardiopulmonary bypass and a left-sided modified Blalock-Taussig shunt. The mortality
rate of these procedures is less than 5%. For infants with an adequate RV size (i.e.,

tripartite RV), pulmonary valvotomy alone is recommended by some centers. The mortality rate, however, is greater than 50%.

2. A two-ventricular repair is not possible for patients with monopartite RV. Therefore a systemic-PA shunt without the RV outflow patch is recommended. A Fontan operation can be performed at a later time.

3. Patients who have rudimentary RV and sinusoidal channels as the the major source of coronary circulation, which is perfused by desaturated blood, represent a special problem. Decompression of the RV by valvotomy or an outflow patch may result in a reversal of coronary flow into the RV, thereby producing myocardial ischemia.

   a. If coronary anomalies are identified by an aortogram, the sinusoids are left alone, and a systemic-PA shunt is performed for a future Fontan-type operation. After the Fontan operation, the sinusoids are perfused by highly oxygenated blood.

   b. If the aortogram does not show evidence of stenosis or interruption of the coronary system in a patient with an extremely small RV, sinusoidal ligation or closure of the tricuspid valve (i.e., thromboexclusion of the RV) may be performed. This may prevent progressive myocardial ischemia and increase the suitability for an eventual Fontan operation.

Follow-up procedures.
1. For patients who had a transannular patch or a closed pulmonary valvotomy, cardiac catheterization is performed within 4 to 12 months after the initial surgery to determine whether the surgical procedures have increased the RV size. An arterial oxygen saturation greater than 70%, a greater RV volume, and evidence of forward flow through the pulmonary valve are all positive signs.

   a. For patients who received an RV outflow patch and a shunt procedure with substantial growth of the RV cavity, the shunt is surgically closed if the patient tolerates the balloon occlusion of the shunt during cardiac catheterization.

   b. After a pulmonary valvotomy and a Gore-Tex shunt, if the RV and the tricuspid valve annulus have grown to an adequate size, an RV outflow tract reconstruction (with placement of a transannular patch) and closure of the ASD are carried out under cardiopulmonary bypass. The Gore-Tex shunt is closed at the time of surgery. The mortality rate is about 15%.

   c. A two-ventricular repair is not possible for patients who continue to have hypoplasia of the RV and tricuspid valve annulus. A Fontan-type operation is performed at a later date (see Fig. 14-35).

   d. An additional shunt operation may be necessary for patients whose condition makes it impossible for any of these procedures to be performed.

2. For those patients with rudimentary RV and/or coronary sinusoids, Fontan operation is performed at a later date.

Postoperative follow-up.
1. Most patients require close follow-up because none of the surgical procedures available are curative.

2. Antibiotic prophylaxis against SBE is recommended.

EBSTEIN'S ANOMALY

Prevalence
Ebstein's anomaly of the tricuspid valve occurs in fewer than 1% of all CHDs.

Pathology
1. There is a downward displacement of the septal and the posterior leaflets of the

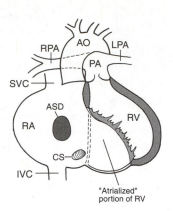

FIG. 14–41
Diagram of Ebstein's anomaly of the tricuspid valve. There is a downward displacement of the tricuspid valve, usually the septal and posterior leaflets, into the RV. Part of the RV is incorporated into the RA ("atrialized" portion of the RV). Regurgitation of the tricuspid valve results in RA enlargement. An ASD is usually present. *CS,* coronary sinus.

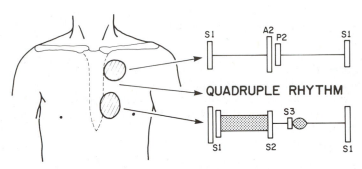

FIG. 14–42
Cardiac findings of Ebstein's anomaly. Quadruple rhythm and a soft, regurgitant systolic murmur are characteristic of the defect.

tricuspid valve into the RV cavity so that a portion of the RV is incorporated into the *atrialized* RV and functional hypoplasia of the RV results (Fig. 14-41). Tricuspid valve regurgitation is usually present, and the RA is dilated and hypertrophied.

2. An interatrial communication (e.g., PFO, true ASD) with a right-to-left shunt is present in all patients.

3. The RV free wall is often dilated and thin. Fibrosis is present in both RV and LV free walls; this may be responsible for severe symptoms early in life and LV dysfunction in later life.

4. WPW syndrome is frequently associated with the anomaly and predisposes the patient to tachyarrhythmias.

5. PS, pulmonary atresia, TOF, VSD, and other defects are occasionally associated with the anomaly.

Clinical Manifestations
   History.

1. In severe cases, cyanosis and CHF develop during the first few days of life. Some subsequent improvement coincides with the reduction of the PVR.

2. Children with milder cases may complain of dyspnea, fatigue, cyanosis, or palpitation on exertion.

3. A history of SVT is occasionally present.

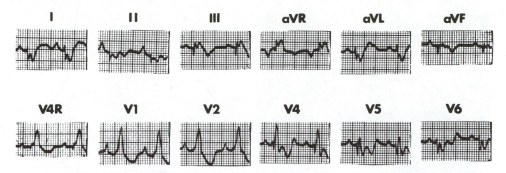

FIG. 14–43
Tracing from a 5-year-old child with Ebstein's anomaly. The tracing shows RAH, right bundle branch block, and first-degree AV block.

Physical examination.

1. Mild to severe cyanosis is present, as well as clubbing of fingers and toes in older infants and children.

2. Characteristic triple or quadruple rhythm is audible. This rhythm has a widely split S2, in addition to split S1, S3, and S4. A soft, systolic regurgitant murmur of TR is usually audible at the LLSB (Fig. 14-42). A soft, scratchy, middiastolic murmur is present at this same location.

3. Hepatomegaly is usually present.

Electrocardiography.

1. Characteristic ECG findings of RBBB and RAH are present in most patients with this condition (Fig. 14-43).

2. First-degree AV block is frequent, occurring in 40% of patients. WPW syndrome is present in 20% of patients with occasional episodes of SVT.

X-ray study. In mild cases the heart is almost normal in size and has normal PVMs. In severe cases an extreme cardiomegaly (principally involving the RA) with a "balloon-shaped" heart and decreased PVMs are present. Some of the largest heart sizes are found in newborns with this condition (Fig. 14-44).

Echocardiography. Two-dimensional echo with color-flow Doppler study is the procedure of choice for morphologic and functional assessment of Ebstein's anomaly. An echo can replace cardiac catheterization and angiography.

1. Apical displacement of the septal leaflet of the tricuspid valve is the most diagnostic feature of the anomaly (Fig. 14-45). A diagnosis of Ebstein's anomaly is made when the tricuspid valve is displaced toward the apex by more than 8 mm/m^2 from the mitral valve insertion. This displacement is seen in the apical four-chamber view. An elongated, somewhat redundant, anterior leaflet with its whiplike motion is also imaged.

2. A large RA, including the atrialized RV, and a small functional RV represent anatomic severity. Evidence of tricuspid valve regurgitation and TS is present. An interatrial communication is imaged.

Natural History

1. Cyanosis tends to improve as the PVR falls during the newborn period. Cyanosis may reappear later.

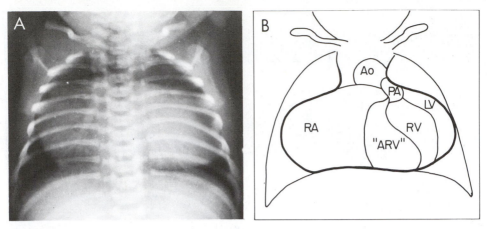

FIG. 14–44
A posteroanterior view **(A)** and a diagram **(B)** of chest roentgenogram from a 2-week-old infant with severe Ebstein's anomaly. Note extreme cardiomegaly involving primarily the RA and diminished pulmonary vascularity. *Ao,* Aorta; *ARV,* atrialized right ventricle.

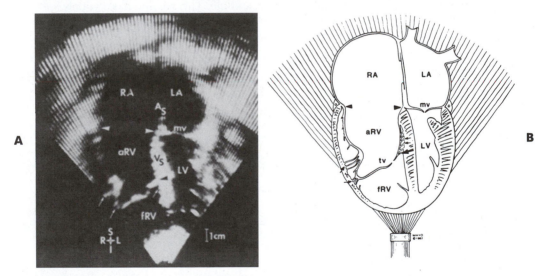

FIG. 14–45
Actual echo **(A)** and diagram **(B)** of an apical four-chamber view in a patient with Ebstein's anomaly. The septal leaflet is displaced into the RV *(large dark arrow)* and thus formed atrialized RV *(aRV)*. Anterior tricuspid leaflet is elongated. Both leaflets are tethered to underlying myocardium *(small arrows)*. Tricuspid annulus and the RA are dilated. (From Shiina A, Serwer JB, Edwards WD et al: Two-dimensional echocardiographic spectrum of Ebstein's anomaly: detailed anatomic assessment, *J Am Coll Cardiol* 3:356-370, 1984.)

2. Patients with a less severe anomaly may be either asymptomatic or mildly symptomatic.

3. Some 18% of symptomatic newborns die in the neonatal period; 30% of patients die before the age of 10 years, usually from CHF. The median age at death is about 20 years old.

4. Hemodynamic deterioration with increasing cyanosis, CHF, and LV dysfunction develop later in life. These developments foretell early death.

5. Attacks of SVT with associated WPW syndrome are common, in that they occur in 15% of all patients. Sudden, unexpected death can occur, probably as a result of arrhythmias.

6. Other possible complications include infective endocarditis, brain abscess, and/or cerebrovascular accident.

Management
Medical.

1. Patients with mild Ebstein's anomaly are asymptomatic and only require regular observation.

2. If CHF develops, anticongestive measures with digoxin and diuretics are indicated.

3. In severely cyanotic newborns, intensive treatment with prostaglandin E_1 infusion, inotropic agents, and correction of metabolic acidosis may be necessary before proceeding with emergency surgery.

4. SVT may be treated with digoxin alone or with propranolol or other antiarrhythmic agents.

5. Maintenance of good dental hygiene and antibiotic prophylaxis for SBE are important.

6. Varying degrees of activity restriction may be necessary for children with this condition.

Surgical.
Indications. Although surgical indications for Epstein's anomaly are not completely defined, they may include the following:

1. Critically ill neonates who show symptoms within the first week of life may be operated on after a period of intensive medical treatment.

2. Activity limited severely (i.e., functional classes III and IV) (see Appendix A, Table A-4).

3. Occurrence of moderate to severe cyanosis, CHF, and RV outflow tract obstruction by redundant tricuspid valve.

4. Repeated, life-threatening arrhythmias in patients with associated WPW syndrome.

Procedures. Controversy exists concerning the type and timing of surgical procedures.

1. The preferred operation is the repair of the tricuspid valve and closure of ASD.

   a. Danielson technique. For the repair of the tricuspid valve, this technique is the most desirable and best tested, although it is frequently limited by anatomy. This technique can be applied in about 60% of the patients (Fig. 14-46). This technique plicates the atrialized portion of the RV, narrows the tricuspid orifice in a selective manner, and results in a monoleaflet valve (by the anterior leaflet of the tricuspid valve). Two other leaflets are often severely hypoplastic and cannot be made to function as a leaflet. The mortality rate is about 5%, which is lower than that for valve replacement.

   b. Carpentier technique. As an alternative, reconstructive surgery of Carpentier may be used. This repair also plicates the atrialized portion of the RV and the tricuspid annulus but in a direction that is at right angles to that used by Danielson. This

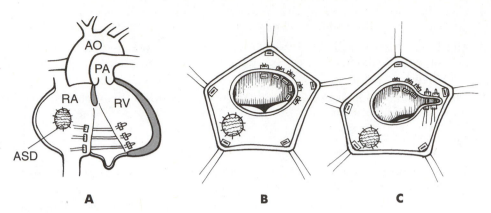

FIG. 14–46
Danielson technique for tricuspid valve repair. **A,** A series of interrupted mattress sutures are placed to obliterate the atrialized portion of the RV. **B,** As the sutures are tied, the atrialized portion of the RV is obliterated (seen through a right atriotomy). **C,** Sutures are placed to further narrow the tricuspid orifice. The valve is now a monocusp valve (anterior leaflet of the tricuspid valve) that is mobile and opens widely during diastole.

repair can be applied in most patients with Ebstein's anomaly. The surgical mortality rate is 15%.

2. Tricuspid valve replacement and closure of ASD is a less desirable surgical approach but may be necessary for 20% to 30% of the patients with Ebstein's anomaly who cannot be candidates for reconstructive surgery. The replacement valve of choice is a stented, antibiotically treated, semilunar valve allograft or a heterograft valve. A pulmonary allograft valve mounted in a short Dacron sleeve can be used in younger children. The surgical mortality rate ranges from 5% to 20%.

3. The Fontan procedure is advocated in patients with severe hypoplasia of the functioning RV (see Fig. 14-35).

4. For a critically ill neonate, the Starnes operation may be performed on an urgent basis after intensive medical treatment. This operation closes the tricuspid valve with autologous pericardium, enlarges the ASD, and creates a modified Blalock-Taussig shunt using a 4 mm tube. A Fontan-type operation is later performed.

5. For patients with WPW syndrome and recurrent SVT, surgical interruption of the accessory pathway is recommended at the time of surgery.

Complications.

1. Complete heart block is a rare complication.

2. Supraventricular arrhythmias persists in 10% to 20% of patients after surgery.

Postoperative follow-up

1. Continued, frequent follow-up is necessary because of the persistence of arrhythmias after surgery, which occurs in 10% to 20% of patients and because of possible problems associated with tricuspid valve surgery that require reoperation.

2. Antibiotic prophylaxis against SBE should be observed.

3. The patient should not participate in competitive or strenuous sports.

PERSISTENT TRUNCUS ARTERIOSUS
Prevalence
Persistent truncus arteriosus occurs in fewer than 1% of all CHDs.

Pathology
1. Only a single arterial trunk with a truncal valve leaves the heart and gives rise to the pulmonary, systemic, and coronary circulations. A large perimembranous VSD is present directly below the truncus (Fig. 14-47). The truncal valve may be bicuspid, tricuspid, or quadricuspid, and it is often incompetent.

2. This anomaly is divided into four types according to Collett and Edwards' classification (Fig. 14-47). The PBF increases in type I, remains normal in types II and III, and decreases in type IV. Type I and II comprise 85% of cases. Type IV is not a true persistent truncus arteriosus; rather, it is a severe form of TOF and pulmonary atresia (i.e., pseudo–truncus arteriosus) with aortic collaterals supplying the lungs.

3. Coronary artery abnormalities are quite common and may contribute to the high surgical mortality. The anomalies include stenotic coronary ostia, high and low take-off of coronary arteries, and abnormal branching and course of the coronary arteries.

4. A right aortic arch is present in 30% of patients. Interrupted aortic arch is seen in 10% of the cases.

5. Evidence of Di George syndrome with hypocalcemia is present in 33% of patients.

Clinical Manifestations
History.
1. Cyanosis may be seen immediately after birth.

2. Signs of CHF develop within several days or weeks after birth.

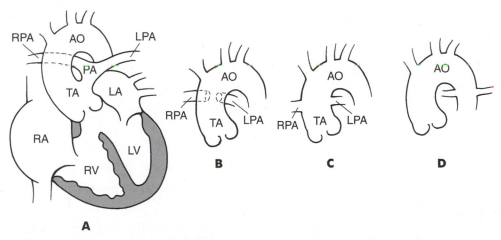

FIG. 14–47
Anatomic types of persistent truncus arteriosus. **A,** In persistent truncus arteriosus, there is a large, single arterial trunk leaving the heart and giving rise to the systemic, pulmonary, and coronary (not shown) circulations. A large perimembranous infundibular VSD is directly under the truncal valve. Branching pattern of the PA is different according to the type. In type I **(A),** the MPA arises from the truncus and then divides into the RPA and LPA. In type II **(B),** the PAs arise from the posterior aspect of the truncus. In type III **(C),** the PAs arise from the lateral aspects of the truncus. In type IV **(D)** or pseudotruncus arteriosus, arteries arising from the descending aorta supply the lungs.

3. History of dyspnea with feeding, failure to thrive, and frequent respiratory infections are usually present in infants.

Physical examination.

1. Varying degrees of cyanosis and signs of CHF with tachypnea and dyspnea are usually present.

2. The peripheral pulses are bounding with a wide pulse pressure.

3. A systolic click is frequently audible at the apex and ULSB. The S2 is single. A harsh (grade 2-4/6), systolic regurgitant murmur, which suggests VSD, is usually audible along the LSB. An apical rumble with or without gallop rhythm may be present when the PBF is large. A high-pitched, early diastolic decrescendo murmur of truncal valve regurgitation may be audible. Rarely is a continuous murmur heard over either side of the chest.

Electrocardiography. The QRS axis is normal (+50 to +120 degrees). CVH is present in 70% of cases; RVH or LVH is less common. LAH is occasionally present.

X-ray study. Cardiomegaly is usually present with increased pulmonary vascularity. A right aortic arch is seen in 30% of the cases.

Echocardiography. Two-dimensional and Doppler echo show the following three diagnostic findings:

1. A large VSD is imaged directly under the truncal valve, similar to TOF.

2. A large, single great artery arises from the heart (i.e., truncus arteriosus). The type of persistent truncus arteriosus can be identified; the size of the PAs can be determined. An artery, branching posteriorly from the truncus, is the PA.

3. The pulmonary valve cannot be imaged; only one semilunar valve (i.e., truncal valve) is imaged.

Natural History

1. Most infants die of CHF within 6 to 12 months. Longer survival is seen in types with normal PBF.

2. Clinical improvement occurs if the infant develops PVOD, which may occur by 3 to 4 months of age. Death occurs around the third decade of life.

3. Truncal valve insufficiency worsens with time.

Management
Medical.

1. Vigorous anticongestive measures with digitalis and diuretics should be pursued.

2. Prophylaxis against SBE should be observed when indications arise.

Surgical.
Palliative procedures. PA banding may be performed in small infants with large PBF and CHF. The banding can produce distortion of the PAs and does not necessarily prevent PVOD. Therefore primary repair of the defect is recommended by many centers. The mortality rate of the banding procedure may be as high as 30% in early infancy.

Definitive procedure.

1. Various modifications of the Rastelli procedure are performed. The VSD is closed in such a way that the LV ejects into the truncus. For type I, a valved or valveless conduit, preferably aortic homograft, is placed between the RV and the PA (Fig. 14-48). A circumferential band of the truncus, which contains both PA orifices, is

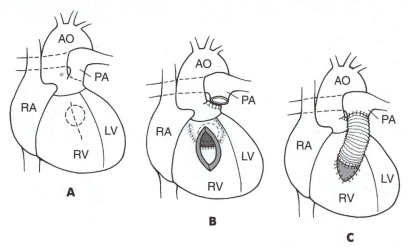

FIG. 14–48
Operative technique for type I truncus arteriosus. **A,** Truncus arteriosus type I is shown with a large VSD *(broken circle)* directly under the truncal valve. The vertical broken line on the RV is the site of the right ventriculotomy. **B,** The pulmonary trunk *(PA)* has been cut away from the truncal artery, and the opening in the truncal artery is sutured. Patch closure of the VSD, which is visible through the ventriculotomy, is completed. **C,** The allograft valved cylinder is anastomosed to the pulmonary trunk. The posterior half of the proximal cylinder is anastomosed to the upper end of the ventriculotomy. A small pericardial patch is trimmed and sutured into place to fill the defect between the allograft and the lower end of the right ventriculotomy.

removed for types II and III. This cuff is tailored and then connected to the RV by the use of a valved or valveless Dacron tube. Aortic continuity is restored with a tubular Dacron graft (Fig. 14-49). The surgical mortality rate is 10% to 30%. Careful investigation of coronary artery anomalies and avoidance of surgical interruption of the coronary arteries are important. The optimal age for this corrective surgery is before the age of 3 months, which is before the PVOD develops. Patients who had PA banding may be operated on at a slightly older age.

2. Barbero-Marcial operation. In this procedure, autologous tissue is used to correct type I truncus (Fig. 14-50). The operation should be performed before 3 months of age.

3. Truncal valve replacement is indicated if there is significant truncal valve insufficiency. It has an extremely high mortality rate of 50% or greater.

Postoperative follow-up

1. Continued, frequent follow-up every 4 to 12 months is required for various reasons to detect late complications, either natural or postoperative.

   a. Progressive truncal valve insufficiency may develop. Truncal valve replacement may be needed for this insufficiency.

   b. A small conduit needs to be changed to a large size, usually by 2 to 3 years of age.

   c. Calcification of the valve in the conduit may occur within 1 to 5 years, which requires reoperation.

   d. Ventricular arrhythmias may develop because of right ventriculotomy.

2. SBE prophylaxis should be observed on indications.

3. The patient should not participate in competitive, strenuous sports.

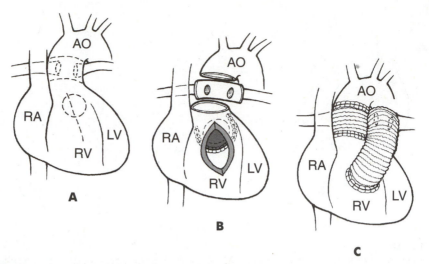

FIG. 14–49
Operative technique for type II and III truncus arteriosus. **A,** Two broken lines on the
truncal artery indicate the sites of excision of the PAs. The vertical broken line is the site
of the right ventriculotomy. A VSD is under the truncal valve *(broken circle).* **B,** The VSD
is closed with patch through right ventriculotomy (which is visible through the
ventriculotomy). The cuff of truncal tissue, including the PA orifices, has been excised
and trimmed. **C,** Continuity of the truncal artery, which is now the aorta, has been
restored with a Dacron graft. The lower end of a Dacron conduit containing a
heterograft valve has been anastomosed to the right ventriculotomy, and the upper end
of the conduit to the PA.

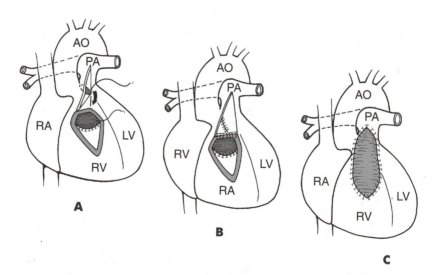

FIG. 14–50
Barbero-Marcial operation for type I truncus arteriosus. **A,** A longitudinal incision is
made from the PA to the left sinus of Valsalva. Through the incision the orifice of the
pulmonary trunk (partially shown) will be closed. A right ventriculotomy is made, and the
VSD has been closed with a patch through the ventriculotomy. **B,** Suturing of the
inferior flap of the PA incision and the superior aspect of the right ventriculotomy is
completed. This becomes the posterior wall of the RV-PA pathway to be created.
Completed suture line of the pulmonary trunk orifice is visible. **C,** Autograft or bovine
pericardial patch is sutured to form the anterior wall of the RV-PA pathway.

SINGLE VENTRICLE

Prevalence

Single ventricle (double inlet ventricle) occurs in fewer than 1% of all CHDs.

Pathology

1. Both AV valves are connected to a main, single ventricular chamber (i.e., double-inlet ventricle), and the main chamber is in turn connected to a rudimentary chamber through the bulboventricular foramen. One great artery arises from the main chamber, the other arises from the rudimentary chamber (Fig. 14-51). In about 80% of the cases the main ventricular chamber has anatomic characteristics of the LV (i.e., double-inlet LV). Occasionally, the main chamber has anatomic characteristics of the RV (i.e., double-inlet RV). Rarely does the ventricle have an intermediate trabecular pattern without a rudimentary chamber (i.e., common ventricle). Also, both atria rarely empty via a common AV valve into the main ventricular chamber with either LV or RV morphology (i.e., common-inlet ventricle).

2. TGA, of either the D-form or L-form, is present in 85% of the cases. The most common form of single ventricle is double-inlet LV with L-TGA and with the aorta arising from the rudimentary chamber in 70 to 75% of cases (Fig. 14-51). The mitral valve is right-sided; the tricuspid valve is left-sided. PS or pulmonary atresia is present in about 50% of cases. COA and interrupted aortic arch are also common. Less commonly, D-TGA is present with the aorta arising from the right and anterior rudimentary chamber.

3. The bulboventricular foramen is frequently obstructive. Anomalies of the AV valves, which includes stenosis, in addition to overriding or straddling, are frequent.

4. In double-inlet RV either right or left atrial isomerism and straddling and/or overriding of the AV valves are common. The most frequently encountered ventriculoarterial connection is a double-outlet from the main chamber. PS is frequently found.

Pathophysiology

1. Since there is almost complete mixing in the single ventricle, the systemic arterial saturation is primarily determined by the amount of PBF. With PS, cyanosis is present. Cyanosis is intense at birth with pulmonary atresia. When the pulmonary valve is not stenotic, the PBF is large and signs of CHF develop within days or weeks with either minimal or no cyanosis.

2. An obstructed bulboventricular foramen may occur either naturally with growth or, for unknown reasons, develop after a PA banding. This condition occurs in 70% to 85% of banded patients. The occurrence of an obstructed foramen has a profound

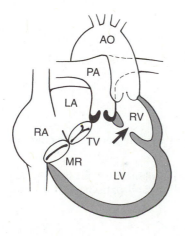

FIG. 14–51

Diagram of the most common form of single ventricle. The single ventricle is an anatomic LV. The great arteries are transposed with the aorta anterior to and left of the PA and arises from the rudimentary RV. Stenosis of the pulmonary valve is present in about 50% of cases (shown as thick valves). This type accounts for 70% to 75% of cases of single ventricle.

hemodynamic effect, in addition to major surgical implications in patients with the aorta arising from the anterior rudimentary chamber. The obstruction increases PBF and decreases systemic perfusion. The banding also causes excessive hypertrophy of the left ventricle, resulting in a decreased compliance of the ventricle, which places the patient at risk for a future Fontan operation.

Clinical Manifestations
History.

1. Cyanosis of varying degrees is present from birth.

2. History of a failure to thrive, signs of heart failure, or pneumonias may be present.

Physical examination. Physical findings depend on the magnitude of PBF.

1. With *increased PBF*, physical findings resemble those of TGA and VSD or even of large VSD:

   a. Mild cyanosis and CHF with growth retardation are present in early infancy.

   b. The S2 is single or narrowly split with a loud P2. A grade 3-4/6 long systolic murmur is audible along the LSB. A loud S3 or an apical diastolic rumble may also be audible.

   c. A diastolic murmur of PR may be present along the ULSB as a result of pulmonary hypertension.

2. With *decreased PBF*, physical findings resemble those of TOF.

   a. Moderate to severe cyanosis is present. CHF is not present. Clubbing may be seen in older infants and children.

   b. The S2 is loud and single. A grade 2-4/6 ejection systolic murmur may be heard at the URSB or ULSB.

Electrocardiography.

1. Unusual ventricular hypertrophy pattern with similar QRS complexes across most or all precordial leads is common (e.g., RS, rS, QR pattern).

2. Abnormal Q waves (representing abnormalities in septal depolarization) are also common and take one of the following forms: Q waves in the right precordial leads, no Q waves in any precordial leads, or Q waves in both the right and left precordial leads.

3. Either first- or second-degree AV block may be present.

4. Arrhythmias occur (e.g., SVT, wandering pacemaker, and so on).

X-ray Study.

1. With increased PBF, the heart size enlarges and the pulmonary vascularity increases.

2. When PBF is normal or decreased, the heart size is normal and the pulmonary vascularity is normal or decreased.

3. Narrow upper mediastinum that suggests TGA may be present.

Echocardiography.

1. The most important diagnostic sign is the presence of a single ventricular chamber into which two AV valves empty.

2. The following anatomic and functional information is important from the surgical point of view and should be systematically obtained in each patient with a single ventricle:

a. Morphology of the single ventricle should be determined (e.g., double-inlet LV? double-inlet RV?).

b. Location of the rudimentary outflow chamber, which is usually left and anterior.

c. The size of the bulboventricular foramen and whether there an obstruction should be determined. Obstruction of the foramen is present if the pressure gradient across the foramen is greater than 10 mm Hg, or if the area of the foramen is less than 2 cm^2/m^2. The foramen, which is nearly as large as the aortic annulus, is considered ideal.

d. The presence or absence of D-TGA or L-TGA, stenosis of the pulmonary or aortic valve, and the size of the PAs.

e. The anatomy of the AV valves should be observed. The position of the mitral and tricuspid valves, in addition to the presence of stenosis, regurgitation, hypoplasia, or straddling, should be checked.

f. The size of atrial septal defect should be determined.

g. Associated defects such as COA, interrupted aortic arch, or PDA should be sought.

Natural History

1. CHF and growth failure develop in early infancy. Without surgery, about 50% of the patients die before reaching 1 year of age.

2. Clinical improvement occurs if PVOD develops.

3. Cyanosis increases if PS worsens.

4. If the aorta arises from the rudimentary chamber, the bulboventricular foramen is often small or becomes obstructed. This results in increased PBF and decreased systemic perfusion.

5. Complete heart block develops in about 12% of patients, but most of them tolerate it well.

6. SBE or cerebral complication may develop, as in TOF.

Management
   Medical.

1. Newborns with severe PS or pulmonary atresia, as well as those with interrupted aortic arch or coarctation, require prostaglandin E$_1$ infusion and other supportive measures before surgery.

2. Anticongestive measures with digoxin and diuretics should be taken if CHF develops.

Surgical.
Palliative Procedures.

1. Systemic-PA shunt is necessary for patients with PS or pulmonary atresia and severe cyanosis (Fig. 14-20). The mortality rate remains low.

2. For infants with CHF and pulmonary edema resulting from increased PBF, PA banding can be considered, although banding carries an unacceptably high mortality rate, which is between 25% and 50%. The major risk factor is the presence or development of an obstructed bulboventricular foramen. Most infants with obstructed foramen do not tolerate the banding well, so the following may be done:

a. If the bulboventricular foramen is *normal* or *unobstructed*, PA banding is performed, but the patient should be watched for the development of subaortic stenosis after the banding.

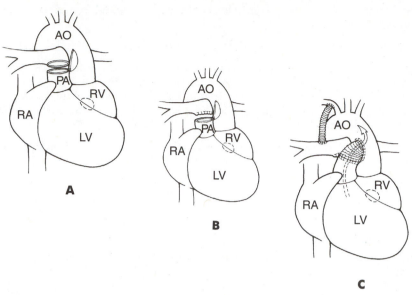

FIG. 14–52
Damus-Kaye-Stansel anastomosis for single ventricle and subaortic stenosis. **A,** The PA is transected proximal to the bifurcation. An appropriately positioned and sized incision is made in the ascending aorta. **B,** The distal end of the PA is oversewn and the proximal end of the PA is anastomosed to the opening in the aorta. **C** An appropriately shaped hood (Dacron tube, pericardium, allograft or Gore-Tex) is added to the anastomosis. A systemic-PA shunt has been completed.

  b. If the foramen too *small*, one of the following two alternative procedures may be performed, although a high mortality rate remains:

   1) Damus-Kaye-Stansel operation is the prefered procedure. This procedure involves a PA-aorta anastomosis, which is accomplished by the transection of the MPA and anastomosis of the proximal PA to the ascending aorta, in addition to a systemic-PA shunt or a cavopulmonary shunt (Fig. 14-52). A Fontan-type operation can be performed later (see Fig. 14-35).

   2) Another procedure involves the enlargement of the bulboventricular foramen by a transaortic approach and without cardiopulmonary bypass. This procedure is performed especially when PS is present. The surgical mortality rate is about 15%.

3. Surgery for interrupted aortic arch or coarctation should be performed, if present.

Definitive procedures.

1. The Fontan-type operation is performed at 3 to 4 years of age and certainly before the age of 10. Most of these children had either a PA band or a Damus-Kaye-Stansel operation. PA distortion in children younger than 3 years old are high risk factors. However, the age must be weighed against the deleterious effects of a systemic-PA shunt, which may result in PA distortion and/or depressed ventricular function. If an AV valve is incompetent, it may need to be closed during surgery. The surgical mortality has recently been reduced to about 10%, similar to that for tricuspid atresia.

2. Attempts at septating the single ventricle are usually unsuccessful. The overall hospital mortality for this procedure has been as high as 30% to 40%.

Postoperative follow-up

1. Most survivors of surgery are symptomatic with cyanosis, dyspnea as a result of ventricular dysfunction, and arrhythmias. These symptoms require regular follow-up.

2. Antibiotic prophylaxis against SBE should be observed whenever necessary.

DOUBLE-OUTLET RIGHT VENTRICLE

Prevalence

DORV occurs in fewer than 1% of all CHDs.

Pathology (Fig. 14-53)

1. Both the aorta and PA arise from the RV. The only outlet from the LV is a large VSD.

2. The great arteries usually lie side by side. The aorta is usually to the right of the PA, although one of the great arteries may be more anterior than the other. The aortic and pulmonary valves are at the same level. Conus septum is present between the aorta and the PA. The subaortic and subpulmonary conuses separate the aortic and pulmonary valves from the tricuspid and mitral valves, respectively. This means there is no fibrous continuity between the semilunar valves and the AV valves. In a normal heart, the aortic valve is lower than the pulmonary valve, and the aortic valve is in fibrous continuity with the mitral valve.

3. The position of the VSD and the presence or absence of PS influence hemodynamic alterations and form the basis for dividing the defect into the following types of DORV:

   a. Subaortic VSD (Fig. 14-53, A and C) — The VSD is closer to the aortic valve than to the pulmonary valve and lies to the right of the conus septum. This is the most common type, in that it occurs in 60% to 70% of the cases. PS is common, especially the infundibular type, and it occurs in about 50% in this type of DORV.

   b. Subpulmonary VSD (i.e., Taussig-Bing anomaly) (Fig. 14-53, B) — The VSD is closer to the pulmonary valve than to the aortic valve, and it usually lies above the crista supraventricularis and to the left of the conus septum. This type accounts for approximately 10% of cases.

   c. Doubly committed VSD — The VSD is closely related to both semilunar valves and is usually above the crista supraventricularis.

   d. Remote VSD — The VSD is clearly away from the semilunar valves. It most commonly represents the AV canal-type VSD and occasionally is an isolated muscular VSD. Atrial isomerism is commonly seen with this type.

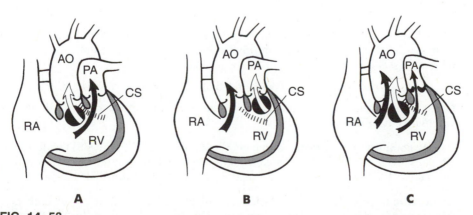

FIG. 14–53
Diagram of three representative types of DORV, viewed with the RV free wall removed. **A,** Subaortic VSD. **B,** Subpulmonary VSD (Taussig-Bing anomaly). **C,** Subaortic VSD with PS. Doubly committed and remote VSDs are not shown. *Ao,* Aorta; *CS,* crista supraventricularis.

Pathophysiology and Clinical Manifestations

Pathophysiology and clinical manifestations of DORV are primarily determined by the position of the VSD and the presence or absence of PS. Each representative type is presented separately.

Subaortic ventricular septal defect without pulmonary stenosis. In subaortic VSD, oxygenated blood *(open arrow)* from the LV is directed to the aorta (AO) and desaturated systemic venous blood *(solid arrow)* is directed to the PA, thereby producing mild or no cyanosis (Fig. 14-53, A). The PBF increases in the absence of PS or PVOD, which results in CHF. Therefore clinical pictures of this type resemble those of a large VSD with pulmonary hypertension and CHF.

1. Growth retardation, tachypnea, and other signs of CHF are usually present. A hyperactive precordium, a loud S2, and a VSD-type (regurgitant) systolic murmur are present. An apical diastolic rumble may be audible.

2. The ECG often resembles that of complete ECD. Superior QRS axis (i.e., −30 to −170 degrees) may be found in this type. RVH or CVH, as well as LAH are common. Occasionally, first-degree AV block is present.

3. Chest x-ray images show cardiomegaly with increased PVMs and a prominent MPA segment.

Subpulmonary ventricular septal defect (Taussig-Bing malformation). In subpulmonary VSD, or Taussig-Bing malformation, oxygenated blood from the LV is directed to the PA, and desaturated blood from the systemic vein is directed to the aorta. This results in severe cyanosis (Fig. 14-53, B). The PBF increases with the fall of the PVR. Clinical pictures resemble those of TGA.

1. Growth retardation and severe cyanosis with or without clubbing are common findings. The S2 is loud, and a grade 2-3/6 systolic murmur is audible at the ULSB. An ejection click and an occasional PR murmur as a result of pulmonary hypertension may be audible.

2. The ECG shows RAD, RAH, and RVH. LVH may be seen during infancy.

3. Chest x-ray images show cardiomegaly with increased PVMs and a prominent MPA segment.

Fallot-type double-outlet right ventricle with pulmonary stenosis. Even though the VSD is subaortic, in the presence of PS (i.e., Fallot type), some desaturated blood goes to the aorta. This causes cyanosis and a decrease in PBF. Clinical pictures resemble those of TOF (Fig. 14-53, C).

1. Growth retardation, cyanosis, and clubbing are all common. The S2 is loud and single. A grade 2-4/6 ejection systolic murmur along the LSB is present either with or without a systolic thrill.

2. The ECG shows RAD, RAH, RVH, or RBBB. First-degree AV block is frequent.

3. Chest x-ray images show normal heart size with an upturned apex. Pulmonary vascularity decreases.

Doubly committed or remote ventricular septal defect. With the VSD close to both semilunar valves, called *doubly committed VSD* or remotely located from these valves, called *remote VSD,* cyanosis of a mild degree is present and the PBF increases.

Echocardiography. Three diagnostic signs of DORV are the origin of both great arteries from the anterior RV, the absence of LV outflow other than the VSD, and the discontinuity of the mitral and semilunar valves.

1. In the parasternal long-axis view all three diagnostic features of DORV are imaged.

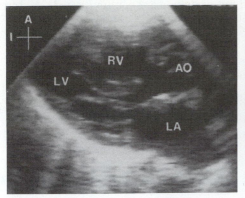
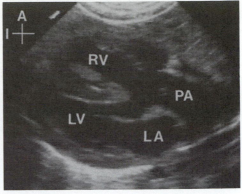

FIG. 14–54

Parasternal long-axis view of DORV. **A,** Subaortic VSD. The VSD is closely related to the aorta. The marked separation between the anterior mitral valve leaflet and the aortic valve can be seen. The aorta overrides the ventricular septum by more than 50%.
B, Subpulmonary VSD. The great artery which is closely related to the VSD has an immediate posterior sweep, suggesting that it is a PA. Note the separation between the anterior mitral leaflet and the pulmonary valve. The PA overrides the ventricular septum by more than 50%. (**A** from Snider AR, Serwer GA: *Echocardiography in pediatric heart disease,* St Louis, 1990, Mosby; **B** from Snider AR: Two-dimensional and Doppler echocardiographic evaluation of heart disease in the neonate and fetus, *Clin Perinatol* 15:523-565, 1988.)

Typical subaortic or subpulmonary VSD can be demonstrated in this view for most patients (Fig. 14-54, *A* and *B*). No great artery is seen to arise from the posterior ventricle. The great arteries arising from the anterior ventricle are seen in parallel orientation. In addition, a mass of echopositive tissue, usually greater than 5 mm in length, is present between the mitral valve annulus and the semilunar valve (i.e., mitral-semilunar discontinuity).

2. In the parasternal short-axis view a *double circle,* rather than the normal *circle and sausage* appearance of the great arteries, may be seen. The great arteries are either side by side with the aorta to the right, or the aorta is anterior and slightly to the right of the PA.

3. The size and position of the VSD should be determined in relation to the great arteries.

    a. Typical subpulmonary or subaortic VSD can be demonstrated by the parasternal long-axis scanning in most patients (Fig. 14-54, *A* and *B*).

    b. In the subcostal four-chamber view the subaortic VSD is located to the right of the conus septum just beneath the aortic valve. The subpulmonary VSD is located to the left of the conus septum just beneath the pulmonary valve.

    c. Doubly committed VSD is recognized in the parasternal or the apical long-axis view.

    d. Remote VSDs, either endocardial cushion type or apical muscular VSD, are best recognized in the apical four-chamber view.

4. Associated anomalies such as valvar and/or subvalvar PS, occurring in 60% of cases, and other left-to-right shunt lesions (e.g., ASD, PDA) should be looked for.

5. Occasionally, differentiation of DORV from TOF with a marked overriding of the aorta or from TGA is necessary. There is mitral-semilunar continuity in TOF and TGA

(i.e., mitral-aortic continuity in TOF, and mitral-pulmonary continuity in TGA), but no mitral-semilunar continuity is present in DORV.

Natural History

1. Infants without PS may develop severe CHF, and later PVOD, if left untreated. Spontaneous closure of VSD, which is fatal, is rare.

2. When PS is present, complications common to cyanotic CHD (e.g., polycythemia, cerebrovascular accident) may develop.

3. In patients with the Taussig-Bing malformation, severe PVOD develops early in life. Associated anomalies (e.g., COA, LV hypoplasia) also contributes to the poor prognosis.

Management
Medical.

1. Treatment of CHF with digoxin and diuretics are needed.

2. Antibiotic prophylaxis against SBE should be observed on indications.

Surgical.
Palliative procedures.

1. PA banding for symptomatic infants with increased PBF and CHF is occasionally performed. However, this procedure is not recommended for infants with subaortic VSD or doubly committed VSD. Primary repair is a better choice.

2. For infants with Taussig-Bing type, enlarging the interatrial communication is important for better mixing and for decompressing the LA. Balloon atrial septostomy, blade atrial septostomy, and even the Blalock-Hanlon operation (i.e., surgical atrial septectomy) should be considered.

3. In infants with PS and decreased PBF with cyanosis a systemic-PA shunt procedure is needed. The mortality rate is low.

Definitive surgeries.

SUBAORTIC VSD OR DOUBLY COMMITTED VSD. Creation of an intraventricular tunnel between the VSD and the subaortic outflow tract by means of a Dacron patch is performed early in life, at least by 6 months of age, without preliminary PA banding. The mortality rate is less than 5% for simple subaortic VSD; it is slightly higher for doubly committed VSD.

TAUSSIG-BING ANOMALY (I.E., SUBPULMONARY VSD). There are three possible surgical approaches. These operations should be carried out at 3 to 4 months or sooner because of a rapid development of the PVOD.

1. An intraventricular tunnel between the VSD and the PA with the arterial switch operation is the procedure of choice. The operation should be performed during the first month of life. The mortality rate is between 10% and 15%.

2. An intraventricular tunnel between the VSD and the PA along with the Senning operation is a less desirable approach. This procedure has a high mortality rate (i.e., > 40%) and a higher late complication rate.

3. An intraventricular tunnel between the VSD and the aorta is desirable but often technically impossible. The surgical mortality rate is about 15%.

FALLOT TYPE.

1. An intraventricular tunnel between the VSD and the aorta, in addition to relief of PS by a patch graft is carried out between 6 months and 2 years of age. This procedure is similar to the Lecompte operation for patients who have the combination of TGA, VSD, and PS (see Fig. 14-11). The surgical mortality rate is 10% to 15%.

2. If preoperative studies indicate the need for a homograft valved extracardiac conduit, the corrective repair is deferred until age 4 or 5 years old, with a shunt operation performed in infancy.

REMOTE VSD. The surgery may be delayed until 2 to 3 years of age. The PA banding is usually needed in infancy to control CHF. The following are three possible options:

1. When possible, an intraventricular tunnel procedure between the AV canal type VSD and the aorta is preferred, but the mortality rate is high (i.e., 30% to 40%).

2. The Senning operation, VSD repair, and LV-to-PA valved extracardiac conduit is an alternative. The mortality rate is relatively low (i.e., about 15%).

3. If the above procedures are not possible, a Fontan-type operation, which has a recent mortality rate of less than 5%, is performed.

Postoperative follow-up

Long-term, regular follow-up at the interval of 6 to 12 months is necessary to detect and manage late complications of surgery for the defect.

1. In general, patients who had subaortic VSD without PS have an extremely good, long-term outlook.

2. Ventricular arrhythmia should be treated, since it may cause sudden death.

3. Occasionally, patients require reoperation of the intraventricular tunnel (i.e., about 20%).

4. Continued SBE prophylaxis is necessary for most patients who had repair of DORV.

SPLENIC SYNDROMES

There is a failure of differentiation into the right-side and left-sided organs in splenic syndromes with resulting congenital malformations of multiple organ systems. Asplenia syndrome (i.e. Ivemark's syndrome, right atrial isomerism) is associated with the absence of the spleen, which is a left-sided organ, and a tendency for bilateral right-sidedness. In polysplenia syndrome (i.e., left atrial isomerism), multiple splenic tissues are present with a tendency for bilateral left-sidedness. There is a striking tendency for symmetric development of normally asymmetric organs or pairs of organs. Members of paired organs, such as the lungs, commonly show pronounced isomerism; unpaired organs, such as the stomach, seem to be located in a random fashion. Although the type and severity of cardiovascular malformations differ between the two syndromes, the same types of defects may be present in both.

Asplenia Syndrome

Prevalence. Asplenia syndrome occurs in 1% of newborns with symptomatic CHDs. This syndrome occurs more often in males (60% of asplenia syndrome cases).

Pathology.

1. The spleen is absent in asplenia syndrome. Since the spleen is a left-sided organ, a striking tendency for bilateral right-sidedness characterizes malformations of the major organ systems. Bilateral, three-lobed right lungs with bilateral, eparterial bronchi (Fig. 14-55); various gastrointestinal malformations (occurring in 20% of cases); a symmetric, midline liver; and malrotation of the intestines are all present. The stomach may be located on either the right or the left.

2. Complex cardiac malformations are always present. Cardiovascular malformations involve all parts of the heart, systemic veins and pulmonary veins, and the great arteries. Two sinoatrial nodes are present. Table 14-1 summarizes and compares

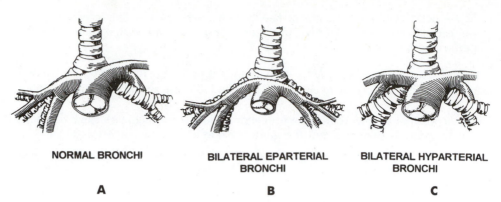

A   **B**   **C**

FIG. 14–55
Diagram of normal bronchi **(A)**; bilateral eparterial bronchi, usually seen in asplenia syndrome **(B)**; and bilateral hyparterial bronchi, usually seen in polysplenia syndrome **(C)**. (From Fyler DC, ed: *Nadas' pediatric cardiology,* St Louis, 1992, Mosby.)

TABLE 14–1.

Cardiovascular Malformations in Asplenia and Polysplenia Syndromes

Structures	Asplenia Syndrome	Polysplenia Syndrome
Systemic veins	Bilateral SVC; single SVC usually right (35%)	Bilateral SVC (33%); single SVC right or left (66%)
	Normal IVC in all, but may be left-sided (35%); azygos continuation rarely seen	*Absent hepatic segment of IVC with azygos continuation right or left (85%)
	Juxtaposition of IVC and aorta common	Juxtaposition of IVC and aorta occasionally
	Normal hepatic veins to IVC (75%)	Bilateral, common hepatic vein to RA
Pulmonary veins	*TAPVR with extracardiac connection (75%) and often with PV obstruction	†Normal PV return (50%); right PVs to right-sided atrium and left PVs to left-sided atrium (50%)
Atrium and atrial septum	Bilateral right atria (with bilateral sinus node)	Bilateral, left atria
	Absent coronary sinus	Absent coronary sinus
	†Primum ASD (100%), secundum ASD (66%)	Single atrium, primum ASD (60%), or secundum ASD (25%)
AV valve	*Single AV valve (90%)	Normal AV valve (50%); single AV valve (15%)
Ventricles and cardiac apex	†Single ventricle (50%) usually morphologic RV or undetermined; two ventricles (in 50%)	*Two ventricles usually present; VSD (65%); DORV (20%)
	Left apex (60%); right apex (40%)	Left apex (60%); right apex (40%)
Great arteries	*Either D- or L-transposition (70%)	†Normal great arteries (85%); transposition (15%)
	†Stenosis (40%) or atresia (40%) of pulmonary valve	Normal pulmonary valve (60%); PS or pulmonary atresia (40%)
ECG	Normal P axis or in the +90 to +180 degree quadrant	†Superior P axis (70%)

* Extremely important differentiating points.
† Important differentiating points.

these malformations with those of polysplenia syndrome. Cardiovascular anomalies that help distinguish asplenia syndrome from polysplenia syndrome include the following:

a. TGA with PS or pulmonary atresia occurs in about 80% of asplenia syndrome cases, thereby producing severe cyanosis during the newborn period. TGA is present in only 15% of patients with polysplenia syndrome.

b. Single ventricle and common AV valve occur with greater frequency in asplenia syndrome. In polysplenia syndrome two ventricles are usually present.

c. TAPVR to *extracardiac* structures occurs in more than 75% of cases, although it is difficult to diagnose.

Pathophysiology.

1. Complete mixing of systemic and pulmonary venous blood usually occurs because of the multiple cardiovascular abnormalities associated with this syndrome.

2. PBF is reduced because of stenosis or atresia of the pulmonary valve. This results in severe cyanosis shortly after birth.

3. Although rare, the absence of PS may result in CHF early in life.

Clinical manifestations.
Physical examination.

1. Cyanosis is usually the presenting sign and is often severe.

2. Auscultation of the heart is nonspecific. Heart murmurs of PS and VSD are frequently audible.

3. A symmetric liver (midline liver) is palpable.

Electrocardiography.

1. A *superior* QRS axis is present, resulting from the presence of ECD.

2. The P axis is either normal (0 to +90 degrees) or alternating between the left lower and right lower quadrants. This occurs because two sinus nodes alternate the pacemaker function.

3. RVH, LVH, or CVH is usually present.

X-ray study.

1. The heart size is usually normal or slightly increased with decreased PVM.

2. The heart is in the right chest, left chest, or midline (i.e., mesocardia).

3. A symmetric liver is a striking feature (see Fig. 28-1).

4. Tracheobronchial symmetry with bilateral, eparterial bronchi is usually identified.

Echocardiography. When the systematic approach is used, two-dimensional echo and color-flow Doppler studies can detect all or most of the anomalies described in the section on pathology. The anatomy of the IVC and great arteries and the presence or absence of PS or pulmonary atresia are important in differentiating the two splenic syndromes.

Laboratory studies.

1. Howell-Jolly and Heinz bodies seen on the peripheral smear suggest asplenia syndrome. However, these bodies may be found in some normal newborns and septic infants, too.

2. A splenic scan may be useful in older infants but is of limited value in the extremely ill neonates.

Natural history. Without palliative surgical procedures, more than 95% of patients with asplenia syndrome die within the first year of life. Fulminating sepsis is one cause of death.

Management.
Medical.

1. In severely cyanotic newborns, prostaglandin E_1 infusion is given to reopen the ductus.

2. The risk of fulminating infection, especially by pneumococcus, is high. Continuous antibiotic therapy with amoxicillin (20 to 25 mg/kg/day, divided into two doses) should be given to patients until 2 years of age.

3. Immunization with polyvalent pneumococcal vaccine (Pneumovax 23) and quadrivalent vaccine are recommended at 2 years of age. Hemophillus B-conjugate vaccine is recommended for patients who are 18 months old and older. More than 50% of patients fail to adequately respond after the pneumococcal vaccine, therefore their antibody responses should be monitored. Revaccination after 3 to 5 years of age should be considered for children with asplenia syndrome.

Surgical.

1. A systemic-PA shunt is usually necessary during either the newborn period or infancy. The surgical mortality for the shunt is higher in asplenia patients than in other defects, and it is probably related to the regurgitation of the common AV valve and undiagnosed obstructive TAPVR.

   a. Patients with common AV valve, especially those with regurgitation of the valve, do not tolerate the volume overload that results from the shunt.

   b. Patients with the obstructive type of TAPVR may show evidence of the anomalous return with signs of pulmonary edema only after the systemic-PA shunt. Surgical mortality for both the shunt and repair of the TAPVR is unacceptably high, in that death occurs in more than 90% of all cases.

   c. Identification of infants with obstructive TAPVR by pulmonary angiography with prostaglandin E_1 infusion before surgery is important. In infants with the infracardiac type of TAPVR, a successful connection can be made between the pulmonary venous confluence and the RA with the use of a partial exclusion clamp and without cardiopulmonary bypass.

2. Although complete anatomic correction of the defect is impossible, a Fontan-type operation can be performed (after 3 years of age). The overall mortality rate for Fontan-type surgery is as high as 65%. A regurgitation of the AV valve is a high-risk factor, requiring repair or replacement of the valve.

Polysplenia Syndrome

Prevalence. Polysplenia syndrome (i.e. left atrial isomerism) occurs in fewer than 1% of all CHDs. It occurs more often in females (70% of all cases).

Pathology.

1. Multiple splenic tissues are present. Since the spleen is a left-sided organ, a tendency for bilateral left-sidedness characterizes this syndrome. Noncardiovascular malformations include bilateral, bilobed lungs (i.e., two left lungs), bilateral, hyparterial bronchi (Fig. 14-55), symmetric liver (25%), occasional absence of gallbladder, and some degree of intestinal malrotation (80%).

2. Cardiovascular malformations are similar to those seen in asplenia syndrome but have a lower frequency of pulmonary valve stenosis or atresia. A normal heart or minimal malformation of the heart is present in as many as 25% of patients with polysplenia

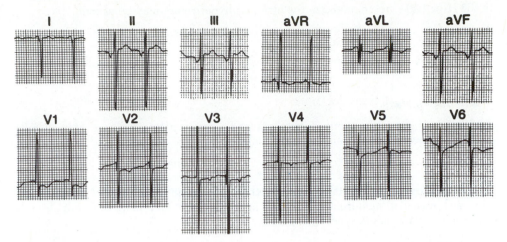

FIG. 14–56
Tracing from a 1-week-old neonate with polysplenia syndrome. Both the P and QRS axes are in the left upper quadrant (−45 and −80 degrees, respectively). Thus the ECG shows an ectopic atrial rhythm and a superior QRS axis. The QRS voltages indicate RVH and probable additional LVH.

syndrome. Cardiovascular malformations are summarized and compared with those of asplenia syndrome in Table 14-1.

Important features of polysplenia syndrome that distinguish it from asplenia syndrome include the following:

a. The absence of the hepatic segment of the IVC with azygos (right side) or hemiazygos (left side) continuation is seen in 85% of the patients. This abnormality is rarely present in asplenia syndrome.

b. Two ventricles are usually present. A single ventricle with a common AV valve is common in asplenia syndrome.

c. TGA, PS or pulmonary atresia, and TAPVR occur less often than they do in asplenia syndrome.

d. The ECG shows a superiorly oriented P axis (i.e., ectopic atrial rhythm), resulting from the absence of the sinus node (Fig. 14-56).

e. Polysplenia syndrome occurs more often in females (70%).

Pathophysiology. Since PS or pulmonary atresia occurs less frequently, cyanosis is not intense, if it is present at all. Rather, CHF often develops because of an increased PBF.

Clinical manifestation.
Physical examination.

1. Cyanosis is either absent or mild. Signs of CHF may develop during the neonatal period.

2. Heart murmur of VSD may be audible. A symmetric liver is usually palpable.

Electrocardiography (Fig. 14-56).

1. A superiorly oriented P axis (−30 to −90 degrees) is seen in more than 70% of patients, since there is no sinus node in a situation in which two left atria are present.

2. A superior QRS axis is present as a result of the presence of ECD.

3. RVH or LVH are common, but ventricular hypertrophy may be absent.

4. Complete heart block occurs in about 10% of patients.

X-ray study. Mild to moderate cardiomegaly with increased PVMs; midline liver (see Fig. 28-1); and bilateral, hyparterial bronchi may be present.

Laboratory study.

1. Some patients with splenic hypoplasia and hypofunction may have Howell-Jolly bodies, however, not in an excessive number.

2. The radioactive splenic scan may show multiple splenic tissues.

Echocardiography. Two-dimensional and Doppler-echo studies reveal all or most of the cardiovascular malformations listed in Table 14-1 and help differentiate this syndrome from asplenia syndrome.

Natural history.

1. The first year mortality rate is 60%, in comparison with more than 95% as in asplenia syndrome.

2. Most infants with severe cardiac malformation die within the first year without surgical palliation or repair.

3. The heart rate is lower than in normal children. Excessive nodal bradycardia may develop, resulting in CHF.

Management.
Medical.

1. If present, CHF should be treated.

2. PA banding should be performed if intractable CHF develops with large PBF.

Surgical.

1. Occasionally, pacemaker therapy is required for children with excessive AV nodal bradycardia and CHF.

2. Total correction of the defect is possible in some children. If total correction is not possible, at least a Fontan-type operation can be performed. The surgical mortality rate of the Fontan-type operation in this group of children is about 25%, which is lower than that for asplenia but higher than that for tricuspid atresia.

Postoperative follow-up

Periodic, regular follow-up is necessary because of continuing medical and surgical problems.

1. Although most patients are in the New York Heart Association class I or class II (see Appendix A, Table AA-4), persistent ascites or edema are frequent and require medications such as digoxin and diuretics several years after the Fontan-type operation.

2. Cardiac arrhythmias, usually supraventricular, are present in 25% of the patients. Some require antiarrhythmic medications.

15 / Vascular Ring

Prevalence

Vascular ring reportedly represents less than 1% of all congenital cardiovascular anomalies, but this may be an underestimate because some conditions are asymptomatic.

Pathology

1. *Vascular ring* refers to a group of anomalies of the aortic arch that cause respiratory symptoms or feeding problems. A rare anomaly of the left PA that causes symptoms is also included in this group. The vascular ring may be divided into two groups: complete (or true) and incomplete.

    a. *Complete vascular ring* refers to conditions in which the abnormal vascular structures form a complete circle around the trachea and esophagus. These include double aortic arch and right aortic arch with left ligamentum arteriosum.

    b. *Incomplete vascular ring* refers to vascular anomalies that do not form a complete circle around the trachea and esophagus but do compress the trachea or esophagus. These include anomalous innominate artery, aberrant right subclavian artery, and anomalous left PA ("vascular sling").

2. Double aortic arch is the most common vascular ring (40%) (Fig. 15-1). This anomaly is due to a failure of the regression of both the right and left fourth branchial arches, resulting in right and left aortic arches, respectively. These two arches completely encircle and compress the trachea and esophagus, producing respiratory distress and feeding problems in early infancy. The right arch gives off two arch vessels, the right common carotid and the right subclavian, whereas the left arch gives off the left common carotid and left subclavian arteries. The right aortic arch is usually larger than the left arch, but on rare occasions partial obstruction or complete atresia of the left arch may exist. Double aortic arch is commonly an isolated anomaly but is occasionally associated with a variety of CHDs, such as TGA, VSD, persistent truncus arteriosus, TOF, and COA.

3. Right aortic arch with left ligamentum arteriosum is the second most common vascular ring (30%) (see Fig. 15-1). This results from persistence of the right fourth branchial arch (forming the right aortic arch). When this structure is combined with the left-sided ligamentum arteriosum or PDA, a constricting ring results and compresses the trachea and esophagus. The ductus may be attached to the left subclavian artery or to a retroesophageal, descending aortic diverticulum. The aortic arch usually shows mirror-image branching; the first branch is the (left) innominate artery, followed by the right common carotid and right subclavian arteries. This condition is highly associated with CHDs (98% of cases), particularly TOF (48% of cases). Approximately 25% of patients with cyanotic CHD and right aortic arch have left ligamentum arteriosum.

4. Anomalous innominate artery occurs in about 10% of patients with vascular ring (see Fig. 15-1). If the innominate artery takes off too far to the left from the aortic arch or more posteriorly, it may compress the trachea, producing mild respiratory symptoms. This anomaly is commonly associated with other CHDs, such as VSD.

5. Aberrant right subclavian artery accounts for 20% of the cases of vascular ring, but

245

	Anatomy	Ba-Esophagogram	Other X-ray Findings	Symptoms	Treatment
Double aortic arcc	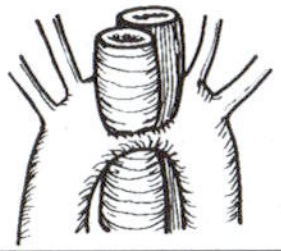	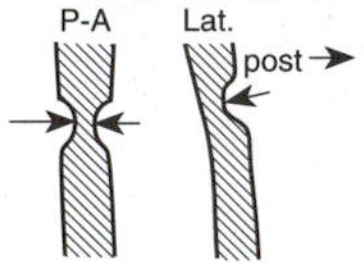	Anterior compression of trachea	Respiratory difficulty (onset < 3 mos.) Swallowing dysfunction	Surgical division of a smaller arch
Right aortic arch with left lig. arteriosuo	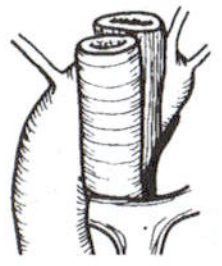	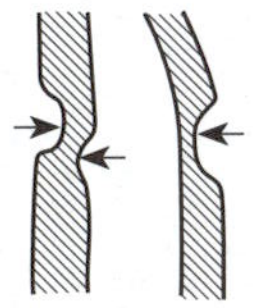		Mild respiratory difficulty (onset > 1 year) Swallowing dysfunction	Surgical division of the lig. arteriosum
Anomalous innominate artery	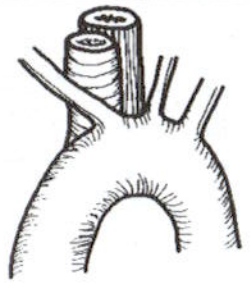	Normal	Anterior compression of trachea	Stridor and/or cough in infancc	Conservative management, or surgical suturing of the artery to the sternuu
Aberrant right subclavian artery	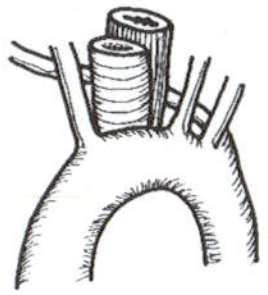	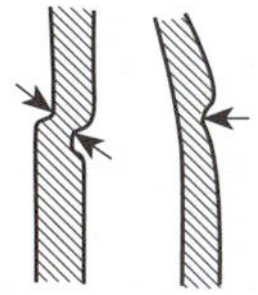		Occasional swallowing dysfunction	Usually no treatment is necessary
"Vascular sling"	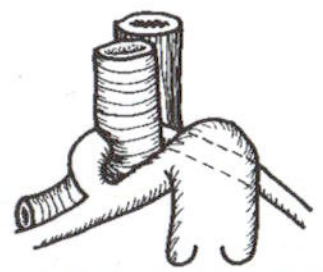	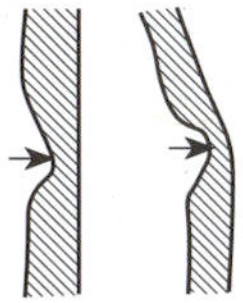	Right-sided emphysema or atelectasis. Posterior compression of trachea or rt. main stem bronchuu	Wheezing and cyanotic episodes since birth	Surgical division of the anomal. LPA (from the RPA) and anastomosis to the MPA

FIG. 15–1.
Summary and clinical features of vascular ring. *PA*, posteroanterior view; *Lat*, Lateral view.

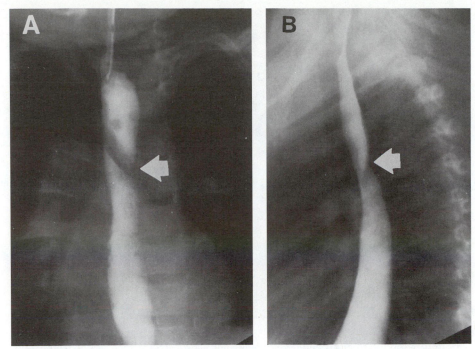

FIG. 15–2.
Barium esophagogram in a child with aberrant right subclavian artery. **A,** Anteroposterior view showing an oblique indentation at the level slightly higher than the carina *(arrow)* produced by the subclavian artery. The indentation proceeds upward and to the right toward the right shoulder. **B,** Lateral projection showing a relatively shallow, long retroesophageal impression produced by the aberrant artery.

its true prevalence is probably much higher if asymptomatic patients are included. When the right subclavian artery arises independently from the descending aorta, it courses behind the esophagus, compressing the posterior aspect of the esophagus and producing mild feeding problems (Figs. 15-1 and 15-2). Often, a larger compression is found behind the esophagus by an aortic diverticulum that is found at the take-off of the right subclavian artery. This anomaly usually is an isolated anomaly but may be associated with TOF with left aortic arch, COA, or interrupted aortic arch.

6. Anomalous left PA ("vascular sling") is a rare anomaly in which the left PA arises from the RPA (Figs. 15-1 and 15-3). To reach the left lung, the anomalous artery courses over the proximal portion of the right main stem bronchus, behind the trachea, and in front of the esophagus to the hilum of the left lung. Therefore both respiratory symptoms and feeding problems (such as coughing, wheezing, stridor, and episodes of choking, cyanosis, or apnea) may occur. This anomaly is associated with other cardiac defects, such as PDA, VSD, ASD, AV canal, single ventricle, and aortic arch anomalies, in more than half of all cases.

Clinical Manifestations
  History.

1. Inspiratory stridor and feeding problems of varying severity are present, beginning at a varying age. In double aortic arch, symptoms tend to appear in the newborn period or in early infancy (less than 3 months of age), and they are more severe than in right aortic arch with left ligamentum arteriosum. Symptoms often are made worse

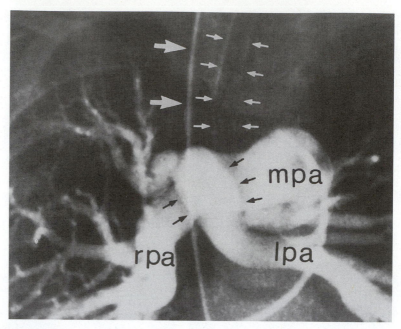

FIG. 15–3.
Pulmonary arteriogram in an infant with "vascular sling." The left PA arises from the postosuperior aspect of the RPA *(black arrows)*, rather than from the MPA. The origin of the LPA is to the right of the trachea, which is easily identifiable by an endotracheal tube *(white arrows)*. The esophagus is directly behind the proximal portion of the aberrent LPA, which caused an anterior indentation on the barium esophagogram. The esophagus is identifiable by an orogastric tube which was inserted at the time of cardiac catheterization *(large white arrows)*.

by feeding. Affected infants frequently hyperextend their necks to reduce tracheal compression.

2. Respiratory symptoms or feeding problems are milder with incomplete forms of vascular ring than with the complete form.

3. A history of pneumonia frequently is elicited.

4. A history of atelectasis, emphysema, or pneumonia of the right lung is found with "vascular sling."

Physical Examination.

1. Physical examination is not revealing, except for a varying degree of rhonchi when the vascular ring is an isolated anomaly.

2. Cardiac examination is usually normal, except in about 25% of patients in whom associated cardiac anomalies are present.

Electrocardiography.

ECG is normal.

X-ray Study.

1. Compression of the air-filled trachea may be visible on posteroanterior and lateral chest x-ray films. Aspiration pneumonia or atelectasis may be present.

2. Barium esophagogram is usually diagnostic, except in anomalous innominate artery (see Fig. 15-1).

a. In double aortic arch, two large indentations are present in both sides (with the right one usually larger) in the posteroanterior view, and a posterior indentation is seen on the lateral view.

b. In right aortic arch with left ligamentum arteriosum, a large right-sided indentation and a much smaller left-sided indentation are present. A posterior indentation, either small or large, also is present on the lateral view.

c. Barium esophagogram is normal in anomalous left innominate artery.

d. In aberrant right subclavian artery, there is a small oblique indentation extending toward the right shoulder on the posteroanterior view. There is a small posterior indentation on the lateral view (see Figs. 15-1 and 15-2). Indentations may be large if the compression is made by an aortic diverticulum.

e. In vascular sling, an anterior indentation of the esophagus seen in the lateral view at the level of the carina is characteristic. This is the only vascular ring that produces an anterior esophageal indentation. A right-sided indentation usually is seen on the posteroanterior view. The right lung is either hyperlucent or atelectatic with pneumonic infiltrations.

Echocardiography.

Echo is helpful, both for excluding intracardiac defects and for diagnosing the vascular ring. One should perform a careful segmental investigation of the aortic arch and arch vessels. The SSN views are especially useful in establishing the diagnosis.

Diagnosis

1. Vascular ring is suspected based on clinical symptoms.

2. Barium esophagogram is probably the most useful noninvasive diagnostic tool (see Fig. 15-1).

3. Echo studies can allow the diagnosis of vascular ring (and intracardiac defects), although the studies may not always provide detailed anatomic information about the vascular anomaly.

4. Angiography usually is indicated to confirm the diagnosis and to prepare for surgery. However, in selected cases of critically ill infants, the combination of barium esophagogram and echo findings can substitute for the angiography.

5. Other modalities that have been used to diagnose the vascular ring are digital subtraction angiography, computed tomographic scanning, and magnetic resonance imaging.

6. The diagnostic procedures of tracheography and bronchoscopy usually add little information and may be hazardous in some patients. However, these tests may be useful in delineating tracheobronchial abnormalities in some patients, such as those with double aortic arch or vascular sling.

Management
Medical.

1. Asymptomatic patients need no surgical treatment, even when the anomalies are found incidentally.

2. Medical management for infants with mild symptoms includes careful feeding with soft foods and aggressive treatment of pulmonary infections.

Surgical.
Indications and timing. Respiratory distress and a history of recurrent pulmonary infections and apneic spells are indications for surgical intervention. The timing of surgery depends on the severity of symptoms, and surgery may be performed during infancy.

Procedures and mortality.

DOUBLE AORTIC ARCH. Division of the smaller of the two arches (usually the left) is performed through a left thoractomy. The surgical mortality rate is less than 5%.

RIGHT AORTIC ARCH AND LEFT LIGAMENTUM ARTERIOSUM. Division of the ligamentum is performed through a left thoracotomy. The mortality rate is less than 5%.

ANOMALOUS INNOMINATE ARTERY. Surgical suturing of the innominate artery to the sternum rarely is indicated.

ABERRANT RIGHT SUBCLAVIAN ARTERY. Surgical interruption of the artery rarely is performed in symptomatic patients with dysphagia.

ANOMALOUS LEFT PA. Surgical division and reimplantation of the LPA is performed. The surgical mortality rate may be as high as 50%.

Complications. In infants who have had surgery for severe symptoms, airway obstruction may persist for weeks or months; this obstruction is caused by preexisting tracheomalacia and requires careful respiratory management in the postoperative period. This complication is more likely in patients who have had double aortic arch, vascular sling, or right aortic arch with left ligamentum arteriosum.

16 / Chamber Localization and Cardiac Malposition

In this chapter, clinical methods of locating cardiac chambers using chest x-ray films, ECGs, and physical examination will be briefly discussed. This will be followed by application of a principle that may aid in anatomic diagnosis of the heart in the right chest (dextrocardia) or in the midline (mesocardia). Although these methods are valid, many false-positive and false-negative results are possible. Two-dimensional echo usually reveals the correct diagnosis, but occasionally cardiac catheterization and angiography may be needed.

CHAMBER LOCALIZATION

The heart and great arteries can be viewed as three separate segments: the atria, the ventricles, and the great arteries. These three segments can vary from their normal positions either independently or together, resulting in many possible sets of abnormalities. The *segmental approach* of Van Praagh is very useful in determining the relationship at each segment. This approach also simplifies the description of complex cardiac defects and abnormal positions of the heart (e.g., dextrocardia, levocardia, mesocardia).

Localization of the Atria

The atria can be localized accurately by three noninvasive methods: chest x-ray films, ECG, and echo. The x-ray method relies on the fact that the atrial situs is almost always the same as the type of visceral situs; the RA is on the same side as the liver or on the opposite side of the stomach bubble. The ECG method is based on the principle that the sinus node is always located in the RA and that the site of the sinus node can be determined by the P axis. Echo clarifies the relationship between systemic veins and pulmonary veins and the atria.

Chest x-ray films. The clinician should locate the liver shadow and the stomach bubble.

1. Right-sided liver shadow and left-sided stomach bubble (situs solitus) indicate situs solitus of the atria (the RA on the right of the LA, as in normal) (Fig. 16-1, *A*). Left-sided liver shadow and right-sided stomach bubble (situs inversus) indicate situs inversus of the atria (the RA on the left side of the LA) (Fig. 16-1, *B*).

2. A midline (symmetric) liver shadow with a variable location of stomach bubble suggests splenic syndromes in which either two RA or two LA (situs ambiguus) and other complex cardiac anomalies are present (Fig. 16-1, *C*) (see also sections on splenic syndromes in Chapter 14).

Electrocardiography. The sinus node is always located in the RA. Therefore the P axis of the ECG can be used to locate the atria; the RA is located in the opposite side of the P axis.

1. When the P axis is in the left lower quadrant of the hexaxial reference system (0 to +90 degrees), the RA is on the right side (the RA to the right of the LA, or situs solitus of the atria) (Fig. 16-2).

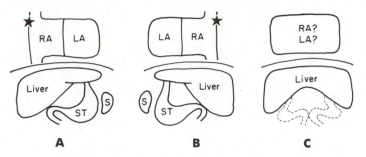

FIG. 16–1.
The visceroatrial relationship. *(A)* Situs solitus; *(B)* Situs inversus. *(C)* Situs ambiguous.
The RA is either on the same side as the liver or on the opposite side of the stomach.
The SA node *(star)* is always in the RA. *ST,* Stomach; *S,* Spleen.

FIG. 16–2.
Locating the atria by the use of the P axis.
When the RA is on the right side, the P axis
is in the left lower quadrant (0 to +90
degree). When the RA is on the left side,
the P axis is in the right lower quadrant
(+90 to +180 degree). (From Park MK,
Guntheroth WG: *How to read pediatric
ECGs,* ed 3, St Louis, 1992, Mosby.)

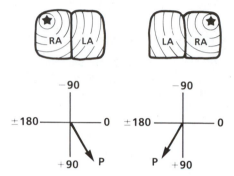

2. When the P axis is in the right lower quadrant (+90 degrees to +180 degrees), the RA is on the left side (the RA on the left of the LA, or situs inversus of the atria) (Fig. 16-2).

3. With splenic abnormalities, the P axis may be superiorly directed (polysplenia syndrome) or may change between the left lower quadrant and the right lower quadrant from time to time (asplenia syndrome).

Two-dimensional echocardiography and other methods. Two-dimensional echo identifies the IVC and/or pulmonary veins. The atrial chamber that is connected to the IVC is the RA, and the atrium that receives the pulmonary veins is the LA. Angiocardiogram, surgical inspection, or autopsy findings aid further in the diagnosis of atrial situs.

Localization of the Ventricles

Ventricles can be localized noninvasively by the ECG and two-dimensional echo (or invasively by angiocardiograms).

Electrocardiography. The ECG method of localizing the ventricle is based on the fact that the depolarization of the ventricular septum moves from the embryonic LV to the RV. This produces Q waves in the precordial leads that lie over the anatomic LV.

1. If Q waves are present in V5 and V6 (as well as I) but not in V1, D-loop of the ventricle, as in the normal person, is likely (Fig. 16-3, *A*).

2. If Q waves are present in V4R, V1, and V2 but not in V5 and V6, L-loop of the ventricles is likely (ventricular inversion) (Fig. 16-3, *B*).

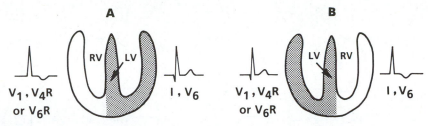

FIG. 16–3.
Locating the ventricles from the ECG. The LV is usually located on the same side as the precordial leads that show Q waves. If V6 shows a Q wave, the LV is on the left side. If V4R and V1 shows a Q wave, the LV is to the right of the anatomic RV. Note that Q waves are also present in V1 in severe RVH. (From Park MK, Guntheroth WG: *How to read pediatric ECGs,* ed 3, St Louis, 1992, Mosby.)

Two-dimensional echocardiography. The anatomic RV and LV are identified by the facts that the tricuspid valve leaflet usually inserts on the interventricular septum in a more apical position than the mitral septal leaflet and that the LV is invariably attached to the mitral valve and the RV to the tricuspid valve. A ventricular chamber that has two papillary muscles is the LV.

Ventriculograms. The anatomic RV is coarsely trabeculated and triangular, and the anatomic LV is finely trabeculated and ellipsoidal.

Localization of the Great Arteries

One can accurately determine the relationship between the two great arteries and the relationship of the great arteries to the ventricles noninvasively through echo (and invasively through angiocardiography). The ECG and chest x-ray films are not very helpful in determining the relationship between the great arteries and the ventricles. In many cases, however, one can deduce the relationship through the *loop rule* (of Van Praagh). The loop rule states that the D-loop of the ventricle (with the anatomic RV to the right of the LV) usually is associated with normally related great arteries or with D-TGA. The L-loop of the ventricle (with the anatomic RV to the left of the anatomic LV) usually is associated with the mirror image of normally related great arteries or with L-TGA. There are four types of relationships between the two great arteries: (1) solitus, (2) inversus, (3) D-transposition, and (4) L-transposition (Fig. 16-4). One can deduce the relationship of the great artery. For example, when the situs solitus of the atria and the D-loop of the ventricle are confirmed, a situs solitus relationship is present if the patient is not cyanotic; if the patient is cyanotic, a DTGA is present.

Segmental Expression

The following symbols are used in describing the segmental relationship:

1. Visceroatrial relationship: S (solitus), I (inversus), or A (ambiguus)

2. Ventricular loop: D (D-loop), L (L-loop), or X (uncertain or indeterminate)

3. Great arteries: S (solitus), I (inversus), D (D-transposition), or L (L-transposition)

With these symbols, the segmental relationship of the heart can be expressed by three letters. The first letter signifies the visceroatrial relationship; the second letter, the ventricular loop; and the third letter, the relationship of the great arteries. The segmental approach to the diagnosis of cardiac malposition is independent of the location of the cardiac apex. Consequently, this approach applies to normally located hearts (levocardia in situs solitus) as well as to the abnormally located hearts, such as dextrocardia and

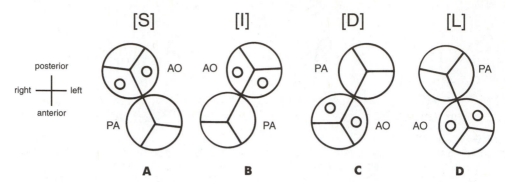

FIG. 16–4.
Four types of relationships between the great arteries, viewed in the horizontal section. **A,** Solitus *(S)* relationship is present when the aortic valve is posterior and rightward to the pulmonary valve. **B,** In inversus *(I)* relationship, the aortic valve is posterior and leftward to the pulmonary valve (mirror-image of normal). **C,** D-transposition *(D)* is present when the aortic valve is anterior and to the right of the pulmonary valve. **D,** L-transposition *(L)* is present when the aortic valve is anterior and to the left of the pulmonary valve.

mesocardia. A few examples of normal and well-known abnormal segmental relationships can be expressed as follows:

Normal heart with situs solitus: (S, D, S)

Normal heart with situs inversus (mirror image of normal): (I, L, I)

Complete transposition of the great arteries (D-TGA): (S, D, D)

D-TGA with situs inversus: (I, L, L)

Congenitally corrected TGA (L-TGA) with situs solitus: (S, L, L)

Normally formed heart that is displaced to the right side of the chest secondary to hypoplasia of the right lung ("dextroversion"): (S, D, S)

DEXTROCARDIA AND MESOCARDIA

Dextrocardia refers to a condition in which the heart is located on the right side of the chest. *Mesocardia* indicates that the heart is located approximately on the midline of the thorax; that is, the heart lies predominantly neither to the right nor to the left on the posteroanterior chest x-ray film. The terms *dextrocardia* and *mesocardia* express the position of the heart as a whole but do not specify the segmental relationship of the heart.

The four common types of heart in the right chest (dextrocardia) are (1) classic mirror-image dextrocardia (Fig. 16-5, *A*), (2) normal heart displaced to the right side of the chest (Fig. 16-5, *B*), (3) congenitally corrected TGA (Fig. 16-5, *C*), and (4) single ventricle. Less commonly, asplenia and polysplenia syndromes with situs ambiguus and complicated cardiac defects cause dextrocardia (Fig. 16-5, *D*). All of these abnormalities may result in mesocardia.

With chest x-ray studies and the ECG, one can deduce the location of the atria and the ventricles in dextrocardia (as well as in mesocardia). One can gain a more conclusive diagnosis of the segmental relationship through two-dimensional echo and angiocardiography.

1. Classic mirror-image dextrocardia (I, L, I) (see Fig. 16-5, *A*) will show:

   a. The liver shadow on the left and the stomach bubble on the right on x-ray film

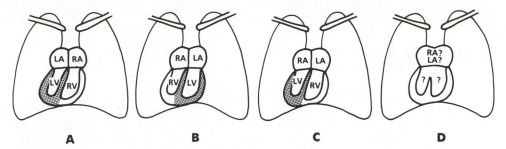

FIG. 16–5.
Examples of common conditions when the apex of the heart is in the right chest.
A, Classic mirror-image dextrocardia. **B,** Normally formed heart shifted toward the right side of the chest. **C,** L-TGA with situs solitus. **D,** Situs ambiguus seen with splenic syndromes. (From Park MK, Guntheroth WG: *How to read pediatric ECGs,* ed 3, St Louis, 1992, Mosby.)

and the P axis between +90 degrees and +180 degrees on the ECG (situs inversus)

  b. Q waves in V5R and V6R (V5R and V6R are right-sided precordial leads, mirror-image positions of V5 and V6, respectively)

2. Normal heart shifted toward the right side of the chest with the normal right-to-left relationship maintained (dextroversion) (S, D, S) (see Fig. 16-5, *B*) will show:

  a. The liver shadow on the right and the stomach bubble on the left on x-ray film and the P axis between 0 and +90 degrees on the ECG (situs solitus)

  b. Q waves in V5 and V6

3. Congenitally corrected TGA (L-TGA) with situs solitus (S, L, L) (see Fig. 16-5, *C*) will show:

  a. Situs solitus of abdominal viscera on x-ray film and the P axis in the normal quadrant (0 to +90 degrees) on the ECG

  b. Q waves in V5R and V6R

4. Undifferentiated cardiac chambers (see Fig. 16-5, *D*) often are associated with complicated cardiac defects and may show:

  a. Midline liver on the x-ray film and shifting P axis or superiorly oriented P axis on the ECG

  b. Abnormal Q waves in the precordial leads (similar to those described for single ventricle; see Chapter 14).

17 / Miscellaneous Congenital Cardiac Conditions

In this chapter, CHD with relatively low incidence, which has not been discussed previously, will be presented briefly.

ANEURYSM OF THE SINUS OF VALSALVA

In aneurysm of the sinus of Valsalva (congenital aortic sinus aneurysm), there is a gradual downward bulge of a sinus of Valsalva, usually the right coronary sinus, herniating into the RA or RV. Associated CHD is common and includes VSD, bicuspid aortic valve, and COA.

Unruptured aneurysm produces no symptoms or signs. The aneurysm ruptures during the third and fourth decade, usually into the RA or RV. The rupture is characterized by sudden onset of chest pain, dyspnea, a continuous heart murmur over the RSB or LSB and bounding peripheral pulses. Severe CHF eventually develops. Chest x-ray films show cardiomegaly and increased pulmonary vascularity. The ECG may show CVH, first- or second-degree AV block, or AV nodal rhythm.

Small to moderate-sized unruptured aneurysm probably does not need surgery. Unruptured aneurysms of the sinus of Valsalva that produce hemodynamic derangement should be repaired. When the aneurysm of the congenital sinus of Valsalva has ruptured or is associated with a VSD or a VSD and AR, prompt operation is advisable.

ANOMALOUS ORIGIN OF THE LEFT CORONARY ARTERY FROM THE PULMONARY ARTERY

In anomalous origin of the left coronary artery from the PA (Bland-White-Garland syndrome, ALCAPA syndrome), the left coronary artery arises abnormally from the PA. The patients usually are asymptomatic in the newborn period until the PA pressure falls to a critical level after birth. The direction of blood flow is from the right coronary artery, through intercoronary collaterals, to the left coronary artery, and into the PA. This results in LV insufficiency or infarction.

Symptoms appear at 2 to 3 months of age and consist of recurring episodes of distress (anginal pain), marked cardiomegaly, and CHF. Significant heart murmur usually is absent. The ECG shows an anterolateral myocardial infarction pattern consisting of abnormally deep and wide Q waves, inverted T waves, and ST-segment shift in leads I and aVL and precordial leads (see Fig. 27-5) (see Appendix A, Fig. AA-3).

All patients with the diagnosis need operation. The optimal operation in infancy remains controversial.

Palliative Surgery

In critically ill infants, simple ligation of the anomalous left coronary artery close to its origin from the PA may be performed to prevent steal into the PA. This should be followed by a later elective bypass procedure. Even in critically ill infants, many centers prefer to create a two-coronary system through one of the following three procedures: tunnel repair, implantation of the left coronary artery to the ascending aorta, and anastomosis of the left subclavian to the left coronary artery.

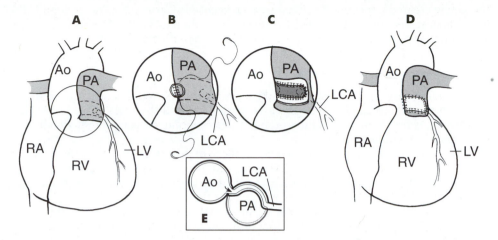

FIG. 17–1.
Intrapulmonary artery tunnel repair for anomalous origin of the left coronary artery from the PA (Takeuchi repair). **A,** Two dashed lines on the anterior wall of the PA are the proposed incision sites to create a flap of the PA. **B,** An aortopulmonary shunt is being created, after making a punch hole (5 to 6 mm in size) in the contiguous wall of the aorta and PA. **C,** The flap of the PA is sutured into place to form the convex roof of a tunnel through which aortic blood passes to the anomalous orifice of the left coronary artery. **D,** A piece of pericardium is used to close the opening in the anterior wall of the PA. **E,** Cross-sectional view of the tunnel operation when completed.

Definitive Surgery

Intrapulmonary tunnel operation (Takeuchi repair). Intrapulmonary tunnel operation is the most popular among two-coronary repair surgeries (Fig. 17-1). Two circular openings are made in the contiguous wall of the aorta and the pulmonary trunk, and a 5- to 6-mm aortopulmonary window is created by suturing together these two openings. Two horizontal incisions are made in the anterior wall of the PA directly over the aortopulmonary window to create the flap of PA wall. The flap is sutured in the posterior wall of the PA, and a tunnel is created that connects the opening of the aortopulmonary window and the orifice of the anomalous left coronary artery. The opening in the anterior wall of the PA is closed by a piece of pericardium. The mortality rate ranges from 0% to as high as 40%. This operation has the inherent disadvantage of late obstruction of the tunnel or obstruction of the MPA.

Left coronary artery implantation. Left coronary artery implantation with direct transfer of the anomalous left coronary artery into the aortic root, appears to be the most advisable procedure, but it is not always possible. The anomalous coronary artery is excised from the PA along with a button of PA wall, and the artery is reimplanted into the anterior aspect of the ascending aorta. The early surgical mortality rate is 15% to 20%.

Subclavian–left coronary artery anastomosis. In subclavian–left coronary artery anastomosis, the end of the left subclavian artery is turned down and anastomosed end-to-end to the anomalous left coronary artery. Aortic cross-clamping, which could be the source of ventricular impairment with postoperative low cardiac output and a high mortality rate, is avoided.

Tashiro repair. Tashiro et al (1993) reported a new two-coronary artery repair technique that was performed in adult patients. In this procedure, a narrow cuff of the MPA, including the orifice of the left coronary artery, is transected; the upper and lower edges of the cuff are closed to form a new left main coronary artery; and the aorta and the newly creased left coronary artery are anastomosed side-to-side. The divided MPA is anastomosed end-to-end. This will create no obstruction to the PA. This technique has a potential application in the pediatric population, including small infants.

AORTOPULMONARY SEPTAL DEFECT

In aortopulmonary septal defect (aortopulmonary window, aortopulmonary fenestration), a large defect is present between the ascending aorta and the MPA (Fig. 17-2). This condition results from the failure of the spiral septum to completely divide the embryonic truncus arteriosus.

Hemodynamic abnormalities are similar to those of persistent truncus arteriosus and are more severe than those of PDA. CHF and pulmonary hypertension appear in early infancy. Peripheral pulses are bounding, but the heart murmur usually is of the systolic ejection type (rather than continuous murmur) at the base.

The natural history of this defect is similar to that of a large untreated VSD, with development of pulmonary vascular disease in surviving patients. This defect has no known tendency to close spontaneously. Prompt surgical closure of the defect under cardiopulmonary bypass is indicated when the diagnosis is made. The surgical mortality rate is very low.

FIG. 17–2.
Diagrammatic drawing of aortopulmonary window **(A)** and persistent truncus arteriosus **(B)**. These two conditions are similar from a hemodynamic point of view. Anatomically, however, there are two separate semilunar valves (AoV, PV) in aortopulmonary window, whereas there is only one truncal valve (TV) with associated VSD in persistent truncus arteriosus. AO, Aorta.

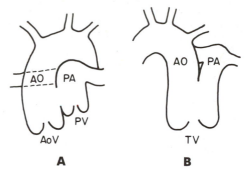

ARTERIOVENOUS FISTULA, CORONARY

Coronary artery fistulae are the most common congenital anomalies of the coronary artery. In the majority of cases (60%), the fistulae arise from the right coronary artery. The left coronary artery is the site of aneurysm in about 30%, with the remainder arising from both right and left coronary arteries or from a single coronary artery.

These fistulae occur in one of two patterns. They may represent a branching tributary from a coronary artery coursing along a normal anatomic distribution ("true" coronary arteriovenous fistulae), occurring in only 7% of cases (Fig. 17-3). In the majority of the cases, the fistulae result from an abnormal coronary artery system with aberrant termination (coronary artery fistulae). In more than 90% of reported cases, the fistulae terminate in the right side of the heart (40% in the RV, 25% in the RA, and 20% in the PA). It rarely terminates in the left side of the heart, with the majority of cases entering the LA.

The patients usually are asymptomatic. A continuous murmur, similar to the murmur of PDA, is audible over the precordium, rather than in the left infraclavicular area. The ECG usually is normal but may show RVH or LVH if the fistula is large. Chest x-ray films usually show a normal heart size. Echo studies usually suggest the site and type of the fistulae.

Elective surgery is indicated as soon as the diagnosis is made because SBE, fistula rupture, and myocardial infarction are significant risk factors. Using cardiopulmonary bypass, the fistulous point is closed nearest to the entry into the cardiac chamber, without compromising the coronary circulation. The surgical mortality rate can be as high as 5%.

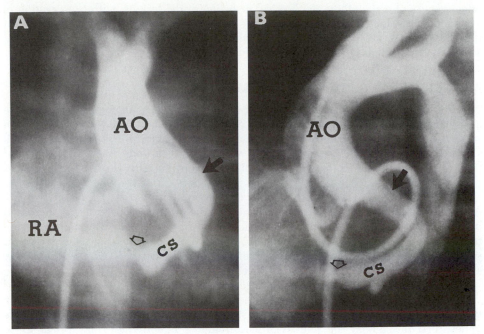

FIG. 17–3.
Aortogram showing coronary arteriovenous fistula in the distribution of the left circumflex artery *(solid arrows)*. **A,** The AP projection. **B,** The lateral projection. The fistula empties through the coronary sinus *(cs)* and eventually into the RA. The point of entry into the RA is marked by an open arrow.

Successful nonsurgical closure of the fistula with the use of Gianturco coils or a double-umbrella device recently was reported in selected patients.

ARTERIOVENOUS FISTULA, PULMONARY

The PAs and pulmonary veins communicate directly, bypassing the pulmonary capillary circulation. The fistulae may take the form of either multiple tiny angiomas (telangiectasis) or a large PA-to-pulmonary vein communication. About 60% of patients with pulmonary arteriovenous fistulae have Rendu-Osler-Weber syndrome (see Table 1-1). Rarely, chronic liver disease may be the cause of the fistula, but the mechanism of this remains an enigma. Desaturated systemic blood from the PAs reaches the pulmonary veins, bypassing the lung tissue and resulting in systemic arterial desaturation and cyanosis. The PBF and pressure remain unchanged, and there is no volume overload to the heart.

Physical examination may reveal cyanosis and clubbing. The peripheral pulses are not bounding. A faint systolic or continuous murmur may be audible over the affected area in about 50% of patients. Polycythemia usually is present, and arterial oxygen saturation runs between 50% and 85%. Chest x-ray films show normal heart size. One or more rounded opacities of variable size may be present in the lung fields. The ECG usually is normal. Occasional complications include stroke, brain abscess, rupture of the fistula with hemoptysis or hemothorax, and SBE.

Although pulmonary angiography remains the definitive method for locating pulmonary AV fistula, the diagnosis can be made through contrast two-dimensional echo by the appearance of microcavitations in the LA. The echo study can identify the site of appearance of microcavitations in the LA, and it can be used to monitor the effectiveness of embolotherapy. Surgical resection of the lesions, with preservation of as much healthy lung tissue as possible, may be attempted in symptomatic children, but the progressive nature of the disorder calls for a conservative approach. Recently, selective embolotherapy has been proposed as an alternative to surgical resection.

ARTERIOVENOUS FISTULA, SYSTEMIC

There is direct communication (either a vascular channel or angiomas) between the artery and a vein without the interposition of the capillary bed. The two most common sites of systemic AV fistulaes are the brain and liver. Because of decreased peripheral vascular resistance, an increase in stroke volume (with a wide pulse pressure) and tachycardia result, leading to increased cardiac output, volume overload to the heart, and even CHF.

Physical examination reveals a systolic or continuous murmur over the affected organ. An ejection systolic murmur may be present over the precordium because of increased blood flow through the semilunar valves. The peripheral pulses may be bounding during the high-output state but weak when CHF develops. A gallop rhythm may be present with CHF. Chest x-ray films show cardiomegaly and increased PVM. The ECG may show hypertrophy of either or both ventricles.

Most patients with large cerebral AV fistulae and CHF die in the neonatal period, and surgical ligation of the affected artery to the brain rarely is possible without infarcting the brain. Surgical treatment of hepatic fistulae often is impossible because they are widespread throughout the liver. Corticosteroids or radiotherapy may prove to be effective.

CERVICAL AORTIC ARCH

In this rare anomaly, the aortic arch is elongated, usually into the neck just above the clavicle. The aortic arch is almost always right-sided. A pulsating mass with associated thrill is present in the right supraclavicular fossa. An aortogram may assist in making an accurate diagnosis.

COMMON ATRIUM

In common atrium (single atrium, cor triloculare biventriculare), either the atrial septum is completely absent, or only the vestigial element of poorly developed atrial septum is present. This is a form of ECD with cleft mitral valve, producing a superiorly oriented QRS axis (left anterior hemiblock) on the ECG. An rsR' pattern is present in the RPLs as in ASD. This condition is most commonly seen with Ellis–van Creveld syndrome (see Table 1-1). Successful creation of polyvinyl septum is possible.

COR TRIATRIATUM

Cor triatriatum is a rare congenital cardiac anomaly in which the LA is divided into two compartments by an abnormal fibromuscular septum with a small opening (Fig. 17-4, A), producing obstruction of pulmonary venous return. Pulmonary venous and pulmonary arterial hypertension result. Embryologically, this condition results from the failure of the incorporation of the embryonic common pulmonary vein into the LA. Therefore the upper compartment (accessory LA) is a dilated common pulmonary vein, and the lower compartment is the true LA. Hemodynamic abnormalities of this condition are similar to those of MS in that both conditions produce pulmonary venous and pulmonary arterial hypertension (see Chapter 10).

Important physical findings include dyspnea, basal pulmonary rales, loud S2, and a nonspecific systolic murmur. The ECG shows RAD and severe RVH and occasional RAH. Chest x-ray films show evidence of pulmonary venous congestion or pulmonary edema, prominent MPA segment, and right-sided heart enlargement. Echo demonstrates a linear structure within the LA cavity (Fig. 17-4, B). Surgical correction is always

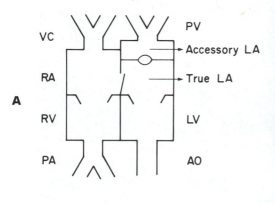
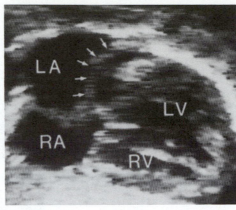

FIG. 17–4.
Cor triatriatum. **A,** Diagrammatic drawing. **B,** Subcostal four-chamber view of an echo demonstrating a membrane *(small arrows)* in the LA.

indicated. Pulmonary hypertension regresses rapidly in survivors if the correction is made early.

DOUBLE-CHAMBER RIGHT VENTRICLE

Double-chamber RV (anomalous muscle bundle of the RV) is characterized by aberrant hypertrophied muscle bands that divide the RV cavity into a proximal high-pressure chamber and a distal low-pressure chamber. In the majority of the patients, VSD or pulmonary valve stenosis also is present.

Clinical manifestations closely resemble those of pulmonary valvular or infundibular stenosis: a loud, grade 3-5/6 SEM along the ULSB and MLSB is present. Surgical resection of the bundle, as well as repair of other anomalies, usually is indicated as soon as the diagnosis is made.

ECTOPIA CORDIS

In this extremely rare condition, the heart is partially or totally outside the thorax. Most reported cases of ectopia cordis are either thoracic (60%) or thoracoabdominal (40%); rarely a case may be cervical or abdominal. The thoracic type is characterized by a sternal defect, absence of the parietal pericardium, cephalic orientation of the cardiac apex, epigastric omphalocele, and a small thoracic cavity. The thoracoabdominal type has partial absence or cleft of the lower sternum, an anterior diaphragmatic defect through which a portion of the ventricle protrudes into the abdominal cavity, a defect of parietal pericardium, and an omphalocele. Intracardiac abnormalities are very common but not invariable, and ASD, VSD, TOF, and tricuspid atresia are the most common intracardiac defects. One reported case of the abdominal type (1806) was a healthy French soldier, the father of three children, who died of pyelonephritis.

The treatment and prognosis of the defect are determined by the location of the defect, the extent of the cardiac displacement, and the presence or absence of intracardiac anomalies. Simple sternal cleft with minimal cardiac protrusion can be successfully treated in early infancy. However, in more severe cases, most surgical efforts to put the heart into the thorax have failed because of smallness of the thorax and kinking of the blood vessels. Patients without omphalocele or intracardiac defects may remain largely asymptomatic and can undergo surgical repair later in childhood.

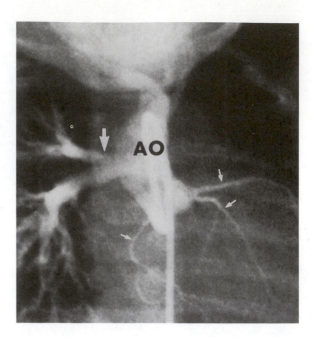

FIG. 17–5.
Hemitruncus. Aortogram
showing the RPA *(large arrow)*
originating anomalously from
the ascending aorta *(AO)*.
Coronary arteries are also
opacified *(small arrows)*.

HEMITRUNCUS ARTERIOSUS

In hemitruncus arteriosus (origin of one PA from the ascending aorta), one of the PAs, usually the RPA, arises from the ascending aorta (Fig. 17-5). Associated defects such as PDA, VSD, and TOF occasionally are present. Hemodynamically, one lung receives blood directly from the aorta, as in PDA, with resulting volume and/or pressure overload, and the other lung receives the entire RV output, resulting in volume overload of that lung. Therefore pulmonary hypertension of both lungs develops. CHF develops early in infancy, with respiratory distress and poor weight gain. A continuous murmur and bounding pulses may be present. The ECG shows CVH, and chest x-ray films show cardiomegaly and increased PVMs. Early surgical correction (anastomosis of the anomalous PA to the MPA) is indicated.

IDIOPATHIC DILATATION OF THE PULMONARY ARTERY

In idiopathic dilation of the PA (congenital pulmonary insufficiency), PR is present in the absence of pulmonary hypertension in asymptomatic children or adolescents. Many regard this as a mild pulmonary valve stenosis with resulting poststenotic dilatation and subsequent decrease in the murmur of PS.

A characteristic auscultatory finding is a grade 1-3/6 low-frequency, decrescendo diastolic murmur at the ULSB and MLSB. The S2 is normal. The ECG usually is normal, but occasional RBBB is present. Chest x-ray films show a prominent MPA segment with normal peripheral pulmonary vascularity. The prognosis is generally good, but right-sided heart failure may occur in adult life.

KARTAGENER'S SYNDROME

Kartagener's syndrome consists of the triad of situs inversus (with dextrocardia), paranasal sinusitis, and bronchiectasis. This disorder is inherited as an autosomal recessive trait; males and females are affected with equal frequency. The dextrocardia is a mirror image of normal and is functionally normal. Bronchiectasis is believed to result from a functional defect of the mucociliary epithelium with immotility of the cilia. In addition, affected males are infertile as a result of immobile spermatozoa.

MITRAL REGURGITATION, CONGENITAL

Congenital MR is extremely rare as an isolated defect. It is most frequently found in association with other CHDs. A regurgitant holosystolic murmur is audible at the apex with radiation to the left axilla and left back. An apical rumble and a loud S3 may be present. The ECG and chest x-ray films may show hypertrophy and enlargement of the LA and LV. Medical management should be tried initially. In patients unresponsive to medical management, mitral valvuloplasty or anuloplasty should be attempted to preserve the valve. If this is not possible, valve replacement is performed.

MITRAL STENOSIS, CONGENITAL

The onset of symptoms or signs depends on the severity of the stenosis: onset is neonatal with severe stenosis and later with less severe stenosis. Symptoms and signs are related to pulmonary venous congestion or pulmonary edema, eventually leading to pulmonary hypertension and right-sided heart failure (see Chapter 10). COA and AS are commonly associated anomalies, and LV endocardial fibroelastosis also is common.

Physical examination reveals an increased RV impulse and an apical middiastolic murmur. Other findings may include presystolic accentuation, loud S1, and opening snap. The ECG shows RVH and CAH, and chest x-ray films show enlargement of the LA, MPA, and RV. Kerley's B lines may be present in severe cases. Echo is diagnostic of the condition.

Conservative management with diuretics and digoxin is recommended. For severe obstruction, surgical relief by closed or open valvotomy or placement of a prosthetic valve may be indicated but carries significant mortality and morbidity. In selected children without a parachute deformity of the mitral valve (see later discussion) and in those with a hypoplastic mitral annulus, balloon valvuloplasty may be an attractive alternative before mitral valve replacement surgery. MR may result from the balloon procedure.

Parachute mitral valve is characterized by insertion of all the chordae tendineae into a single papillary muscle group, producing MS. This can be suspected by two-dimensional echo on the parasternal views. Commonly associated conditions include supravalvular mitral ring, subvalvular and/or valvular AS, and COA; all are components of the "Shone complex."

PATENT FORAMEN OVALE

PFO is a patent tunnel between the septum secundum and the superior margin of the septum primum. The septum secundum is a thick, concave, muscular structure that expands from the posterosuperior wall and partially partitions the atria. The septum primum extends inferiorly to the endocardial cushion tissue. In prenatal life, this tunnel is open and allows a direct flow of oxygenated blood from the placenta via the ductus venosus into the LA.

Postnatally, when the pressure in the LA exceeds that of the RA, the thin flap of the superior end of the septum primum is forced to shut against the septum secundum, thereby resulting in functional closure of the foramen. In most individuals, the foramen ovale is sealed immediately after birth. However, if for some reason the pressure in the RA is higher than that in the LA, the foramen ovale may remain patent. Probe patency of a competent foramen ovale is found in 25% of normal adults. Coughing or Valsalva's maneuver can produce a higher pressure in the RA, and a transient right-to-left shunt is possible. In some adult patients with idiopathic cerebrovascular accident, a competent PFO was found, through which a right-to-left shunt could be demonstrated to occur by contrast echo. Abnormally high atrial pressures (in either the RA or LA) cause the two septa to pull apart, transforming the competent foramen ovale to an open hole. A bidirectional shunt in this case is possible.

PERICARDIAL DEFECT, CONGENITAL

This rare congenital anomaly of the pericardium may be partial or complete. The majority of these cases occur on the left side (85%), and they are more often complete (65%) than partial. From 30% to 50% of the cases are associated with congenital anomalies of the heart (PDA, ASD, TOF, MS), lung, chest wall, or diaphragm. Pleural defect almost always is present.

Unless an associated cardiac anomaly is present, most patients are asymptomatic. Occasionally, a partial defect may produce chest pain, syncope, or systemic embolism secondary to herniation and strangulation of the LA appendage. A complete defect may produce vague positional discomfort in the supine or left lateral positions. Congenital pericardial defects are difficult to diagnose preoperatively. Occasionally, chest x-ray films may show a prominence of the left hilum or the PA caused by herniation of these structures. Complete absence of the left pericardium may be characterized by leftward displacement of the heart and aortic knob, or a prominent PA. Traditionally, the appearance of pneumopericardium after the introduction of air into the left pleural cavity was diagnostic. Recently, noninvasive procedures, such as two-dimensional echo, computed tomography, and magnetic resonance imaging, have been successfully applied for the diagnosis of the condition. Surgical treatment is recommended only for symptomatic patients.

Surgical procedures used in this condition include longitudinal pericardiotomy, partial pericardiectomy, primary closure, partial appendectomy (of the LA appendage), and pericardioplasty with pleural flaps, Teflon, or porcine pericardium.

PSEUDOCOARCTATION OF THE AORTA

Pseudocoarctation of the aorta is a condition in which the distal portion of the aortic arch and the proximal portion of the descending aorta are abnormally elongated and tortuous, giving the x-ray film the appearance of COA. Physical examination and the ECG are normal, but some cases might progress to show substantial pressure difference between the arms and legs.

PULMONARY ARTERY STENOSIS

The stenosis of the PA occurs most frequently near the bifurcation, but occasionally it may involve further peripheral branches. This may be an isolated anomaly or may be seen in association with rubella syndrome, Williams' syndrome, and other conditions. This condition should be distinguished from the normally small PA branches (with a relatively large MPA) seen in normal newborn infants, which produce the innocent pulmonary flow murmur of the newborn. Mild stenosis of the PAs causes no hemodynamic abnormalities. If the stenosis is severe, the RV may hypertrophy.

An ejection systolic murmur grade 2-3/6, is audible at the ULSB, with good transmission to the axillae and back. Occasionally, a continuous murmur is audible. The S2 is either normal or more obviously split. The murmur is louder than the innocent pulmonary flow murmur of the newborn and persists beyond 6 months of age. The ECG is normal with mild stenosis, but it shows RVH with severe stenosis. Chest x-ray films usually are normal. The echo may show stenosis in the MPA or near the bifurcation. Stenosis of the peripheral PA branches can be demonstrated only by an angiography.

No treatment is necessary for isolated mild PA stenosis. The central (extraparenchymal) type is surgically correctable, but the multiple peripheral (intraparenchymal) type is not amenable to surgery. In some cases, an intravascular stent can be placed successfully.

RUBELLA SYNDROME

Rubella syndrome is caused by intrauterine infection of the fetus by rubella virus during the first trimester of pregnancy. The triad of this syndrome is deafness, cataracts, and cardiac defects. Other malformations include intrauterine growth retardation, micro-cephaly, microphthalmia, hepatitis, and neonatal thrombocytopenic purpura. The most common cardiac malformations are PDA and stenoses of the PAs. Other intracardiac defects, such as TOF, VSD, ASD, and TGA, are found in 5% to 10% of cases.

SCIMITAR SYNDROME

All or some of the pulmonary veins from the lower lobe and sometimes the middle lobe of the right lung drain anomalously into the IVC, making a peculiar scimitar-shaped vertical radiographic shadow along the right lower cardiac border.

In symptomatic infants, associated anomalies (such as ASD, PDA, hypoplasia of the right lung and RPA, pulmonary venous obstruction, and systemic arterial supply to the lung) are frequent. Left-sided obstructive lesions (such as hypoplastic LV, subaortic stenosis, and aortic arch obstruction) also are frequently present. These anomalies are found less frequently in asymptomatic children than in symptomatic infants. Anomalous systemic arterial supply originates in the descending aorta, usually supplies the right lung, and rarely supplies the left lung (bronchopulmonary sequestration). Dextrocardia also is frequently found.

In symptomatic infants, embolization or ligation of systemic arterial supply to the right lung, if present, may result in improvement of pulmonary hypertension and signs of CHF. Most symptomatic infants require additional surgery for associated defects with a high surgical mortality rate (near 50%). Children and adults with the syndrome are either minimally symptomatic or asymptomatic, probably because they have a low incidence of associated anomalies. For older children, the anomalous pulmonary venous return can be redirected to the LA, but in patients with associated bronchopulmonary sequestration, the involved lobes of the right lung may need to be resectioned.

SYSTEMIC VENOUS ANOMALIES

A wide variety of abnormalities appear in the systemic venous system; some of these have little physiologic importance, and others produce cyanosis. Recent developments in the diagnosis and treatment of cardiovascular disorders have brought these anomalies

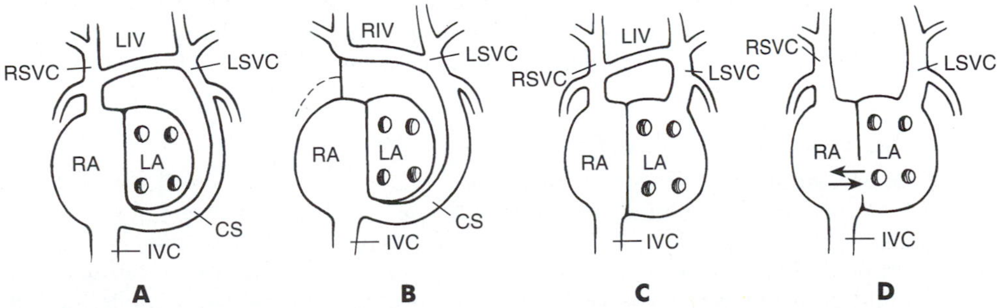

FIG. 17–6.
Schematic diagram of persistent left SVC (LSVC). **A,** Left SVC drains via coronary sinus (CS) into the RA. The left innominate vein (LIV) and the right SVC (RSVC) are adequate. **B,** Uncommonly, the RSVC may be atretic. The coronary sinus (CS) is large because it receives blood from both the right and left upper parts of the body. **C,** The coronary sinus is absent, and the LSVC drains directly into the LA. The atrial septum is intact. **D,** The LSVC connects to the LA, and there is a posterior ASD, which allows a predominant left-to-right atrial shunt.

to the attention of the cardiologist and thoracic surgeon. Some of these abnormalities produce difficulties in the manipulation of catheters during cardiac catheterization, and preoperative knowledge of systemic venous anomalies is important in cardiac surgery. Therefore the search for common abnormalities of the systemic veins has become routine in the evaluation of pediatric cardiac patients during echo and cardiac catheterization.

Two well-known anomalies of systemic veins are persistent left SVC and infrahepatic interruption of the IVC with azygos continuation. Rarely, either persistent left SVC or interrupted IVC can drain into the LA, producing cyanosis.

Anomalies of Superior Vena Cava

Persistent left SVC occurs in 3% to 5% of children with CHDs. The persistent left SVC is connected to the RA in 92% of cases and to the LA (producing cyanosis) in the remainder.

Persistent left superior vena cava draining into the right atrium. In the most common type, the left SVC is connected to the coronary sinus (Fig. 17-6, A). As a rule, persistent left SVC is part of a bilateral SVC, but rarely the right SVC is absent (Fig. 17-6, B). A bridging innominate vein is present in 60% of cases.

Isolated persistent left SVC (Fig. 17-6, A and B) does not produce symptoms or signs. Cardiac examination is entirely normal. Chest x-ray films may show the shadow of the left SVC along the left upper border of the mediastinum. A high prevalence of leftward P axis (+ 15 degrees or less) has been reported on the ECG. The enlarged coronary sinus may be imaged by an echo study. Although two-dimensional echo usually images the persistent left SVC, angiocardiography confirms the diagnosis. Treatment for isolated persistent left SVC is not necessary.

Persistent left superior vena cava draining into the left atrium. Rarely (8% of the cases), persistent left SVC drains into the LA, resulting in systemic arterial desaturation (Fig. 17-6, C and D). This is due to the failure of invagination between the left sinus horn and LA, and therefore the coronary sinus is absent. Associated cardiac anomalies almost invariably are present. Complex defects, such as cor biloculare, conotruncal abnormalities, and asplenia syndrome, most commonly are found. Defects of the atrial septum (single atrium, secundum ASD, primum ASD) also are frequently found.

Clinical manifestations are dominated by the associated complex cardiac defects. In the absence of complex defects, cyanosis is more marked when there is no atrial communication (Fig. 17-6, C) than when there is an ASD. When there is an ASD (Fig. 17-6, D), clinical findings resemble those of ASD with left-to-right shunt, with only mild arterial desaturation. Surgical correction is necessary. When there is an adequate-size bridging vein that connects two SVCs, simple ligation of the left VSC is performed. If the right SVC is absent or a bridging vein is inadequate, the left SVC is transposed to the RA.

Anomalies of the Inferior Vena Cava

Many abnormalities in the formation of the IVC have been reported. Among the significant anomalies are infrahepatic interruption of the IVC with azygos continuation and anomalous drainage of the IVC into the LA, producing cyanosis (Fig. 17-7).

Interrupted IVC with azygos continuation (Fig. 17-7, A) has been reported in about 3% of children with CHDs. The IVC below the level of the renal veins is normal, but the hepatic portion of the IVC is absent. Instead of receiving the hepatic veins and entering the RA, the IVC drains via an enlarged azygos system into the right SVC and eventually to the RA. The hepatic veins connect directly to the RA. Bilateral SVC also is common. Azygos continuation of the IVC often is associated with complex cyanotic heart defects, such as polysplenia syndrome, DORV, cor biloculare, and anomalies of pulmonary venous return. Less often, a simple cardiac defect is associated. No case has been reported in association with asplenia syndrome. This defect creates difficulties

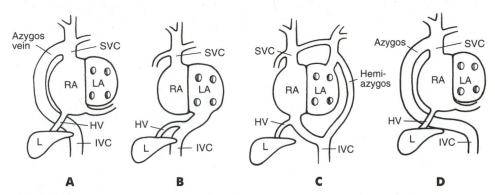

FIG. 17–7.
Schematic diagram of selected abnormalities of the IVC. **A,** Interrupted IVC with azygos continuation, the most common abnormality of the IVC. The hepatic veins *(HV)* connect directly to the RA. **B,** Right IVC draining into the LA. **C,** Absence of the lower right IVC. The IVC drains into the LA through the left SVC, and the RA through the hepatic portion of the IVC. **D,** Complete absence of the right IVC with communicating vein draining to the azygos vein.

during cardiac catheterization and can complicate surgical correction of an underlying cardiac defect. This venous anomaly does not require surgical correction.

IVC connecting to the LA is an extremely rare condition in which the IVC receives the hepatic veins, curves toward the LA, and makes a direct connection with the chamber (Fig. 17-7, *B*). Pathologic persistence of the eustachian valve can result in a clinically similar situation in which a membrane completely excludes the IVC from the RA, with the IVC blood shunted to the LA through either an ASD or a PFO (not shown in Fig. 17-7).

Two other extremely rare cases of IVC abnormalities also are shown in Fig. 17-7. In one of them, the lower end of the right IVC is absent, and the dominant left IVC drains into the LA (producing cyanosis) through the (left-sided) hemiazygos system and persistent left SVC (Fig. 17-7, *C*). In the other case, the lower end of the right IVC is absent, and the left IVC drains through the (right-sided) azygos system (Fig. 17-7, *D*).

TAUSSIG-BING MALFORMATION

Taussig-Bing malformation is a form of DORV (see Chapter 14) in which the VSD is subpulmonic and PS is absent. Because the VSD is closely related to the PA, oxygenated blood from the LV goes to the lungs, and desaturated blood from the venae cavae goes to the aorta, producing marked cyanosis. Because there is no PS, early CHF develops in these infants. Therefore clinical pictures resemble those of D-TGA with VSD. Two-dimensional echo, cardiac catheterization, and angiocardiography are required for diagnosis.

PART V

Acquired Heart Disease

Among acquired heart diseases, emphasis will be placed on the more common pediatric diseases, such as cardiomyopathies; cardiovascular infections, including myocarditis and infective endocarditis; acute rheumatic fever; and valvular heart disease. Although the etiology of Kawasaki's disease is not entirely clear, it will be discussed in the section on cardiovascular infection. Mitral valve prolapse (MVP) will be discussed in the section on valvular heart disease. A brief list of cardiac involvements in some systemic diseases also is presented.

18 / Primary Myocardial Disease

Primary myocardial disease or cardiomyopathy is a disease of the heart muscle itself, not associated with congenital, valvular, or coronary heart disease or systemic disorders. It is distinct from the specific heart muscle diseases of known cause. Cardiomyopathy has been classified into three types based on anatomic and functional features: (1) hypertrophic, (2) dilated (or congestive), and (3) restrictive (Fig. 18-1).

1. In hypertrophic cardiomyopathy, there is a massive ventricular hypertrophy with a smaller-than-normal ventricular cavity. Contractile function of the ventricle is enhanced, but ventricular filling is impaired by relaxation abnormalities.

2. Dilated (or congestive) cardiomyopathy is characterized by a decreased contractile function of the ventricle associated with ventricular dilatation. Endocardial fibroelastosis (seen in infancy) and doxorubicin cardiomyopathy (seen in children who have received chemotherapy for malignancies) have clinical features similar to those of dilated cardiomyopathy.

3. Restrictive cardiomyopathy denotes a restriction of diastolic filling of the ventricles caused by endocardial or myocardial disease (usually infiltrative disease), and contractile function of the ventricle may be normal.

The three types of cardiomyopathies are functionally different from one another, and the demands of therapy also are different. Table 18-1 summarizes clinical characteristics of the three types of cardiomyopathy.

HYPERTROPHIC CARDIOMYOPATHY

Pathology and Pathophysiology

1. The most characteristic abnormality is the hypertrophied LV, with the ventricular cavity usually small or normal in size. Although asymmetric septal hypertrophy (ASH), a condition formerly known as idiopathic hypertrophic subaortic stenosis (IHSS) (Fig. 18-2), is most common, the hypertrophy may be concentric or localized to a small segment of the septum (Fig. 18-3). Microscopically, an extensive disarray of hypertrophied myocardial cells, myocardial scarring, and abnormalities of the small intramural coronary arteries are present.

2. In some patients, an intracavitary pressure gradient develops during systole partly because of systolic anterior motion (SAM) of the mitral valve against the hypertrophied septum, which is called hypertrophic obstructive cardiomyopathy (HOCM) (see Fig. 18-2). The SAM probably is created by the high outflow velocities and Venturi forces.

3. The myocardium itself has an enhanced contractile state, but diastolic ventricular filling is impaired by abnormal stiffness of the LV, which may lead to LA enlargement and pulmonary venous congestion, producing congestive symptoms (exertional dyspnea, orthopnea, paroxysmal nocturnal dyspnea).

4. In about 60% of cases, hypertrophic cardiomyopathy appears to be genetically transmitted as an autosomal dominant trait, and in the remainder, it occurs sporadically. It may be seen in children with LEOPARD syndrome (see Table 1-1).

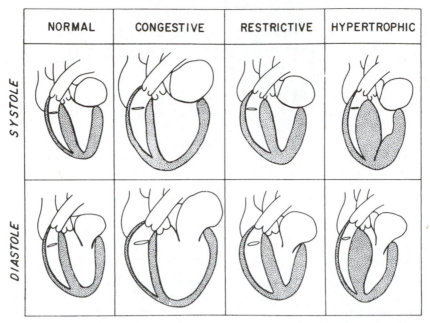

FIG. 18–1.
Diagram of the 50-degree left anterior oblique view of the heart in different types of cardiomyopathy at end-systole and end-diastole. "Congestive" corresponds to "dilated" cardiomyopathy as used in the text. (From Goldman MR, Boucher CA: Values of radionuclide imaging techniques in assessing cardiomyopathy, *Am J Cardiol* 46:1232-1236, 1980.)

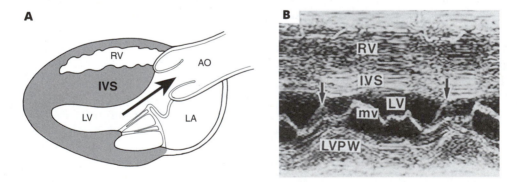

FIG. 18–2.
Systolic anterior motion of the mitral valve. **A,** Diagrammatic illustration of systolic anterior motion in the presence of an asymmetric septal hypertrophy. The Venturi effect may be important in the production of systolic anterior motion. **B,** M-mode echo of the mitral valve in a patient with hypertrophic cardiomyopathy. Systolic anterior motion of the anterior leaflet of the mitral valve is indicated by arrows.

5. A unique aspect of HOCM is the variability of the degree of obstruction from moment to moment. Because the obstruction of the LV outflow tract results from systolic anterior motion of the mitral valve against the hypertrophied ventricular septum, any influence that reduces the LV systolic volume (such as positive inotropic agents, reduced blood volume, or lowering of the SVR) increases the obstruction, and any

TABLE 18–1.

Summary of Clinical Characteristics of Cardiomyopathies

Clinical Features	Hypertrophic	Dilated	Restrictive
Etiology	Inherited (AD in 60%) Sporadic (new mutation ±)	Pleuricausal (e.g., toxic, metabolic, infectious, alcohol, doxorubicin)	Myocardial fibrosis, hypertrophy, or infiltration (amyloid)
Hemodynamic dysfunction	Diastolic dysfunction (with normal systolic function) (abnormally stiff LV with impaired ventricular filling)	Systolic contractile dysfunction ($\downarrow$ cardiac output, $\downarrow$ stroke volume, $\uparrow$LVEDP)	Diastolic dysfunction (rigid ventricular walls impede ventricular filling)
Echo (morphology)	Thickened LV (and RV) wall Small or normal LV chamber dimension Supernormal LV contractility HOCM and/or ASH	Biventricular dilatation ($\uparrow$LVDD, $\uparrow$LVSD) Atrial enlargement in proportion to ventricular enlargement Decreased LV contractility Apical thrombus (±)	Biatrial enlargement Normal LV and RV volume Normal LV systolic function until advanced stage Atrial thrombus (±)
Doppler	Reduced relaxation pattern (see Fig. 18-6)	Reduced relaxation pattern (see Fig. 18-6)	"Restrictive" pattern (see Fig. 18-6)
Treatment	β-Adrenoreceptor blockers Calcium antagonists (Digitalis/catechols and nitrates contraindicated) (Diuretics may worsen sxs)	Vasodilator therapy Digitalis plus diuretics β-Adrenoceptor blockers (±) Anticoagulants Antiarrhythmics (±) Cardiac transplant (±)	Diuretics Anticoagulants (±) Corticosteroids (±) Permanent pacemaker for advanced heart block (±) Cardiac transplant (±)

AD, Autosomal dominance; *LVEDP,* LV end-diastolic pressure; *ASH,* asymmetric septal hypertrophy; *LVDD,* LV diastolic dimenison; *LVSD,* LV systolic dimension.

influence that increases the systolic volume (such as negative inotropic agents, leg raising, blood transfusion, or increasing SVR) lessens the obstruction.

6. A large portion of the stroke volume (about 80%) is ejected during the early part of systole when there is little or no obstruction, producing a sharp upstroke in the arterial pulse, a characteristic finding of HOCM. The obstruction occurs late in systole, producing a late systolic murmur. Because of the variable degree of obstruction, the intensity of the heart murmur varies from time to time.

7. Patients with severe hypertrophy and obstruction may experience anginal chest pain, lightheadedness, near syncope, or syncope. Patients also are prone to develop arrhythmias, which may lead to sudden death (presumably from ventricular tachycardia and/or fibrillation).

Clinical Manifestations
History.

1. Hypertrophic cardiomyopathy usually is seen in adolescents and young adults, with equal gender distribution.

2. Family history is positive for the disease in 30% to 60% of patients.

3. Easy fatigability, dyspnea, palpitation, or anginal pain may be present.

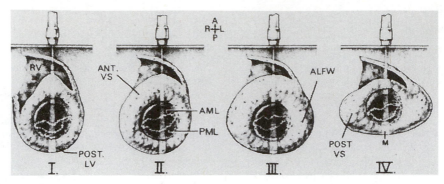

FIG. 18–3.
Morphologic variability in hypertrophic cardiomyopathy seen on parasternal short-axis view of two-dimensional echo. In type I hypertrophy, relatvely mild LV hypertrophy confined to the anterior portion of the ventricular septum *(VS)* is present. In type II, hypertrophy of anterior and posterior septum is present in the absence of free wall thickening. In type III, there is diffuse hypertrophy of substantial portions of both the ventricular septum and anterolateral free wall *(ALFW)*. In type IV, the M-mode echo beam *(M)* does not traverse the thickened portions of LV in posterior septum and anterolateral free wall. *AML,* Anterior mitral leaflet; *A* or *ANT,* anterior; *L,* left; *LVFW,* LV free wall; *P* or *POST,* posterior; *PML,* posterior mitral leaflet; *R,* right. (From Maron BJ: Asymmetry in hypertrophic cardiomyopathy: the septal to free wall thickness ratio revisited, *Am J Cardiol* 55:835-838, 1985 [Editorial].)

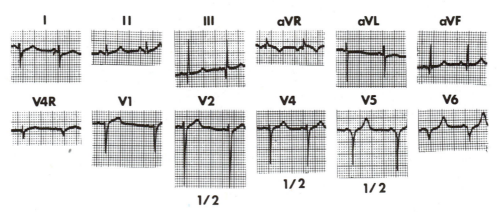

FIG. 18–4.
Tracing from a 17-year-old girl with HOCM with marked septal hypertrophy. Note prominent Q waves with absent R waves in V5 and V6.

Physical examination.

1. A sharp upstroke of the arterial pulse is characteristic (in contrast to a slow upstroke seen with fixed AS). A left-ventricular lift and a systolic thrill at the apex or along the LLSB may be present.

2. The S2 is normal, and an ejection click generally is absent. A grade 1-3/6 SEM of medium pitch is most audible at the MLSB and LLSB or at the apex. A soft holosystolic murmur of MR often is present. The intensity and even the presence of the murmur vary from examination to examination.

Electrocardiography. The ECG is abnormal in the majority of patients. Common ECG abnormalities include LVH by voltage criteria, ST-T changes, abnormally deep Q waves (owing to septal hypertrophy) with diminished or absent R waves in the LPLs (Fig. 18-4), and arrhythmias.

X-ray study. Mild LV enlargement with a globular-shaped heart may be present. The pulmonary vascularity is normal.

Echocardiography.

1. Echo is diagnostic. Two-dimensional echo demonstrates the wide morphologic spectrum of the disease, including concentric hypertrophy (Fig. 18-5), localized segmental hypertrophy, and asymmetric septal hypertrophy (see Fig. 18-3).

2. M-mode echo may demonstrate an asymmetric septal hypertrophy of the interventricular septum (with the septal thickness 1.4 times greater than the posterior LV wall) and occasionally systolic anterior motion of the anterior mitral valve leaflet in the obstructive type (see Fig. 18-2).

3. Mitral inflow Doppler tracing demonstrates decreased E wave velocity, increased deceleration time, and decreased ration of E wave to A wave velocity (Fig. 18-6).

Natural History

1. The obstruction may be absent, stable, or slowly progressive. Genetically predisposed individuals often show striking increases in wall thickness during childhood.

2. Sudden death may occur most commonly in patients between 10 and 35 years of age, particularly during exercise, even in patients with only mild obstruction. The incidence of sudden death is 4% to 6% a year in children and adolescents and 2% to 4% a year in adults. Even brief episodes of asymptomatic ventricular tachycardia on ambulatory ECG monitoring may be a risk factor.

3. Atrial fibrillation results in clinical deterioration, resulting from loss of the atrial "kick" needed for filling the thick LV.

4. In a minority of patients, heart failure with cardiac dilatation ("burned out" phase of the disease) may develop later in life.

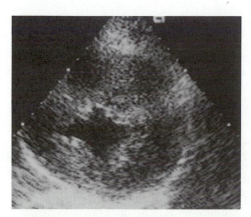 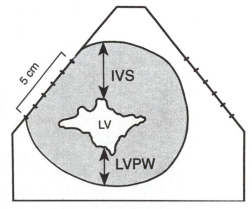

FIG. 18-5.
Parasternal short-axis view of a 14-year-old boy with hypertrophic cardiomyopathy. Marked hypertrophy of the interventricular septum *(IVS)* as well as the posterior wall of the left ventricle *(LVPW)* is present. The LV cavity is small. The interventricular septum is approximately 39 mm, and the LV posterior wall is 26 mm in thickness. The thickness of both structures does not exceed 10 mm in normal persons.

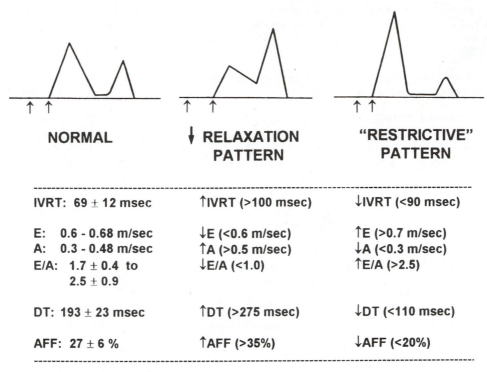

NORMAL	↓ RELAXATION PATTERN	"RESTRICTIVE" PATTERN
IVRT: 69 ± 12 msec	↑IVRT (>100 msec)	↓IVRT (<90 msec)
E: 0.6 - 0.68 m/sec	↓E (<0.6 m/sec)	↑E (>0.7 m/sec)
A: 0.3 - 0.48 m/sec	↑A (>0.5 m/sec)	↓A (<0.3 m/sec)
E/A: 1.7 ± 0.4 to 2.5 ± 0.9	↓E/A (<1.0)	↑E/A (>2.5)
DT: 193 ± 23 msec	↑DT (>275 msec)	↓DT (<110 msec)
AFF: 27 ± 6 %	↑AFF (>35%)	↓AFF (<20%)

FIG. 18–6.
Examples of diastolic dysfunction seen in various forms of cardiomyopathy. (See chapter 6 for further discussion.) *A,* A wave (the velocity of a second wave that coincides with atrial contraction); *AFF,* atrial filling fraction; *DT,* deceleration time; *E,* E wave (the velocity of an early peak); *E/A,* ratio of E wave to A wave velocity; *IVRT,* isovolumic relaxation time.

5. SBE may affect the mitral valve.

6. Pregnancy is usually well-tolerated.

Management
   Medical.

1. Moderate restriction of physical activity is recommended.

2. Prophylactic therapy with either β-adrenergic blockers or the calcium channel blocker verapamil is controversial. Some favor prophylactic administration of these drugs to prevent sudden death or to delay progression of the disease process, and others limit prophylactic drug therapy to young patients with a family history of premature sudden death and those with particularly marked LVH.

3. A β-adrenergic blocker (such as propranolol, atenolol, or metoprolol) is the drug of choice in the obstructive subgroup. This drug reduces the degree of outflow tract obstruction, decreases the incidence of anginal pain, and has antiarrhythmic effects.

4. Calcium channel blockers (principally verapamil) may be equally effective. These agents reduce hypercontractile systolic function and improve diastolic filling.

5. Ventricular arrhythmias may be treated with propranolol, amiodarone, and other standard antiarrhythmic agents guided by serial ambulatory ECG monitoring.

6. Digitalis is contraindicated because it increases the degree of obstruction. Other

cardiotonic drugs and vasodilators should be avoided because they tend to increase the pressure gradient.

7. Diuretics usually are ineffective and can be harmful. However, judicious use can help improve congestive symptoms (e.g., exertional dyspnea, orthopnea) by reducing LV filling pressure.

8. Prophylaxis against SBE is indicated.

Surgical.

Indications. Operative management remains an important therapeutic alternative for symptomatic patients who do not respond to medical management and who have severe obstruction with a resting pressure gradient of greater than 50 mm Hg.

Procedures.

MORROW'S MYOTOMY-MYECTOMY. Transaortic LV septal myotomy-myectomy (Morrow's operation) is the procedure of choice. This operation is performed through an aortotomy without the benefit of complete direct visualization. Two vertical and parallel incisions are made (about 1 cm apart, 1.0 to 1.5 cm deep) into the hypertrophied ventricular septum. A third transverse incision connects the two incisions at their distal extent, and the bar of a rectangular septal muscle is excised. The mortality rate is 3% to 5%. Symptoms improve in most patients, but patients later die of congestive symptoms and arrhythmias caused by the cardiomyopathy. Postoperative annual mortality rate remains about the same (1.8%). Serious complications of the surgery include complete heart block (3% to 5%) and surgically induced VSD (3%).

MITRAL VALVE REPLACEMENT. Mitral valve replacement with a low-profile prosthetic valve may be indicated in selected patients in whom the basal anterior septum is relatively thin (less than 18 mm), the region of greatest septal thickness is inaccessible to a transaortic myotomy-myectomy, or there is severe mitral regurgitation. The operative mortality is about 6%. About 70% of the patients show symptomatic improvement, but complications related to the prosthetic valve occur.

DILATED OR CONGESTIVE CARDIOMYOPATHY

Pathology and Pathophysiology

1. In dilated cardiomyopathy, a weakening of systolic contraction is associated with dilatation of all four cardiac chambers. Dilatation of the atria is in proportion to ventricular dilatation. The ventricular walls are not thickened, although heart weight is increased.

2. Intracavitary thrombus formation is common in the apical portion of the ventricular cavities and in atrial appendages and may give rise to pulmonary and systemic emboli.

3. Histologic examination reveals extensive small areas of degeneration and necrosis. Inflammatory cells usually are absent. These hearts are distinguished from primary endocardial fibroelastrosis by the absence of diffuse endocardial thickening, and from myocarditis by the absence of myocardial inflammation. However, a varying incidence of inflammatory myocarditis has been reported in patients with clinical findings of dilated cardiomyopathy. Many cases of unexplained dilated cardiomyopathy may, in fact, result from myocarditis.

4. Dilated cardiomyopathy may represent the end result of myocardial damage produced by a variety of infectious, toxic, or metabolic agents or immunologic defects. Doxorubicin (Adriamycin) toxicity is the most common cause of dilated cardiomyopathy in children (see later section on Doxorubicin cardiomyopathy). Occasionally, pheochromocytoma produces (a reversible) dilated cardiomyopathy.

5. Rarely, more than one family member has been reported to have dilated cardiomyopathy (occurring in up to 20% of patients with this disease).

Clinical Manifestations

History.

1. A history of fatigue, weakness, and symptoms of left-sided heart failure (dyspnea on exertion, orthopnea) may be elicited.

2. A history of prior viral illness occasionally is obtained.

Physical examination.

1. Signs of CHF (tachycardia, pulmonary rales, weak peripheral pulses, distended neck veins, hepatomegaly) are present. The apical impulse usually is displaced to the left and inferiorly.

2. The S2 may be normal or narrowly split with accentuated P2 if pulmonary hypertension develops. A prominent S3 is present with or without gallop rhythm. A soft regurgitant systolic murmur (caused by mitral or tricuspid regurgitation) may be present.

Electrocardiography.

1. Sinus tachycardia, LVH, and ST-T changes are the most common findings. LAH or RAH may be present. Rarely, a healed anterior myocardial infarction pattern may be present.

2. Atrial or ventricular arrhythmias and AV conduction disturbances may be seen.

X-ray study. Generalized cardiomegaly usually is present with or without signs of pulmonary venous hypertension or pulmonary edema.

Echocardiography. Echo is the most important tool in the diagnosis of the condition and is important in the longitudinal follow-up of patients.

1. The LV and RV are enlarged. The end-diastolic and end-systolic dimensions of the LV are increased, with a reduced fractional shortening and ejection fraction (Fig. 18-7).

2. Pericardial effusion and intracavitary thrombus may be seen.

3. Mitral inflow Doppler tracing demonstrates a reduced E velocity and a decreased E/A ratio (ratio of E wave to A wave velocity) compared with normal subjects (see Fig. 18-6).

Natural History

1. Progressive deterioration is the rule rather than the exception. About two thirds of patients die from intractable heart failure within 4 years after the onset of symptoms of CHF.

2. Atrial and ventricular arrhythmias develop with time (in about 50% of patients studied by 24-hour Holter monitor) but are not predictive of outcome.

3. Systemic and pulmonary embolism resulting from dislodgment of intracavitary thrombi occurs in the late stages of the illness.

4. Causes of death are CHF, sudden death resulting from arrhythmias, and massive embolization.

Treatment

1. Treatment has consisted of the aggressive management of CHF with digoxin and diuretics. Vasodilators (e.g., captopril, enalapril, hydralazine) are an integral part of therapy, as well as bed rest or restriction of activity.

2. Anticoagulants (coumadin or heparin) are recommended because of the frequency of embolization.

3. Patients with arrhythmias may be treated by the addition of amiodarone or other antiarrhythmic agents or a pacemaker. An automatic implantable cardioverter-defibrillator may be considered but has limited experience in children.

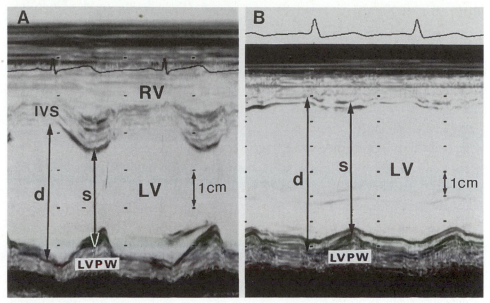

FIG. 18–7.
M-mode echo in a child with dilated cardiomyopathy. **A,** M-mode echo from a 9-year-old normal child. The LV diastolic dimension *(d)* is 36 mm, and the LV systolic dimension *(s)* is 24 mm, with resulting fractional shortening of 33%. **B,** M-mode echo from an 8-year-old child with dilated cardiomyopathy with a markedly decreased LV contractile function. The LV diastolic dimension (62 mm) and LV systolic dimension (52 mm) are markedly increased with a marked decrease in the fractional shortening (16%). *IVS,* Interventricular septum; *LVPW,* LV posterior wall.

4. Beneficial effects of β-Adrenergic blocking agents (somewhat heretical given poor contractility) are under investigation. Recent evidence suggests that activation of the sympathetic nervous system may have deleterious cardiac effects (rather than being an important compensatory mechanism as traditionally thought). β-Adrenergic blockers may exert beneficial effects by negative chronotropic effect with reduced oxygen demand, reduction in catecholamine toxicity, inhibition of sympathetically mediated vasoconstriction, or reduction of potentially lethal ventricular arrhythmias.

5. Many of these children may become candidates for cardiac transplantation.

ENDOCARDIAL FIBROELASTOSIS

Prevalence

The prevalence of the nonfamilial form of endocardial fibroelastosis is extremely rare. The prevalence has declined in the past 2 decades for unknown reasons, it was 4% of cardiac autopsy cases in children.

Pathology

1. Endocardial fibroelastosis is a form of dilated cardiomyopathy seen in infants and children. The condition is characterized by diffuse changes in the endocardium with a white, opaque, glistening appearance. The heart chambers, primarily the LA and LV, are notably dilated and hypertrophied. Involvement of the right-sided heart chambers is rare. Deformities and shortening of the papillary muscles and chordae tendineae (resulting in MR) often are present late in the course. Similar pathology appears secondary to severe congenital obstructive lesions of the left heart, such as AS, COA, and HLHS (called *secondary fibroelastosis*).

2. The cause of primary fibroelastosis is not known. It may be the result of a process of reaction to many different insults, rather than a specific disease. Viral myocarditis and a sequel to interstitial myocarditis have received more attention than other proposed etiologies, including systemic carnitine deficiency and genetic factors.

Clinical Manifestations

History. Symptoms and signs of CHF (feeding difficulties, tachypnea, sweating, irritability, pallor, failure to thrive) develop in the first 10 months of life.

Physical examination.

1. Patients have tachycardia and tachypnea.

2. No heart murmur is audible in the majority of patients, although a gallop rhythm usually is present. Occasionally, a heart murmur of MR is audible.

3. Hepatomegaly frequently is present.

Electrocardiography. LVH with "strain" is typical of the condition. Occasionally, myocardial infarction patterns, arrhythmias, and varying degrees of AV block may be seen.

X-ray study. Marked generalized cardiomegaly with normal or congested pulmonary vascularity usually is present.

Echocardiography. A markedly dilated and poorly contracting LV in the absence of structural heart defects is characteristic. The LA also is markedly dilated. Bright endocardial echoes are typical of the condition.

Treatment

1. Early diagnosis and long-term (for years) treatment with digoxin, diuretics, and afterload-reducing agents are mandatory. Digoxin is continued for a minimum of 2 to 3 years and then gradually is discontinued if symptoms are absent, heart size is normal, and the ECG has reverted to normal.

2. An afterload-reducing agent (hydralazine up to 4.0 mg/kg/day, in 4 divided doses) has been reported to be beneficial.

3. SBE prophylaxis should be observed on indications, especially when MR is present.

Prognosis

When proper treatment is instituted, about one third of patients deteriorate and die of CHF. Another one third survive but experience persistent symptoms. The remaining one third exhibit complete recovery. Operative procedures are not available.

Differential Diagnosis

Infants with cardiomegaly and no heart murmur often present a diagnostic challenge. The cardiomegaly may result from diseases that affect primarily myocardium or coronary arteries CHDs with severe CHF, respiratory diseases, or other miscellaneous conditions. The box lists differential diagnoses of cardiomegaly without heart murmur in infants and young children. All of these conditions show cardiomegaly on chest roentgenograms, usually with, but occasionally without, signs of CHF. Conditions listed under myocardial diseases and coronary artery diseases in the box on p. 281 will be briefly discussed in this chapter.

Myocarditis. Viral myocarditis caused by coxsackievirus B carries a high mortality (70%) in the newborn period. Myocarditis caused by other viruses occurs more frequently in infants older than 1 year.

Acute myocarditis may manifest with a history of a recent upper respiratory infection and signs of CHF (e.g., tachycardia, dyspnea, wheezing, pulmonary edema, cardiomegaly, gallop rhythm). Heart murmur usually is absent. The ECG often shows low QRS

Differential Diagnosis of Cardiomegaly Without Heart Murmur in Pediatric Patients

Myocardial Diseases

Endocardial fibroelastosis
Myocarditis (viral or idiopathic)
Glycogen storage disease

Coronary Artery Diseases Resulting in Myocardial Insufficiency

Anomalous origin of the left coronary artery from the PA
Collagen disease (periarteritis nodosa)
Kawasaki's disease (mucocutaneous lymph node syndrome)

CHD With Severe Heart Failure

COA in infants
Ebstein's anomaly (a soft TR murmur frequently is present)

Miscellaneous Conditions

CHF secondary to respiratory disease (upper airway obstruction, chronic alveolar hypoxia such as seen
    with bronchopulmonary dysplasia, extensive pneumonia)
SVT with CHF
Pericardial effusion
Severe anemia
Tumors of the heart
Neonatal thyrotoxicosis
Malnutrition (infantile beriberi, protein calorie malnutrition)
Toxicity (drugs, such as doxorubicin [Adriamycin], or radiation)

---

voltages (rather than LVH as in endocardial fibroelastosis) and prolongation of the PR interval, QRS duration, or QT interval. Flat or inverted T waves may be present in leads representing the LV.

Clinical manifestations vary with the stage of the disease. Subacute or chronic myocarditis is characterized by persistent cardiomegaly with or without signs of CHF, and the ECG findings of LVH or CVH with strain pattern. Therefore clinical pictures of subacute or chronic myocarditis are indistinguishable from those of endocardial fibroelastosis or dilated cardiomyopathy.

Treatment consists of anticongestive and supportive measures (see also the section on myocarditis in Chapter 19).

Glycogen storage disease. The classic glycogen storage disease that causes heart failure in infancy is Pompe's disease (Cori's type II), which is due to deficiency of α-1,4-glycosidase. This is a familial disease characterized by generalized muscle weakness, macroglossia, hepatomegaly, and signs of CHF or severe arrhythmias. The onset of CHF is around 2 to 3 months of age, with fatal outcome usually during infancy. The ECG may show a short PR interval, LVH in the majority of patients, occasional CVH, and ST-T changes in the LPLs. Excessive glycogen deposits in a skeletal muscle biopsy specimen are diagnostic. No treatment is available, but genetic counseling should be provided for the family.

Anomalous left coronary artery from the pulmonary artery. In anomalous left coronary artery from the PA, signs and symptoms of myocardial infarction and CHF may be manifested around 2 to 3 months of age. The ECG typically shows evidence of anterolateral myocardial infarction (see also Chapter 17).

Kawasaki's disease. Mucocutaneous lymph node syndrome of Kawasaki may present with evidence of coronary insufficiency and heart failure during the subacute phase of the disease. It usually involves children younger than 4 years. Signs of cardiac involvement are preceded by characteristic clinical pictures of the disease by a week or two (see Chapter 19).

Other rare conditions that involve coronary arteries include periarteritis nodosa, calcification of coronary arteries, and medial necrosis of coronary arteries. Overlap seems likely among the four arterial disorders.

DOXORUBICIN CARDIOMYOPATHY

Prevalence

Doxorubicin cardiomyopathy is becoming the most common cause of chronic CHF in children. Its prevalence is nonlinearly dose-related, occurring in 2% to 5% of patients who have received a cumulative dose of 400 to 500 mg/m^2 and up to 50% of patients who have received more than 1000 mg/m^2 of doxorubicin (Adriamycin).

Etiology

1. Doxorubicin, which is commonly used in pediatric oncologic disorders, is the cause of the cardiomyopathy. C-13 anthracycline metabolites, which are inhibitors of adenosinetriphosphatases of sarcoplasmic reticulum, mitochondria, and sarcolemma, have been implicated in the mechanism of cardiotoxicity.

2. Risk factors include age younger than 4 years, a cumulative dose exceeding 400 to 600 mg/m^2, and a dosing regimen with larger and less frequent doses.

Pathology and Pathophysiology

1. Dilated LV, decreased contractility, elevated filling pressures of the LV, and reduced cardiac output characterize pathophysiologic features.

2. Microscopically, interstitial edema without evidence of inflammatory changes, loss of myofibrils within the myocyte, vacuolar degeneration, necrosis, and fibrosis are present.

Clinical Manifestations

1. Patients are usually asymptomatic until signs of heart failure develop. Patients have a history of having received doxorubicin, with the onset of symptoms 2 to 4 months, and rarely years, after completion of therapy. Tachypnea and dyspnea made worse by exertion are the usual presenting complaints. Occasionally palpitation, cough, or substernal discomfort are complaints.

2. Signs of CHF are present, with hepatomegaly and distended neck veins. Gallop rhythm may be present with occasional soft murmur of MR or TR.

3. X-ray films show cardiomegaly with or without pulmonary congestion or pleural effusion.

4. The ECG shows sinus tachycardia with ST-T changes in a small number of patients (2% to 8%). A progressive increase in the basal (early morning) heart rate is reported.

5. Echo studies reveal the following:

    a. The size of the LV is slightly increased, and the thickness of the LV wall is decreased.

    b. The LV contractility (either ejection fraction or fractional shortening) is decreased.

    c. Dobutamine stress echo is reported to be more sensitive than routine echo in examining the cardiac status of asymptomatic doxorubicin-treated patients.

Management

1. Anticongestive measures with inotropic agents (digoxin), diuretics, and afterload-reducing agents (captopril) are useful.

2. Risk factors of doxorubicin cardiotoxicity should be avoided or closely monitored:

    a. Continuous infusion therapy can reduce cardiac injury.

b. Restriction of the total cumulative dose to 400 to 500 mg/m² will reduce the incidence of CHF to 5%, but this dose may not be effective in treating some malignancies.

c. Some have recommended close monitoring for signs of cardiomyopathy by serial echo, radionuclide angiocardiography, and even cardiac catheterization and endomyocardial biopsy.

3. The advisability of modifying anthracycline therapy is controversial. The Cardiology Committee of Children's Cancer Study Group (Steinherz, 1992) recommended either withholding anthracycline therapy or subsequently reducing the dose if the above tests show abnormalities of LV systolic function (e.g., fractional shortening less than 29% by echo or LV ejection fraction less than 55% by radionuclide angiocardiography and other tests). These recommendations recently were challenged (Lipshultz, 1994) on the grounds that (1) the studies cited in the committee's recommendations are not convincing, (2) the methods of screening for anthracycline cardiotoxicity have not been shown to be adequately predictive of cardiac outcome, and (3) modification of anthracycline therapy may result in increased death from malignancies while potentially reducing the cardiotoxicity. This group therefore recommends dose modification only when clinical evidence of cardiotoxicity is present. Further controlled studies are needed to settle the debate.

4. Cardiac transplantation may be an option for selected patients.

Prognosis

Symptomatic cardiomyopathy carries a high mortality rate. The 2-year survival rate is about 20%, and all patients die by 9 years after onset of the illness.

RESTRICTIVE CARDIOMYOPATHY

Prevalence

Restrictive cardiomyopathy, an extremely rare cardiomyopathy in children, is the least common of the three types of cardiomyopathy in adults in North America.

Pathology and Pathophysiology

1. This condition is characterized by abnormal diastolic ventricular filling resulting from excessively stiff ventricular walls. The ventricles are neither excessively dilated nor hypertrophied, and contractile function is normal. The atria are enlarged out of proportion to the ventricular dimension. Therefore they resemble constrictive pericarditis in clinical presentation and hemodynamic abnormalities.

2. There are areas of myocardial fibrosis and hypertrophy of myocytes, or the myocardium may be infiltrated by various materials. Infiltrative restrictive cardio-myopathy may be due to conditions such as amyloidosis, sarcoidosis, hemochroma-tosis, glycogen deposit, Fabry's disease (with deposition of glycosphingolipids), or neoplastic infiltration.

Clinical Manifestations (see Table 18-1)

1. The patient may have a history of exercise intolerance, weakness and dyspnea, or chest pain.

2. Jugular venous distention, gallop rhythm, and a systolic murmur of AV valve regurgitation may be present.

3. Chest x-ray films show cardiomegaly, pulmonary congestion, and pleural effusion. The ECG may show atrial fibrillation and paroxysms of SVT.

4. Echo reveals characteristic biatrial enlargement with normal cavity size of the LV and RV. LV systolic function (ejection fraction) is normal until the late stages of the disease. Atrial thrombus may be present.

5. Mitral inflow Doppler tracing shows an increased E velocity with decreased deceleration time, and increased E/A ratio (see Fig. 18-6).

Treatment

1. Diuretics are beneficial, but digoxin is not indicated because systolic function is unimpaired.

2. Anticoagulants (warfarin) and antiplatelet drugs (aspirin and dipyridamole) may help prevent thrombosis.

3. Corticosteroids and immunosuppressive agents have been suggested.

4. A permanent pacemaker is indicated for complete heart block.

5. Cardiac transplantation may be considered.

RIGHT VENTRICULAR DYSPLASIA

Pathology

1. RV dysplasia, which is also called RV cardiomyopathy, is a rare abnormality of unknown etiology in which the myocardium of the RV is partially or totally replaced by fibrous or adipose tissue. The RV wall may assume a paper-thin appearance because of the total absence of myocardial tissue, but in others, RV wall thickness is normal or near normal. The LV usually is spared.

2. Most cases appear to be sporadic, although familial occurrences have been reported. Whether the disease is congenital or acquired is unknown, although recent evidence favors an acquired degenerative process. The disease appears to be prevalent in northern Italy.

Clinical Manifestations

1. The onset is in infancy, childhood, or adulthood (but usually before the age of 20), with a history of palpitation, syncopal episodes, or both. Sudden death may be the first sign of the disease.

2. Presenting manifestations may be arrhythmias (ventricular tachycardia, supraventricular arrhythmias) or signs of CHF.

3. Chest x-ray films usually show cardiomegaly, and the ECG most often shows tall P waves in lead II (RAH) and decreased RV potentials.

4. Echo shows selective RV enlargement and often areas of akinesia or dyskinesia.

5. A substantial portion of patients die before 5 years of age from CHF and intractable ventricular tachycardia.

Treatment

1. Various antiarrhythmic agents may be tried, but they often are unsuccessful in abolishing ventricular tachycardia.

2. Surgical intervention (ventricular incision or disconnection of the RV free wall) may be tried if antiarrhythmic therapy is unsuccessful.

19 / Cardiovascular Infections

INFECTIVE ENDOCARDITIS

Prevalence

Infective endocarditis accounts for 0.5 to 1 per 1000 hospital admissions, excluding postoperative endocarditis.

Pathogenesis

1. Two factors are important in the pathogenesis of infective endocarditis: the presence of structural abnormalities of the heart or great arteries with a significant pressure gradient or turbulence (with resulting endothelial damage and platelet-fibrin thrombus formation) and bacteremia, even transient.

2. Almost all patients who develop infective endocarditis have a history of CHD or acquired heart disease, although patients with bicuspid aortic valve may not have been diagnosed with the defect before the onset of the endocarditis. Drug addicts may develop endocarditis in the absence of known cardiac anomalies.

3. All CHDs, with the exception of secundum-type ASD, predispose to endocarditis. More frequently encountered defects are TOF, VSD, and aortic valve disease. Rheumatic valvular disease, particularly mitral insufficiency, is responsible in a small number of patients. Those with a prosthetic heart valve or prosthetic material in the heart are at particularly high risk of developing endocarditis. Patients with MVP (with MR) and HOCM (IHSS) also are vulnerable to infective endocarditis.

4. Any localized infection (e.g., abscesses, osteomyelitis, pyelonephritis) can seed organisms into the circulation. Bacteremia frequently results after dental procedures, especially in children who have carious teeth or disease of the gingiva. Bacteremia also occurs with activities such as chewing or brushing the teeth. Chewing with diseased teeth or gums may be the most frequent cause of bacteremia. (Therefore good dental hygiene is more important in prevention of infective endocarditis than antibiotic coverage before dental procedures.)

Pathology

Vegetation of infective endocarditis is found usually in the low-pressure side of the defect, either around the defect or on the opposite surface of the defect where an endothelial damage is established by the jet effect of the defect. For example, vegetations are found in the PA in PDA or systemic-PA shunts, on the atrial surface of the mitral valve in MR, on the ventricular surface of the aortic valve and mitral chordae in AR, and on the superior surface of the aortic valve or at the site of a jet lesion in the aorta in patients with AS.

Microbiology

1. *Streptococcus viridans*, enterococci (*Streptococcus faecalis, faecium,* and *durans*), and *Staphylococcus aureus* are responsible for over 90% of the cases. Less commonly encountered organisms include pneumococcus, *Haemophilus influenzae, Pseudomonas* organisms, *Escherichia coli, Proteus* organisms, *Aerobacter* organisms, and *Listeria* organisms.

2. α-Hemolytic streptococci (*S. viridans*) are the most common cause of endocarditis in patients who had dental procedures or in those with carious teeth or periodontal disease.

3. The enterococcus is the organism most often found after genitourinary or gastrointestinal surgery or instrumentation.

4. The organism most commonly found in postoperative endocarditis and in intravenous drug abusers is the *Staphylococcus.*

5. Candidal endocarditis may occur in patients who are receiving long-term antibiotic or steroid therapy.

Clinical Manifestations
History.

1. Most patients have a history of underlying heart defect.

2. A history of a recent dental procedure or tonsillectomy occasionally is present, but a history of toothache (from dental or gingival disease) is more frequent than a history of a procedure.

3. Insidious onset, with fever, fatigue, loss of appetite, and pallor, is common.

Physical examination.

1. Heart murmur is universal (100%). The appearance of a new heart murmur and an increase in the intensity of an existing murmur are important. However, many innocent heart murmurs also are of new onset.

2. Fever is common (80% to 90%). Fever fluctuates between 101° and 103° F (38.3° and 39.4° C).

3. Splenomegaly is common (70%).

4. Skin manifestations (50%), probably secondary to microemboli, are present in the following forms:

   a. Petechiae on the skin, mucous membrane, or conjunctivas are the most frequent skin lesions.

   b. Osler's nodes (tender red nodes at the ends of the fingers) are rare in children.

   c. Janeway's lesions (small, painless, hemorrhagic areas on the palms or soles) are rare.

   d. Splinter hemorrhage (linear hemorrhagic streaks beneath the nails) also are rare.

5. Embolic phenomena to other organs are present in 50% of cases:

   a. Pulmonary emboli in patients with VSD, PDA, or a systemic-PA shunt.

   b. Seizures and hemiparesis are the result of embolization to the central nervous system (20%) and more common with left-sided defects such as aortic and mitral valve disease or with cyanotic heart disease.

   c. Hematuria and renal failure.

   d. Roth spot (oval, retinal hemorrhage with a pale center located near the optic disc) occurs in fewer than 5% of patients.

6. Carious teeth or periodontal or gingival disease are frequently present.

7. Clubbing of fingers in the absence of cyanosis develops rarely in more chronic cases.

Laboratory studies.

1. Positive blood cultures are found in more than 90% of patients in the absence of previous antimicrobial therapy.

2. A complete blood cell count shows anemia, with hemoglobin levels lower than 12 g/100 ml (present in 80% of patients), and leukocytosis with shift to the left. Patients with polycythemia preceding the onset of infective endocarditis may have normal hemoglobin.

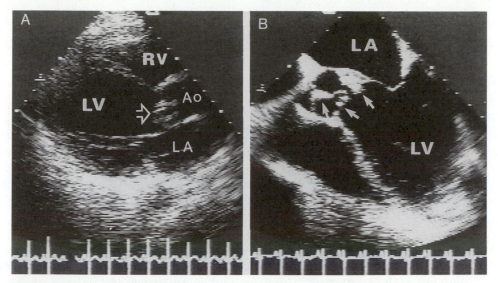

FIG. 19–1.
Echos of aortic valve vegetation. **A;** A parasternal long-axis view of a young adult patient with bicuspid aortic valve demonstrating a vegetation on the aortic valve *(arrow)*. Severe AR was present with dilated LV. **B;** Five-chamber transverse plane of a TEE on the same patient that demonstrates vegetations and aortic valve anatomy more clearly than the ordinary two-dimensional echo.

3. The sedimentation rate is increased unless there is polycythemia.

4. Microscopic hematuria is found in 30% of patients.

   Echocardiography. Two-dimensional echo actually may demonstrate the vegetation (Fig. 19-1). Vegetations over 3 mm in diameter will be imaged by two-dimensional echo. TEE has a better resolution. Negative echo does not rule out infective endocarditis; repeated echo studies are indicated when infective endocarditis is suspected. A false-positive diagnosis also is possible, especially with abnormal valves or improper gain of the echo machine. Echo evidence of vegetation may persist for months or years after bacteriologic cure.

Diagnosis

A *presumptive* diagnosis of infective endocarditis is made when a patient with an underlying heart lesion has a fever of unknown origin of several days' duration and when any of the physical findings or laboratory changes are present. A *definitive* diagnosis is made by positive blood cultures. Demonstration of the vegetation by two-dimensional echo provides a conclusive anatomic diagnosis.

Management

1. Four to six blood cultures are drawn in succession over 24 to 48 hours, unless the patient is very ill. Blood cultures need not be obtained during febrile periods.

2. Treatment is started with intravenous penicillin or oxacillin plus gentamicin or intramuscular streptomycin while awaiting the results of blood cultures:

   a. Penicillin G, 200,000 U/kg/day (maximum of 20 million U) in an intravenous bolus in six divided doses, is given every 4 hours.

   b. Oxacillin, 150 to 200 mg/kg/day (maximum of 12 g/day) intravenously in six divided doses is given every 4 hours.

   c. Gentamicin, 7 mg/kg/day (maximum of 240 mg/day) intravenously, is given in three divided doses.

   d. Streptomycin 30 mg/kg/day (maximum of 1000 mg/day), intramuscularly given in one to two divided doses.

3. The final selection of antibiotics depends on the organism isolated and the result of an antibiotic sensitivity test. In general, however, when S. *viridans* is the causative agents, intravenous penicillin for 4 weeks is recommended. Enterococcus-caused endocarditis usually requires a combination of intravenous penicillin for 4 weeks and intravenous gentamicin or intramuscular streptomycin for 2 weeks. The drug of choice for staphylococcal endocarditis is one of the semisynthetic penicillinase-resistant penicillins, such as oxacillin, methicillin, or cloxacillin, given for 4 to 6 weeks. Penicillin-allergic individuals may be treated with intravenous vancomycin, 40 mg/kg/day (maximum of 2 g/day) in four divided doses for the same duration as penicillin.

4. Patients with prosthetic valve endocarditis should be treated for 4 to 6 weeks based on the organism isolated and the results of the sensitivity test. Operative intervention may be necessary before the antibiotic therapy is completed if the clinical situation warrants (such as progressive CHF, significant malfunction of prosthetic valves, persistently positive blood cultures after 2 weeks' therapy). Bacteriologic relapse after an appropriate course of therapy also calls for operative intervention.

Prognosis

The overall recovery rate is 80% to 85%; 90% or better for S. *viridans* and enterococcus and about 50% for *Staphylococcus* organisms.

Prevention

More important than the diagnosis and treatment of infective endocarditis is its prevention. Moreover, maintenance of good oral hygiene is more important than antibiotic prophylaxis. The following is an excerpt of *Prevention of Bacterial Endocarditis: Recommendations by the American Heart Association* (December, 1990). The "Prevention of Bacterial Endocarditis" wallet card is reproduced in Appendix A, Fig. AA-1 by permission of the American Medical Association.

   Indications and nonindications. Endocarditis prophylaxis is recommended for certain cardiac conditions and procedures, but it is not recommended for other conditions and procedures. The box on p. 289 summarizes these conditions and procedures.

   Antibiotic recommendations. The antibiotic prophylaxis is started 1 hour, *not several days,* before a procedure.

Dental, oral, or upper respiratory tract procedures.

1. Standard prophylaxis. (oral): amoxicillin 50 mg/kg (adults, 3.0 g) orally 1 hour before procedure and then a half dose 6 hours after the initial dose.

2. For patients *allergic* to penicillin, ampicillin, or amoxicillin (penicillins): erythromycin 20 mg/kg, (adults, ethylsuccinate 0.8 g or stearate 1.0 g) orally 2 hours before the procedure and a half-dose 6 hours after the initial dose, or clindamycin 10 mg/kg (adults, 300 mg) orally 1 hour before the procedure and then a half-dose 6 hours after the initial dose.

3. For patients unable to take oral medications: ampillicin, 50 mg/kg (adults, 2.0 g) intravenously or intramuscularly, 30 minutes before the procedure and then a half-dose 6 hours after the initial dose. For patients *allergic* to penicillins. clindamycin 10 mg/kg (adults, 300 mg) intravenously or imtramuscularly 30 minutes before the procedure and then a half-dose (intravenous or orally) 6 hours after the initial dose.

Indications and Nonindications for Infective Endocarditis Prophylaxis
_____

Cardiac Conditions and Procedures for Which the Prophylaxis _is_ Indicated

Cardiac conditions:
  Most CHDs
  Rheumatic and other valvular diseases
  Hypertrophic cardiomyopathy
  MVP with MR
  Prosthetic cardiac valves, including bioprosthetic and homograft valves
  Systemic-PA shunts
  Patients with a history of previous infective endocarditis, even in the absence of heart disease
Procedures:
  Dental procedures known to induce gingival or mucosal bleeding, including routine professional
    dental cleaning
  Tonsillectomy and adenoidectomy, surgical procedures of the respiratory tract, bronchoscopy with a
    rigid bronchoscope
  Esophageal dilatation
  Gallbladder or gastrointestinal surgery
  Urethral dilatation, cystoscopy, urethral catheterization or urinary tract surgery (when associated
    with urinary tract infection), and prostatic surgery
  Incision and drainage of infected tissue
  Vaginal hysterectomy and vaginal delivery in the presence of infection

Cardiac Conditions and Procedures for Which Prophylaxis is _not_ Indicated

Cardiac conditions:
  Isolated secundum ASD
  Surgical repair without residua beyond 6 months of secundum ASD, VSD, or PDA
  Previous coronary artery bypass surgery
  MVP without MR
  Innocent heart murmurs
  Previous Kawasaki's disease without valvular dysfunction
  Previous rheumatic fever without valvular disease
  Cardiac pacemakers and implanted defibrillators
Procedures:
  Shedding of primary teeth, simple adjustment of orthodontic appliances, filling above the gum line,
    and injection of intraoral anesthetic
  Tympanostomy tube insertion
  Endotracheal intubation, bronchoscopy with a flexible bronchoscope, with or without biopsy
  Cardiac catheterization
  Endoscopy with or without gastrointestinal biopsy
  Cesarean section
  In the absence of infection for urethral catheterization, dilatation and curettage, uncomplicated
    vaginal delivery, therapeutic abortion, sterilization procedures, or insertion or removal of intra-
    uterine devices
_____

4. For high-risk patients (ampicillin plus gentamicin, followed by amoxicillin): ampicillin, 50 mg/kg (adults, 2.0 g), plus gentamicin, 2.0 mg/kg (adults, 1.5 mg/kg, maximum 80 mg) intravenously or intramuscularly 30 minutes before the procedure followed by amoxicillin, 25 mg/kg (adults, 1.5 g) orally 6 hours after the initial dose. Alternatively, the parenteral regimen may be repeated 8 hours after the initial dose.

5. For high-risk patients _allergic_ to penicillins: vancomycin, 20 mg/kg (adults, 1.0 g) intravenously over 1 hour, starting 1 hour before procedure; no repeated dose necessary.

6. For those patients taking oral penicillin for secondary prevention of rheumatic fever, one should select either erythromycin or one of the alternative regimens listed previously.

Genitourinary and gastrointestinal procedures.

1. Standard regimen: ampicillin, 50 mg/kg (adults, 2.0 g) plus gentamicin, 2.0 mg/kg (adults, 1.5 mg/kg, maximum 80 mg), intravenously or intramuscularly 30 minutes before the procedure, followed by amoxicillin, 25 mg/kg (adults, 1.5 g) orally 6 hours after the initial dose. Alternatively, the parenteral regimen may be repeated once 8 hours after the initial dose.

2. For patients allergic to penicillins: vancomycin, 20 mg/kg (adults, 1.0 g) intravenously over 1 hour, plus gentamicin, 2.0 mg/kg (adults, 1.5 mg/kg, maximum 80 mg) intravenously or intramuscularly 1 hour before the procedure; it may be repeated once 8 hours after the initial dose.

3. Alternative low-risk patients: amoxicillin 50 mg/kg (adults 3.0 g) orally 1 hour before the procedure; then a half-dose 6 hours after the initial dose.

MYOCARDITIS

Prevalence

Myocarditis severe enough to be recognized clinically is rare, but the prevalence of mild and subclinical cases is probably much higher.

Pathology

1. The principal mechanism of cardiac involvement in viral myocarditis is believed to be a cell-mediated immunologic reaction, not merely myocardial damage from viral replication. Isolation of virus from the myocardium is unusual at autopsy.

2. The inflamed myocardium is soft, flabby, and pale with areas of scarring on gross examination. Microscopic examination reveals patchy infiltrations by plasma cells, mononuclear leukocytes, and some eosinophils during the acute phase and giant cell infiltration in the later stages.

Etiology

1. In North America, viruses are probably the most common causes of myocarditis. Among viruses, coxsackieviruses and echoviruses are the most common agents. Many other viruses (such as poliomyelitis, mumps, measles, rubella, cytomegalovirus, human immunodeficiency virus, arboviruses, adenovirus, and influenza) can cause myocarditis. In South America, Chagas' disease (caused by *Trypanosoma cruzi,* a protozoa) is far more common. Rarely, bacteria, rickettsia, fungi, protozoa, and parasites are the causative agents.

2. Immune mediated diseases, including acute rheumatic fever and Kawasaki's disease, may be the cause.

3. Collagen vascular diseases occur.

4. Toxic myocarditis (drug ingestion, diphtheria exotoxin, and anoxic agents) occur.

Clinical Manifestations
History.

1. Older children may have a history of an upper respiratory infection.

2. The illness may have a sudden onset in newborns and small infants, with anorexia, vomiting, lethargy, and occasionally circulatory shock.

Physical examination.

1. Signs of CHF may be present; these include poor heart tone, tachycardia, gallop rhythm, tachypnea, and rarely, cyanosis.

2. A soft, systolic heart murmur and hepatomegaly may be audible.

3. Irregular rhythm caused by supraventricular or ventricular ectopic beats may be present.

Electrocardiography. Any one or a combination of the following may be seen: low QRS voltages, ST-T changes, prolongation of the QT interval, and arrhythmias, especially premature contractions.

X-ray studies. Cardiomegaly of varying degrees is the most important clinical sign of myocarditis.

Echocardiography. Echo reveals cardiac chamber enlargement and impaired LV function, often regional in nature. Occasionally, increased wall thickness and LV thrombi are found.

Other laboratory findings. Radionuclide scanning (after the administration of gallium-67 or technetium-99m pyrophosphate) may identify inflammatory and necrotic changes characteristic of myocarditis.

Natural History

1. The majority of patients, especially those with only mild inflammation, recover completely.

2. Some patients develop subacute or chronic myocarditis with persistent cardiomegaly with or without signs of CHF and ECG evidence of LVH or CVH. Clinically, these patients are indistinguishable from those with dilated cardiomyopathy or endocardial fibroelastosis.

Management

1. One should attempt virus identification by viral cultures from the blood, stool, or throat washing. Acute and convalescent sera should be compared for serologic titer rise.

2. Bed rest and limitation in activities are recommended during the acute phase (because exercise intensifies the damage from myocarditis in experimental animals).

3. Anticongestive measures include the following:

   a. Rapid-acting diuretics (furosemide or ethacrynic acid, 1 mg/kg, each one to three times a day).

   b. Rapid-acting inotropic agents, such as isoproterenol, dobutamine, or dopamine, are useful in a critically ill child.

   c. Oxygen and bed rest are recommended. "Cardiac chair" or "infant seat" relieves respiratory distress.

   d. Digoxin may be given cautiously, using half of the usual digitalizing dose (see Table 30-3), because some patients with myocarditis are exquisitely sensitive to the drug.

4. Recently, beneficial effects of high-dose gamma globulin (2 g/kg, over 24 hours) have been reported. The gamma globulin was associated with better survival during the first year after presentation, echo evidence of smaller LV diastolic dimension, and higher fractional shortening than the control group. Myocardial damage in myocarditis is mediated in part by immunologic mechanisms, and a high dose of gamma globulin is an immunomodulatory agent, shown to be effective in myocarditis secondary to Kawasaki's disease.

5. The role of corticosteroid is unclear at this time except in the treatment of severe rheumatic carditis (see Chapter 20).

6. ACE inhibitors, such as captopril, may prove beneficial in the acute phase (as demonstrated in animal experiments).

7. Specific therapies include antitoxin in diphtheric myocarditis and gamma globulin and salicylates in Kawasaki's myocarditis.

PERICARDITIS

Etiology

1. Viral infection is probably the most common cause, particularly in infancy. Many viruses similar to those listed in the section on myocarditis can cause pericarditis.

2. Acute rheumatic fever is a common cause of pericarditis, especially in certain parts of the world (see also Chapter 20).

3. Bacterial infection (purulent pericarditis) is common. Commonly encountered are *S. aureus, S. pneumoniae, H. influenzae, Neisseria meningitidis,* and streptococci.

4. Tuberculosis is an occasional cause of constrictive pericarditis, with insidious onset.

5. Heart surgery (postpericardiotomy syndrome, Chapter 36) is a possible cause.

6. Collagen disease such as rheumatoid arthritis (see Chapter 23) can cause pericarditis.

7. Pericarditis can be a complication of oncologic disease or its therapy, including radiation.

8. Uremia (uremic pericarditis) is a possible cause.

Pathology

The parietal and visceral surfaces of the pericardium are inflamed. Pericardial effusion may be serofibrinous, hemorrhagic, or purulent. Effusion may be completely absorbed or may result in pericardial thickening or chronic constriction (constrictive pericarditis).

Pathophysiology

The pathogenesis of symptoms and signs of pericardial effusion is determined by two factors: the speed of fluid accumulation and the competence of the myocardium. A rapid accumulation of a large amount of pericardial fluid produces more serious circulatory embarrassment. A slow accumulation of a relatively small amount of fluid may result in serious circulatory embarrassment (cardiac tamponade) if the extent of myocarditis is significant. Slow accumulation of a large amount of fluid may be well tolerated if the myocardium is intact.

With the development of pericardial tamponade, several compensatory mechanisms are triggered: systemic and pulmonary venous constriction to improve diastolic filling, an increase in SVR to raise falling blood pressure, and tachycardia to improve cardiac output.

Clinical Manifestations

History.

1. The patient may have a history of upper respiratory tract infection.

2. Precordial pain (dull, aching, or stabbing) with occasional radiation to the shoulder and neck may be a presenting complaint. The pain may be relieved by leaning forward and may be made worse by supine position or deep inspiration.

3. Fever of varying degree may be present.

Physical examination.

1. Pericardial friction rub (a grating to-and-fro sound, in phase with the heart sounds) is the cardinal physical sign.

2. The heart is quiet and hypodynamic in the presence of cardiomegaly.

3. Heart murmur usually is absent, although it may be present in acute rheumatic fever (see Chapter 20).

4. In children with *purulent pericarditis,* septic fever (101° to 105° F), tachycardia, chest pain, and dyspnea almost always are present.

5. Signs of *cardiac tamponade* may be present: distant heart sounds, tachycardia, pulsus paradoxus, hepatomegaly, venous distention, and occasional hypotension with peripheral vasoconstriction. Cardiac tamponade occurs more commonly in purulent pericarditis than in other forms of pericarditis.

Electrocardiography.

1. The low-voltage QRS complex caused by pericardial effusion is characteristic but not a constant finding.

2. The following time-dependent changes secondary to myocardial involvement may occur (see Fig. 27-3):

   a. Initial ST segment elevation

   b. Return of the ST segment to the baseline with inversion of T waves (2 to 4 weeks after onset)

X-ray studies.

1. A varying degree of cardiomegaly is present.

2. A pear-shaped or water-bottle–shaped heart is characteristic of large effusion.

3. PVMs may be increased if cardiac tamponade develops.

Echocardiography.

1. Echo is the most useful tool in establishing the diagnosis of pericardial effusion. Effusion is usually seen both anteriorly and posteriorly.

2. Echo is very helpful in detecting *cardiac tamponade.* Helpful two-dimensional echo findings are as follows:

   a. Collapse of the RA in late diastole (Fig. 19-2)

   b. Collapse or indentation of the RV free wall, especially the outflow tract

Management

1. Pericardiocentesis or surgical drainage to identify the etiology of the pericarditis is mandatory, especially when purulent pericarditis or tuberculous pericarditis is suspected.

2. There is no specific treatment for viral pericarditis.

3. Treatment focuses on the basic disease itself (e.g., uremia, collagen disease).

4. Salicylates are given for precordial pain with nonbacterial pericarditis and rheumatic fever.

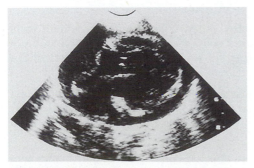 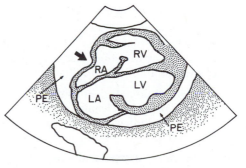

FIG. 19–2.
Subcostal four-chamber view demonstrating pericardial effusion *(PE)* and collapse of the right atrial wall *(arrow),* a sign of cardiac tamponade.

5. Corticosteroid therapy may be indicated in children with severe rheumatic carditis or postpericardiotomy syndrome.

6. For cardiac tamponade, urgent decompression by surgical drainage or pericardiocentesis is indicated. In preparation for pericardial drainage, fluid push with plasmanate to increase central venous pressure is indicated; this helps to improve cardiac filling.

7. Urgent surgical drainage of the pericardium is indicated when purulent pericarditis is suspected. This must be followed by intravenous antibiotic therapy for 4 to 6 weeks.

8. Digitalis is contraindicated in cardiac tamponade because it blocks tachycardia, the compensatory response to impaired venous return.

CONSTRICTIVE PERICARDITIS

A fibrotic, thickened, and adherent pericardium restricts diastolic filling of the heart. Although rare in children, it may be associated with an earlier idiopathic or viral pericarditis, tuberculosis, incomplete drainage of purulent pericarditis, hemopericardium, mediastinal irradiation, neoplastic infiltration, or connective tissue disorders.

Diagnosis of constrictive pericarditis is suggested by the following clinical findings:

1. Signs of elevated jugular venous pressure occur.

2. Hepatomegaly with ascites and systemic edema may be present.

3. Diastolic pericardial knock, which resembles the opening snap, is often heard along the LSB in the absence of heart murmur

4. Calcification of the pericardium, enlargement of the SVC and the LA, and pleural effusion are common on chest x-ray film.

5. The ECG may show low QRS voltages, T-wave inversion or flattening, and LAH. Atrial fibrillation occasionally is seen.

6. M-mode echo may reveal two parallel lines representing the thickened visceral and parietal pericardia or multiple dense echoes. Two-dimensional echo shows an immobile and dense appearance of the pericardium, abrupt displacement of the interventricular septum during early diastolic filling ("septal bounce"), and dilatation of the hepatic veins and IVC.

Cardiac catheterization may document the presence of constrictive physiology. The treatment for constrictive pericarditis is complete resection of the pericardium; symptomatic improvement occurs in 75% of patients.

KAWASAKI'S DISEASE

Etiology and Epidemiology

1. The etiology of Kawasaki's disease (also called mucocutaneous lymph node syndrome) is not known. Most investigators believe the disease is related to, if not caused by, an infectious disease. The disease then is probably driven by abnormalities of the immune system initiated by the infectious insult.

2. An environmental toxin could be an important cofactor. Associations of this illness with rug or carpet cleaning (which may possibly liberate or aerosolize infective agents with 13 to 30 days incubation) and with residence near bodies of water have been reported.

3. Children of all racial and ethnic groups are affected, although it is more common in Asians. The male-to-female ratio is 1.5:1. It peaks in winter and spring.

4. It occurs primarily in young children; 80% of patients are younger than 4 years of age, and 50% are younger than 2 years of age; cases in children older than 8 years rarely are reported.

Pathology

1. This generalized febrile illness is accompanied by significant pathologies of the heart. There is vasculitis of the coronary artery with aneurysm formation, which may lead to scar formation and calcification of the artery. Occasionally, myocardial infarction may result in death (see Chapter 27 for ECG changes and Appendix A, Fig. AA-3).

2. The elevated platelet count seen in this condition contributes to coronary thrombosis.

Clinical Manifestations

The clinical course of the disease may be divided into three phases: acute, subacute, and convalescent. Each phase of the disease is characterized by unique symptoms and signs.

Acute phase (first 10 days).

1. Six signs that compose the diagnostic criteria for Kawasaki's disease are present during the acute phase (see box below).

2. Other frequently associated findings include sterile pyuria (70%); arthritis (40%); gastrointestinal symptoms, including diarrhea, vomiting, abdominal pain, hydrops of the gallbladder (25%); and aseptic meningitis (in almost all patients).

3. Occasionally, a distinctive perineal rash develops 3 to 4 days after the onset of the illness and desquamates in all instances by days 5 to 7.

4. Cardiovascular abnormalities (gallop rhythm, cardiomegaly, ECG changes, pericardial effusion, coronary aneurysm, and decreased LV contractility) may appear during the acute phase (see later discussion).

Subacute phase (11 to 25 days after onset).

1. Desquamation of the tips of the fingers and toes is characteristic.

2. Rash, fever, and lymphadenopathy disappear.

3. Significant cardiovascular changes, including coronary aneurysm, pericardial effusion, CHF, and myocardial infarction occur in this phase. Approximately 20% of patients manifest coronary artery aneurysm on echo.

4. Thrombocytosis also occurs during this period, peaking at 2 weeks or more after the onset of the illness (which is not very helpful in early diagnosis).

Convalescent phase (until elevated erythrocyte sedimentation rate and platelet count return to normal). Deep transverse grooves (Beau's lines) may appear across the fingernails and toenails.

Diagnostic Criteria for Kawasaki's Disease

1. Fever, spiking up to 40° C and persisting more than 5 days
2. Bilateral conjunctival injection (without exudate)
3. Changes in the mouth and lips: strawberry tongue, diffuse reddening of oral cavity, and erythema and cracking of the lips
4. Changes in the hands and feet: erythema and edema of the hands and feet
5. Polymorphous exanthem
6. Cervical lymphadenopathy (greater than 1.5 cm in diameter), usually unilateral

When fever and four of the remaining five criteria are present, the diagnosis of Kawasaki's disease is probable. The presence of coronary artery pathology may be diagnostic even when fewer than four criteria are present.

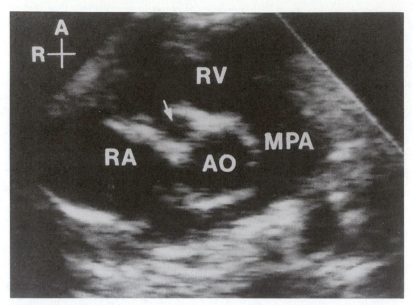

FIG. 19–3.
Parasternal short-axis view from a patient with Kawasaki's disease. There is a large circular aneurysm *(arrow)* of the right coronary artery (From Snider AR, Serwer GA: *Echocardiography in pediatric heart disease,* Chicago, 1990, Mosby.)

Echocardiography. The main purpose of an echo study is to detect coronary artery aneurysm and other reported cardiac dysfunction. For the initial examination, sedation with chloral hydrate (65 to 100 mg/kg, maximum 1000 mg) or other short-acting sedative or hypnotic agents is recommended.

1. Multiple echo views should be obtained to visualize all major coronary artery segments; examination of the main coronary arteries alone is not adequate. Configuration (saccular, fusiform, ectatic), size, number, and the presence or absence of intraluminal or mural thrombi should be assessed. The normal caliber of the coronary arteries is 2 mm in infants and 5 mm in teenagers in the proximal 10 mm of the arteries, and normal coronary arteries are uniform in caliber. Figure 19-3 shows a large aneurysm of the right coronary artery.

2. Depressed LV function (with diminished fractional shortening, increased LV diastolic and systolic dimensions, and decreased rate-corrected velocity of shortening [Vcf]) may be present.

3. Regurgitation of the tricuspid, mitral, and aortic valves occurs in about 50% of patients during the acute phase, presumably from myocarditis, myocardial infarction, or coronary artery occlusion.

4. Pericardial effusion occasionally is present.

Electrocardiography.

1. The ECG may show reduced QRS voltages, ST-T changes, and a prolonged PR interval (occurring in up to 60% of patients).

2. Abnormal Q waves (wide and deep) in the limb leads or precordial leads suggest myocardial infarction (see Chapter 27).

X-ray studies. Chest x-ray films may show cardiomegaly if myocarditis or significant coronary artery abnormality or valvular regurgitation is present.

Laboratory studies.

1. Marked leukocytosis with a shift to the left is common. Neutrophils with vacuoles and toxic granules are common in the first week of the disease.

2. Acute phase reactant levels (C-reactive protein levels, α_1-antitrypsin levels, and erythrocyte sedimentation rate) typically are elevated during the acute phase.

3. Thrombocytosis occurs during the subacute phase (600,000 to more than 1 million/mm^3).

4. Normocytic normochromic anemia (with values below 2 standard deviation) is common (about 50% of patients).

5. Pyuria is common on microscopic examination.

6. Liver enzymes are elevated, and mild hyperbilirubinemia may develop.

7. Elevated myocardial enzyme levels (such as serum creatine phosphokinase MB fraction) suggest myocardial infarction (see Appendix A, Fig. AA-3).

8. Lipid abnormalities are common. Significantly low levels of high-density lipoprotein are present during the illness and follow-up (for more than 3 years), especially in patients with persistent coronary artery abnormalities. The total cholesterol level is normal, but the triglyceride level tends to be high. (Repeat measurement is recommended a year later in patients with abnormal lipid profiles.)

Natural History

Kawasaki's disease is a self-limited disease for most patients. Cardiovascular involvement is the most serious complication of the disease.

1. Coronary aneurysm occurs in 15% to 25% of patients and is responsible for myocardial infarction (less than 5%) and mortality (1% to 5%). More than 70% of myocardial infarctions occur in the first year after onset of the disease without warning symptoms or signs. The mortality from the first myocardial infarction is about 20%. Of survivors of a first myocardial infarction 16% develop a second myocardial infarction, with a mortality rate of more than 60%. Giant aneurysm (greater than 8 mm) is associated with a greater morbidity and mortality (because of thrombotic occlusion or stenotic obstruction and subsequent myocardial infarction). Significantly higher temperature (greater than 38.5° C on days 9 to 12) and longer duration of fever (more than 14 days) appear to be risk factors for coronary aneurysm.

2. Coronary aneurysm tends to regress within 1 year in about 50% of patients, but in some patients, stenosis of the coronary artery results.

3. If the coronary arteries remain normal throughout the first month after the onset, subsequent development of a new coronary lesion is extremely unusual.

4. Involvement of the aorta and other peripheral arteries (cervical, axillary, renal, hepatic, iliac) has been reported.

Diagnosis

1. The diagnosis of Kawasaki's disease is based on clinical findings. There are no consistently reliable laboratory tests for this disease. Fever and at least four of the remaining five diagnostic criteria are required to make the diagnosis (see box on p. 295). However, patients with fever and fewer than four criteria can be diagnosed as having Kawasaki's disease when coronary artery abnormality is detected. More than 90% of patients have the first five signs listed in the box on p. 295, and about 70% have lymphadenopathy.

2. One must rule out diseases with similar manifestations through appropriate cultures and the use of laboratory tests. Measles and group A β-hemolytic streptococcal infection most closely mimic Kawasaki's disease. Children with Kawasaki's disease are extremely irritable (often inconsolable). In addition, they are less likely to have exudative conjunctivitis or pharyngitis, generalized lymphadenopathy, and discrete intraoral lesions and are more likely to have a perineal distribution of their rash. Other diseases with findings similar to Kawasaki's disease, such as viral exanthems, sepsis, drug reactions, juvenile rheumatoid arthritis, and Rocky Mountain spotted fever, require differentiation.

Treatment

No specific therapy is available. Two goals of therapy are reduction of inflammation within the coronary artery and in the myocardium and prevention of thrombosis by inhibition of platelet aggregation. Aspirin has antiinflammatory effects at high doses and an antithrombotic effect at low doses. Intravenous gamma globulin, given within the first 10 days of illness, significantly reduces the prevalence of short- and long-term coronary artery abnormalities, results in a more rapid defervescence and resolution of laboratory indices of inflammation, and resolves more rapidly the impaired cardiac function. An earlier study indicates that corticosteroids are contraindicated because they may increase the incidence of coronary aneurysm.

1. Single-dose intravenous gamma globulin (at a dose of 2 g/kg/day) with aspirin (80 to 100 mg/kg/day), given within 10 days after the onset of illness, now is considered the treatment of choice. The single-dose intravenous gamma globulin results in a more rapid resolution of fever and laboratory indices of acute inflammation (C-reactive protein and α_1-antitrypsin) than the 4-day schedule (400 mg/kg/day for 4 days). Some children may require more than 100 mg/kg/day of aspirin to achieve an antiinflammatory serum concentration of salicylate because of impaired absorption and increased renal clearance of the drug.

2. Aspirin is reduced to 3 to 10 mg/kg/day (antiplatelet dose) in single dose on about day 14 of the illness. Aspirin should be discontinued by 6 to 8 weeks after the onset of illness if no coronary artery abnormalities show up on echo. Some Japanese authorities recommend the antiplatelet dose of aspirin from the onset, because the high dose may inhibit prostacyclin production (a compound with a potent vasodilating effect and a platelet-aggregation inhibitory effect) and result in increased frequency of hepatotoxicity, gastrointestinal irritation and bleeding and Reye's syndrome.

3. Serial echo follow-up is important for evaluation of the cardiac status. The recommendation of the Committee on Rheumatic Fever, Endocarditis, and Kawasaki Disease, American Heart Association (Dajani et al: *Circulation* 1994), is summarized in Table 19-1.

   a. An echo is indicated as soon as the patient is suspected of having Kawasaki's disease. In the absence of giant coronary artery aneurysm, follow-up echoes are indicated in 6 to 8 weeks and 6 to 12 months after the onset. If significant abnormalities of the coronary vessels, LV dysfunction, or valvular regurgitation is found, echo should be repeated at more frequent intervals (see Table 19-1).

   b. Occasionally, coronary angiography may be indicated in infants with a very large ("giant") aneurysm and in patients with symptoms suggestive of ischemia with positive exercise tests or thallium studies and/or with evidence of myocardial infarction. See Table 19-1 for specific recommendations according to the degree of coronary artery involvement.

4. On rare occasions, coronary artery bypass surgery may be indicated.

TABLE 19–1.

Follow-up Recommendations According to the Degree of Coronary Artery Involvement

Risk Level	Pharmacologic Therapy	Physical Activity	Follow-up and Diagnostic Testing	Invasive Testing
I (no coronary artery changes at any stage of illness)	Aspirin for initial 6-8 wk only	No restrictions beyond initial 6-8 wk	None occurs beyond first year unless cardiac disease suspected	None recommended
II (transient coronary artery ectasia that disappears during acute phase)*	Aspirin for initial 6-8 wk only	No restrictions beyond initial 6-8 wk	None occurs beyond first year unless cardiac disease suspected. Physician may choose to see patient at 3- to 5-yr intervals	None recommended
III (small to medium solitary coronary artery aneurysm)†	Aspirin, 3-5 mg/kg/day, at least until abnormalities resolve	For patients ≤ 10 yr, no restrictions beyond initial 6-8 wk For patients > 10 yr, physical activity guided by stress testing every other year. Competitive contact athletics with endurance training is discouraged.	Annual follow-up is done with echo and possibly ECG until 10 yr of age	Angiography, if stress testing or echo suggests stenosis
IV (one or more giant coronary artery aneurysms, or multiple small to medium aneurysms, without obstruction)†	Long-term aspirin (3-5 mg/kg/day) with or without warfarin (international normalized ratio of 2.0-3.0)	For patients ≤ 10 yr, no restriction beyond initial 6-8 wk For patients > 10 yr, recommendations guided by annual stress testing. Strenuous athletics are strongly discouraged. If stress test rules out ischemia, noncontact recreational sports allowed.	Annual follow-up is done with echo, possibly ECG, and possibly chest x-rays. Additional ECG at 6-mo intervals may be advisable. For patients ≤ 10 yr, pharmacologic stress testing should be considered.	Angiography, if stress testing or echo suggests stenosis; possible elective catheterization in certain circumstances.

Continued.

TABLE 19–1.
Continued

Risk Level	Pharmacologic Therapy	Physical Activity	Follow-up and Diagnostic Testing	Invasive Testing
V (coronary artery obstruction)	Long-term aspirin (3-5 mg/kg/day) with or without warfarin (international normalized ratio of 2.0-3.0) Possible use of calcium channel blockers to reduce myocardial oxygen consumption	Contact sports, isometrics, and weight training, avoided. Other physical activity recommendations guided by outcome of stress testing or myocardial perfusion scan.	Echo and ECG are done at 6-mo intervals, and annual Holter and stress testing are performed.	Angiography recommended for some patients to aid in selecting therapeutic options; repeat angiography with new onset or worsening ischemia.

*Ectasia is present when the coronary artery diameter is larger than normal, but a segmental aneurysm is not apparent.
†Aneurysms are classified as small (<5 mm in internal diameter), medium (5-8 mm), or giant (>8 mm).
Modified from Dajani AS, Taubert KA, Takahashi M, et al: Guidelines for long-term management of patients with Kawasaki's disease, *Circulation* 89:916-922, 1994.

LYME CARDITIS

Prevalence

Lyme carditis occurs in about 10% of patients with lyme disease.

Etiology and Pathology

1. Lyme disease is the leading tick-born illness in North America and Europe. The disease is endemic in three U.S. regions: the Northeast, most commonly in coastal areas from Maryland to northern Massachusetts; the upper Midwest, in Wisconsin and Minnesota; and the Far West, in California and Oregon. The disease has been reported from every part of the world, including most of the United States.

2. It is caused by the spirochete *Borrelia burgdorferi,* carried by hard-bodied ticks (e.g., Ixodes dammini). The spirochete initially produces a characteristic skin lesion and then spreads through the lymphatics and blood stream and disseminates to other organs, including the heart.

3. The organism can be found in the heart and other parts of the body and is responsible for clinical symptoms and signs.

Clinical Manifestations

1. Most cases are identified during the summer months, and a history of tick bites may be elicited.

2. Lyme disease can be divided into three stages.

   a. *Stage 1* (localized erythema migrans) begins 3 to 30 days after the tick bite with the onset of influenza-like symptoms (fever, headache, myalgia, arthalgias, malaise) and the characteristic rash, ***erythema chronicum migrans.*** The skin lesion, seen in 60% to 80% of patients at the site of the tick bite, begins as a macule or papule followed by progressive expansion of an erythematous ring over approximately 7 days. The ring is as large as 15 cm with red borders and central clearing, most often appearing on the thigh, groin, or axilla. Even in untreated patients, erythema migrans lesions usually fade within 3 to 4 weeks, but they may recur.

b. *Stage 2* (disseminated infection) starts 2 to 12 weeks after the tick bite and includes neurologic (10% to 15%) and cardiac (10%) manifestations. The classic triad of Lyme neuroborreliosis is aseptic meningitis, cranial nerve palsies (most commonly, unilateral or bilateral Bell palsy), and peripheral radiculoneuropathy. The most common cardiac manifestation is fluctuating AV block (see later discussion), although myocarditis, pericarditis, and LV dysfunction can occur.

c. *Stage 3* (persistent infection) manifests as large-joint arthritis, weeks to years after stage 2, and is seen in about 50% of the patients not previously treated. In general, joint manifestation is self-limited but may recur in patients who do not receive appropriate antibiotic therapy.

3. Cardiac manifestations occur in about 10% of cases. They generally appear 4 to 8 weeks after the initial illness, but their appearance can vary from 4 days to 7 months. The most common cardiac manifestation is varying levels of AV block, occurring in up to 87% of cases. Over 95% of these show first-degree AV block at some time in their course. Up to 50% develop complete heart block, some of them permanent block. First-degree AV block can change to complete heart block within minutes.

Diagnosis

1. Diagnosis is suggested by the presence of the distinctive erythema chronicum migrans and other features of Lyme disease. A history of tick exposure (e.g., travel to an endemic area) and any of the manifestations of stages 2 and 3 are important clues to the disease. The presence of an AV block alone is not specific for Lyme carditis; it can be caused by other infective agents, such as viral infections (coxsackie A and B, echovirus, mumps, polio), rickettsial infections, *Treponema pallidum*, *Yersinia enterocolitica*, toxoplasmosis, diphtheria, and Chagas's disease.

2. Although cultivation or visualization of *Borrelia burgdorferi* is the most reliable technique to confirm the diagnosis, this test is rarely positive.

3. Enzyme-linked immunosorbent assays (ELISAs) are probably more accurate than indirect immunofluorescence assays. The diagnosis of Lyme disease is confirmed if there is a single titer greater than 1:256 or a fourfold increase in antibody titer over time and compatible clinical symptoms. A positive serologic test alone, in the absence of compatible clinical symptoms, should not be used indiscriminately to diagnose Lyme disease (or as the sole basis for administration of antibiotic therapy).

4. Serologic tests, however, have limitations and they often add diagnostic confusion rather than clarity. Recently, the detection of *B. burgdorferi* deoxyribonucleic acid (DNA) by the polymerase chain reaction in the joint fluid of patients has been suggested to be a better diagnostic test.

Treatment

1. Either amoxicillin or penicillin probably is the drug of choice. Tetracycline is the alternative agent for older children and adults, and erythromycin is the alternative for younger children.

2. If antibiotic therapy is begun in stage 1, the duration of the skin lesion is shortened and subsequent complications can be averted. Antibiotic treatment also improves cardiac and neurologic symptoms.

3. Heart blocks respond to antibiotic treatment, usually within 6 weeks, and have a good prognosis.

4. For high-level AV block, temporary pacing may be indicated (in up to one third of patients).

20 / Acute Rheumatic Fever

PREVALENCE

Acute rheumatic fever is relatively uncommon in the United States but is a common cause of heart disease in underdeveloped countries. In recent years, new small outbreaks of this disease have been reported in the United States.

ETIOLOGY

1. Acute rheumatic fever is believed to be an immunologic lesion that occurs as a delayed sequela of group A streptococcal infection of the pharynx but not of the skin. The attack rate of acute rheumatic fever after streptococcal infection varies with the severity of the infection, ranging from 0.3% to 3.0%.

2. Important predisposing factors include family history of rheumatic fever, low socioeconomic status (poverty, poor hygiene, medical deprivation), and age between 6 and 15 years (with peak incidence at 8 years of age).

PATHOLOGY

1. The inflammatory lesion is found in many parts of the body, most notably in the heart, brain, joints, and skin. Valvular damage most frequently involves the mitral, less commonly the aortic, and rarely the tricuspid and pulmonary valves.

2. Aschoff bodies in the atrial myocardium are believed to be characteristic of rheumatic fever. These consist of inflammatory lesions associated with swelling, fragmentation of collagen fibers, and alterations in the staining characteristics of connective tissue.

CLINICAL MANIFESTATIONS

Acute rheumatic fever is diagnosed by the use of revised Jones criteria (updated in 1992) (see box on p. 303). The criteria are three groups of important clinical and laboratory findings: (1) five major manifestations, (2) four minor manifestations, and (3) supporting evidence of an antecedent group A streptococcal infection. These and other important clinical findings are presented here.

History

1. Streptococcal pharyngitis, 1 to 5 weeks (average, 3 weeks) before the onset of symptoms is common. The latent period may be as long as 2 to 6 months (average, 4 months) in cases of isolated chorea.

2. Pallor, malaise, easy fatigability, and other history such as epistaxis (5% to 10%) and abdominal pain may be present.

3. Family history of rheumatic fever frequently is positive.

Major Manifestations

Arthritis. Arthritis, the most common manifestation of acute rheumatic fever (70% of cases), usually involves large joints (e.g., knees, ankles, elbows, wrists). Often more than one joint, either simultaneously or in succession, is involved, with a characteristic migratory nature of the arthritis. Swelling, heat, redness, severe pain, tenderness, and

Guidelines for the Diagnosis of Initial Attack of Rheumatic Fever (Jones Criteria, Updated 1992)

Major Manifestations	Minor Manifestations
Carditis	*Clinical findings*
Polyarthritis	Arthralgia
Chorea	Fever
Erythema marginatum	*Laboratory findings*
Subcutaneous nodule	Elevated acute phase reactants
	(erythrocyte sedimentation rate C-reactive protein)
	Prolonged PR interval

Plus

Supporting evidence of antecedent group A streptococcal infection

Positive throat culture or rapid streptococcal antigen test
Elevated or rising streptococcal antibody titer

If supported by evidence of preceding group A streptococcal infection, the presence of two major manifestations or of one major and two minor manifestations indicates a high probability of acute rheumatic fever.
From Special Writing Group of the Committee on Rheumatic Fever, Endocarditis, and Kawasaki's Disease of the Council of Cardiovascular Disease in the Young, American Heart Association: *Circulation* 87:302-307, 1993.

limitation of motion are common. The arthritis responds dramatically to salicylate therapy; if patients treated with salicylates (with documented therapeutic levels) do not improve in 48 hours, the diagnosis of acute rheumatic fever probably is incorrect. Such patients have been categorized as having "poststreptococcal reactive arthritis"; the relationship of this disease to acute rheumatic fever remains undetermined.

Carditis. Carditis occurs in 50% of patients. Signs of carditis include some or all of the following, in increasing order of severity:

1. Tachycardia (out of proportion for the degree of fever) is common; its absence makes the diagnosis of myocarditis unlikely.

2. A heart murmur of valvulitis (caused by MR and/or AR) is almost always present; without the murmurs of MR and/or AR, carditis should not be diagnosed. Echo has added a new dimension in the evaluation of patients with rheumatic fever. It is capable of evaluating the severity of myocarditis, the presence and degree of MR and AR, and the presence of pericardial effusion. However, the presence of MR or AR by echo and Doppler studies, without accompanying auscultatory findings, cannot be taken as the sole criterion for valvulitis.

3. Pericarditis (friction rub, pericardial effusion, chest pain, and ECG changes) may be present.

4. Cardiomegaly on chest x-ray films is indicative of pericarditis, pancarditis, or CHF.

5. Signs of CHF (gallop rhythm, distant heart sounds, cardiomegaly) are indications of severe carditis.

Erythema marginatum. Erythema marginatum occurs in fewer than 10% of patients with acute rheumatic fever. The characteristic nonpruritic serpiginous or annular erythematous rashes are most prominent on the trunk and the inner proximal portions of the extremities; they are never seen on the face. The rashes are evanescent, disappearing on exposure to cold and reappearing after a hot shower or when the patient is covered with a warm blanket. They seldom are detected in air-conditioned hospital rooms.

Subcutaneous nodules. Subcutaneous nodules are found in 2% to 10% of cases, particularly in those with recurrences. They are hard, painless, nonpruritic, freely movable, swelling, and 0.2 to 2.0 cm in diameter. They usually are found symmetrically, singly or in clusters, on the extensor surfaces of both large and small joints, over the scalp, or along the spine. They are not transient, lasting for weeks, and have a significant association with carditis.

Sydenham's chorea. Sydenham's chorea (St. Vitus' dance) is found in 15% of patients with acute rheumatic fever. It occurs more often in prepubertal girls (8 to 12 years) than in boys. It begins with emotional lability and personality changes, and these soon are replaced by loss of motor coordination. Characteristic spontaneous, purposeless movement then develops, followed by motor weakness. Recently, the presence of two behavioral symptom complexes of attention deficit hyperactivity disorder and obsessive-compulsive disorder has been identified shortly before the onset of the choreiform movement. Antineuronal antibodies are present in more than 90% of patients. This may be related to dysfunction of basal ganglia and cortical neuronal components. The adventitious movements, weakness, and hypotonia continue for an average of 7 months (and up to 17 months) before slowly waning in severity.

Minor Manifestations

1. Arthralgia refers to joint pain without the objective changes of arthritis. It must not be considered a minor manifestation when arthritis is present.

2. Fever (with a temperature usually of at least 39° C) generally is present early in the course of untreated rheumatic fever.

3. In laboratory findings, elevated acute-phase reactants (elevated C-reactive protein levels and elevated erythrocyte sedimentation rate) are objective evidence of an inflammatory process.

4. A prolonged PR interval on the ECG is neither specific for acute rheumatic fever, nor an indication of active carditis.

Evidence of Antecedent Group A Streptococcal Infection

1. A history of sore throat or of scarlet fever unsubstantiated by laboratory data is not adequate evidence of recent group A streptococcal infection.

2. Positive throat cultures or rapid streptococcal antigen tests for group A streptococci are less reliable than antibody tests because they do not distinguish between recent infection and chronic pharyngeal carriage. Antigen detection tests are very specific but not very sensitive; a negative test result should be confirmed by a conventional throat culture.

3. Streptococcal antibody tests are the most reliable laboratory evidence of antecedent streptococcal infection capable of producing acute rheumatic fever. The onset of the clinical manifestations of acute rheumatic fever coincides with the peak of the streptococcal antibody response.

   a. Antistreptolysin O (ASO) titer is well standardized and therefore is the most widely used test. It is elevated in 80% of patients with acute rheumatic fever and 20% of normal individuals. Antistreptolysin O titers greater than 320 Todd units in children and greater than 240 Todd units in adults are considered significant. A single, low ASO titer does not exclude acute rheumatic fever. If three other antistreptococcal antibody tests (antideoxyribonuclease B, antistreptokinase, and antihyaluronidase tests) are obtained, a titer for at least one antibody test is elevated in about 95% of patients.

   b. The antideoxyribonuclease B test is favored over other tests. Titers of 240 Todd units or greater in children and 120 Todd units or greater in adults are considered elevated.

    c. The Streptozyme test (Wampole Laboratories) is a relatively simple slide agglutination test, but it is less standardized and less reproducible than the other antibody tests. It should not be used as a definitive test for evidence of antecedent group A streptococcal infection.

Other Clinical Features

1. Abdominal pain, rapid sleeping heart rate, tachycardia out of proportion to fever, malaise, anemia, epistaxis, and precordial pain are relatively common but not specific.

2. A positive family history of rheumatic fever also may heighten the suspicion but cannot be used as a diagnostic manifestation.

DIAGNOSIS

1. The revised Jones criteria are used for the diagnosis of acute rheumatic fever (see box). Only the major and minor criteria and evidence of an antecedent group A streptococcal infection are included in the criteria, although other findings play a supporting role. A diagnosis of acute rheumatic fever is highly probable when either two major manifestations or one major plus two minor manifestations, plus evidence of antecedent streptococcal infection is present. The absence of supporting evidence of a previous group A streptococcal infection makes the diagnosis doubtful (see later discussion for exceptions).

2. Exceptions to the Jones criteria include the following three specific situations:

    a. Chorea may occur as the only manifestation of rheumatic fever.

    b. Indolent carditis may be the only manifestation in patients who come to medical attention months after the onset of rheumatic fever.

    c. Occasionally, patients with rheumatic fever recurrences may not fulfill the Jones criteria.

3. The following tips help in applying the Jones criteria:

    a. Two major manifestations always are stronger than one major plus two minor manifestations.

    b. Arthralgia or a prolonged PR interval cannot be used as a minor manifestation in the presence of arthritis or carditis, respectively.

    c. A history of rheumatic fever or rheumatic heart disease no longer is considered a minor manifestation (a change from the last revised Jones criteria, 1984).

    d. The absence of evidence of an antecedent group A streptococcal infection is a warning sign against acute rheumatic fever (except when chorea is present).

    e. The vibratory innocent (Still's) murmur frequently is misinterpreted as a murmur of MR and thereby is a frequent cause of misdiagnosis (or overdiagnosis) of acute rheumatic fever. The murmur of MR is a *regurgitant*-type systolic murmur (starting with the S1), but the innocent murmur is low pitched and an *ejection* type. A cardiology consultation during the acute phase minimizes the frequency of misdiagnosis.

    f. The possibility of the early suppression of full clinical manifestation should be sought during the history taking. Subtherapeutic doses of aspirin or salicylate-containing analgesics (e.g., Bufferin, Anacin) may suppress full manifestations.

DIFFERENTIAL DIAGNOSIS

1. Juvenile rheumatoid arthritis often is misdiagnosed as acute rheumatic fever. The following findings suggest juvenile rheumatoid arthritis rather than acute rheumatic

fever: (1) involvement of peripheral small joints, (2) symmetric involvement of large joints without migratory arthritis, (3) pallor of the involved joints, (4) a more indolent course, (5) no evidence of preceding streptococcal infection, and (6) the absence of prompt response to salicylate therapy within 24 to 48 hours.

2. Other collagen vascular diseases (systemic lupus erythematosus, mixed connective tissue disease); reactive arthritis, including poststreptococcal arthritis; serum sickness; and infectious arthritis (such as gonococcal) occasionally require differentiation.

3. Virus-associated acute arthritis (rubella, parvovirus, hepatitis B virus, herpes viruses, enteroviruses) is much more common in adults.

4. Hematologic disorders, such as sicklemia and leukemia, should be considered in the differential diagnosis.

CLINICAL COURSE

1. Only carditis can cause permanent cardiac damage. A mild carditis disappears rapidly in weeks, but severe carditis may last for 2 to 6 months.

2. Arthritis subsides within a few days to several weeks, even without treatment, and does not cause permanent damage.

3. Chorea gradually subsides in 6 to 7 months or longer and usually does not cause permanent neurologic sequelae.

MANAGEMENT

1. When acute rheumatic fever is suggested by history and physical examination, one should obtain the following laboratory studies: (1) complete blood count, (2) acute-phase reactants (erythrocyte sedimentation rate and C-reactive protein), (3) throat culture, (4) antistreptolysin O titer (and a second antibody titer, particularly with chorea), (5) chest x-ray films, and (6) ECG. Cardiology consultation is indicated to clarify whether there is cardiac involvement; two-dimensional echo and Doppler studies usually are performed at that time.

2. Benzathin penicillin G, 0.6 to 1.2 million units intramuscularly, is given to eradicate streptococci. This serves as the first dose of penicillin prophylaxis as well (see later discussion of prophylaxis). In patients allergic to penicillin, erythromycin at 40 mg/kg/day in two to four doses for 10 days, may be substituted for penicillin.

3. Antiinflammatory or suppressive therapy with salicylates or steroids must not be started until a definite diagnosis is made. Early suppressive therapy may interfere with a definite diagnosis of acute rheumatic fever by suppressing full development of joint manifestations and suppressing acute-phase reactants.

4. When the diagnosis of acute rheumatic fever is confirmed, one must educate the patient and parents about the need to prevent subsequent streptococcal infection through continuous antibiotic prophylaxis. In patients with cardiac involvement, the need for prophylaxis against infective endocarditis also should be emphasized.

5. Bed rest of varying duration is recommended. The duration depends on the type and severity of the manifestations and may range from a week (for isolated arthritis) to weeks for severe carditis. Bed rest is followed by a period of indoor ambulation of varying duration before the child is allowed to return to school. The erythrocyte sedimentation rate is a helpful guide to the rheumatic activity and therefore to the duration of restriction of activities. Full activity is allowed later when the erythrocyte sedimentation rate returns to normal, except in children with significant cardiac involvement. Table 20-1 is a conservative guide to the period of bed rest and activities.

TABLE 20–1.

General Guidelines for Bed Rest and Ambulation

Arthritis Alone	Minimal Carditis*	Moderate Carditis*	Severe Carditis*
Bed rest			
1-2 wk	2-3 wk	4-6 wk	2-4 mo
Indoor ambulation			
1-2 wk	2-3 wk	4-6 wk	2-3 mo
Outdoor activity (school)			
2 wk	2-4 wk	1-3 mo	2-3 mo
Full activity			
After 4-6 wk	After 6-10 wk	After 3-6 mo	Variable

*Minimal carditis, Questionable cardiomegaly; moderate carditis, definite but mild cardiomegaly; severe carditis, marked cardiomegaly or CHF.

TABLE 20–2.

Recommended Antiinflammatory Agents

	Arthritis Alone	Minimal Carditis	Moderate Carditis	Severe Carditis
Prednisone	0	0	2-4 wk*	2-6 wk*
Aspirin	1-2 wk	2-4 wk†	6-8 wk	2-4 mo

Dosages: Prednisone: 2 mg/kg/day, in four divided doses.

Aspirin: 100 mg/kg/day, four to six divided doses.

*The dose of prednisone should be tapered and aspirin started during the final week.
†Aspirin may be reduced by 60/mg/kg day after 2 weeks of therapy.

6. Therapy with antiinflammatory agents should be started as soon as acute rheumatic fever has been diagnosed.

   a. Prednisone (2 mg/kg/day in four divided doses for 2 to 6 weeks) is indicated only in cases of severe carditis (see Table 20-2).

   b. For mild to moderate carditis, aspirin alone is recommended in a dose of 90 to 100 mg/kg/day in four to six divided doses. An adequate blood level of salicylates is 20 to 25 mg/100 ml. This dose is continued for 4 to 8 weeks, depending on the clinical response. On improvement, the therapy is withdrawn gradually over the following 4 to 6 weeks while one monitors acute-phase reactants.

   c. For arthritis, aspirin therapy is continued for 2 weeks and gradually withdrawn over the following 2 to 3 weeks. Rapid resolution of joint symptoms with aspirin within 24 to 36 hours is supportive evidence of the arthritis of acute rheumatic fever.

7. Treatment of CHF includes some or all of the following (see also Chapter 30):

   a. Complete bed rest with orthopneic position, and moist, cool oxygen

   b. Morphine sulfate, 0.2 mg/kg, at 4-hour intervals for severe CHF with respiratory distress

   c. Restriction of sodium and fluid intake

d. Prednisone for severe carditis of recent onset (see Table 20-2)

e. Digoxin (used with caution, because certain patients with rheumatic carditis are supersensitive to digitalis), beginning with half of the usual recommended dose (see Table 30-2)

f. Furosemide, 1 mg/kg every 6 to 12 hours, if indicated

8. Management of Sydenham's chorea:

a. Reduce physical and emotional stress and use protective measures as indicated.

b. Give benzathine penicillin G, 1.2 million, initially for eradication of *streptococcus* and also every 28 days for prevention of recurrence, just as in patients with other rheumatic manifestations. Without the prophylaxis, about 25% of patients with isolated chorea (without carditis) develop rheumatic valvular heart disease in 20-year follow-up.

c. Antiinflammatory agents are not needed in patients with isolated chorea.

d. For severe cases, any of the following drugs may be used: phenobarbital (15 to 30 mg every 6 to 8 hours), haloperidrol (starting at 0.5 mg and increasing to 2.0 mg every 8 hours), valproic acid, chlorpromazine (Thorazine), diazepam (Valium), or steroids.

e. Plasma exchange and IV immunoglobulin therapy (because of the presence of antineuronal antibodies) are in the experimental stage, but the preliminary results are promising in reducing the duration of chorea (Swedo et al: *Pediatrics* 1993).

PROGNOSIS

The presence or absence of permanent cardiac damage determines the prognosis. The development of residual heart disease is influenced by the following three factors:

1. Cardiac status at the start of treatment: The more severe the cardiac involvement at the time the patient first is seen, the greater the incidence of residual heart disease.

2. Recurrence of rheumatic fever: The severity of valvular involvement increases with each recurrence.

3. Regression of heart disease: Evidence of cardiac involvement at the first attack may disappear in 10% to 25% of patients 10 years after the initial attack. Valvular disease resolves more frequently when prophylaxis is followed.

PREVENTION

Population

Patients with documented histories of rheumatic fever, including those with isolated chorea and those without evidence of rheumatic heart disease, must receive the prophylaxis.

Duration

Ideally, patients should receive prophylaxis indefinitely. However, many cardiologists recommend discontinuing the prophylaxis at the age of 21 to 25 provided that the patient does not have evidence of valvular involvement and the patient is not in a high-risk occupation (e.g., school teachers, physicians, nurses). If the patient has rheumatic valvular disease, the prophylaxis should be continued longer, possibly for life. The chance of recurrence is highest in the first 5 years after the acute rheumatic fever.

Methods

The method of choice for secondary prevention is benzathine penicillin G, 600,000 units for patients weighing less than 60 lb (27 kg) and 1.2 million units for patients weighing more than 60 lb, given intramuscularly every 28 days (not once a month). Alternative methods, although not as effective, are:

1. Oral penicillin V, 125 to 250 mg, twice daily

2. Oral sulfadiazine, 0.5 g once a day for children weighing less than 60 lb, and 1.0 g once a day for children weighing more than 60 lb (Note that the sulfonamides are not effective for the prophylaxis of infective endocarditis.)

Primary prevention

Primary prevention of rheumatic fever is possible with a 10-day course of penicillin therapy for streptococcal pharyngitis. However, the primary prevention is not possible in patients who develop subclinical pharyngitis and therefore do not seek medical treatment (30%) and in patients who develop acute rheumatic fever without symptoms of streptococcal pharyngitis (30%).

21 / Valvular Heart Disease

Valvular heart disease is congenital or acquired. The pathophysiology and clinical manifestations are similar for both entities. Congenital abnormalities of cardiac valves have been discussed. Stenoses of the aortic and pulmonary valves are discussed in the section on obstructive lesions in Chapter 13, and congenital mitral valve abnormalities are discussed in Chapter 17 in the section on miscellaneous congenital cardiac conditions.

This chapter discusses acquired valvular heart disease. Almost all acquired valvular heart diseases are rheumatic in origin. Mitral valve involvement occurs in about three fourths, and aortic valve involvement in about one fourth, of all cases of rheumatic heart disease. Stenosis and regurgitation of the same valve usually occur together. Isolated aortic stenosis of rheumatic origin without mitral valve involvement is extremely rare. Rheumatic involvement of the tricuspid valve is very rare, and that of the pulmonary valve almost never occurs. Therefore only MS, MR, and AR of rheumatic origin are discussed in this chapter. Although the etiology of MVP is not entirely clear, it is discussed in this chapter because it involves a cardiac valve.

MITRAL STENOSIS

Prevalence

Although MS of rheumatic origin is rare in children (because it requires 5 to 10 years from the initial attack to develop), it is the most common valvular involvement in adult rheumatic patients. In certain parts of the world where rheumatic fever is prevalent, severe MS occurs in children under age of 15 years.

Pathology

1. Thickening of the leaflets and fusion of the commissures dominate the pathologic findings. Calcification with immobility of the valve results over time.

2. The LA and right-sided heart chambers become dilated and hypertrophied (see Chapter 10).

3. In patients with severe pulmonary venous hypertension, pulmonary congestion and edema, and fibrosis of the alveolar walls, hypertrophy of the pulmonary arterioles and loss of lung compliance result.

Clinical Manifestations

History.

1. Patients with mild MS are asymptomatic.

2. Dyspnea with or without exertion is the most common symptom. Orthopnea, nocturnal dyspnea, or palpitation is present in more severe cases.

Physical examination (Fig. 21-1).

1. An increased RV impulse is palpable along the LSB. Peripheral pulses may be weak with narrow pulse pressure. Neck veins are distended if right-sided heart failure supervenes.

2. A loud S1 at the apex and a narrowly split S2 with accentuated P2 are audible if pulmonary hyptertension is present. An opening snap (a short snapping sound accompanying the opening of the mitral valve) is followed by a low-frequency mitral

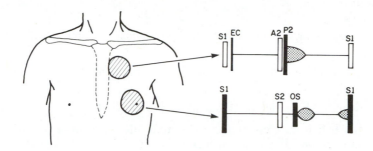

FIG. 21–1.
Cardiac findings of MS. Abnormal sounds are shown in black and include a loud S1, an ejection click *(EC)*, a loud S2, and an opening snap *(OS)*. Also note the middiastolic rumble and presystolic murmur. The murmur of pulmonary insufficiency indicates long-standing pulmonary hypertension.

diastolic rumble at the apex (see Fig. 21-1). A crescendo presystolic murmur may be audible at the apex. Occasionally, a high-frequency diastolic murmur of PR (Graham Steell's murmur) is present at the ULSB, but it is difficult to distinguish from AR.

Electrocardiography. RAD, LAH, and RVH (caused by pulmonary hypertension) are common. Atrial fibrillation is rare in children.

X-ray study.

1. The LA and RV usually are enlarged and the MPA segment usually is prominent.

2. Lung fields show pulmonary venous congestion, interstitial edema shown as Kerley's B lines (dense, short, horizontal lines most commonly seen in the costophrenic angles), and redistribution of PBF (with increased pulmonary vascularity) to the upper lobes.

Echocardiography. Echo is the most accurate noninvasive tool for the detection of MS.

1. M-mode echo may show a diminished E to F slope (reflecting a slow diastolic closure of the anterior mitral leaflet), anterior movement of the posterior leaflet during diastole, multiple echoes from thickened mitral leaflets, and large LA dimension.

2. Two-dimensional echo shows doming of thick mitral leaflets, a small mitral valve orifice inscribed by the thickened valve, and a dilated LA. The MPA, RV, and RA also are dilated.

3. Doppler studies can estimate the pressure gradient across the mitral valve and the level of PA pressures (by the modified Bernoulli's equation).

Natural History

1. Most children with MS are asymptomatic but become symptomatic with exertion. Recurrence of rheumatic fever worsens the stenosis.

2. Atrial flutter or fibrillation and thromboembolism (related to the chronic atrial arrhythmias) are rare in children.

3. SBE can occur, but it is rare.

4. Hemoptysis can develop from the rupture of small vessels in the bronchi as a result of long-standing pulmonary venous hypertension.

Management
  Medical.

1. Good dental hygiene and antibiotic prophylaxis against SBE are important.

2. Recurrence of rheumatic fever is prevented with penicillin or sulfonamide (see Chapter 20).

3. Varying degrees of restriction of activity may be indicated.

4. If atrial fibrillation develops (rare in children), digoxin should be used to control ventricular response. All patients with MS should receive anticoagulation therapy. If the patient develops pulmonary edema from atrial fibrillation, cardioversion should be attempted. The patient ideally should receive anticoagulation therapy for 3 to 4 weeks, and quinidine should be started 2 days before the procedure.

5. Limited experience with balloon valvuloplasty suggests that it is an alternative to surgical closed commissurotomy and may delay surgical intervention. The results are comparable with those of closed mitral commissurotomy. Ideal candidates may be symptomatic patients with a body surface area greater than 0.5 m², a transvalvular pressure gradient greater than 10 mm Hg, stenosis resulting from rheumatic heart disease, and mobile leaflets with no more than mild MR.

Surgical.
Indications.

1. Symptomatic patients (dyspnea on exertion, pulmonary edema, paroxysmal dyspnea) may be candidates for surgery.

2. Recurrent atrial fibrillation, thromboembolic phenomenon, and hemoptysis may be indications for surgery.

Procedures and mortality.

1. Closed mitral commissurotomy remains the procedure of choice for those with a pliable mitral valve without calcification or MR. The operative mortality rate is less than 1%.

2. Open mitral commissurotomy can be performed, with the hospital mortality rate of less than 1% in the adult and slightly higher in children.

3. Valve replacement may be indicated in patients with calcified valves and those with MR. The hospital mortality rate is 2% to 7%. Prosthetic valves (Starr-Edwards, Bjork-Shiley, St. Jude) have the advantage of longer durability but require long-term anticoagulation therapy with their attendant risks (bleeding, thrombus formation, mechanical dysfunction). The bioprostheses (porcine valve, heterograft valve) do not require anticoagulation therapy but tend to deteriorate more rapidly in the young.

Complications.

1. Postoperative CHF is the most common cause of early postoperative death.

2. Arterial embolization and postperfusion syndrome (see Chapter 36) are rare complications.

3. Bleeding diathesis is possible with anticoagulation therapy for an implanted prosthetic valve.

MITRAL REGURGITATION
Prevalence

MR is the most common valvular involvement in children with rheumatic heart disease.

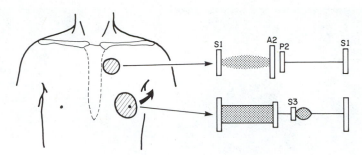

FIG. 21–2.
Cardiac findings of MR. Arrow near the apex indicates the direction of radiation of the murmur toward the axilla.

Pathology

1. Mitral valve leaflets are shortened because of fibrosis.

2. When the degree of MR increases, dilatation of the LA and LV results, and the mitral valve ring may become dilated.

Clinical Manifestations
History.

1. Patients usually are asymptomatic during childhood (because MR does not produce pulmonary congestion in the early phase).

2. Rarely, fatigue (caused by reduced forward cardiac output) and palpitation (caused by atrial fibrillation) develop.

Physical examination (Fig. 21-2).

1. The jugular venous pulse is normal in the absence of CHF. A heaving, hyperdynamic apical impulse is palpable in severe MR.

2. The S1 is normal or diminished. The S2 may split widely as a result of shortening of the LV ejection and early aortic closure. The S3 commonly is present and loud. The hallmark of MR is a regurgitant systolic murmur starting with S1, grade 2-4/6, at the apex, with good transmission to the left axilla (best demonstrated on left decubitus position). A short, low-frequency diastolic rumble may be present at the apex (see Fig. 21-2).

Electrocardiography.

1. ECG is normal in mild cases.

2. LVH or LV dominance, with or without LAH, is usually present.

3. Atrial fibrillation is rare in children but often develops in the adult.

X-rays study (Fig. 21-3).

1. The LA and LV are enlarged varying degrees.

2. Pulmonary vascularity usually is within normal limits, but a pulmonary venous congestion pattern may develop if CHF supervenes.

Echocardiography.

1. Two-dimensional echo shows dilated LA and LV, and the degree of dilatation is related to the severity of MR.

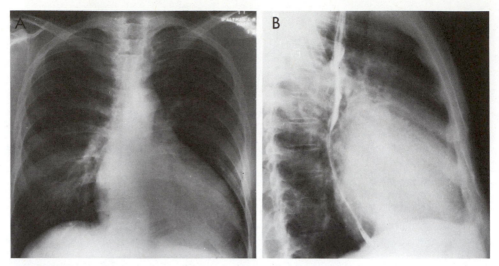

FIG. 21–3.
PA **(A)** and lateral **(B)** views of chest roentgenogram in a patient with moderately severe MR of rheumatic origin. The lateral view was obtained with barium swallow. The cardiothoracic ratio is increased (0.64), and the apex is displaced downward and laterally in the PA view. The lateral view shows an indentation of the barium-filled esophagus by an enlarged LA, and the LV is displaced posteriorly.

2. Color-flow mapping of the regurgitant jet into the LA and Doppler studies can assess the severity of the regurgitation.

Natural History

1. Patients are relatively stable for a long time, but MS eventually supervenes in some patients.

2. Infective endocarditis is a rare complication.

3. LV failure and consequent pulmonary hypertension may occur in adult life.

Management
Medical.

1. Preventive measures against SBE (see Chapter 19) and prophylaxis against recurrence of rheumatic fever (see Chapter 20) are important.

2. Activity need not be restricted in most mild cases.

3. Afterload-reducing agents are useful in maintaining the forward stroke volume.

4. Anticongestive measures (with diuretics and digoxin) are provided if CHF develops.

5. If atrial fibrillation develops (rare in children), digoxin is indicated to slow the ventricular response.

Surgical.
Indications. The indications for surgery are not clearly defined, but intractable CHF, progressive cardiomegaly with symptoms, and pulmonary hypertension may be indications. In adults, the LV diastolic dimension of 60 mm has been proposed as an indication for mitral valve replacement.

Procedures and mortality. Mitral valve repair or valve replacement is performed under cardiopulmonary bypass. Valve repair surgery is preferred over valve replacement in children as long as the valve is pliable. Valve repair has a lower mortality rate (less than 1%), and anticoagulation is not necessary. Valve replacement is necessary if the valve is thick, scarred, and grossly deformed. Frequently used low-profile prostheses are the Bjork-Shiley tilting disc and the St. Jude pyrolite carbon valve. The surgical mortality rate is 2% to 7% for valve replacement. If a prosthetic valve is used, anticoagulation therapy must be continued.

Complications. Complications are similar to those listed for MS.

AORTIC REGURGITATION

Prevalence

AR is less common than MR. Most patients with AR have associated mitral valve disease.

Pathology

Semilunar cusps are deformed and shortened, and the valve ring is dilated so that the cusps fail to appose tightly. The commissures usually are fused to a varying degree.

Clinical Manifestations
History.

1. Patients with mild regurgitation are asymptomatic.

2. Exercise tolerance is reduced with more severe AR or CHF.

Physical examination (Fig. 21-4).

1. The precordium may be hyperdynamic with a laterally displaced apical impulse. A diastolic thrill occasionally is present at the 3LICS. A wide pulse pressure and a bounding water-hammer pulse may be present with severe AR.

2. The S1 is decreased in intensity. The S2 may be normal or single. A high-pitched diastolic decrescendo murmur, best audible at the 3LICS or 4LICS, is the auscultatory hallmark. This murmur is more easily audible with the patient sitting and leaning forward. The longer the murmur, the more severe the regurgitation (see Fig. 21-4). A systolic murmur of varying intensity may be present at the 2RICS because of relative AS caused by an increased stroke volume. The combination of the diastolic and systolic murmurs gives rise to a to-and-fro murmur. A middiastolic mitral rumble (Austin Flint murmur) occasionally is present at the apex when the AR is severe.

Electrocardiography. The ECG may be normal in mild cases. In severe cases, LVH usually is present. LAH may be present in long-standing cases.

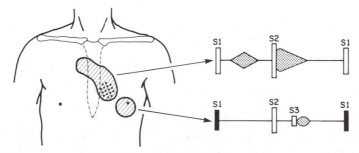

FIG. 21—4.
Cardiac findings of AR. The S1 is abnormally soft *(black bar)*. The predominant murmur is a high-pitched, diastolic decrescendo murmur at 3LICS.

X-ray study. Cardiomegaly involving the LV is present. A dilated ascending aorta and/or a prominent aortic knob frequently are present. Pulmonary venous congestion develops if LV failure supervenes.

Echocardiography. The LV dimension is increased, but the LA remains normal in size. Color-flow and Doppler examination can be used to estimate the severity of the regurgitation.

Natural History

1. The patient remains asymptomatic for a long time, but if symptoms begin to develop, many patients deteriorate rapidly.

2. Anginal pain, CHF, and multiple PVCs are unfavorable signs.

3. Infective endocarditis is a rare complication.

Management
Medical.

1. Good oral hygiene and antibiotic prophylaxis against SBE are important.

2. Prophylaxis should be continued against the recurrence of rheumatic fever with penicillin or sulfonamides (see Chapter 20).

3. Activity need not be restricted in mild cases, but varying degrees of restriction are indicated in more severe cases.

4. If CHF develops, digoxin, diuretics, and afterload-reducing agents may be beneficial, but benefits rarely are maintained.

Surgical.

Indications. A major clinical decision in AR is the timing of aortic valve replacement. Ideally, it should be performed before irreversible dilatation of the LV develops, but there is no reliable method of detecting that point. The following findings have been used as indications for valve replacement therapy:

1. Symptoms such as anginal pain or dyspnea on exertion are indications.

2. Even in asymptomatic patients, significant cardiomegaly (cardiothoracic ratio greater than 55% on chest x-ray films), ejection fraction less than 40%, or stress-test–induced symptoms may be an indication.

Procedure and mortality. Aortic valve replacement is performed under cardiopulmonary bypass. The mortality rate (for the first three valve replacement surgeries) is about 2% to 5%.

1. The antibiotic-sterilized aortic homograft has been widely used and appears to be the device of choice.

2. The porcine heterograft has the risk of accelerated degeneration.

3. The Bjork-Shiley and St. Jude prostheses require anticoagulation therapy and are less suited for young patients.

4. A pulmonary-root autograft (Ross procedure) may be an attractive alternative (see Fig. 13-10) in selected adolescents and young adults. In this procedure, the patient's own pulmonary valve and the adjacent PA are used to replace the diseased aortic valve and the adjacent aorta. The coronary arteries are detached from the aorta and implanted into the PA. The surgical mortality rate is near zero. This procedure does not require anticoagulant therapy, and the autograft may last longer than a porcine bioprosthesis.

Complications.

1. Postoperative acute cardiac failure is the most common cause of death.

2. Thromboembolism, chronic hemoptysis, and anticoagulant-induced hemorrhage may occur with a prosthetic valve.

3. Porcine valve tends to develop early calcification in children.

4. Prosthetic valve endocarditis is a rare complication.

Postoperative Follow-Up

1. Patients who receive a prosthetic valve should be treated with coumadin (Warfarin), and the patient's prothrombin time should be maintained at 2.5 to 3.5 international normalized ratio (INR).

2. One should emphasize the importance of maintaining good oral hygiene and antibiotic prophylaxis against SBE.

MITRAL VALVE PROLAPSE

Prevalence

A reported incidence of MVP of 5% in the pediatric population probably is an overestimate. This condition usually occurs in older children and adolescents (it is more common in adults), and has a female preponderance (M:F ratio of 1:2).

Pathology

1. Thick and redundant mitral valve leaflets bulge into the mitral annulus (caused by myxomatous degeneration of the valve leaflets and/or the chordae).

2. The posterior leaflet is more commonly and more severely affected than the anterior leaflet.

Etiology

1. MVP is idiopathic in more than 50% of cases.

2. CHD is present in one third of patients with MVP. Secundum ASD is the most common defect, and VSD and Ebstein's anomaly are found rarely.

3. Of patients with MVP, 4% have Marfan's syndrome, and nearly all patients with Marfan's syndrome have MVP. MVP may be seen in association with other connective tissue disorders.

4. MVP is familial in the primary form (with an autosomal-dominant mode of inheritance).

Clinical Manifestations
  History.

1. MVP usually is asymptomatic, but a history of nonexertional chest pain, palpitation, and, rarely, syncope may be elicited.

2. The patient occasionally has a family history of MVP.

  Physical examination (Fig. 21-5).

1. An asthenic build with a high incidence of thoracic skeletal anomalies (80%), including pectus excavatum (50%), straight back (20%), and scoliosis (10%), is common. (*Straight-back syndrome* is a condition where the normal dorsal curvature of the spine is lost, resulting in a shortening of the chest's anteroposterior diameter.)

2. The midsystolic click with or without a late systolic murmur is the hallmarks of this syndrome and is best audible at the apex (see Fig. 21-5). The presence or absence

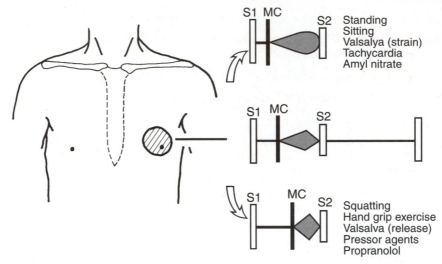

FIG. 21–5.
Diagram of auscultatory findings in MVP and the effect of various maneuvers on the
timing of the midsystolic click *(MC)* and the murmur. The maneuvers that reduce
ventricular volume enhance leaflet redundancy and move the click and murmur earlier
in systole. An increase in LV dimension has the opposite effect.

of the click and murmur, as well as their timing, vary from one examination to
the next.

a. The click and murmur may be brought out by held expiration, left decubitus
position, sitting, standing, or leaning forward. They may disappear on inspiration.

b. Various maneuvers can alter the timing of the click and the murmur:

  1) The click moves toward the S1 and the murmur lengthens with maneuvers that
  decrease the LV volume, such as standing, sitting, Valsalva's strain phase,
  tachycardia, and the administration of amyl nitrite.

  2) The click moves toward the S2, and the murmur shortens with maneuvers that
  increase the LV volume, such as squatting, hand grip exercise, Valsalva's
  release phase, bradycardia, and the administration of pressor agents or
  propranolol.

Electrocardiography.

1. A superiorly directed T vector (flat or inverted T waves in II, III, and aVF) occurs
in 20% to 60% of patients (Fig. 21-6).

2. Arrhythmias are relatively uncommon and include SVT, PACs, and PVCs.

3. Conduction disturbances (first-degree AV block, WPW syndrome or its variants,
prolonged QT interval, or RBBB) occasionally are reported.

4. LVH or LAH rarely is present.

X-ray study.

1. X-ray films are unremarkable except for LA enlargement in patients with severe MR.

2. Thoracoskeletal abnormalities (e.g., straight back, pectus excavatum, scoliosis) may
be present.

Echocardiography. Echo findings for adult patients with MVP have been established,
but for those for pediatric patients are not clearly defined.

1. M-mode echo shows posterior motion of the posterior and/or anterior leaflets of the mitral valve.

2. Two-dimensional echo is more reliable and shows prolapse of the mitral valve leaflet(s) superior to the plane of the mitral valve. The parasternal long-axis view is most reliable. The superior displacement seen only on the apical four-chamber view is not diagnostic because more than 30% of preselected normal children show this finding. The "saddle-shaped" mitral valve ring explains the superior displacement of the mitral valve seen in normal people in the apical four-chamber view.

3. The mitral valve leaflets are thick, and MR occasionally is demonstrable by color-flow mapping and Doppler examination.

4. Many children with classic midsystolic clicks (usually without late systolic murmur) fail to show the displacement of the mitral valve leaflets superior to the mitral valve plane in the parasternal long-axis view, although thickened leaflets and the bowing of the leaflets within the LV cavity frequently are found. The absence of the adult echo criteria for MVP in children may be explained by the fact that MVP is a progressive disease with a less-than-full manifestation in children.

Natural History

1. The majority of patients are asymptomatic, particularly during childhood.

2. Complications that are reported in adult patients, although rare in childhood, include sudden death (probably from ventricular arrhythmias), SBE, spontaneous rupture of chordae tendineae, progressive MR, CHF, and arrhythmias and conduction disturbances.

Management

1. Asymptomatic patients require no treatment or restriction of activity.

2. Preventive measures against SBE, especially when MR is present, are recommended.

3. Patients who are symptomatic (with palpitation, lightheadedness, dizziness, or syncope) or who have arrhythmias should undergo ambulatory ECG monitoring and/or treadmill exercise testing. Propranolol (or another β-adrenergic blocker) is the drug of choice for ventricular arrhythmias. Other drugs, such as calcium blockers, quinidine, or Pronestyl, may prove to be effective in some patients.

4. Chest pain may be treated with propranolol. (It is not relieved by nitroglycerin but may worsen.)

5. Reconstructive surgery or mitral valve replacement rarely may be indicated in patients with severe MR.

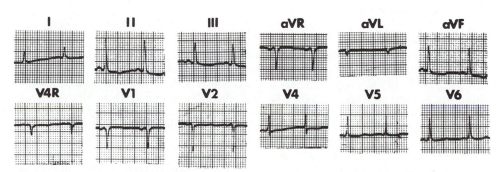

FIG. 21–6.
Tracing from a 14-year-old girl with MVP. The T wave in aVF is inverted.

22 / Cardiac Tumors

PREVALENCE

Cardiac tumors in the pediatric age group are extremely rare. A primary cardiac tumor was diagnosed in 0.001% to 0.003% of admissions at large children's referral centers. The male-to-female distribution is equal.

PATHOLOGY

1. The most common cardiac tumor in the pediatric age group is rhabdomyoma. In infants less than 1 year old, more than 75% of tumors are rhabdomyomas and teratomas, and in children 1 to 15 years of age, 80% of cardiac tumors are rhabdomyomas, fibromas, and myxomas (Table 22-1). More than 90% of primary tumors are benign.

2. Primary malignant tumors are extremely rare in infants and children. Malignant teratoma, rhabdomyosarcoma, fibrosarcoma, and neurogenic sarcoma have been reported.

3. Secondary malignant tumors also are rare in children. Solid tumors and lymphosarcomas are the most common lesions. Persistent pericardial effusion, often bloodstained, is a common finding.

4. Brief descriptions of the pathologies of common primary pediatric cardiac tumors follow (Armed Forces Institute of Pathology, 1978).

Rhabdomyomas

Rhabdomyomas are by far the most frequent tumors in the pediatric age group, accounting for about half the cases of cardiac tumors. They usually are multiple, ranging in size from several millimeters to several centimeters. The most common location is in the ventricular septum, but they may appear in the wall of any of the chambers or in the atrial septum. More than half the cases with multiple rhabdomyomas have tuberous sclerosis (e.g., with adenoma of the sebaceous glands, mental retardation, seizures). The tumors may produce symptoms of obstruction to blood flow, arrhythmias (usually ventricular tachycardia, occasionally SVT), or sudden death. The tumor itself may be the cause of WPW syndrome. Surgical treatment is indicated if the tumors produce hemodynamic derangement, but complete removal is not always possible. Spontaneous regression has been reported.

Fibroma

Cardiac fibromas usually occur as a single solid tumor, most commonly in the ventricular septum, although they may occur in the wall of any cardiac chamber. The size of the tumor varies from several millimeters to centimeters. Occasionally the tumor calcifies. The tumor may obstruct blood flow and disturb atrioventricular or ventricular conduction. In some cases, the tumor can be removed completely, but in others the tumor intermingles with myocardial tissue so that complete resection is not possible.

Teratoma

Teratomas contain elements from all three germ layers. Most of the tumors are intrapericardial and are attached to the root of the arterial pedicles in the base of the heart. Surgical excision usually is possible.

TABLE 22–1.

Relative Incidence of Cardiac Tumors in Infants and Children*

Tumor	Incidence
Infants (less than 12 months) (total 47 cases)	
Benign tumors (96%)	
Rhabdomyoma	60%
Teratoma	19%
Fibroma	13%
Others	4%
Malignant (4%)	
Fibrosarcoma	2%
Rhabdomyosarcoma	2%
Children (1 to 15 years) (total of 86 cases)	
Benign tumors (91%)	
Rhabdomyoma	41%
Fibroma	14%
Myxoma	14%
Teratoma	13%
Hemangioma	5%
Others	5%
Malignant tumors (9%)	
Malignant teratoma	5%
Rhabdomyosarcoma	2%
Others	2%

*From a series of 444 primary tumors of the heart and pericardium in which 133 cases were from infants and children less than 15 years of age.

Adopted from McAllister HA, Fenoglio JJ Jr: Tumors of the cardiovascular system, *Atlas of tumor pathology,* second series, Washington, DC, 1978, Armed Forces Institute of Pathology.

Myxoma

Myxomas are the most common type of cardiac tumors in adults, accounting for about 30% of all primary cardiac tumors, but they are very rare in infants and children. The majority of myxomas arise in the LA, 25% arise in the RA, and very few arise in the ventricles. Myxomas can produce hemodynamic disturbances, commonly interfering with mitral valve function or producing thromboembolic phenomenon in the systemic circulation. With RA myxoma, similar effects on the tricuspid valve and thromboembolic phenomenon in the pulmonary circulation may be found. Rarely, patients may have symptoms while sitting and standing, but their symptoms improve when they lie down, because of the intermittent protrusion of the tumor through the mitral valve. Surgical removal usually is successful.

CLINICAL MANIFESTATIONS

1. Syncope or chest pain may be a presenting complaint. Sudden unexpected death may be the first manifestation. Rarely symptoms vary with posture in cases of pedunculated tumors.

2. Clinical manifestations of cardiac tumors often are nonspecific and vary primarily with the location of the tumor.

   a. Tumors near cardiac valves may produce heart murmurs of stenosis or regurgitation of valves. So-called tumor plop may occur with a pedunculated and sessile tumor, such as LA myxoma.

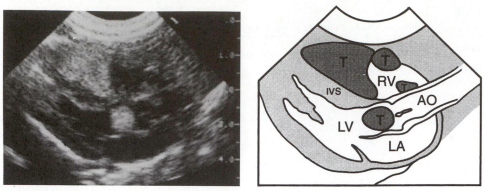

FIG. 22–1.
Parasternal long-axis view showing multiple rhabdomyomas *(T)* in a newborn. There is a round, mobile mass in the LV outflow tract, with resulting obstruction of the LV. One large and at least two other smaller tumor masses are imaged in the RV. The tumor in the LV outflow tract was surgically removed because of the obstructive nature of the mass.

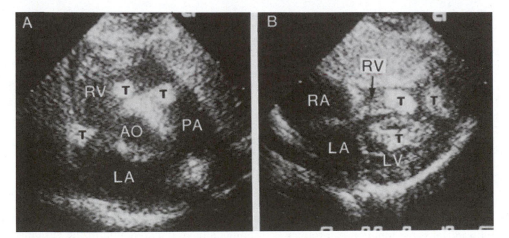

FIG. 22–2.
Parasternal short-axis view **(A)** and subcostal four-chamber view **(B)** showing multiple rhabdomyomas *(T)* in a newborn infant.

b. Tumors involving the conduction tissue may manifest with arrhythmias or conduction disturbances.

c. Intracavitary tumors may produce inflow or outflow obstruction, with clinical findings similar to those of mitral or semilunar valve stenosis or thromoembolic phenomenon.

d. Involvement of the myocardium (mural tumors) may result in heart failure or cardiac arrhythmias.

e. Pericardial tumors, which may signal a malignant nature of the tumor, may

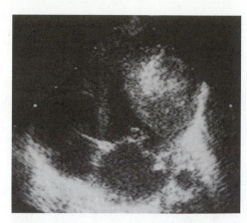 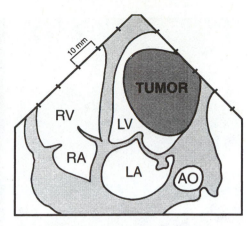

FIG. 22–3.
Apical four-chamber (apex-up) view showing a large solitary tumor *(TUMOR)* in the LV cavity in a newborn. The mass is attached to the LV free wall. Because of symptoms, surgical attempt was made to remove the mass, but the infant died. Pathologic examination revealed the mass to be fibroma.

produce pericardial effusion and cardiac tamponade or features simulating infective pericarditis.

3. Fragmentation of intracavitary tumors may lead to embolism of the pulmonary or systemic circulations.

4. Occasionally, for unknown reasons, fever and general malaise may manifest, especially with myxomas.

5. The ECG may show nonspecific ST-T changes, an infarctlike pattern, low-voltage QRS complexes, or preexcitation. Various arrhythmias and conduction disturbances have been reported.

6. Chest x-ray films occasionally may reveal altered contour of the heart, with or without changes in PVMs.

7. Echo and Doppler studies allow accurate determination of the presence, extent, and location of the tumor. These studies also determine the hemodynamic significance of the lesion. Cardiac tumors usually are found on a routine echo study when the diagnosis is not suspected, especially in small infants (Figs. 22-1 through 22-3).

   a. Multiple intraventricular tumors in infants and children most likely are rhabdomyomas (Figs. 22-1 and 22-2).

   b. A solitary tumor of varying size, arising from the ventricular septum or the ventricular wall, is likely to be a fibroma (Fig. 22-3).

   c. LA tumors, especially when pedunculated, usually are myxomas (Fig. 22-4).

   d. An intrapericardial tumor arising near the great arteries most likely is a teratoma.

   e. Pericardial effusion suggests a secondary malignant tumor.

8. Abnormal laboratory findings, such as an elevated sedimentation rate, hypergammaglobulinemia, thrombocytosis or thrombocytopenia, polycythemia or anemia, and leukocytosis, have been reported.

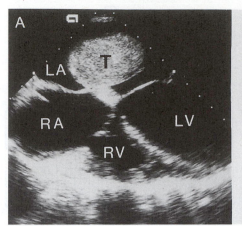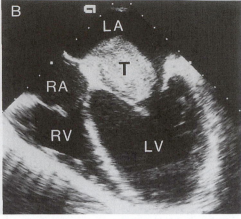

FIG. 22–4.
The four-chamber view of the transverse plane of a TEE from a 54-year-old man with LA myxoma *(T)*. **A,** A systolic freeze frame showing a large oval mass in the LA. This mass is attached to the atrial septum. The primum atrial septum is also thickened. **B,** During diastole, the myxoma protrudes through the mitral valve.

TREATMENT

Surgery is the only treatment for cardiac tumors that require intervention. Surgery is indicated in cases with symptoms of cardiac failure or ventricular arrhythmias refractory to medical treatment and in patients with inlet or outlet obstruction.

1. A successful complete resection of a fibroma is possible.

2. In asymptomatic patients with multiple rhabdomyomas, surgery should be delayed because of the possibility of spontaneous regression of the tumor.

3. Surgical removal is a standard procedure for myxomas and has a favorable outcome. The stalk of the tumor should be removed completely to prevent recurrence.

4. If myocardial involvement is extensive, surgical treatment is not possible. Cardiac transplantation may be an option in such cases.

23 / Cardiac Involvement in Systemic Diseases

Many collagen, neuromuscular, endocrine, and other systemic diseases may have important cardiovascular manifestations. The involvement of the cardiovascular system usually becomes evident when the diagnosis of the primary disease is well established, but occasionally cardiac manifestations may precede evidence of the basic disease. Cardiac manifestations of selected systemic diseases are briefly described here.

MUCOPOLYSACCHARIDOSES

The mucosaccharidoses are a diverse group of inherited metabolic disorders in which excessive amounts of mocopolysaccharides are stored in various tissues, including the myocardium and coronary arteries. Included in this group are syndromes of Hurler, Hunter, Scheie, Sanfilippo, Morquio, and others.

More than half of the cases show evidence of cardiac involvement. Regurgitation of cardiac valves, especially of the mitral, aortic, and tricuspid valves, is common. Occasionally systemic hypertension is present. Rarely, myocardial infarction can occur. Chest x-ray films may show cardiomegaly in severe cases of cardiac valve regurgitation. The ECG may show a prolonged QT interval, RVH, LVH, or LAH.

PERIARTERITIS NODOSA

This disease manifests with persistent fever, rash, and conjunctivitis. Periarteritis nodosa is seen more commonly in men, and its peak frequency is in the third to fifth decade. The majority of the cases demonstrate coronary arteritis, myocardial infarction, pericarditis, or cardiac hypertrophy, alone or in combination with minimal, if any, myocarditis. When periarteritis nodosa occurs in infants and children, it has a more fulminant course, and it can resemble Kawasaki's disease. In fact, periarteritis nodosa and Kawasaki's disease may have a similar, if not the same, etiology.

Hypertension, tachycardia, and heart failure are common findings. Heart murmurs are not common, and pericardial friction rub rarely is audible. The most common ECG abnormality is nonspecific T-wave changes, and occasionally arrhythmias are seen.

SYSTEMIC LUPUS ERYTHEMATOSUS

Cardiovascular manifestations occur in about 40% of the patients with systemic lupus erythematosus, a higher rate than with other connective tissue diseases. Pericarditis and pericardial effusion are the most common. The classical atypical verrucous endocarditis (Libman-Sacks) may be found on both surfaces of all four cardiac valves. The demonstration of lupus erythematosus cells in the pericardial fluid in association with low complement is important in the diagnosis of the disease.

Apical systolic murmur of MR frequently is found, but pericardial friction rub rarely is audible. The ECG shows nonspecific ST-T changes, arrhythmias, or conduction disturbances. With pericarditis, T-wave inversion and ST-segment elevation may develop.

RHEUMATOID ARTHRITIS

Pericarditis is the most common finding, occurring in 30% of the clinical population and 45% of autopsy cases. Occasionally, constrictive pericarditis may result. The endocardium rarely is involved, with thickening of mitral and aortic valve edges (20%), but the myocardium usually is spared. Rarely, MR, coronary arteritis, focal or diffuse myocarditis, and involvement of the conduction system with heart block can occur.

Tachycardia and nonspecific ejection systolic murmurs commonly are present. Chest pain and friction rub signify pericarditis. Occasionally, a regurgitant systolic murmur of MR may be audible. ECG abnormalities occur in 20% of cases, with the most common findings being nonspecific ST-T changes.

FRIEDREICH'S ATAXIA

Hypertrophy of ventricles, especially the LV, commonly is found, but the endocardium and cardiac valves usually are not involved. Microscopically, diffuse, interstitial fibrosis and fatty degeneration of the myocardium with compensatory hypertrophy of remaining cells frequently are found. A varying degree of atheromatous involvement of the coronary arteries is common. CHF is the terminal event in 70% of patients.

Cardiac symptoms (e.g., dyspnea, chest pain) are common, usually appearing in individuals with clear neurologic changes. Because of physical disability, cardiac problems may not be recognized until arrhythmias or signs of CHF develop. A systolic murmur may be audible at the ULSB, attributable to increased blood flow through the pulmonary valve or muscular subaortic stenosis. ECG abnormalities are very common. The most common finding is the T-vector change in the limb leads and/or LPLs. Occasionally, LVH, RVH, or abnormal Q waves are found. Chest x-ray films usually are normal, but rarely moderate cardiomegaly is seen. Echo studies reveal evidence of cardiomyopathy in more than 30% of cases; concentric hypertrophy of the LV is the most common finding. Asymmetric septal hypertrophy, systolic anterior motion of the mitral valve, or globally decreased LV function also are present.

MUSCULAR DYSTROPHY

Duchenne's muscular dystrophy is a sex-linked recessive disease. Involvement of the pelvic muscles leads to lordosis, waddling gait, a protuberant abdomen, and difficulty in rising. Significant cardiac involvement is seen only in Duchenne's type of muscular dystrophy and manifests clinically during adolescence. Cardiac enlargement, with occasional endocardial thickening of the LV and LA, is found on gross examination. Fatty degeneration and lymphocytic infiltration are found on the microscopic examination. Dystrophic changes in the papillary muscles may be evident, with MR or mitral valve prolapse. The coronary arteries, cardiac valves, and pericardium are normal.

Exertional dyspnea and tachypnea are common symptoms. The P2 may be loud if pulmonary hypertension is present. CHF is an ominous terminal sign. One may hear either a nonspecific systolic ejection murmur at the base or a regurgitant apical systolic murmur of MR caused by dystrophic changes in the papillary muscles. ECG abnormalities occur in 90% of teenagers with Duchenne's type, and RVH and RBBB are the most common abnormalities. Deep Q waves frequently are seen in the LPLs. T-vector changes may be seen in the limb leads or LPLs. Echo studies may show normal contractile function of the LV but reduced diastolic relaxation, which appears to be a sensitive indicator of early cardiac involvement. Echo features of MVP may be seen.

MARFAN SYNDROME

Marfan syndrome is a generalized connective tissue disease with clinical features involving skeletal, cardiovascular, and ocular systems. It is inherited as an autosomal dominant pattern with variable expressivity. A spectrum of cardiovascular abnormalities is recognized in this syndrome. Clinically evident cardiovascular involvement occurs in over 50% of patients by the age of 21. Microscopic changes probably are present in almost all patients, even during infancy and childhood. The common cardiovascular abnormalities include aneurysmal dilatation of the ascending aorta with or without dissection or rupture, enlargement of the sinus of Valsalva, AR, aneurysm of the PA, and dilatation of the mitral annulus with resulting MR. Rarely, myocardial fibrosis and infarction, rupture of chordae tendineae, aneurysm of the abdominal aorta, and aneurysmal dilatation of the proximal coronary arteries have been reported. Dilatation of the ascending aorta begins in the sinus of Valsalva and results in AR. The mitral valve and LA endocardium often undergo a fibromyxoid degeneration, resulting in MR and MVP. Microscopic examination of the proximal aorta (and the proximal coronary arteries) reveals disruption of the elastic media, with fragmentation and disorganization of the elastic fibers. Large accumulations of dermatan sulfate or heparan sulfate and chondroitin sulfate also have been reported in the media of the aorta.

In children and young adults, clinical findings of mitral valve involvement are more common than aortic lesions. Auscultatory findings of MR and MVP appear in more than 50% of patients (see Chapter 21). Rarely, the murmur of AR is audible. The S2 may be accentuated in many patients, especially in those with thin chest walls or dilated PAs. The ECG findings may include LVH; T-wave inversion in II, III, aVF, and LPLs, and first-degree AV block. Chest x-ray films may show cardiomegaly, either generalized or involving only the LV and LA or a prominence of the ascending aorta, aortic knob, or MPA. Echo shows an increased dimension of the aortic root with or without AR and/or MVP with thickened valve leaflets and MR.

A recent study suggested that prophylactic β-adrenergic blockers (propranolol or atenolol) is effective in slowing the rate of aortic dilatation and reducing the development of aortic complication in some patients with Marfan syndrome (Shores J et al: *N Engl J Med*, 330:1335, 1994).

ACUTE GLOMERULONEPHRITIS

Significant myocardial damage is found in 10% of postmortem examinations. Clinically evident myocardial involvement is found in 30% to 40% of patients. Pulmonary edema, systemic venous congestion, and cardiomegaly also are common. Systemic hypertension, sometimes appearing with hypertensive encephalopathy, is a frequent manifestation and may be responsible for signs of CHF in some, but not all, of the patients. Although hypertension probably reflects fluid expansion (secondary to impaired salt and water excretion), peripheral resistance has been found to be elevated. Increased renin activity may be responsible for the latter.

HYPERTHYROIDISM, CONGENITAL AND JUVENILE

The thyroid hormones increase oxygen consumption, stimulate protein synthesis and growth, and affect the metabolism of carbohydrates. Congenital hyperthyroidism most often is caused by increased thyroid-stimulating immunoglobulin in infants of mothers who had Graves' disease during pregnancy. Juvenile hyperthyroidism is believed to be caused by thyroid-stimulating antibodies and often is associated with lymphocytic thyroiditis and other autoimmune disorders.

Thyroid hormones may influence the cardiovascular system by increasing the demand for cardiac output by increasing oxygen use and metabolic consumption. These hormones also may increase myocardial sensitivity to catecholamines. A newborn infant with congenital hyperthyroidism often is premature and usually has a goiter. The baby appears anxious, restless, alert, and irritable. The eyes are widely open and appear exophthalmic. The incidence of juvenile hyperthyroidism peaks during adolescence, with females affected more often than males. The children become hyperactive, irritable, and excitable. The thyroid gland is enlarged.

Tachycardia, full and bounding pulses, and increased systolic and pulse pressures are common. A nonspecific systolic murmur may be audible. Bruits may be audible over the enlarged thyroid in children but not in the newborn. In severely affected patients, cardiac enlargement and cardiac failure may develop. These have a grave prognosis and require prompt recognition and treatment. Chest x-ray films usually are normal but may show cardiomegaly and increased pulmonary vascularity, especially in the presence of heart failure. ECG abnormalities include sinus tachycardia and peaked P waves. Various arrhythmias (SVT, nodal rhythm), complete heart block, RVH, LVH, and CVH are common in congenital hyperthyroidism, but arrhythmias are rare in juvenile hyperthyroidism. Echo studies reveal a hyperkinetic state with increased fractional shortening. In severely affected patients, a β-adrenergic blocker, such as propranolol, is indicated to reduce the effect of catecholamines.

HYPOTHYROIDISM, CONGENITAL OR JUVENILE

Congenital hypothyroidism most often is caused by a developmental defect of the thyroid gland. The typical picture of hypothyroidism may not be apparent until 3 months of age. The picture includes a protuberant tongue, cool and mottled skin, subnormal temperature, carotenemia, and myxedema. Untreated children become mentally retarded and slow in physical development. Acquired hypothyroidism most often results from lymphocytic thyroiditis (Hashimoto's disease or autoimmune thyroiditis). Rarely, amiodarone, an antiarrhythmic agent, can cause hypothyroidism. Serum levels of thyroxine and triiodothyronine are low or borderline.

The heart rate is relatively slow, and the heart sounds may be soft. PDA and PS are cardiac defects frequently associated with congenital hypothyroidism. ECG abnormalities occur in over 90% of cases and consist of some or all of the following: (1) low QRS voltages, especially in the limb leads; (2) low T-wave amplitude, not affecting the T axis; (3) prolongation of PR and QT intervals; and (4) dome-shaped T wave with an absent ST segment ("mosque" sign) (Fig. 23-1). Chest x-ray films may show cardiomegaly caused by cardiac enlargement or pericardial effusion. Echo studies frequently show pericardial effusion and asymmetric septal hypertrophy. The ECG, chest x-ray, and echo findings of juvenile hypothyroidism are the same as for congenital hypothyroidism, described previously.

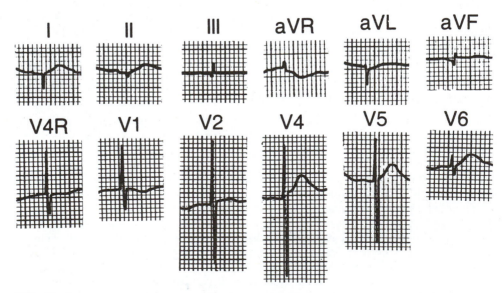

FIG. 23–1.
Tracing from a 3-month-old infant with congenital hypothyroidism. Note low QRS voltages in the limb leads, relatively low T-wave amplitude, and dome-shaped T wave with an absent ST segment in V6.

SICKLE CELL ANEMIA

In sickle cell anemia, erythrocytes become rigid and "sickle," leading to capillary occlusion and sickle cell "crisis." The increased stroke volume of the heart compensates for anemia, and the heart gradually dilates and hypertrophies. Heart failure may be a late complication.

The arterial pulse is brisk, and the precordium is hyperactive. The diastolic pressure is low with a wide pulse pressure. An ejection systolic murmur usually is audible along the ULSB and URSB. Rarely, one may hear an apical rumble and a gallop rhythm. ECG abnormalities may include first-degree AV block, LVH, and nonspecific T-wave changes. Chest x-ray films show generalized cardiomegaly in nearly all patients. Echo findings include increased LV dimension and vigorous LV contraction, but the ejection fraction and systolic time intervals are within normal limits.

PART VI

Electrocardiography II

Chapter 3 discusses steps in routine interpretation of an ECG and two common ECG abnormalities in children, hypertrophy and ventricular conduction disturbances. This section discusses arrhythmias, AV conduction disturbances, pacemaker ECGs, and ECG abnormalities involving ST segments and T waves.

24 / Cardiac Arrhythmias

The frequency and clinical significance of arrhythmias differ in children and adults. Although dysrhythmias are relatively infrequent in infants and children, the common practice of monitoring of cardiac rhythm in children requires primary care physicians and intensivists to be able to recognize and manage common arrhythmias.

The normal heart rate varies with age: The younger the child, the faster the heart rate. Therefore the definitions of *bradycardia* (fewer than 60 beats/min) and tachycardia (more than 100 beats/min) used for adults do not apply to infants and children. *Tachycardia* is defined as a heart rate beyond the upper limit of normal for the patient's age, and *bradycardia* is defined as a heart rate slower than the lower limit of normal. Normal resting heart rates by age are presented in Table 24-1.

This chapter discusses basic arrhythmias according to the origin of their impulse. Each arrhythmia is described along with its causes, significance, and treatment.

RHYTHMS ORIGINATING IN THE SINUS NODE

All rhythms that originate in the SA node (sinus rhythm) have two important characteristics (Fig. 24-1). Both are required to be called sinus rhythm.

1. P waves precede each QRS complex with a regular PR interval. (The PR interval may be prolonged, as in first-degree AV block).

2. The P axis falls between 0 and +90 degrees, an often neglected criterion. This produces upright P waves in II and inverted P waves in aVR. (See Chapter 3 for a detailed discussion of sinus rhythm.)

Regular Sinus Rhythm
Description. The rhythm is regular and the rate is normal for age. The two characteristics of sinus rhythm described previously are present (see Fig. 24-1).

Significance. Rhythm is normal at any age.

Treatment. No treatment is required.

Sinus Tachycardia
Description. Characteristics of sinus rhythm are present (see previous description). The rate is faster than the upper limit of normal for age (see Table 24-1). A rate greater than 140 beats/min in children and greater than 160 beats/min in infants may be significant. The heart rate usually is lower than 200 beats/min in sinus tachycardia (see Fig. 24-1).

Causes. Anxiety, fever, hypovolemia or circulatory shock, anemia, CHF, administration of catecholamines, thyrotoxicosis, and myocardial disease are possible causes.

Significance. Increased cardiac work is well tolerated by healthy myocardium.

Treatment. The underlying cause is treated.

Sinus Bradycardia
Description. The characteristics of sinus rhythm are present (see previous description), but the heart rate is slower than the lower range of normal for the age (see

TABLE 24–1.

Normal Ranges of Resting Heart Rate.

Age	Beats/Min
Newborn	110-150
2 yr	85-125
4 yr	75-115
Over 6 yr	60-100

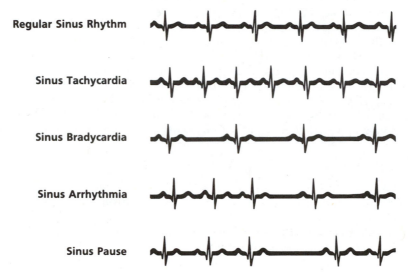

FIG. 24–1.

Normal and abnormal rhythms originating in the SA node. (From Park MK, Guntheroth WG: *How to read pediatric ECGs,* ed 3, St. Louis, 1992, Mosby.)

Table 24-1). A rate slower than 80 beats/min in newborn infants and slower than 60 beats/min in older children may be significant (see Fig. 24-1).

Causes. Sinus bradycardia may occur in normal individuals and trained athletes and with vagal stimulation, increased intracranial pressure, hypothyroidism, hypothermia, hypoxia, hyperkalemia, and administration of drugs such as digitalis and β-adrenergic blockers.

Significance. In some patients, marked bradycardia may not maintain normal cardiac output.

Treatment. The underlying cause is treated.

Sinus Arrhythmia
Description. Sinus arrhythmia is a phasic variation in the heart rate. The heart rate increases during inspiration and decreases during expiration. Arrhythmia occurs, with maintenance of characteristics of sinus rhythm (see Fig. 24-1).

Causes. This is a normal phenomenon and is due to phasic variation in the firing rate of cardiac autonomic nerves with the phases of respiration.

Significance. Sinus arrhythmia has no significance because it is a normal finding in children and a sign of good cardiac reserve.

Treatment. No treatment is indicated.

Sinus Pause

Description. In *sinus pause*, the sinus node pacemaker momentarily ceases activity, resulting in the absence of the P wave and QRS complex for a relatively short time (see Fig. 24-1). *Sinus arrest* is of longer duration and usually results in an escape beat (see later discussion) by other pacemakers, such as the nodal tissue (nodal escape).

Cause. Increased vagal tone, hypoxia, digitalis toxicity, and sick sinus syndrome are possible causes.

Significance. Sinus pause usually has no hemodynamic significance but may reduce cardiac output.

Treatment. Treatment is rarely indicated except in sick sinus syndrome (see later discussion) and digitalis toxicity (see Chapter 30).

Sick Sinus Syndrome

Description. The sinus node fails to function as the dominant pacemaker of the heart or performs abnormally slowly, resulting in a variety of arrhythmias. The arrhythmias include profound sinus bradycardia, sinus node exit block, sinus arrest with junctional escape, SVT, ectopic atrial or nodal rhythm, and bradytachyarrhythmia.

Causes.

1. Extensive cardiac surgery, particularly involving the atria, such as the Mustard or Senning procedure, is a possible cause.

2. Rarely, arteritis or focal myocarditis is a cause.

3. Sick sinus syndrome is occasionally idiopathic, involving an otherwise normal heart without structural defect.

Significance. Bradytachyarrhythmia is the most worrisome. Profound bradycardia after a period of tachycardia (overdrive suppression) can cause syncope and even death.

Treatment.

1. Antiarrhythmic drugs such as propranolol or quinidine are given to suppress tachycardia (see Appendix D).

2. Symptomatic patients with episodes of extreme bradycardia may require demand ventricular pacemakers.

RHYTHMS ORIGINATING IN THE ATRIUM

Rhythms that originate in the atrium (ectopic atrial rhythm) are characterized by the following (Fig. 24-2):

1. P waves of unusual contour, which are caused by an abnormal P axis, and/or an abnormal number of P waves per QRS complex

2. QRS complexes are usually of normal configuration, but occasional bizarre QRS complexes caused by aberrancy may occur (see later discussion)

Premature Atrial Contraction

Description. The QRS complex appears prematurely. The P wave may be upright in lead II when the ectopic focus is high in the atrium. The P wave is inverted when the ectopic focus is low in the atrium ("coronary sinus rhythm"). The compensatory pause is incomplete; that is, the length of two cycles, including one premature beat, is less than the length of two normal cycles (see Fig. 24-2). An occasional PAC is not followed by a QRS complex (a nonconducted PAC) (see Fig. 24-2).

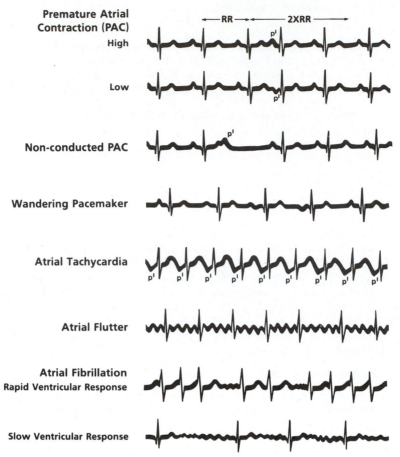

FIG. 24–2.
Arrhythmias originating in the atrium. (From Park MK, Guntheroth WG: *How to read pediatric ECGs,* ed 3, St. Louis, 1992, Mosby.)

Causes. PAC appears in healthy children, including newborns. It also may appear after cardiac surgery and with digitalis toxicity.

Significance. PAC has no hemodynamic significance.

Treatment. Usually no treatment is indicated, except in digitalis toxicity.

Wandering Atrial Pacemaker

Description. Wandering atrial pacemaker is characterized by gradual changes in the shape of P waves and PR intervals (see Fig. 24-2). The QRS complex is normal.

Causes. Wandering atrial pacemaker is seen in otherwise healthy children. It is the result of a gradual shift of the site of impulse formation in the atria through several cardiac cycles.

Significance. Wandering atrial pacemaker is a benign arrhythmia and has no clinical significance.

Treatment. No treatment is indicated.

Atrial Tachycardia

Atrial tachycardia is difficult to separate from the rarer nodal tachycardia. This has led to the use of the term *supraventricular tachycardia (SVT)* to describe both atrial and nodal tachycardias. Therefore atrial tachycardia is discussed in the section on supraventricular tachycardia (see later discussion).

Atrial Flutter

Description. The pacemaker lies in an ectopic focus, and "circus movement" in the atrium is the mechanism of this arrhythmia. Atrial flutter is characterized by an atrial rate (F wave with "saw-tooth" configuration) of about 300 beats/min, a ventricular response with varying degrees of block (e.g., 2:1, 3:1, 4:1), and normal QRS complexes (see Fig. 24-2).

Causes. Possible causes are structural heart disease with dilated atria, myocarditis, previous surgery involving atria (Mustard's procedure, Fontan operation, or ASD repair), and digitalis toxicity.

Significance. The ventricular rate determines eventual cardiac output; a too-rapid ventricular rate may decrease cardiac output. Atrial flutter usually suggests a significant cardiac pathology.

Treatment.

1. Digitalization is provided if the arrhythmia is not the result of digitalis toxicity; digitalis increases the AV block and thereby slows the ventricular rate.

2. Propranolol (1.0 to 4.0 mg/kg/day orally in three or four doses) may be added.

3. Electric cardioversion may be required. Digitalis should be discontinued for at least 48 hours before cardioversion. Coumadin is recommended by some physicians before cardioversion to prevent embolization.

4. Rapid atrial pacing with a catheter in the esophagus or the RA can be effective when cardioversion is contraindicated (e.g., digitalized patients).

5. Quinidine may prevent recurrence (see Appendix D).

Atrial Fibrillation

Description. The mechanism of this arrhythmia is "circus movement," as in atrial flutter. Atrial fibrillation is characterized by an extremely fast atrial rate (f wave at a rate of 350 to 600 beats/min) and an irregularly irregular ventricular response with normal QRS complexes (see Fig. 24-2).

Causes. Atrial fibrillation usually is associated with structural heart disease including dilated atria, myocarditis, digitalis toxicity, or previous intraatrial surgery.

Significance.

1. The rapid ventricular rate, in addition to the loss of coordinated contraction of the atria and ventricles, decreases the cardiac output, as occurs in atrial tachycardia.

2. Atrial fibrillation usually suggests a significant cardiac pathology.

Treatment.

1. Digoxin is provided to slow the ventricular rate (see Table 30-3 for dosage).

2. Propranolol (1.0 to 4.0 mg/kg/day orally in three or four divided doses) may be added if necessary.

3. Cardioversion may be indicated, but recurrence is common. When atrial thrombus is present or suspected, coumadin is recommended before and after cardioversion for 3 to 4 weeks each.

4. Quinidine is provided to prevent recurrence (see Appendix D).

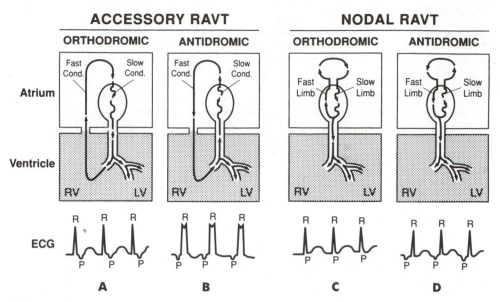

FIG. 24–3.

Diagram showing the mechanism of reciprocating AV tachycardia *(RAVT)* in relation to ECG findings. **A,** Orthodromic accessory RAVT is the most common mechanism of SVT in patients with WPW syndrome. Antegrade conduction through the normal, slow AV node produces a normal QRS complex, and the retrograde conduction through the bypass tract creates inverted P waves after the QRS complex (with a short RP interval). **B,** In antidromic accessory RAVT, the antegrade conduction through the bypass tract produces a wide QRS complex. Retrograde P waves precede the wide QRS complex with a short PR interval (and a long RP interval). **C,** In the orthodromic nodal RAVT (common form), the retrograde P waves are usually concealed in the QRS complex of normal duration. The ECG is similar to that of orthodromic accessory RAVT, and differentiation between these two is possible only when the tachyarrhythmia terminates by the presence of preexcitation in the accessory RAVT. **D,** In the antidromic nodal RAVT (uncommon), narrow QRS complexes are preceded by retrograde P waves, with a short PR interval. The ECG is similar to that of ectopic atrial tachycardia. (From Park MK, Guntheroth WG, *How to read pediatric ECGs,* ed 3, St. Louis, 1992, Mosby).

Supraventricular Tachycardia

Description. Three groups of tachycardia are included in SVT: atrial tachycardia (ectopic or nonreciprocating atrial tachycardia), nodal (or AV junctional) tachycardia, and AV reentrant (or reciprocating) tachycardia. The majority of SVTs are due to reentry AV tachycardia rather than rapid firing of a single focus in the atria (nonreciprocating atrial tachycardia) or in the AV node (nodal tachycardia).

The heart rate is extremely rapid and regular (usually 240 ± 40 beats/min). The P wave usually is invisible but when visible, has an abnormal P axis and either precedes or follows the QRS complex (see Figs. 24-2 and 24-3). The QRS duration usually is normal, but occasionally aberrancy increases the QRS duration, making differentiation from ventricular tachycardia difficult (see later discussion).

AV reentrant (or reciprocating) tachycardia is not only the most common mechanism of SVT, but also the most common tachyarrhythmia seen in the pediatric age group. This arrhythmia was formerly called *paroxysmal atrial tachycardia (PAT)* because the onset and termination of this arrhythmia were characteristically abrupt. In SVT caused by reentry, two pathways are involved; at least one of these is the AV node, and the other is an accessory pathway. The accessory pathway may be an anatomically separate bypass tract, such as the bundle of Kent (which produces *accessory reciprocating AV tachycardia,* Fig. 24-3, *A* and *B*), or only a functionally separate bypass tract, such as in a dual AV node pathway (which produces *nodal reciprocating AV tachycardia,* Fig. 24-3, *C* and *D*). Patients with accessory pathways frequently have preexcitation (or WPW) syndrome.

Fig. 24-3 shows the mechanism of reciprocating AV tachycardia in relation to ECG findings. If a PAC occurs, the prematurity of the extrasystole may find the accessory bundle refractory, but the AV node may conduct, producing a normal QRS complex; when the impulse reaches the bundle of Kent from the ventricular side, the bundle will have recovered and allows reentry into the atrium, producing a superiorly directed P wave that is difficult to detect. In turn, the cycle is maintained by reentry into the AV node, with a very fast heart rate. When there is an antegrade conduction through the AV node (slow pathway), the rhythm is called *orthodromic reciprocating AV tachycardia* (Fig. 24-3, *A*). Less common is a widened QRS complex with antegrade conduction into the ventricle via the accessory (fast) pathway and retrograde conduction through the (slower) AV node (*antidromic reciprocating AV tachycardia,* Fig. 24-3, *B*). A PVC could initiate this arrhythmia if the recovery time of the two limbs is ideal for the initiation of the reentry.

Dual pathways in the AV node are more common than accessory bundles, at least as functional entities. For SVT to occur, the two pathways would have to have, at least temporarily, different conduction and recovery rates, creating the substrate for a reentry tachycardia. When the normal, slow pathway through the AV node is used in antegrade conduction to the bundle of His *(orthodromic),* the resulting QRS complex is normal with an abnormal P vector but is unrecognizable because it is superimposed on the QRS complex (Fig. 24-3, *C*). The resulting tachycardia could be the same as seen with SVT associated with WPW syndrome. The two can be differentiated only after conversion from the SVT; after conversion, the patient with accessory bundle would have preexcitation. In *antidromic* nodal reentrant AV tachycardia (Fig. 24-3, *D*), which is uncommon, the fast tract of the AV node transmits the antegrade impulse to the bundle of His, and the normal, slow pathway of the AV node transmits the impulse retrogradely. The resulting SVT demonstrates normal QRS duration, a short PR interval, and an inverted P wave.

Any type of AV block is incompatible with reentrant tachycardia; AV block would abruptly terminate the tachycardia, at least temporarily. This is the reason that adenosine works well for this type of arrhythmia.

Ectopic or nonreciprocating atrial tachycardia is a rare mechanism of SVT in which rapid firing of a single focus in the atrium is responsible for the tachycardia. Unlike reciprocating atrial tachycardia, in ectopic atrial tachycardia, the heart rate varies substantially during the course of a day, and second-degree AV block may develop.

Nodal tachycardia may superficially resemble atrial tachycardia because the P wave is buried and becomes invisible in the T waves of the preceding beat, but the rate of nodal tachycardia is relatively slower (120 to 200 beats/min) than the rate of atrial tachycardia.

Causes.

1. No heart disease (idiopathic) is found in about half of patients. The idiopathic type occurs more commonly in young infants than in older children.

2. WPW syndrome is present in 10% to 20% of cases and is evident only after conversion to sinus rhythm.

3. Some CHDs (Ebstein's anomaly, single ventricle, L-TGA) are more prone to this arrhythmia.

Significance.

1. SVT may decrease cardiac output and result in CHF.

2. Many infants tolerate SVT well for 24 hours, but within 48 hours, about 50% of patients develop heart failure.

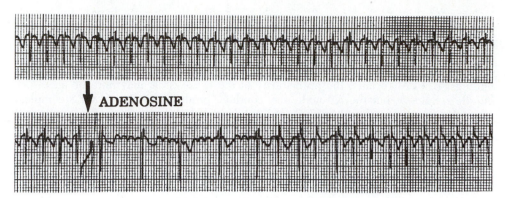

FIG. 24–4.
Adenosine uncovering of the mechanism of an SVT. A 3-month-old infant developed an extremely fast, narrow QRS complex tachycardia and a heart rate of 220 beats/min after insertion of a central line through a jugular vein. Adenosine produced a transient AV block and unmasked very rapid atrial fibrillation waves (570 beats/min).

3. Clinical manifestations of CHF include irritability, tachypnea, poor feeding, and pallor. When CHF develops, the infant's condition can deteriorate rapidly.

Treatment.

1. Vagal stimulatory maneuvers (carotid sinus massage, gagging, pressure on an eyeball) may be effective in older children but rarely are effective in infants.

2. Placing an icebag on the face (up to 10 seconds) often is effective in infants.

3. Adenosine, an endogenous nucleoside, has negative chronotropic, dromotropic, and inotropic actions of very short duration (with a half-life < 1.5 sec), with minimal hemodynamic consequences. It transiently blocks the AV conduction and sinus node pacemaking activity. Adenosine may be the drug of choice in the treatment of SVT because it terminates almost all SVT in which the AV node forms part of the reentry circuit. Adenosine also has a differential diagnostic ability with both narrow- and wide-complex *regular* tachycardia because of its absence of adverse hemodynamic effects. (It is not recommended for the management of irregular tachycardias.) It terminates SVT with aberration but is not effective with nonreciprocating atrial tachycardia, atrial flutter/fibrillation, and ventricular tachycardia. Its transient AV block may unmask atrial activities by slowing the ventricular rate and help clarify the mechanism of certain supraventricular arrhythmias (Fig. 24-4). Adenosine is given by rapid intravenous bolus followed by a saline flush, starting at 50 μg/kg and increasing in increments of 50 μg/kg every 1 to 2 minutes (maximum 250 μg/kg). The usual effective dose in children is 100 to 150 μg/kg. Digitalization follows in small children to prevent recurrence of the tachycardia.

4. If adenosine is not available, initial cardioversion may be performed in infants with CHF. The initial dose of 0.5 joules/kg may be increased in steps up to 2 joules/kg. This is followed by digitalization.

5. Digitalization may be used in infants without CHF and those with mild CHF (see Chapter 30). Cardioversion may induce ventricular tachycardia in patients who have been digitalized. Thus an initial cardioversion is preferred in patients with CHF.

6. If the patient is not in CHF, adenosine is not available, and digitalis is not effective, intravenous infusion of phenylephrine may be tried when a rapid conversion to sinus rhythm is desirable. Phenylephrine raises blood pressure abruptly and converts the tachycardia by reflex increase in vagal tone. This method is not recommended in

infants with CHF because increasing the afterload may be detrimental to a failing heart. A total of 10 mg of phenylephrine is added to 200 ml of intravenous solution, and drips are administered rapidly while the physician frequently monitors blood pressure. The systolic pressure should not exceed 150-170 mm Hg.

7. Intravenous administration of propranolol or verapamil may be tried, but they are not the treatment of choice. These drugs may produce extreme bradycardia and hypotension in infants younger than 1 year of age and should be avoided when possible. The clinician should administer these drugs in small doses, carefully monitor vital signs, and be ready to respond to adverse effects.

8. Overdrive suppression by transesophageal pacing in the intensive care unit or by atrial pacing in the cardiac catheterization laboratory may be indicated in children who already have undergone digitalization.

9. The recurrence of SVT should be prevented with a maintenance dose of digoxin (see Table 30-3) for 3 to 6 months. In children over 8 years old with WPW syndrome, propranolol or atenolol may be preferable to digoxin.

10. Occasionally, catheter ablation or surgical interruption of accessory pathways should be considered if medical management fails.

RHYTHMS ORIGINATING IN THE AV NODE

Rhythms that originate in the AV node are characterized by the following findings (Fig. 24-5):

1. The P wave may be absent, or inverted P waves may follow the QRS complex.

2. The QRS complex usually is normal in duration and configuration.

Only the lower part (NH region) of the AV node has pacemaker ability. The upper (AN region) and middle (N region) parts do not function as pacemakers, but delay the conduction of an impulse, either antegrade or retrograde.

Nodal Premature Beats

Description. A normal QRS complex occurs prematurely. P waves usually are absent, but inverted P waves may follow QRS complexes (see Fig. 24-5). The compensatory pause may be complete or incomplete.

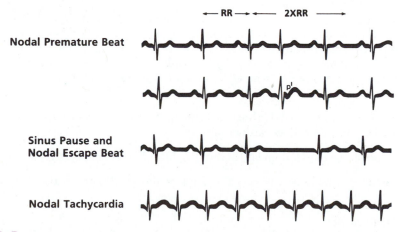

FIG. 24–5.
Arrhythmias originating in the AV node. (From Park MK, Guntheroth WG: *How to read pediatric ECGs,* ed 3, St. Louis, 1992, Mosby.)

Causes. Nodal premature beats usually are idiopathic in an otherwise normal heart; they may result from cardiac surgery and digitalis toxicity.

Significance. Nodal premature beats usually have no hemodynamic significance.

Treatment. Treatment is not indicated unless the cause is digitalis toxicity.

Nodal Escape Beats

Description. When the SA node impulse fails to reach the AV node, the NH region of the AV node initiates an impulse (nodal or junctional escape beat). The QRS complex occurs later than the anticipated normal beat. The P wave may be absent, or an inverted P wave follows the QRS complex (see Fig. 24-5). The duration and configuration of QRS complexes are normal.

Causes. Nodal escape beats may occur after cardiac surgery involving the atria (the Mustard or Senning procedure) or in otherwise healthy children.

Significance. Nodal escape beats have little hemodynamic significance.

Treatment. Generally no specific treatment is required.

Nodal or Junctional Rhythm

Description. If the SA node consistently fails, the AV node may function as the main pacemaker of the heart, producing a relatively slow rate (40 to 60 beats/min). Nodal rhythm is characterized by no P waves or inverted P waves after QRS complexes, and normal QRS complexes with a rate of 40 to 60 beats/min.

Causes. Nodal or junctional rhythm may occur in an otherwise normal heart, as a result of cardiac surgery, increased vagal tone (increased intracranial pressure, pharyngeal stimulation), and digitalis toxicity.

Significance. The slow heart rate may significantly decrease cardiac output and produce symptoms.

Treatment.

1. Known causes such as digitalis toxicity should be treated.

2. No treatment is indicated if the patient's condition is asymptomatic.

3. Atropine or electric pacing is indicated if the patient is symptomatic.

Accelerated Nodal Rhythm

Description. When the patient has a normal sinus rate and AV conduction and the AV node (NH region) has enhanced automaticity and captures the pacemaker function at a faster rate than normal junctional rate (60 to 120 beats/min), the rhythm is called *accelerated nodal* (or *AV junctional) rhythm.* Either P waves are absent, or inverted P waves follow QRS complexes. The QRS complex is normal, and the heart rate is 60 to 120 beats/min.

Causes. Accelerated nodal rhythm may be idiopathic, may result from digitalis toxicity or myocarditis, or may follow cardiac surgery.

Significance. Accelerated nodal rhythm has little hemodynamic significance.

Treatment. No treatment is necessary unless the condition is caused by digitalis toxicity.

Nodal Tachycardia

Description. The ventricular rate varies from 120 to 200 beats/min. Either the P waves are absent, or inverted P waves follow QRS complexes (see Fig. 24-5). The QRS complex is usually normal, but *aberration* may occur on rare occasions, as in atrial tachycardia. Nodal tachycardia is difficult to separate from atrial tachycardia. Therefore both arrhythmias are grouped under SVT (see previous discussion).

Causes. Causes are similar to those of atrial tachycardia.

Significance. The significance is similar to atrial tachycardia.

Treatment. Treatment is not indicated if the rate is slower than 130 beats/min. Although digoxin is used in the treatment of most cases of SVT of atrial origin, it may be contraindicated in the true form of nodal tachycardia. In this instance, quinidine probably is the drug of choice.

RHYTHMS ORIGINATING IN THE VENTRICLE

Rhythms that originate in the ventricle (ventricular arrhythmias) are characterized by (Fig. 24-6) the following:

1. Bizarre and wide QRS complexes

2. T waves pointing in directions opposite of QRS complexes

3. QRS complexes randomly related to P waves, if visible

Premature Ventricular Contraction
Description.

A bizarre, wide QRS complex appears earlier than anticipated, and the T wave points in the opposite direction. A full compensatory pause usually appears; that is, the length of two cycles, including the premature beat, is the same as that of two normal cycles (see Fig. 24-6). The appearance of a full compensatory pause indicates that the sinus node is not prematurely discharged by the PVC. If the retrograde impulse discharges and resets the sinus node prematurely, it produces a pause that is not fully compensatory. PVCs may be classified into the following types, depending on their interrelationship, similarities, timing, and coupling intervals.

Interrelationship.
1. Ventricular *bigeminy* or *coupling:* Each abnormal QRS complex regularly alternates with a normal QRS complex.

2. Ventricular *trigeminy:* Each abnormal QRS complex regularly follows two normal QRS complexes.

3. *Couplets:* Two abnormal QRS complexes appear in sequence.

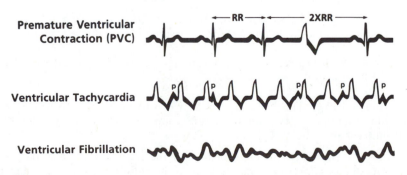

FIG. 24–6.
Ventricular arrhythmias. (From Park MK, Guntheroth WG: *How to read pediatric ECGs,* ed 3, St. Louis, 1992, Mosby.)

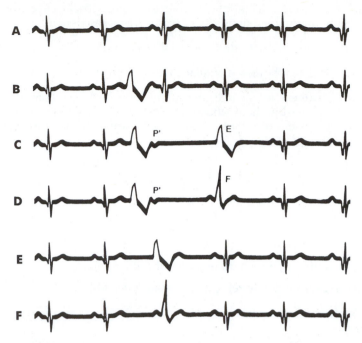

FIG. 24–7.
Types of PVCs according to timing in the cardiac cycle. **A,** Regular sinus rhythm. **B,** Interpolated PVC followed by a slightly prolonged PR interval. **C,** Early PVC, which results in a retrogradely conducted P wave (P′) with a less-than-full compensatory pause. The first postectopic beat is a ventricular escape beat *(E)*. **D,** Early PVC with a retrogradely conducted P wave (P′) with a less-than-full compensatory pause. A ventricular fusion beat *(F)* resumes the cardiac cycle. **E,** Late PVC, which results in a full compensatory pause; presumably retrograde discharge of the sinus node did not occur. **F,** Ventricular fusion beat with a full compensatory pause.

    4. *Triplets:* Three abnormal QRS complexes appear in sequence. Three or more successive PVCs arbitrarily are termed *ventricular tachycardia.*

Similarities among abnormal QRS complexes. Depending on the similarities of the bizarre QRS complex, PVCs may be classified into the following types:

    1. Uniform (or unifocal) PVCs: Abnormal QRS complexes have the same configuration in a single lead. They are assumed to originate from a single focus.

    2. Multiform (or multifocal) PVCs: Abnormal QRS complexes have different configurations in a single lead. They are assumed to originate from different foci.

Timing in the cardiac cycle. Depending on their timing in the cardiac cycle, PVCs may be classified into several types (Fig. 24-7).

    1. Interpolated PVC: The PVC appears between two conducted sinus beats. Sinus rhythm is not interrupted, and there is no compensatory pause after the PVC. The PR interval after the PVC is slightly increased (Fig. 24-7, *B*).

    2. Early PVC: The PVC appears shortly after the normal T wave of the preceding beat. A compensatory pause may appear. If the sinus rate is slow and a retrograde atrial conduction prematurely discharges the sinus node, a noncompensatory pause results. Either a ventricular escape beat or a fusion beat resumes the cardiac cycle (Fig. 24-7, *C* and *D*).

3. Late PVC: The PVC appears slightly before the normal P wave of the next beat. A full compensatory pause results (Fig. 24-7, *E*).

4. *Fusion beats:* The PVC occurs so late in the cardiac cycle that a normal sinus pacemaker impulse already has penetrated the AV node and has started to depolarize the ventricle. The resulting QRS complex appears midway between the patient's normal conducted beat and the pure ectopic ventricular beat because it is produced partly by a normally conducted supraventricular impulse and partly by an ectopic ventricular impulse. The presence of a "fusion" complex is a reliable sign of PVC and helps differentiate the PVC from a supraventricular arrhythmia with aberrant ventricular conduction (see later discussion).

Coupling interval.

Fixed coupling. PVCs appear at a constant interval after the QRS complex of the previous cardiac cycle. This suggests ventricular *reentry* within the Purkinje system as the underlying mechanism. Most PVCs in children have a fixed coupling interval and a uniform LBBB morphology.

Varying coupling interval. When coupling intervals vary by more than 80 msec, the PVCs may result from parasystole, a changing conduction in a reentrant circuit, or a changing discharge rate of an abnormal focus. Determining the precise mechanism of the PVC is difficult. However, if the intervals between ectopic beats can be factored so that each interval is a multiple of a single basic interval (within 0.08 sec), ventricular parasystole is diagnosed. (Ventricular parasystole consists of an impulse-forming focus in the ventricle that is independent of the sinus-node-generated impulse and is protected from depolarization (entrance block) by sinus impulses.) PVCs with varying coupling intervals may be more significant than those with fixed coupling.

Causes.

1. PVC may appear in otherwise healthy children. Up to 50% to 70% of normal children may show PVCs on 24-hour ambulatory ECGs.

2. A link has been found between LV false tendon and PVCs (and innocent heart murmurs). More than 50% of healthy people are thought to have demonstrable LV false tendons. These are thin, chordal strands that extend from the ventricular septum to either the LV free wall or an LV papillary muscle; they are detectable by two-dimensional echo (Fig. 24-8). False tendons contain Purkinje fibers, which may be the source of the arrhythmia.

3. Myocarditis and myocardial injury or infarction are possible causes.

4. Cardiomyopathy (dilated or hypertrophic) is a possible cause.

5. Cardiac tumors are possible causes.

6. RV dysplasia (RV cardiomyopathy) may be the cause in children with symptomatic tachycardia (see section on primary myocardial disease in Chapter 18).

7. Long QT syndrome (see section on long QT syndrome in Chapter 35) may be the cause.

8. CHD or acquired heart disease, preoperative or postoperative, is a possible cause.

9. Digitalis toxicity or certain drugs such as catecholamines, theophylline, caffeine, amphetamines, and some anesthetic agents are possible causes.

10. MVP is a possible cause.

Significance.

1. Occasional PVCs are benign in children, particularly if they are uniform and disappear or become less frequent with exercise.

2. PVCs are more significant if the following are true:

    a. They are associated with underlying heart disease (preoperative or postoperative status, MVP, cardiomyopathy).

    b. There is a history of syncope or a family history of sudden death.

    c. They are precipitated by, or become more frequent with, activity.

    d. They are multiform, particularly couplets.

    e. There are runs of PVC with symptoms.

    f. There are incessant or frequent episodes of paroxysmal ventricular tachycardia (more likely myocardial tumors).

3. Ventricular parasystole does not appear to have any consequence in children.

4. The R-on-T phenomenon does not appear to have any prognostic significance, except possibly in children with prolonged QT intervals (see section on long QT syndrome in Chapter 35).

Investigation.

1. In children with otherwise normal hearts, occasional isolated uniform PVCs that are suppressed by exercise probably do not require extensive investigations.

2. Children with uniform PVCs, including ventricular bigeminy and trigeminy, need not be treated or followed by cardiologists if the ECG, echo, and exercise test results are normal.

    a. The physician obtains an ECG to detect ST-T changes and QTc prolongation.

    b. Echo will detect CHD or acquired heart disease, such as hypertrophic cardiomyopathy, MVP, and RV dysplasia. LV false tendons can be imaged through this medium (see Fig. 24-8).

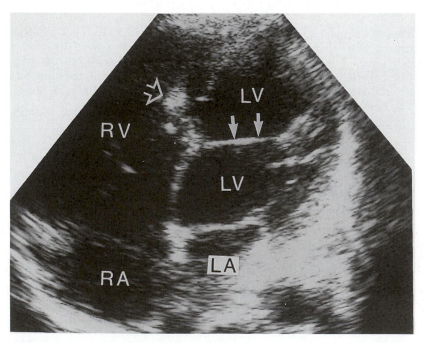

FIG. 24–8.
An apical four-chamber view of echo showing a false tendon *(solid arrows)* in the LV in a 13-year-old boy who had surgical repair of a VSD *(open arrow)*. This patient had a "twanging string" type of systolic murmur.

c. In children, PVCs characteristically are reduced or eliminated by exercise. The induction or exacerbation of arrhythmia with exercise may be an indication of underlying heart disease. Exercise may reveal prolonged QT interval. A QTc interval greater than 0.44 second at 1 minute after cessation of exercise may be significant.

3. Children with multiform PVCs and ventricular couplets should have 24-hour Holter monitoring, even if they have structurally normal hearts, as shown by testing, to detect the severity and extent of ventricular arrhythmias. They also should be followed yearly with echo, exercise tests, and 24-hour Holter monitoring.

4. Symptomatic ventricular arrhythmias or sustained ventricular tachycardia and a seemingly normal heart should undergo cardiac catheterization, (which is better than echo in the diagnosis of RV dysplasia). Occasionally, invasive electrophysiologic studies and RV endomyocardial biopsy may be indicated.

Treatment.

1. PVCs that cause no symptoms and have no hemodynamic consequences in patients with normal hearts do not require treatment.

2. All children with symptomatic ventricular arrhythmias should be treated.

   a. Frequent PVCs occasionally require treatment with an intravenous bolus of lidocaine (1 mg/kg per dose), followed by an intravenous drip of lidocaine (20 to 50 mg/kg/min).

   b. β-Blockers (such as atenolol, 1 to 2 mg/kg orally in a single daily dose) are effective for cardiomyopathy and occasionally for RV dysplasia.

   c. Other antiarrhythmic drugs, such as diphenylhydantoin (Dilantin) and mexiletine may prove effective. Antiarrhythmic agents that prolong the QT interval, such as those of class IA (quinidine, procainamide) and class III (amiodarone, bretylium) should be avoided. (See Appendix A, Table AA-3, and Appendix D).

Ventricular Tachycardia
Description.

1. Ventricular tachycardia is a series of three or more PVCs with a heart rate of 120 to 200 beats/min. QRS complexes are wide and bizarre, with T waves pointing in opposite directions (see Fig. 24-6).

2. The onset may be paroxysmal (sudden) or nonparoxysmal, and ventricular tachycardia may be sustained (lasting > 30 sec) or unsustained.

3. QRS contours during ventricular tachycardia may be unchanging (uniform, monophasic) or may vary randomly (multiform, polymorphous, or pleomorphic). Torsades de pointes (meaning "twisting of the points") is a distinct form of polymorphic ventricular tachycardia, occurring in patients with marked QT prolongation. Torsades de pointes is characterized by a paroxysm of ventricular tachycardia during which there are progressive changes in the amplitude and polarity of QRS complexes separated by a narrow transition QRS complex.

4. Differentiating ventricular tachycardia from SVT with aberrant conduction (see later discussion) sometimes is difficult. However, almost all wide QRS tachycardias are ventricular tachycardia in children. Wide QRS tachycardia in an infant or child must be considered ventricular tachycardia until proved otherwise.

Causes.

1. All the causes listed for PVCs also are causes of ventricular tachycardia, except that ventricular tachycardia does not occur in children with normal hearts.

2. Torsades de pointes may be caused by drugs or chemicals that prolong the QT interval, such as antiarrhythmic drugs, especially class IA (quinidine, procainamide) and class IC (encainide, flacainide) (see Appendix A, Table AA-3 for classification); phenothiazines (Thorazine, Mellaril); tricyclic antidepressants (imipramine, desipramine); certain antibiotics (ampicillin, erythromycin, trimethoprim-sulfa); and organophosphate insecticides. (Class II and IV antiarrhythmic drugs do not prolong the QT interval.)

Significance.

1. Ventricular tachycardia usually signifies a serious myocardial pathology or dysfunction.

2. With a fast heart rate, cardiac output may decrease notably, and the rate may deteriorate to ventricular fibrillation.

Treatment.

1. Ventricular tachycardia must be treated promptly with synchronized cardioversion (0.5 to 1.0 joules/kg) if the patient is unconscious or has cardiovascular instability with clinical evidence of low-cardiac output.

2. If the patient is conscious, an intravenous bolus of lidocaine (1.0 mg/kg/dose over 1 to 2 minutes) followed by an intravenous drip of lidocaine (20 to 50 µg/kg/min) may be effective.

3. If lidocaine is unsuccessful, bretylium tosylate (5 mg/kg intravenously over 8 to 10 minutes) may be tried.

4. Intravenous injection of magnesium sulfate recently was reported to be a very effective and safe treatment for torsades de pointes in adults (2 g in an intravenous bolus). The conventional treatment for torsades de pointes is aimed at shortening the QT interval by increasing the heart rate (by isoproterenol infusion or cardiac pacing).

5. The physician should search for reversible conditions contributing to the initiation and maintenance of ventricular tachycardia (such as hypokalemia, hypoxemia) and should correct the conditions, if possible.

6. Recurrence may be prevented with administration of propranolol, atenolol, diphenylhydantoin, or quinidine (see Appendix D). A combination of 24-hour Holter monitoring and treadmill exercise testing is the best noninvasive means of evaluating drug effectiveness. Complete pharmacologic suppression may not be achieved without serious complications. Therefore controlling the rate to an asymptomatic level may be adequate.

7. If antiarrhythmic control is inadequate, invasive electrophysiologic studies should be considered.

8. Rarely, ventricular or atrial pacing combined with antiarrhythmic agents, an implantable cardioverter/defibrillator, surgical excision, or ablation techniques may be tested in selected patients.

Aberration. When a supraventricular impulse prematurely reaches the AV node or bundle of His, it may find one bundle branch excitable and the other still refractory. Therefore the resulting QRS complex resembles a bundle branch block pattern. The right bundle branch usually has a longer refractory period than the left bundle branch, producing QRS complexes similar to those of RBBB. The following features help in differentiating aberrant ventricular conduction from ectopic ventricular impulses:

1. An rsR′ pattern in V1 that resembles QRS complexes of RBBB suggests aberration. In a ventricular ectopic beat, the QRS morphology is bizarre and does not resemble the classic form of RBBB or LBBB.

2. Occasional wide QRS complexes after P waves with regular PR intervals suggest an aberration.

3. The presence of a ventricular "fusion" complex (see previous discussion) is a reliable sign of ventricular ectopic rhythm.

Ventricular Fibrillation

Description. Ventricular fibrillation is characterized by bizarre QRS complexes of varying sizes and configurations. The rate is rapid and irregular (see Fig. 24-6).

Causes. Possible causes are postoperative state, severe hypoxia, hyperkalemia, digitalis or quinidine toxicity, myocarditis, myocardial infarction, and drugs (e.g., catecholamines, anesthetics).

Significance. Ventricular fibrillation usually is a terminal arrhythmia because it results in ineffective circulation.

Treatment. Treatment is immediate cardiopulmonary resuscitative procedures, including electric defibrillation at the dose of 2 joules/kg.

25 / Disturbances of Atrioventricular Conduction

Atrioventricular (AV) block is a disturbance in conduction between the normal sinus impulse and the eventual ventricular response. The block is assigned to one of three classes, depending on the severity of the conduction disturbance. First-degree AV block is a simple prolongation of the PR interval. In second-degree AV block, some atrial impulses are not conducted into the ventricle. In third-degree AV block, none of the atrial impulses is conducted into the ventricle (complete heart block) (Fig. 25-1).

FIRST-DEGREE AV BLOCK

Description. The PR interval is prolonged beyond the upper limits of normal for the patient's age and heart rate (see Table 3-2 and Fig. 25-1). This is produced by an abnormal delay in conduction through the AV node.

Causes. First-degree AV block can appear in otherwise healthy children. Other causes are acute rheumatic fever, cardiomyopathies, CHDs (e.g., ASD, Ebstein's anomaly, ECD), cardiac surgery, and digitalis toxicity.

Significance. First-degree AV block does not produce symptoms of hemodynamic disturbance. It sometimes progresses to a more advanced AV block.

Treatment. No treatment is indicated, except when the block is caused by digitalis toxicity (see Chapter 30).

SECOND-DEGREE AV BLOCK

Some, but not all, P waves are followed by QRS complexes (dropped beats). There are three types: Mobitz type I (Wenckebach phenomenon), Mobitz type II, and two-to-one (or higher) AV block.

Mobitz Type I
Description. The PR interval becomes progressively prolonged until one QRS complex is dropped completely (see Fig. 25-1).

Causes. Mobitz type I AV block appears in otherwise healthy children. Other causes are myocarditis, cardiomyopathy, myocardial infarction, CHD, cardiac surgery, and digitalis toxicity.

Significance. The block is at the level of the AV node. It usually does not progress to complete heart block.

Treatment. The underlying causes are treated.

Mobitz Type II
Description. The AV conduction is "all or none": AV conduction is either normal or is completely blocked (see Fig. 25-1).

Causes. Causes are the same as for Mobitz Type I.

350

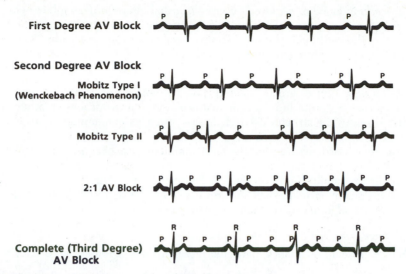

First Degree AV Block

Second Degree AV Block

Mobitz Type I
(Wenckebach Phenomenon)

Mobitz Type II

2:1 AV Block

Complete (Third Degree)
AV Block

FIG. 25–1.
Atriovenricular block. (From Park MK, Guntheroth WG: *How to read pediatric ECGs,*
ed 3, St. Louis, 1992, Mosby.)

Significance. The block is at the level of the bundle of His. It is more serious than type I block because it may progress to complete heart block.

Treatment. The underlying causes are treated. Prophylactic pacemaker therapy may be indicated.

Two-to-One (or Higher) AV Block
Description. A QRS complex follows every second, third, or fourth P wave resulting in 2:1, 3:1, or 4:1 AV block (see Fig. 25-1).

Causes. Causes are similar to those of other second-degree AV blocks.

Significance. The block is usually at the AV nodal level and occasionally at the level of the bundle of His. It occasionally may progress to complete heart block.

Treatment. The underlying causes are treated. Electrophysiologic studies may be necessary to determine the level of the block. Pacemaker therapy occasionally is necessary.

THIRD-DEGREE AV BLOCK
Description. In third-degree AV block (complete heart block), atrial and ventricular activities are entirely independent of one other (see Fig. 25-1).

1. The P waves are regular (regular PP interval) with a rate comparable to the heart rate of the patient's age.

2. The QRS complexes also are regular (regular R-R interval) with a rate much slower than the P rate.

3. In *congenital* complete heart block, the duration of the QRS complex is normal because the pacemaker for the ventricular complex is at a level higher than the bifurcation of the bundle of His. The ventricular rate is faster (50 to 80 beats/min) than that in the acquired type.

4. In *surgically* induced or *acquired* (after myocardial infarction) complete heart block, the QRS duration is prolonged, and the ventricular rate is in the range of 40 to 50 beats/min (idioventricular rhythm). The pacemaker for the ventricular complex is at a level below the bifurcation of the bundle of His.

Causes.

Congenital type. Causes are an isolated anomaly (without associated structural heart defect), maternal systemic lupus erythematosus, Sjögren syndrome or other connective tissue diseases, or structural heart disease, such as congenitally corrected TGA (L-TGA).

Acquired type. Cardiac surgery is the most common cause of acquired complete heart block in children. Other rare causes include severe myocarditis, Lyme carditis, acute rheumatic fever, mumps, diphtheria, cardiomyopathies, tumors in the conduction system, overdoses of certain drugs, and results of myocardial infarction. These causes produce either temporary or permanent heart block.

Significance.

1. CHF may develop in infancy, particularly when there are associated CHDs.

2. Patients with isolated congenital heart block who survive infancy usually are asymptomatic with normal growth and development for 5 to 10 years. Chest x-ray films may show cardiomegaly.

3. Syncopal attacks (Stokes-Adams attack) may occur with the heart rate below 40 to 45 beats/min. A sudden onset of acquired heart block may result in death, unless treatment maintains the heart rate in the acceptable range.

Treatment.

1. No treatment is required for children with asymptomatic congenital complete heart block.

2. Atropine or isoproterenol is indicated in symptomatic children and adults until temporary ventricular pacing is secured.

3. A temporary transvenous ventricular pacemaker is indicated in patients with heart block or is given prophylactically in patients who might develop heart block.

4. A permanent artificial ventricular pacemaker is indicated in patients with surgically induced heart block and in patients with congenital heart block who are symptomatic or have CHF (see Chapter 26). Dizziness or lightheadedness may be an early warning sign of the need of a pacemaker.

5. A variety of problems may arise after a pacemaker is placed in children. Stress placed on the lead system by the linear growth of the child, fracture of the lead system in a physically active child, electrode malfunction (scarring of the myocardium around the electrode, especially in infants), and the limited life span of the pulse generator require follow-up of children with artificial pacemakers.

26 / Pacemakers in Children

Physicians encounter an increasing number of children with either temporary or permanent pacemakers. Basic knowledge about the pacemaker and rhythm strip is essential in taking care of these children. This chapter presents examples of ECG rhythm strips from children with various types of pacemakers and elementary information about pacemaker therapy in children.

Temporary pacing is indicated for (1) advanced second-degree or complete heart block secondary to overdose of certain drugs, myocarditis, or myocardial infarction; (2) patients with a malfunctioning permanent pacemaker before it is replaced by a new permanent pacemaker; and (3) certain patients immediately after cardiac surgery.

Permanent cardiac pacemakers are indicated most frequently for symptomatic bradycardia (with syncope, dizziness, exercise intolerance, or CHF) and complete heart block, either congenital or acquired, including surgically induced heart block (see later discussion).

ECGS OF ARTIFICIAL CARDIAC PACEMAKERS

The need to recognize rhythm strips of artificial pacemakers has increased in recent years, especially in the intensive care and emergency room settings. The position and number of the pacemaker spikes on the ECG rhythm strip are used to recognize different types of pacemakers. Thus a pacemaker may be classified as a ventricular pacemaker, atrial pacemaker, or P-wave–triggered ventricular pacemaker. When the pacemaker stimulates the atrium, the resulting P wave demonstrates an abnormal P axis. When the pacemaker stimulates the ventricle, wide QRS complexes result. The ventricle that is stimulated (or the ventricle on which the pacemaker electrode is placed) can be identified by the morphology of the QRS complexes. With the pacing electrode on the RV, the QRS complex resembles an LBBB pattern; with the pacemaker placed on the LV, an RBBB pattern results.

Ventricular Pacemaker (Ventricular Sensing and Pacing)

This mode of pacing is recognized by vertical pacemaker spikes that initiate ventricular depolarization with wide QRS complexes (Fig. 26-1, *A*). The electronic spike has no fixed relationship with atrial activity (P wave). The pacemaker rate may be fixed (as in Fig. 26-1, *A*), or it may be on a demand (or standby) mode in which the pacemaker fires only after a long pause between the patient's own ventricular beats.

Atrial Pacemaker (Atrial Sensing and Pacing)

The atrial pacemaker is recognized by a pacemaker spike followed by an atrial complex; when AV conduction is normal, a QRS complex of normal duration follows (Fig. 26-1, *B*). This type of pacemaker is indicated in patients with sinus node dysfunction with bradycardia. When the patient has high-degree or complete AV block in addition to sinus node dysfunction, an additional ventricular pacemaker may be required (AV sequential pacemaker, not illustrated in Fig. 26-1). The AV sequential pacemaker is recognized by two sets of electronic spikes, one before the P wave and another before the wide QRS complex.

P-Wave–Triggered Ventricular Pacemaker (Atrial Sensing, Ventricular Pacing)

This pacemaker may be recognized by pacemaker spikes that follow the patient's own P waves at regular PR intervals and with wide QRS complexes (Fig. 26-1, *C*). The

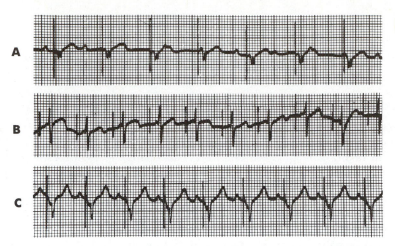

FIG. 26–1.
Examples of some artificial pacemakers. **A,** fixed-rate ventricular pacemaker. Note the regular rate of the electronic spikes with no relationship to the P waves. **B,** Atrial pacemaker. This tracing is from a 2-year-old child in whom extreme, symptomatic bradycardia developed following the Mustard operation. **C,** P-wave–triggered pacemaker. This tracing is from a child in whom surgically induced complete heart block developed after repair of TOF. (From Park MK, Guntheroth WG: *How to read pediatric ECGs,* ed 3, St Louis, 1992 Mosby.)

patient's own P waves are sensed and trigger a ventricular pacemaker after an electronically preset PR interval. This type of pacemaker is most physiologic and is indicated when the patient has an advanced AV block but a normal sinus mechanism. Advantages of this type of pacemaker are that the heart rate varies with physiologic need and the atrial contraction contributes to ventricular filling and improves cardiac output.

PACEMAKER THERAPY IN CHILDREN

Remarkable technologic advances recently have been made in pacemaker design and function. Surgical corrections of cardiac defects and their late sequela have increased the need for the pacemaker therapy in children. New pacemakers (physiologic pacemakers) are capable of closely mimicking normal cardiac rhythm, and most of them are small enough to be implanted in an infant.

A pacemaker is a device that delivers battery-supplied electrical stimuli over leads to electrodes in contact with the heart. The electrical leads are inserted either directly over the epicardium or transvenously. Electronic circuitry regulates the timing and characteristics of the stimuli. The power source usually is a lithium-iodine battery.

Indications

The indications for pacemaker implantation in children are continually evolving as the reliability of pacing systems improves and clinical experience increases. The box on p. 355 lists conditions for which pacemaker therapy is or is not indicated based on a Task Force of the American College of Cardiology and American Heart Association.

Bradycardia is the most common and noncontroversial indication for permanent pacemaker therapy in both children and adults. In children, significant bradycardia with syncope or near syncope results most commonly from surgery involving the atria (such as Senning's operation for TGA, surgery for ASD or TAPVR, and Fontan operation). Another noncontroversial indication is surgically acquired heart block that lasts more than 2 weeks after surgery. The risk of death from surgically acquired heart block is as

Indications and Nonindications for Pacemaker Therapy
_____

Conditions for which Permanent Pacemaker Implantation is Indicated

Second or third-degree AV block with symptomatic bradycardia
Advanced second or third-degree AV block with moderate to marked exercise intolerance
External ophthalmoplegia with bifascicular block (Kearns-Sayre syndrome)[*]
Sinus node dysfunction with symptomatic bradycardia
Congenital AV block with wide QRS escape rhythm or with block below the bundle of His
Advanced second or third-degree AV block persisting 10 to 14 days after cardiac surgery

Conditions for which Pacemakers are Unnecessary

Asymptomatic congenital heart block without profound bradycardia in relation to age
Asymptomatic type I second-degree AV block (Wenckebach phenomenon)
Transient, surgically induced AV block that returns to normal conduction in less than a week
Asymptomatic postoperative bifascicular block
Asymptomatic postoperative bifascicular block with first-degree AV block

Adapted from the Task Force of the American College of Cardiology and American Heart Association: *J Am Coll Cardiol* 18:1-13, 1991.
[*]Kearns-Sayre syndrome is a mitochondrial myopathy characterized by progressive external ophthalmoplegia, pigmentary retinopathy, and heart block. Cardiac involvement affects primarily the specialized conduction pathways. Myocardial involvement is rare; only occasionally one may see dilated cardiomyopathy with CHF. These patients develop gradual progressive impairment of infranodal conduction (left anterior hemiblock, RBBB, and complete heart block).
_____

high as 35% in unpaced patients. Most children with congenital heart block, especially those with additional structural heart defects, require pacemaker therapy.

In other conditions, permanent pacemakers frequently are used, but experts differ in their opinions. For example, some experts have advocated pacemaker implantation in children with congenital complete heart block if the awake ventricular rate drops below a certain level (<55 beats/min in infants, <45 to 50 beats/min in children, and <40 beats/min in adolescents) even without symptoms because CHF is predicted to develop and sudden death is more likely to occur with rates below these. In children with structural heart defects and bradycardia, a ventricular rate 10 beats/min higher than those listed here may be considered significant.

Before implanting a permanent pacemaker, the physician should establish the association of syncope (or other symptoms such as fatigue or palpitation) with bradycardia. Careful history taking and an ambulatory ECG and exercise test are important tools in confirming the need for pacemaker implantation.

1. Syncope or near syncope associated with bradycardia should be documented by a 24-hour ambulatory ECG.

2. Significant exercise intolerance associated with bradycardia should be confirmed by an exercise tolerance test.

3. A history of sleep disturbances (including restless sleep and nightmares) and poor school performance, especially late in the day, may be important.

Types of Pacing Devices

The North American Society of Pacing and Electrophysiology (NASPE) and the British Pacing and Electrophysiology Group (BPEG) devised a generic letter code to describe the types and functions of pacemakers. The letter in the first position identifies the chamber paced, and the second is the chamber sensed (A, atrium, V, ventricle). The third letter corresponds to the response of the pacemaker to an intrinsic cardiac event (I, inhibited; T, triggered). In any position, the letter O denotes the absence of response

TABLE 26–1.

NASPE/BPEG Generic Pacemaker Code

Position	I	II	III	IV	V
Category	Chamber(s) Paced	Chamber(s) Sensed	Response to Sensing	Programmability, Rate Modulation	Antiar-rhythmia Function
	O, None	O, None	O, None	O, None	O, None
	A, Atrium	A, Atrium	T, Triggered	P, Simple pro-grammable	P, Pacing (antitachy-arrhythmia)
	V, Ventricle	V, Ventricle	I, Inhibited	M, Multipro-grammable	S, Shock
	D, Dual (A + V)	D, Dual (A + V)	D, Dual (T + I)	C, Communi-cating	D, Dual (P + S)
				R, Rate mod-ulation	
Manufac-turer's designa-tion only	S, Single (A or V)	S, Single (A or V)			

Adapted from Bernstein AD, et al: The NASPE/BPEG generic pacemaker code for antibradyarrhythmia and adaptive-rate pacing and antitachyarrhythmia device, *PACE*, 10:794-499, 1987.)

(Table 26-1). The last two letters describe newer functions such as programmability, telemetry, rate modulation, and antitachycardia pacing capability. Examples are:

1. A VOO device provides ventricular pacing, no sensing, and no response.

2. A VVI device is ventricle stimulated and ventricle sensed; it inhibits paced output if endogenous ventricular activity occurs (thus preventing competition with native QRS activity).

3. An AAI device paces and senses the atrium and is inhibited by atrial activity.

4. A DDD device is a dual-chamber pacemaker that is capable of pacing either chamber, sensing activity in either chamber, and either triggering or inhibiting paced output (with resulting AV synchrony).

Selection of Pacing Mode

The pacemaker choice is based on several factors, including the presence or absence of underlying cardiac disease, the size of the patient, and the relevant hemodynamic factors (including the need for atrial contribution in cardiac output).

1. The patient who has sinus node dysfunction but an intact AV node function may receive an atrial pacemaker (without dual-chamber pacing) or a ventricular pacemaker.

2. If the sinus node and AV node both are dysfunctional, a dual-chamber device is implanted.

Battery, Leads, and Route

Lithium anode batteries now are used almost exclusively. The most widely used type of lithium battery is the lithium iodide. Battery longevity depends on several factors, such as battery size, stimulation frequency, and output per stimulation. Battery life varies from 3 years for a dual-chamber pacemaker used in a small child to 15 years for a large single-chamber device needed infrequently.

There are two types of leads, unipolar and biopolar. The unipolar lead (in which the tip of the lead is the negative pole and the pacemaker itself is the positive pole) has the advantages of a smaller size and a larger sensing circuit, which amplifies low-voltage P waves. The bipolar lead (which possesses a tip electrode [−] and a ring electrode [+] near the end of the pacing catheter) can screen pectoral muscle "noise", has a lower likelihood of external muscle stimulation, and can function even if the pacemaker is out of contact with the body.

Transvenous implantation is the method of choice and is performed on the side contralateral to the dominant hand. Transvenous implantation has several advantages over epicardial implantation: Both atrial and ventricular capture threshold generally are lower, and pacing problems are significantly fewer than with the epicardial implantation. The epicardial implantation is performed through a xyphoid approach and is chosen when a transvenous implantation is precluded: when the patient is a neonate or a small infant (<10 kg), and when the transvenous approach is not possible (after Fontan operation or SVC obstruction).

27 / ST-Segment and T-Wave Changes

ECG changes involving the ST segment and the T wave are common in adults but relatively rare in children. This is because of a high incidence of ischemic heart disease, bundle branch blocks, myocardial infarction, and other myocardial disorders in adults.

NONPATHOLOGIC ST-SEGMENT SHIFT

Not all ST-segment shifts are abnormal. Slight shift of the ST segment is common in normal children. Elevation or depression of up to 1 mm in the limb leads and up to 2 mm in the precordial leads is within normal limits.

Two common types of nonpathologic ST-segment shift are J-depression and early repolarization. The T vector remains normal in these conditions.

J-Depression

J-depression is a shift of the junction between the QRS and the ST segment (J-point) without sustained ST-segment depression (Fig. 27-1, A). It is a normal ST-segment shift. The J-depression is seen more often in the precordial leads than in the limb leads (and therefore is best shown in the ECG recorded during an exercise test). Fig. 27-2 shows both the J-depression (seen in most of the precordial leads) and early repolarization (seen in the limb leads, see later discussion).

Early Repolarization

In early repolarization, all leads with upright T waves have elevated ST segments, and leads with inverted T waves have depressed ST segments (see Fig. 27-2). The T vector remains normal. This condition, seen in healthy adolescents and young adults, resembles the ST-segment shift seen in acute pericarditis; in the former, the ST segment is stable, and in the latter, the ST segment returns to the isoelectric line.

PATHOLOGIC ST-SEGMENT SHIFT

Abnormal shifts of the ST segment often are accompanied by T-wave inversion. A pathologic ST-segment shift assumes one of the following two forms:

1. Downward slant followed by a diphasic or inverted T wave (see Fig. 27-1, B).

2. Horizontal elevation or depression sustained for over 0.08 second (see Fig. 27,1 C).

Pathologic ST-segment shifts are seen in LVH or RVH with "strain" (see Chapter 3); digitalis effect (see Chap. 30); pericarditis, including postoperative state; myocarditis; myocardial infarction; and some electrolyte disturbances (hypokalemia and hyperkalemia).

T-wave changes usually are associated with the previously mentioned conditions. Other conditions associated with T-wave changes with or without ST-segment shift, discussed in previous chapters, include bundle branch block and ventricular arrhythmias. Only conditions not covered previously are discussed briefly in this chapter.

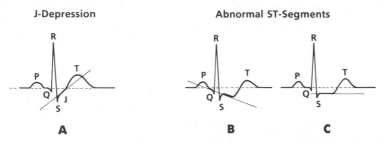

J-Depression

Abnormal ST-Segments

A

B

C

FIG. 27–1.
Nonpathologic (nonischemic) and pathologic (ischemic) ST-segment and T-wave
changes. **A,** characteristic nonischemic ST-segment change called *J-depression;* note
that the ST slope is upward. **B** and **C,** Examples of pathologic ST-segment changes;
note that the downward slope of the ST-segment **(B)** or the horizontal segment is
sustained **(C).** (From Park MK, Guntheroth WG: *How to read pediatric ECGs,* ed 3, St
Louis, 1992, Mosby.)

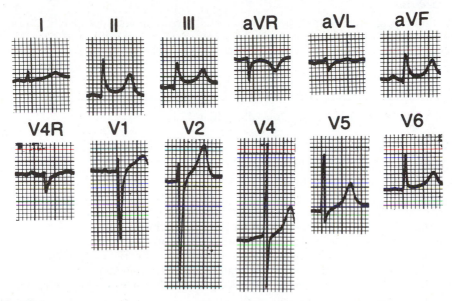

FIG. 27–2.
Tracing from a healthy 16-year-old boy that exhibits early repolarization and
J-depression. The ST-segment is shifted toward the direction of the T wave and is most
marked in II, III, and aVF. J-depression is seen in most of the precordial leads.

Pericarditis

The ECG changes seen in pericarditis are the results of subepicardial myocardial
damage and/or pericardial effusion and consist of the following:

1. Pericardial effusion may produce low QRS voltages (QRS voltages <5mm in every
   one of the limb leads).

2. Subepicardial myocardial damage produces the following time-dependent changes
   in the ST segment and T wave (Fig. 27-3):

   a. ST-segment elevation occurs in the leads representing the LV.

   b. The ST-segment shift returns to normal within 2 to 3 days.

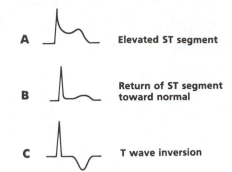

FIG. 27–3.
Time-dependent changes of the ST segment and T wave in pericarditis. (From Park MK, Guntheroth WG: *How to read pediatric ECGs,* ed 3, St Louis, 1992, Mosby.)

      c. T-wave inversion (with isoelectric ST segment) occurs 2 to 4 weeks after the onset of pericarditis.

Myocarditis

ECG findings of myocarditis (rheumatic or viral) are relatively nonspecific and may include changes in all phases of the cardiac cycle. Various arrhythmias also have been associated with myocarditis. One or more of the following changes are seen in myocarditis:

1. Disturbances in AV conduction (first- or second-degree AV block)

2. Low QRS voltages ($\leq$ 5 mm in all six limb leads)

3. Decreased amplitude of the T wave

4. Prolongation of the QT interval

5. Arrhythmias or ectopic beats

Myocardial Infarction

Myocardial infarction is relatively rate in infants and children, but correctly diagnosing the condition is important for the proper care of children. All conditions that have been associated with myocardial infarction in adults have been described as causing myocardial infarction in children, such as atherosclerosis, inflammatory disease of the myocardium, lupus erythematosus, syphilis, polyarteritis nodosa, hypertension, and diabetes mellitus. Uncommon causes of myocardial infarction in pediatric patients include anomalous origin of the left coronary artery from the PA, endocardial fibroelastosis, coronary artery embolization resulting from infective endocarditis or from diagnostic procedures performed in the left side of the heart, and inadvertent surgical interruption of the coronary artery during cardiac surgery. In recent years, early and late sequelae of Kawasaki's disease, surgical complications of the arterial switch operation for TGA, and dilated cardiomyopathy have emerged as important causes of myocardial infarction in the pediatric population.

    The ECG findings of adult myocardial infarction are time dependent and are illustrated in Fig. 27-4. Changes seen during the hyperacute phase are short lived. The more common ECG findings are those of the early evolving phase. These consist of pathologic Q waves (abnormally deep and abnormally wide), ST-segment elevation, and T-wave inversion. The duration of the Q wave is 0.04 second or greater in the adult, and it should be at least 0.03 second in children. During the next few weeks, the elevated ST segment gradually returns toward the baseline, but inverted T waves persist (late evolving phase). The pathologic Q waves persist for years after myocardial infarction (see Fig. 27-4). Leads that show these abnormalities vary with the location of the infarction and are summarized in Table 27-1.

TABLE 27–1.

Leads Showing Abnormal ECG Findings in Myocardial Infarction

	Limb Leads	Precordial Leads
Lateral	I, aVL	V5, V6
Anterior		V1, V2, V3
Anterolateral	I, aVL	V2-V6
Diaphragmatic	II, III, aVF	
Posterior		V1-V3*

*None of the leads is oriented toward the posterior surface of the heart. Therefore in posterior infarction, changes that would have been present in the posterior surface leads are seen in the anterior leads as a mirror image (e.g., tall and slightly wide R waves in V1 and V2, and tall and wide symmetric T waves in V1 and V2).

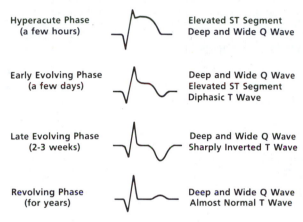

FIG. 27–4.

Sequential changes of the ST segment and T wave in myocardial infarction. (From Park MK, Guntheroth WG: *How to read pediatric ECGs,* ed 3, St Louis, 1992, Mosby.)

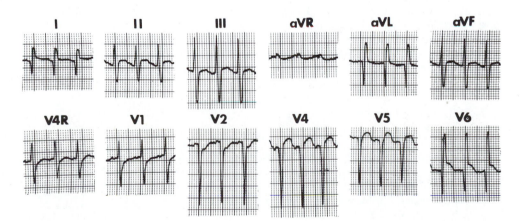

FIG. 27–5.

Tracing from a 2-month-old infant who has anomalous origin of the left coronary artery from the PA. An abnormally deep and wide Q wave (0.04 second) seen in I, aVL and V6 and a QS pattern seen in V2 through V6 are characteristic of anterolateral myocardial infarction.

In most pediatric patients with myocardial infarction the time of onset is not clearly known, and the evolution of the different phases described is difficult to document. Frequent ECG findings in children with acute myocardial infarction include the following (Towbin JA et al: *Am J Cardiol* 69:1545, 1992):

1. Wide Q waves (>0.035 second) with or without Q-wave notching

2. ST-segment elevation (>2 mm)

3. Prolongation of QTc interval (>0.44 second) with accompanying abnormal Q waves

The width of the Q wave is more important than the depth, the depth of the Q wave varies widely in normal children (see Table 3-6).

Fig. 27-5 is an ECG of myocardial infarction in an infant with anomalous origin of the left coronary artery from the PA. The most important abnormality is the presence of a deep and wide Q wave (0.04 second) in I, aVL, and V6. A QS pattern appears in V2 through V5, indicating anterolateral myocardial infarction (see Table 27-1).

ELECTROLYTE DISTURBANCES

Two important serum electrolytes that produce ECG changes are calcium and potassium. Although T-wave changes are not seen with hypocalcemia and hypercalcemia, these conditions are discussed because they change the relative position of the T wave.

Calcium

Calcium ion affects the duration of the ST segment without producing ST-segment shift or changes in the T vector. Hypocalcemia prolongs the ST segment and as a result prolongs the QTc interval (Fig. 27-6). The T-wave duration remains normal. Hypercalcemia shortens the ST segment without affecting the T wave, resulting in shortening of the QTc interval (see Fig. 27-6).

Potassium

Hypokalemia produces one of the least specific ECG changes. When the serum potassium level is below 2.5 mEq/L, ECG changes consist of a prominent U wave with apparent prolongation of the QTc, flat or diphasic T waves, and ST-segment depression (Fig. 27-7). With further lowering of serum potassium levels, the PR interval becomes prolonged, and sinoatrial block may occur.

The earliest ECG abnormality seen in hyperkalemia is a tall, peaked, symmetric T wave with a narrow base, the so called tented T wave. A progressive increase in the serum potassium level (hyperkalemia) produces the following ECG changes, usually seen best in II and III and the LPL:

1. Tall, tented T waves

2. Prolongation of QRS duration (intraventricular block)

3. Prolongation of the PR interval (first-degree AV block)

4. Disappearance of the P wave

5. Wide, bizarre diphasic QRS complex ("sine wave")

6. Eventual asystole

ECG changes associated with a progressive increase in the serum potassium level are shown in Fig. 27-7. With a further increase in serum potassium levels, the patient may develop SA block, second-degree AV block (either Mobitz type I or II), and accelerated junctional or ventricular escape rhythm. Severe hyperkalemia may result in either ventricular fibrillation or arrest.

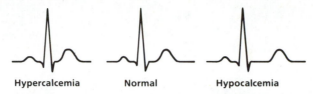

FIG. 27–6.
ECG findings of hypercalcemia and hypocalcemia. Hypercalcemia shortens and hypocalcemia lengthens the ST segment. (From Park MK, Guntheroth WG: *How to read pediatric ECGs,* ed 3, St Louis, 1992, Mosby.)

SERUM K

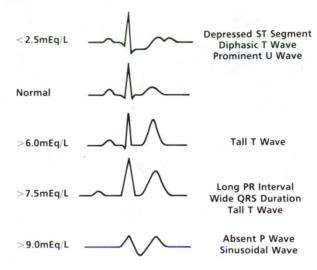

FIG. 27–7.
ECG findings of hypokalemia and hyperkalemia. (From Park MK, Guntheroth WG: *How to read pediatric ECGs,* ed 3, St Louis, 1992, Mosby.)

PART VII

Neonatal Cardiac Problems

The basic tools in the routine evaluation of cardiac patients (history, physical examination, ECGs, chest x-ray films, and flow diagrams), presented in Part I, and the pathophysiology of CHDs, presented in Part III, pertain primarily to older infants and children. In the fetal and perinatal period, however, a unique circulatory physiology and a rapidly changing cardiovascular physiology make physical findings, chest x-ray studies, and ECGs of limited value in the evaluation of the cardiovascular system. Furthermore, these findings change rapidly in the newborn. Thus a noninvasive special tool, such as echo with Doppler examination, plays a vital role in the evaluation of the newborn.

This section presents features unique to the cardiovascular evaluation of the newborn, including the physical examination and the interpretation of the ECG and chest x-ray films. This section also explores topics such as heart murmurs in the newborn, the detection and work-up for cyanosis in the newborn, heart failure in the newborn period, and arrhythmias of the newborn.

28 / Special Features In Cardiac Evaluation of The Newborn

Newborn infants have RV dominance with a thick RV wall and elevated PVR secondary to a thick medial layer of the pulmonary arterioles. The thick PA smooth muscle gradually becomes thinner and by 6 to 8 weeks of age resembles that of the adult. Most perinatal changes in hemodynamics are related to the normal evolution (thinning) of the pulmonary vascular smooth muscle, resulting in a gradual fall in the PVR and a loss of RV dominance of the newborn (see Chapter 8). Premature infants in general have less RV dominance and a lower PVR than full-term neonates, adding variability to this generalization.

This chapter briefly reviews some important aspects of normal and abnormal findings in the physical examination, ECG, and chest x-ray studies of the newborn.

PHYSICAL EXAMINATION
Normal Physical Findings
The following physical findings are common to normal newborn infants:

1. The heart rate generally is faster in the newborn than in older children and adults (the newborn rate usually is over 100 beats/min, with the normal range 70 to 180 beats/min)

2. A varying degree of acrocyanosis is the rule rather than the exception.

3. Mild arterial desaturation with arterial Po_2 as low as 60 mm Hg is not unusual in an otherwise normal neonate. This may be caused by an intrapulmonary shunt through an as-yet unexpanded portion of the lungs or by a RA-to-LA shunt through a PFO.

4. The RV is relatively hyperactive, with the PMI at the LLSB rather than at the apex.

5. The S2 may be single in the first days of life.

6. An ejection click (representing pulmonary hypertension) occasionally is heard in the first hours of life.

7. The newborn may have an innocent heart murmur. The most common innocent heart murmur in this age group is the pulmonary flow murmur of the newborn. This murmur is a grade 1-2/6 systolic ejection murmur and characteristically radiates well to the sides and the back of the chest (see Chapter 29).

8. Peripheral pulses are easily palpable in all extremities, including the foot, in *every* normal infant.

Premature infants have additional features that the physician must remember during the examination:

1. The prevalence and the loudness of the pulmonary flow murmur are greater in

premature than in full-term infants because of the thin chest walls of premature infants.

2. PDA murmur is more common in premature infants.

3. The peripheral pulses normally appear to be bounding because of the normal lack of subcutaneous tissue. One must become familiar with the normal volume of peripheral pulses in premature infants.

Abnormal Physical Findings

The following abnormal physical findings suggest cardiac malformations (see Chapter 29 for further discussion). Repeated examination is important because physical findings change rapidly in normal infants as well as in infants with cardiac problems:

1. Cyanosis, particularly when it does not improve with oxygen administration, suggests a cardiac abnormality.

2. Decreased or absent peripheral pulses in the lower extremities suggest COA. Generally weak peripheral pulses suggest HLHS or circulatory shock. Bounding peripheral pulses suggest aortic run-off lesions, such as PDA or persistent truncus arteriosus.

3. Tachypnea of greater than 60 per minute with or without retraction suggests a cardiac abnormality.

4. Hepatomegaly may suggest a heart defect. A midline liver suggests asplenia or polysplenia syndrome.

5. A heart murmur may be a presenting sign of CHD (see Chapter 29). However, innocent murmurs, such as the pulmonary flow murmur of the newborn, are much more frequent than pathologic murmurs.

6. Irregular rhythm and abnormal heart rate (see Chapters 24 and 29) suggest a cardiac abnormality.

BLOOD PRESSURE MEASUREMENTS

Although blood pressure is not routinely measured in the normal newborn, blood pressure must be measured when one suspects COA, hypertension, or hypotension. The conventional auscultatory method is difficult to apply in the newborn. Therefore electronic devices measure newborns' blood pressures.

Indirect Blood Pressure Methods

Most reported normal blood pressure levels in the newborn are obtained by either Doppler ultrasound or the oscillometric (Dinamap) method. The accuracy of the Doppler ultrasound and the oscillometric methods has been demonstrated in the full-term newborn. Table 28-1 shows selected normative blood pressure levels by these two methods. A blood pressure cuff with a width approximately 50% of the circumference of the extremity is best for both the Doppler and Dinamap methods. Although the accuracy of the oscillometric device in the premature infant is debatable, normative blood pressure levels for the very-low-birth-weight group have been published (Table 28-2).

Direct Blood Pressure Measurements

Many sick full-term and premature newborns require intraarterial recording of blood pressures, but normative blood pressure levels measured directly in newborns of varying ages are not available because of the invasive nature of the measurement. Only direct normative blood pressure levels reported in the newborn are those obtained in the first 24 hours of life (Table 28-3). Blood pressure increases after the first days of life, and these values will give at least some sign of the adequacy of the blood pressure beyond the first day.

TABLE 28–1.

Normative Blood Pressure Values in the Newborn by Doppler and Oscillometric Methods*

Authors	< 6 Days	4 or 6 Weeks	Methods
DeSwiet et al (1980)†	77 ± 10/no diastolic (N = 92)	96 ± 11/no diastolic (N = 594)	Doppler ultrasound
Park et al (1987, 1989)‡	65 ± 8/41 ± 6 MAP: 50 ± 7 (N = 219)	92 ± 8/59 ± 7 MAP: 72 ± 9 (N = 60)	Dinamap oscillometric method

MAP, Mean arterial pressure ± SD (mm Hg); *N*, number of patients.
*Systolic ± SD/Diastolic ± SD (mm Hg).
†De Swiet M et al: *Pediatrics* 65:1028-1035, 1980.
‡Park MK et al: *Pediatrics* 83:240-243, 1989, and *Pediatrics* 79:907-914, 1987.

TABLE 28–2.

Dinamap BP Levels (2 SD) in Very-Low-Birth-Weight Infants (< 1500 g) While Awake*

	Day 1	Day 4	3 Weeks	4 Weeks
Systolic	68 (31)	78 (37)	76 (32)	78 (34)
Diastolic	44 (29)	53 (32)	48 (32)	49 (31)
MAP	58 (32)	65 (35)	60 (32)	65 (34)

*In mm Hg. *BP*, Blood pressure; *SD*, standard deviation; *MAP*, mean arterial pressure.
Adapted from Tan KL: *J Pediatr* 112:266-270, 1988.

TABLE 28–3.

Mean Direct Aortic Pressure (and 95% Confidence Limits) in the First 24 Hours of Life

| Pressure | Weight | | | |
	1000 g	2000 g	3000 g	4000 g
Systolic	49 (39-59)	54 (42-65)	61 (49-72)	69 (58-81)
Diastolic	26 (16-36)	31 (22-41)	36 (27-47)	41 (31-50)
MAP	35 (25-44)	41 (31-50)	48 (37-55)	52 (42-61)

MAP, Mean arterial pressure.
Adapted from Versmold HT et al: *Pediatrics* 67:607-613, 1981.

ELECTROCARDIOGRAPHY

Normal Electrocardiography

The normal ECG of a newborn is different from that of a child or an adult and usually shows the following (also see Chapter 3):

1. Sinus tachycardia with a rate as high as 180 beats/min

2. Rightward deviation of the QRS axis with a mean of +125 degrees and a maximum of +180 degrees

3. Relatively small voltages of the QRS complex and the T wave

4. RV dominance with tall R waves in the RPLs (V4R, V1, and V2)

5. Occasional q waves in V1 (seen in about 10% of normal newborns)

6. Benign arrhythmias (see section on ambulatory electrocardiography in Chapter 6).

In interpreting neonatal ECGs, the clinician must use normal standards for the newborn rather than for older children or adults (see Chapter 3 for normal standards).

Abnormal Electrocardiography

An ECG may be abnormal because of an abnormal P axis, abnormal QRS axis, hypertrophy of the ventricles or atria, ventricular conduction disturbances, or arrhythmias. Because of the wide ranges of normal values, many newborn infants with significant CHDs may have normal ECGs for their age. Arrrhythmias in the newborn are discussed in Chapter 29.

P axis.

1. A P axis in the right lower quadrant (90 to 180 degrees) suggests atrial situs inversus, asplenia syndrome, or incorrectly placed ECG electrodes.

2. A superior P axis suggests ectopic atrial rhythm or polysplenia syndrome.

QRS axis.

1. A superiorly oriented QRS axis between 0 and −150 degrees (left anterior hemiblock) suggests ECD (including splenic syndromes) or tricuspid atresia.

2. A QRS axis less than +30 degrees is abnormal and indicates LAD for the patient's age. The axis between +30 and +60 degrees is unusual and indicates relative LAD. LAD may be seen with LVH.

3. A QRS axis greater than +180 degrees (in the range of −150 to −180 degrees) may indicate RAD. It may occur with RVH or RBBB.

Left ventricular hypertrophy.

1. LAD or relative LAD < +60 degrees) for the newborn suggests LVH.

2. R/S progression in the precordial leads resemble adult R/S progression.

3. QRS voltages demonstrate abnormal leftward and posterior forces or abnormal inferior forces for the patient's age (see Chapter 3 for normal data).

Right ventricular hypertrophy. RVH is difficult to diagnose because of the normal dominance of the RV at this age. However, the following are clues to RVH in the newborn:

1. S waves in I that are 12 mm or greater.

2. Pure R waves (with no S waves) in V1 that are greater than 10 mm.

3. R waves in V1 that are greater than 25 mm, or R waves in aVR that are greater than 8 mm.

4. A qR pattern seen in V1 (this also is seen in 10% of normal newborns).

5. Upright T waves seen in V1 after 3 days of age.

6. RAD with the QRS axis greater than +180 degrees.

Atrial hypertrophy.

1. RAH is revealed by a P-wave amplitude greater than 3 mm in any lead.

2. LAH is revealed by a P-wave duration of 0.08 second or greater (usually with notched P waves in the limb leads and biphasic P waves in V1).

Ventricular conduction disturbances. Ventricular conduction disturbances (e.g., RBBB, LBBB, WPW syndrome) are revealed by a QRS duration of 0.07 second or greater (not ≤ 0.1 second as in the adult). The QRS duration increases with age in normal people (see Table 3-3).

1. RBBB may be associated with Ebstein's anomaly, COA in infants, or ASD. It

sometimes may be seen in otherwise normal neonates. RBBB frequently is misinterpreted as RVH.

2. LBBB is extremely rare in the newborn.

3. Intraventricular block (with a widening of the QRS complex throughout the QRS duration) is more significant than RBBB. It often is associated with significant metabolic abnormalities such as hypoxia, acidosis, hyperkalemia, and diffuse myocardial disease. It may be seen with CHD or as a terminal ECG in a dying patient.

4. WPW syndrome may be an isolated finding or may be associated with CHD, such as Ebstein's anomaly or L-TGA. It is a frequent cause of SVT. In patients with the WPW syndrome, QRS voltages may be large without ventricular hypertrophy (see section on WPW syndrome in Chapter 3).

CHEST ROENTGENOGRAPHY

Normal Chest X-Ray Films

The cardiothoracic ratio of normal newborn infants is greater than 0.5, the normal value in older children and adults. No single figure can be given as a normal cardiothoracic ratio in neonates because multiple variables contribute to an abnormal cardiothoracic ratio. Inadequate inspiratory expansion of the lungs and the large thymic shadow are important contributors to this difficulty. Therefore the evaluation of the heart size should consider the degree of inspiration, judged from the level of the diaphragm.

Thymic shadow may have many different shapes. It may show a classic "sail" sign (see Fig. 4-10) or may have undulant or smooth borders on the upper mediastinum, either unilaterally or bilaterally. The thymus occupies anterosuperior mediastinal space, and the lateral view of the chest x-ray films helps in evaluating the thymus.

The cardiac silhouette is not always as well defined in neonates as in older children. The MPA often does not form a prominence in the left middle cardiac border. The lateral chest x-ray film is sensitive to LV enlargement.

The evaluation of PVMs in the neonate poses a problem similar to that described for cardiac size and silhouette. Increased vascularity is not always apparent in the chest x-ray film when the PBF is large. Distinguishing between increased PBF and pulmonary venous congestion often is difficult. Reduced PBF usually is easier to detect and indicates serious cyanotic CHDs.

Abnormal Chest X-Ray Films

A cardiac problem is suggested by abnormal size, position, or silhouette of the heart, by an abnormal shape or position of the liver, or by increased or decreased pulmonary vascularity on chest x-ray films.

Heart size. Unfortunately, there are no reliable criteria for identifying cardiomegaly in newborn infants. The cardiothoracic ratio, which is useful in identifying cardiomegaly in older children and adults (see Fig. 4-1), is of limited value because the ratio of normal neonates usually is greater than 0.5. Many serious CHDs that eventually result in cardiomegaly may show a normal heart size in the newborn period. Unequivocal cardiomegaly may be due to the following:

1. CHDs such as VSD, PDA, TGA, Ebstein's anomaly, and HLHS

2. Myocarditis or cardiomyopathy

3. Pericardial effusion

4. Metabolic disturbances, such as hypoglycemia, severe hypoxemia, and acidosis

5. Overhydration or overtransfusion

In the newborn who is intubated and on a ventilator, the heart size is greatly influenced by the ventilator setting; that is, a premature infant with a large-shunt PDA may have a normal-sized heart on x-ray films if the ventilator settings, especially the positive end-expiratory pressure, are high.

Abnormal cardiac silhouette. An abnormal heart shape may help identify the correct diagnosis. Three examples follow:

1. The "boot-shaped" heart (coeur en sabot) is seen in TOF and tricuspid atresia (see Figs. 4-3 and 14-18).

2. The "egg-shaped" heart with a narrow waist may be seen in TGA (see Figs. 4-3 and 14-2).

3. A large globular heart is seen with Ebstein's anomaly.

Dextrocardia or mesocardia. When the heart is located predominantly in the right side of the chest (dextrocardia) or in the midline of the thorax (mesocardia), the segmental approach of van Praagh should be used to deduce the nature of the segmental relationship of the atria and ventricles (refer to section on chamber localization in Chapter 16).

Four common situations in which the heart is located in the right side of the chest or in the midline follow (see Fig. 16-5):

1. Situs inversus totalis with normal heart

2. Hypoplasia of the right lung with a rightward displacement of a normally formed heart (dextroversion)

3. Complex cyanotic heart defect including atrial or ventricular inversion

4. Asplenia or polysplenia syndrome with a midline liver

Situs of abdominal viscera. The location of the liver or the stomach bubble and the shape of the liver provide important clues to the nature of the cardiac defect.

1. A midline liver indicates asplenia or polysplenia syndrome with complex cyanotic CHD (Fig. 28-1).

2. A left-sided liver (or right-sided stomach bubble) with the heart in the right side of the chest indicates situs inversus totalis with a mirror-image dextrocardia (normal).

3. The liver and the cardiac apex on the same side usually suggest complex cardiac defects.

Pulmonary vascular markings. The evaluation of PVMs is an integral part of the interpretation of cardiac x-ray films.

1. Increased pulmonary vascularity in a cyanotic infant suggests TGA, persistent truncus arteriosus, or single ventricle. In an acyanotic newborn infant, increased pulmonary vascularity suggests VSD, PDA, or ECD.

2. Decreased pulmonary vascularity with "black" lung fields suggests critical cyanotic heart defects with decreased PBF, such as pulmonary atresia, tricuspid atresia, or TOF with pulmonary atresia. The heart size usually is normal in these conditions. Decreased PVMs with marked cardiomegaly are seen in Ebstein's anomaly.

3. A "ground-glass" appearance or a reticulated pattern of lung fields is characteristic of pulmonary venous obstruction and suggests HLHS (see Fig. 29-3) or TAPVR with obstruction.

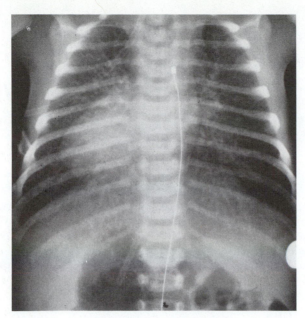

FIG. 28–1.
An x-ray film of the chest and upper abdomen of a newborn infant with polysplenia syndrome. Note a symmetric liver ("midline liver"), a stomach bubble in the midline, dextrocardia, and increased pulmonary vascularity.

29 / Manifestations of Cardiac Problems in The Newborn

Most cardiology consultations are requested during the newborn period because of one or more of these reasons: (1) a heart murmur; (2) cyanosis, or inability to raise oxygen saturation to normal ranges with administration of oxygen; (3) suspected CHF; (4) arrhythmias; (5) abnormal chest x-ray findings; and (6) abnormal ECG findings. The first four conditions are discussed in this chapter. Abnormal ECG and chest x-ray findings are discussed in Chapter 28.

HEART MURMURS

Innocent Heart Murmurs

As in older infants and children, not all heart murmurs in the neonatal period are pathologic. Researchers have reported that more than 50% of full-term newborn infants who were examined frequently were found to have an innocent systolic murmur at some time during the first week of life. The prevalence of heart murmur in premature infants is even higher than in full-term infants. Four common innocent murmurs in the newborn period are: (1) pulmonary flow murmur of the newborn; (2) transient systolic murmur of PDA; (3) transient systolic murmur of TR; and (4) vibratory innocent systolic murmur.

1. Pulmonary flow murmur of the newborn is probably the most common heart murmur in the newborn infant, more common in premature and small for gestational age infants than in full-term infants. It is heard best at the ULSB and transmits well to both sides of the chest, the axillae, and the back. The murmur is soft, usually not louder than a grade 2/6 in intensity. The ECG and chest x-ray films are normal. The murmur is not transient, lasting for weeks or months but usually disappears by 6 months of age (see Chapter 2 for the mechanism of the murmur).

2. Transient systolic murmur of PDA is audible at the ULSB and in the left infraclavicular area on the first day, and it usually disappears shortly thereafter. It is believed to originate from a closing ductus arteriosus. It is a grade 2/6 or less in intensity. It usually is only systolic and crescendic up to the S2.

3. Transient systolic murmur of TR is indistinguishable from that of VSD in that it is regurgitant (starting with the S1) and is maximally audible at the LLSB. It disappears, however, in a day or two. It is believed that a minimal tricuspid valve abnormality produces regurgitation in the presence of high PVR (and high RV pressure), but the regurgitation disappears as the PVR falls. Therefore this murmur is more common in infants who had fetal distress or neonatal asphyxia, because they tend to maintain high PVR for a longer period.

4. Vibratory innocent murmur is a counterpart of Still's murmur in older children (see also section on innocent heart murmur in Chapter 2). It is best audible at the LLSB or near the apex and has a low-frequency, vibratory quality. Therefore differentiation of this murmur from that of VSD may be difficult, but this murmur is an ejection type, rather than a regurgitant type.

374

Pathologic Heart Murmurs

Most pathologic murmurs should be audible during the first month of life, with the exception of an ASD. However, the time of appearance of a heart murmur depends on the nature of the defect.

1. Heart murmurs of stenotic lesions (e.g., AS, PS, COA) are audible immediately after birth and persist, because these murmurs are not affected by the level of PVR.

2. Heart murmurs of left-to-right shunt lesions that depend on the reduction of PVR (dependent shunt) may appear later. For example, a heart murmur of a small VSD (with which the reduction of the PVR is normal) becomes audible shortly after birth, whereas the heart murmur of a large VSD may not become audible until the PVR falls significantly. The appearance of a murmur of large VSD may be delayed until 1 to 2 weeks of age.

3. The continuous murmur of a large PDA may not appear for 2 to 3 weeks. Instead, it is a crescendo systolic murmur with slight or no diastolic component; it is best audible at the left infraclavicular area.

4. The murmur of an ASD appears late in infancy with insidious onset. It becomes loud after a year or two, when the distensibility of the RV becomes maximal. A newborn or a small infant with a large ASD may not have a heart murmur.

Even in the absence of a heart murmur, a newborn infant may have a serious heart defect that requires immediate attention (e.g., severe cyanotic heart defect, such as TGA or pulmonary atresia with a closing PDA). Infants who are in severe CHF may not have a loud murmur until the myocardial function is improved through anticongestive measures.

CYANOSIS IN THE NEWBORN

Most patients with cyanotic heart disease are cyanotic at birth. Early detection of cyanosis in a newborn is crucial. One must look for cyanosis on many parts of the body, including the lips, fingernails, toenails, oral mucous membrane, conjunctivas, and the tip of the nose. The tip of the tongue is a good place to look for cyanosis; it is not affected by race or ethnic background, and the circulation is not sluggish as in the peripheral parts of the body. Cyanosis usually is recognized when the arterial oxygen saturation is 85% or lower. Because the hemoglobin level often is high and the peripheral circulation often is sluggish in the newborn, cyanosis may occur at an oxygen saturation as high as 90% in this age group.

When in doubt, one should obtain arterial oxygen saturation by a pulse oximeter or arterial Po_2 by blood gas determination to confirm or rule out central cyanosis. Normal Po_2 in a 1-day-old infant may be as low as 60 mm Hg. In certain cyanotic CHD with increased PBF the Po_2 may be over 60 mm Hg, and the Po_2 usually does not show a large increase with a hyperoxitest (see later discussion). An arterial oxygen saturation of 90% and above does not completely rule out a cyanotic heart defect. An arterial oxygen saturation of 90% can be seen with a Po_2 of 45 to 50 mm Hg in the newborn because of the normally leftward oxygen hemoglobin dissociation curve (Fig. 29-1). In older children and adults, the Po_2 of 60 to 65 mm Hg is needed to obtain the same level of arterial oxygen saturation.

Etiology

Clinical cyanosis associated with normal arterial oxygen saturation (or normal arterial Po_2) is called *peripheral cyanosis*. Peripheral cyanosis is seen with acrocyanosis or in exposure to cold and has no clinical significance. Central cyanosis associated with decreased arterial oxygen saturation is significant and may be due to central nervous system depression, lung diseases, or cyanotic CHDs. Table 29-1 lists some of the characteristic clinical findings of each type of cyanosis.

TABLE 29–1.
Causes and Clinical Findings of Central Cyanosis

Central Nervous System Depression
Causes
  Perinatal asphyxia
  Heavy maternal sedation
  Intrauterine fetal distress
Findings
  Shallow irregular respiration
  Poor muscle tone
  Cyanosis that disappears when stimulated or oxygen is given to the patient

Pulmonary Disease
Causes
  Parenchymal lung disease (e.g., hyaline membrane disease, atelectasis)
  Pneumothorax or pleural effusion
  Diaphragmatic hernia
  PPHN (or persistent fetal circulation syndrome)
Findings
  Tachypnea and respiratory distress with retraction and expiratory grunting
  Rales and/or decreased breath sounds on auscultation
  Chest x-ray film that may reveal causes (as listed previously)
  Oxygen administration that improves or abolishes cyanosis

Cardiac Disease
Causes
  Cyanotic CHD with right-to-left shunt
Findings
  Tachypnea but usually without retraction
  Lack of rales or abnormal breath sounds unless CHF supervenes
  Heart murmur that may be absent in serious forms of cyanotic CHD
  A continuous murmur (of PDA) that may indicate restricted PBF through the ductus
  Chest x-ray films that may show cardiomegaly, abnormal cardiac silhouette, increased or decreased PVMs
  Little or no increase in Po_2 with oxygen administration

Suggested Approach to Patients With Central Cyanosis

The determination of the arterial blood gas levels clarifies the type of cyanosis (central or peripheral). When the central cyanosis has been confirmed by arterial Po_2, one tests the response of arterial Po_2 to 100% oxygen inhalation (hyperoxitest). This test helps to differentiate cyanosis caused by cardiac disease from that caused by pulmonary disease. Oxygen should be administered through a plastic hood (such as Oxyhood) for at least 10 minutes to replace the alveolar air completely with oxygen (Box on p. 377). With pulmonary disease, arterial Po_2 usually rises to more than 100 mm Hg. When there is a significant intracardiac right-to-left shunt, the arterial Po_2 does not exceed 100 mm Hg, and the rise is not more than 10 to 30 mm Hg. However, some infants with cyanotic CHD with a large PBF, such as with TAPVR, may have a rise in the arterial Po_2 to 100 mm Hg or higher. On the other hand, infants with massive intrapulmonary shunt from a lung disease (but with a normal heart) may not have a rise in arterial Po_2 to 100 mm Hg. Therefore the response of Po_2 to 100% oxygen inhalation should be interpreted in light of the clinical picture, especially the degree of pulmonary pathology seen on chest x-ray films. The box lists suggested steps in the management of cyanotic newborns.

When possible, one should obtain arterial blood samples from the right upper body (right radial, brachial, or temporal artery) to avoid false-low values caused by a right-to-left ductal shunt. If a low arterial Po_2 is obtained from an umbilical artery line or from the lower extremity, another sample from the right upper body should be

Suggested Steps in the Management of Cyanotic Newborns

Chest x-ray films

Chest x-ray films may reveal pulmonary causes of cyanosis and urgency of the problem. They will also hint at the presence or absence and the type of cardiac defects

Arterial blood gases in room air

Arterial blood gases in room air will confirm or reject central cyanosis. An elevated P_{CO_2} suggests pulmonary or central nervous system problems. A low pH may be seen in sepsis, circulatory shock, or severe hypoxemia.

Hyperoxitest

Repeating arterial blood gases while the patient breathes 100% oxygen helps separate cardiac causes of cyanosis from pulmonary or central nervous system causes.

ECG if cardiac origin of cyanosis is suspected

An umbilical artery line

A P_{O_2} value in a preductal artery (such as right radial artery) higher than that in a postductal artery (an umbilical artery line) by 10 to 15 mm Hg suggests a right-to-left ductal shunt. (The umbilical line placed high in the descending aorta can be used for an aortogram during cardiac catheterization, reducing the time spent in the laboratory and eliminating the risk of arterial complications.)

Prostaglandin E_1

If a cyanotic CHD is suspected based on these laboratory tests, Prostin VR Pediatric should be started or made available.

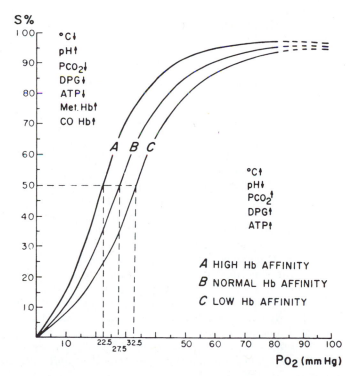

FIG. 29–1.
Factors that influence the position of the oxygen-hemoglobin dissociation curve. Curve B is from a normal adult at 38° C, pH, 7.40, and P_{CO_2} 35.0 mm Hg. Curves A and C illustrate the effect on the affinity for oxygen (P_{50}) of variations in temperature (°C), pH, P_{CO_2}, 2, 3-diphosphoglycerate, adenosine triphosphate, methemoglobin, and carboxyhemoglobin. Curve A is of the newborn. (From Duc G: *Pediatrics* 48:469-481, 1971.)

obtained and compared with a simultaneously obtained sample from the lower part of the body to clarify the presence or absence of a right-to-left ductal shunt. An arterial Po_2 from the right radial artery 10 to 15 mm Hg higher than that from an umbilical artery catheter is significant. In severe cases of a right-to-left ductal shunt, differential cyanosis may be noticeable with a pink upper and a cyanotic lower part of the body. Such a differential cyanosis or differential arterial Po_2 suggests PPHN (persistent fetal circulation syndrome) or obstructive lesions of the left side of the heart (e.g., severe AS, interrupted aortic arch, COA) with a right-to-left ductal shunt.

If cyanotic CHD is suspected, especially a defect that appears to be ductus-dependent (e.g., pulmonary atresia with or without VSD, tricuspid atresia, HLHS, interrupted aortic arch, severe COA), a prostaglandin E_1 (Prostin VR Pediatric) intravenous infusion should be started as soon as the diagnosis is suspected or is established. The starting dose of Prostin is 0.05 to 0.1 μg/kg/min, administered in a continuous intravenous drip. When the desired effects (increased Po_2, increased systemic blood pressure, and improved pH) are achieved, the dose should be reduced step-by-step to 0.01 μg/kg/min. When the initial starting dose has no effect, it may be increased to 0.4 μg/kg/min. Three common side effects of intravenous infusion of Prostin are apnea (12%), fever (14%), and flushing (10%). Less common side effects include tachycardia or bradycardia, hypotension, and cardiac arrest.

If central cyanosis is present or if arterial oxygen saturation cannot be raised to a satisfactory level with administration of oxygen, one should obtain a cardiology consultation. Echo and a Doppler examination will reveal the cause of the central cyanosis.

Although the routine tools of cardiac evaluation (physical examination, ECG, and chest x-ray films) do not help as much in diagnosing a cyanotic defect as in an acyanotic defect, these tools sometimes can be useful, at least in reducing the possibilities. Tables 29-2 and 29-3 summarize the differential diagnosis of cyanotic heart defects, based on PVMs and ECG findings, and further reduce the possibilities by other clinical findings. Note some overlap with Tables 5-1 and 5-2.

Hyperoxitest

A detailed understanding of the hyperoxitest requires an introduction to the hemoglobin dissociation curve. The relationship between the Po_2 and the amount of oxygen bound to hemoglobin and the relationship between the Po_2 and the oxygen dissolved in plasma are different. The relationship is S-shaped (sigmoid) for hemoglobin; the relationship is linear for plasma. For dissolved oxygen in plasma, the solubility coefficient is 0.003 ml/100 ml at a Po_2 of 1 mm Hg at 37° C (or 0.3 ml of oxygen/100 ml plasma at 100 mm Hg of Po_2).

The sigmoid relationship between the Po_2 and the amount of oxygen bound to hemoglobin is expressed by the oxygen-hemoglobin dissociation curve (see Fig. 29-1). The position of the dissociation curve is an expression of the affinity of hemoglobin for oxygen. The Po_2 at which 50% of hemoglobin is saturated has been chosen as the reference point, called P_{50}. The P_{50} averages 27 mm Hg in the adult and 22 mm Hg in the fetus and newborn. The newborn's curve (curve A) with high oxygen affinity favors the extraction of oxygen from the maternal circulation and suits the conditions of the intrauterine environment, but it does not allow the release of as large a proportion of oxygen to tissues as in adults ("stingy" hemoglobin). The adult curve (curve B), with a decreased affinity for oxygen, allows the release of more oxygen to tissues. The adult curve is reached by 3 months of age.

The pH, Pco_2 erythrocyte concentration of 2,3-diphosphoglycerate, adenosine triphosphate (ATP), methemoglobin and carboxyhemoglobin influence the position of the dissociation curve (see Fig. 29-1).

1. A decrease in hydrogen ion concentration (or increased pH), Pco_2, temperature, and 2,3-diphosphoglycerate and ATP concentrations shift the curve to the left (curve A).

2. An increase in the preceding parameters shifts the curve to the right (curve C).

TABLE 29–2.

Differential Diagnosis of Cyanotic Newborns with Increased Pulmonary Vascularity

Conditions	Other Important Clinical Findings
RVH	
D-TGA	Severe cyanosis in a large newborn*
	Male preponderance* (3 : 1)
	Single S2
	Signs of CHF ($\pm$)
	Usually no heart murmur*
	"Egg-shaped" heart with narrow waist (on x-ray film)*
	ECG: Normal or RVH
TAPVR with obstruction	Male preponderance* (4:1)
	Quadruple or quintuple rhythm*
	Usually no heart murmur
	Pulmonary rales ($\pm$)
	Pulmonary venous congestion or pulmonary edema on x-ray film*
	ECG: RVH, Q waves in V1*
DORV with subpulmonary VSD (Taussig-Bing anomaly)	Resembles TGA (severe cyanosis, signs of CHF [$\pm$])*
	Systolic murmur at ULSB, grade 2-3/6*
	ECG: RVH, RAH ($\pm$)
PPHN	Meconium stain or birth asphyxia
	Marked tachypnea + cyanosis*
	Usually no heart murmur
	Differential Po_2 between preductal and postductal arterial sites*
	Cardiomegaly, "ground-glass" appearance, normal vascularity, or lung pathology on x-ray films*
	Normal ECG
LVH or CVH	
Persistent truncus arteriosus (type I)	Mild cyanosis
	Bounding peripheral pulses*
	Systolic ejection click at apex*
	Harsh systolic murmur of VSD
	Early diastolic murmur of truncal valve regurgitation* ($\pm$)
	Signs of CHF ($\pm$)
	Right aortic arch on x-ray film* (30%)
Single ventricle (without PS)	Mild cyanosis
	Signs of CHF and cardiomegaly on x-ray film ($\pm$)
	Loud systolic murmur along LSB
	ECG: (1) no Q waves in precordial leads or Q waves in V4R or V1 and (2) Stereotype QRS (RS, rS, or QR) across most precordial leads
TGA + VSD	Mild cyanosis
	Signs of CHF* ($\pm$)
	Harsh systolic murmur of VSD
Polysplenia syndrome	Mild cyanosis
	Midline liver* (on palpation, x-ray films)
	Superior QRS axis and superior P axis* (ECG)
	ECG: RVH, LVH, or no hypertrophy

*Findings that are particularly important in the diagnosis of the condition.

3. Fetal hemoglobin has about 40% of the affinity for 2,3-diphosphoglycerate as the adult hemoglobin. This makes fetal hemoglobin behave as if 2,3-diphosphoglycerate levels are low; therefore the dissociation curve is shifted to the left (curve *A*).

4. The curve shifts to the right in compensation for high altitude, cyanosis, or anemia, as a result of an increase in the red cell concentration of 2,3-diphosphoglycerate.

TABLE 29–3.
Differential Diagnosis of Cyanotic Newborns with Decreased Pulmonary Vascularity

Conditions	Other Important Clinical Findings
RVH	
TOF	Long systolic murmur, grade 2-3/6, at ULSB*
	Soft continuous murmur in neonates with TOF with pulmonary atresia*
	Concave MPA segment (or "boot-shaped" heart) (on x-ray film)*
	Right aortic arch on x-ray film* (25%)
DORV with PS	Resemblance to TOF*
	Systolic murmur along LSB, grade 3-4/6
	ECG: RVH, first-degree AV block
Asplenia syndrome	Midline liver* (on palpation, x-ray films)
	Superior QRS axis* (ECG)
	ECG: RVH or LVH
	Howell-Jolly body or Heinz body on blood smear
RBBB	
Ebstein's anomaly	Triple or quadruple rhythm*
	Soft TR murmur
	Extreme cardiomegaly with oligemic lung fields (±)* (on x-ray film)
	ECG: RAH, WPW syndrome, first-degree AV block
LVH	
Pulmonary atresia	Severe cyanosis
	Usually no heart murmur, but possible soft PDA murmur*
	ECG: normal QRS axis, LVH, RAH
	X-ray examination: RAE and oligemic lungs
Tricuspid atresia	Severe cyanosis*
	Murmur of VSD or PDA
	Superior QRS axis* (ECG)
	"Boot-shaped" heart* (on x-ray film)
CVH	
TGA + PS	Moderate cyanosis
	No signs of CHF
	Systolic murmur (of PS) at ULSB
Persistent truncus arteriosus (type II or III)	Severe cyanosis
	Systolic ejection click*
	Soft systolic murmur
Single ventricle + PS	Physical findings resembling TOF*
	Systolic murmur along LSB

*Findings that are particularly important to the diagnosis of the condition.

5. Blood stored for more than 1 week loses 2,3-diphosphoglycerate and may not deliver oxygen to tissue optimally until 6 to 24 hours after transfusion.

Fig. 29-2 explains why 100% oxygen breathing does not significantly increase the Po_2 in the presence of a right-to-left intracardiac shunt. Figure 29-2, A is a schematic illustration of the effect of a right-to-left shunt on the Po_2 in room air. Assuming a cardiac output of 2 L/min, 1 L of venous blood is distributed to ventilated alveoli, and 1 L is shunted right-to-left through a cardiac defect. Mixing 1 L of venous blood with an oxygen content of 19.4 ml/100 ml (Po_2 of 30 mm Hg) with 1 L of pulmonary venous blood containing 26.3 ml/100 ml (Po_2 of 100 mm Hg) results in an oxygen content of 22.3 ml/100 ml. The corresponding Po_2 from the dissociation curve is 41.0 mm Hg. Therefore mixing 1 L of blood with a Po_2 of 100 mm Hg with 1 L of blood with a Po_2 of 30 mm Hg results in a Po_2 of 41 mm Hg (Fig. 29-2, A), not an arithmetic average of 65 mm Hg.

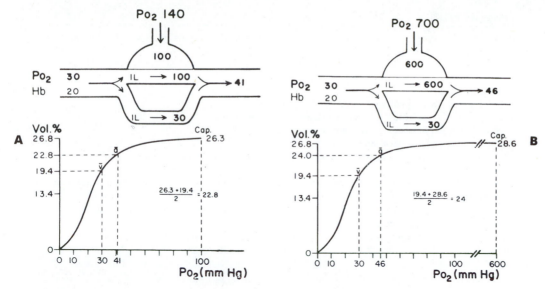

FIG. 29–2.
Result of hyperoxitest in cyanotic heart defects. **A,** Effect of a right-to-left shunt on the arterial Po_2 in room air. The mixing of 1 L blood coming from normal ventilated alveoli (Po_2 of 100 mm Hg) with 1 L of venous blood flowing through the cardiac defect (Po_2 of 30 mm Hg) results in a significant decrease in arterial Po_2 (41 mm Hg). **B,** Effect of a right-to-left shunt on the arterial Po_2 in 100% oxygen. The mixing of 1 L of blood coming from normal ventilated alveoli (Po_2 of 600 mm Hg) with 1 L of venous blood flowing through the shunt (Po_2 of 30 mm Hg) results in arterial Po_2 of 46 mm Hg. Breathing 100% oxygen does not influence significantly the hypoxemia, since the arterial Po_2 increases only from 41 to 46 mm Hg. Note that the oxygen content was calculated using an old number of 1.34 ml (rather than 1.36 ml), which can be bound to 1 g of hemoglobin. See text for the detailed description. (From Duc G: *Pediatrics* 469-481, 1971.)

With the patient breathing 100% oxygen (Fig. 29-2, *B*), the alveolar Po_2 becomes 600 mm Hg (with a corresponding oxygen content of 28.6 ml/100 ml, assuming a hemoglobin count of 20 g/100 ml; this figure is derived from 26.8 mg/100 ml of oxygen bound to hemoglobin plus 1.8 ml of oxygen dissolved in plasma [0.003 × 600]). When 1 L of blood with a Po_2 of 600 mm Hg (oxygen content 28.6 mg/100 ml) is mixed with 1 L of venous blood with a Po_2 of 30 mm Hg (oxygen content of 19.4 ml/100 ml), the resulting oxygen content will be 24 mg/100 ml ([28.6 + 19.4]/2), with a Po_2 of 46 mm Hg (Fig. 29-2, *B*). Thus breathing 100% oxygen does not significantly alter the Po_2 (an increase from 41 to 46 mm Hg) even though the alveolar Po_2 increases from 100 to 600 mm Hg.

Individual cyanotic heart defects are discussed in Chapter 14. However, PPHN is discussed in this section because this condition is one of the most common causes of aortic desaturation demonstrable by an umbilical artery catheter and it mimics cyanotic CHDs.

Persistent Pulmonary Hypertension of the Newborn
   Prevalence. PPHN (persistence of the fetal circulation, PFC syndrome) occurs in approximately 1 in 1500 live births.

   Pathology and pathophysiology.

1. This neonatal condition is characterized by persistence of pulmonary hypertension, which in turn causes a varying degree of cyanosis from a right-to-left shunt through the PDA or the PFO. No underlying CHD is present.

Etiology of PPHN
_____

Pulmonary vasoconstriction in the presence of a normally developed pulmonary vascular bed may be
 caused by or seen in:
  Alveolar hypoxia (meconium aspiration syndrome, hyaline membrane disease, hypoventilation
   caused by central nervous system anomalies)
  Birth asphyxia
  LV dysfunction or circulatory shock
  Infections (such as group B hemolytic streptococcal infection)
  Hyperviscosity syndrome (polycythemia)
  Hypoglycemia and hypocalcemia
Increased pulmonary vascular smooth muscle development (hypertrophy) may be caused by:
  Chronic intrauterine asphyxia
  Maternal use of prostaglandin synthesis inhibitors (aspirin, indomethacin) resulting in early ductal
   closure
Decreased cross-sectional area of pulmonary vascular bed may be seen in association with:
  Congenital diaphragmatic hernia
  Primary pulmonary hypoplasia
_____

2. Various etiologies have been identified, but the etiologies can be divided into three
   groups by the anatomy of the pulmonary vascular bed (see Box above).

   a. *Intense pulmonary vasoconstriction in the presence of a normally developed
      pulmonary vascular bed.* Clinical conditions such as perinatal asphyxia, meconium
      aspiration, ventricular dysfunction, group B streptococcal pneumonia, hypervis-
      cosity syndrome, and hypoglycemia are frequent causes of pulmonary vasocon-
      striction. Alveolar hypoxia and acidosis also are important causes of pulmonary
      vasoconstriction. Thromboxane, vasoconstrictor prostaglandins, leukotrienes, and
      endothelin also may be important causes of PA vasoconstriction.

   b. *Hypertrophy (of the medial layer) of the pulmonary arterioles.* Chronic intrauterine
      hypoxia and maternal ingestion of nonsteroidal antiinflammatory agents may be
      important causes of pulmonary arteriolar hypertrophy.

   c. *Developmentally abnormal pulmonary arterioles with decreased cross-sectional
      area of the pulmonary vascular bed.* Congenital diaphragmatic hernia and primary
      pulmonary hypoplasia are examples.
   In general, pulmonary hypertension caused by the first group is relatively easy to
   reverse, and that caused by the second group is more difficult to reverse than that
   caused by the first group. Pulmonary hypertension caused by the third group is most
   difficult or impossible to reverse.

3. Varying degrees of myocardial dysfunction often occur in association with PPHN,
   manifested by a global decrease in contractility and/or TR. These abnormalities are
   caused by global and/or subendocardial ischemia and are aggravated by hypoglycemia and hypocalcemia.

Clinical manifestations.

1. Symptoms begin 6 to 12 hours after birth, with cyanosis and respiratory difficulties.
   The idiopathic form usually affects full-term or postterm neonates. The patient
   usually has a history of meconium staining or birth asphyxia. A history of maternal
   ingestion of nonsteroidal antiinflammatory drugs (in the third trimester) may be
   elicited.

2. A neonate with a varying degree of cyanosis is tachypneic with retraction and
   grunting.

3. A prominent RV impulse and a single and loud S2 usually are found. Occasional gallop rhythm (from myocardial dysfunction) and a soft regurgitant systolic murmur of TR may be audible. Severe cases of myocardial dysfunction may manifest systemic hypotension.

4. Arterial desaturation is found in blood samples obtained from an umbilical artery catheter. Arterial Po_2 may be lower in the descending aorta (the umbilical artery line) than in the preductal arteries (the right radial, brachial, or temporal artery), because of a right-to-left ductal shunt. In severe cases, differential cyanosis may appear (with a pink upper body and a cyanotic lower half of the body). With a prominent right-to-left intracardiac shunt, usually through the PFO, the preductal and postductal arteries do not show a Po_2 difference.

5. The ECG usually is normal for age, but occasional RVH or T-wave abnormalities may suggest myocardial dysfunction.

6. Chest x-rays may reveal a varying degree of cardiomegaly. The lung fields may be free of abnormal findings or may show hyperinflation and/or atelectasis. The PVMs may appear normal, increased, or decreased.

7. Echo and Doppler studies are indicated to rule out CHD and to identify patients with myocardial dysfunction. The patient has no evidence of cyanotic CHD. The only structural abnormality is the presence of a large PDA with a right-to-left or bidirectional shunt. The RV is enlarged with a flattened interventricular septum. The patient has evidence of increased RA pressures (with the atrial septum bulging toward the left) with or without an interatrial communication, usually a PFO. The aortic arch is normal with no evidence of COA or an interrupted aortic arch. Imaging shows normal drainage of pulmonary veins. The LV dimension may be increased, and its systolic function (fractional shortening or ejection fraction) may be decreased.

8. Cardiac catheterization usually is not indicated. If the diagnosis is unclear or the patient does not respond to therapy, cardiac catheterization and pulmonary arteriography rarely are considered.

Treatment. The goals of therapy are (1) to lower the PVR and PA pressure through the administration of oxygen, the induction of respiratory alkalosis, and the use of pulmonary vasodilators; (2) to correct myocardial dysfunction; and (3) to stabilize the patient and treat associated conditions.

1. General supportive therapy is provided.

    a. Vital signs and oxygen saturations are carefully monitored.

    b. Hypoglycemia, hypocalcemia (defined as ionized calcium levels <3.5 mEq/L), and hypomagnesemia (defined as magnesium levels <1.2 mg/100 ml).

    c. Polycythemia is treated.

    d. Body temperature is maintained between 36.5° and 37.2° C.

2. To achieve arterial Po_2 of 100 mm Hg, 100% oxygen is administered, initially without intubation. If this is not successful, intubation plus continuous positive airway pressure at 2 to 10 cm of water may be effective.

3. Mechanical ventilation is used to improve oxygenation and to produce respiratory alkalosis if the previous measures are not successful. The following ventilator settings are used: fractional inspired oxygen concentration to 1.0, ventilator rate to 40 to 80 breaths/min, peak inspiratory pressure to 40 cm of water, positive end-expiratory pressure to 4 to 10 cm of water, and inspiratory:expiratory time ratio to 1 or less. The patient usually is paralyzed with pancuronium (Pavulon) at 0.1 mg/kg intravenously. When relative normoxemia has been achieved for 12 to 24 hours, careful weaning probably can be begun safely with one ventilator setting at a time.

4. Tolazoline (Priscolin) is infused. One may give a loading dose of 0.5 to 1.0 mg/kg by slow intravenous administration followed by intravenous infusion of 2 to 4 mg/kg/hr. Tolazoline is not a specific pulmonary vasodilator, and it lowers the SVR as well, resulting in systemic hypotension. One must carefully monitor blood pressure and maintain adequate circulating blood volume. Systemic hypotension is treated with volume expanders and dopamine infusion. About two thirds of patients respond with an increase in systemic oxygenation. Side effects of tolazoline include hypotension, increased gastric secretion, gastrointestinal bleeding, decreased platelet counts, and decreased urine output. Cimetidine (a histamine H_2-receptor antagonist) is not recommended because histamine may be important in dilating pulmonary vasculature.

5. For myocardial dysfunction, the following therapy is provided.

   a. Dopamine is used with tolazoline to improve cardiac output. The usual dose of dopamine is 10 mg/kg/min by intravenous infusion.

   b. Dobutamine (a β-adrenergic agent) may be used if signs of CHF are present. The usual starting dose is 5 to 8 mg/kg/min by continuous intravenous infusion.

   c. Correction of acidosis, hypocalcemia, and hypoglycemia helps improve myocardial function.

   d. Diuretics may be included in the regimen. For chronic myocardial dysfunction, digoxin may be added at a later stage.

6. A high-frequency oscillatory ventilator has been shown to be effective in patients with severe PPHN. Through the use of this device, about 40% of patients who would be considered candidates for extracorporeal membrane oxygenation can avoid this procedure.

7. Inhaled nitric oxide is a promising therapy for PPHN. Prolonged low-dose nitric oxide therapy (with 6 ppm) has caused a sustained improvement in oxygenation, leading to recovery without extracorporeal membrane oxygenation therapy. Endothelium-derived relaxing factor has been identified as a nitric oxide or a nitric oxide–containing substance. Inhaled nitric oxide exerts selective pulmonary vasodilatation without causing systemic hypotension. Inhaled nitric oxide diffuses to pulmonary vascular smooth muscle, stimulating cyclic guanosine monophosphate production and causing vasodilatation. Its predilection for the pulmonary circulation is due to the rapid and avid binding of nitric oxide by hemoglobin. Combined treatment with a high-frequency oscillatory ventilator may be more effective.

8. Extracorporeal membrane oxygenation has been shown to be effective in the management of selected patients with severe PPHN. However, this treatment requires ligation of a carotid artery and the jugular vein, and cerebrovascular accidents have been reported.

Prognosis.

1. Prognosis generally is good for neonates with mild PPHN who respond quickly to the therapy. Most of these neonates recover without permanent lung damage or neurologic impairment.

2. For those requiring a maximum ventilator setting for a prolonged time, the chance of survival is smaller, and many survivors develop bronchopulmonary dysplasia and other complications.

3. Patients with developmental decreases in cross-sectional areas of the pulmonary vascular bed usually do not respond to therapy, and their prognosis is poor.

4. Neurodevelopmental abnormalities may manifest. Patients have a high incidence of hearing loss (up to 50%). This is positively related to the degree of alkalosis, the duration of ventilator support, and possibly the use of furosemide and aminoglyco-

sides. An abnormal EEG (up to 80%) and cerebral infarction (45%) have been reported.

HEART FAILURE IN THE NEWBORN

A neonate with CHF usually suffers from a CHD but may have nonstructural heart disease, such as myocardial dysfunction (ischemia, myocarditis) or serious disturbances of heart rate. Metabolic and hematologic abnormalities as well as overtransfusion or overhydration also may be responsible for CHF. (Box below shows causes of CHF in the newborn.)

The clinical picture of CHF in the newborn period may simulate other disorders, such as meningitis, sepsis, pneumonia, or bronchiolitis. Tachypnea, tachycardia, pulmonary rales or rhonchi, hepatomegaly, and weak peripheral pulses are common presenting signs. A detailed discussion of treatment of CHF is presented in Chapter 30.

Two important structural abnormalities of the cardiovascular system that present with CHF in the newborn period are HLHS and large PDAs in premature infants. Three nonstructural heart situations that can present with CHF are transient myocardial ischemia, infants of diabetic mothers, and bronchopulmonary dysplasia. These five conditions are presented in this chapter. Other structural heart defects have been presented under specific conditions in earlier chapters. Arrhythmias that can cause CHF are presented in this chapter in the section on arrhythmias of the newborn.

Hypoplastic Left Heart Syndrome

Prevalence. HLHS occurs in 1% of all CHDs or 9% of CHDs in the newborn. HLHS is the most common cause of death from cardiac defects during the first month of life.

Causes of Heart Failure in the Newborn

Structural Heart Defects

At birth
  HLHS
  Severe TR or PR
  Large systemic AV fistula
First week
  TGA
  Premature infant with large PDA
  TAPVR below diaphragm
1-4 weeks
  Critical AS or PS
  COA

Noncardiac Causes

Birth asphyxia resulting in transient myocardial ischemia
Metabolic: hypoglycemia, hypocalcemia
Severe anemia (as seen in hydrops fetalis)
Overtransfusion or overhydration
Neonatal sepsis

Primary Myocardial Disease

Myocarditis
Transient myocardial ischemia (with or without birth asphyxia)
Cardiomyopathy (seen in infant of diabetic mother)

Disturbances in Heart Rate

SVT
Atrial flutter/fibrillation
Congenital heart block (when associated with CHD)

Pathology.

1. HLHS includes a group of closely related anomalies characterized by hypoplasia of the LV and encompasses atresia or critical stenosis of the aortic and/or mitral valves and hypoplasia of the ascending aorta and aortic arch.

2. The LA is small. The atrial septum may be intact with a normal foramen ovale, or the patient may have a true ASD (15%). A VSD appears in about 10% of patients. COA frequently is an associated finding (up to 75%).

Pathophysiology.

1. During the fetal life, the PVR is higher than the SVR, and the dominant RV maintains normal perfusing pressure in the descending aorta and the placenta through the ductal right-to-left shunt. The proximal aorta and the coronary and cerebral circulations are perfused retrogradely. The fetus tolerates this serious cardiac anomaly well in utero.

2. However, difficulties arise after birth for two reasons: the reversal of the vascular resistance in the two circuits, with higher SVR than the PVR; and the closure of the ductus arteriosus. The result is a marked decrease in systemic cardiac output and aortic pressure, producing circulatory shock and metabolic acidosis.

3. Maintenance of adequate systemic blood flow (and survival of these infants) depends on an adequate size of the ductus arteriosus to permit the RV to send blood to the aorta and an adequate interatrial communication to decompress the LA. In the presence of a large ASD that permits a left-to-right atrial shunt, pulmonary edema is not severe, and the arterial oxygen saturation may be in the 80s. With an intact atrial septum or a small interatrial communication, pulmonary edema is severe, and the arterial oxygen saturation is low. Without treatment, the infant dies shortly after birth.

Clinical manifestations.

1. The neonate with HLHS becomes critically ill within the first few hours to the first few days of life. Tachycardia, dyspnea, pulmonary rales, weak peripheral pulses, and vasoconstricted extremities are characteristic. The patient may not have severe cyanosis.

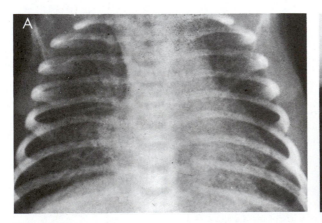 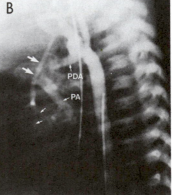

FIG. 29–3.
An AP view of chest film **(A)** and a lateral view of an aortogram **(B)** in a 1-day-old newborn with HLHS. The heart is enlarged, and the pulmonary vascularity is increased, with marked pulmonary venous congestion and pulmonary edema **(A)**. The aortogram, obtained with injection of a radiopaque dye through an umbilical artery catheter, shows a hypoplastic ascending aorta *(thick arrows)* with small coronary arteries *(thin arrows)* filling retrogradely, a large PDA, and PAs.

2. The S2 is loud and single. Heart murmur usually is absent. Occasionally, a grade 1-3/6 nonspecific systolic ejection murmur may be heard over the precordium. Signs of CHF develop with hepatomegaly and gallop rhythm.

3. The ECG almost always shows RVH. Rarely, the ECG suggests LVH: Large R waves may be recorded in V5 and V6 because these leads record over the dilated RV, not over the hypoplastic LV.

4. Chest x-ray films characteristically show pulmonary venous congestion or pulmonary edema (Fig. 29-3, A). The heart is moderately or markedly enlarged.

5. Arterial blood gas levels reveal a slightly decreased Po_2 and a normal Pco_2. Severe metabolic acidosis out of proportion to the Pco_2 (caused by markedly decreased cardiac output) is characteristic of the condition.

6. Echo findings are diagnostic and usually obviate the need for cardiac catheterization and angiocardiography.

   a. The LV cavity is diminutive, but the RV cavity is markedly dilated, and the tricuspid valve is large.

   b. Imaging usually reveals severe hypoplasia of the aorta and aortic annulus and an absent or distorted mitral valve. COA frequently is an associated anomaly.

   c. The patient may have an ASD or a PFO with a left-to-right shunt. The patient occasionally has a VSD with a relatively large LV, aortic annulus, and ascending aorta.

   d. Color-flow mapping and Doppler studies reveal retrograde blood flow in the aortic arch and ascending aorta.

Natural history. Pulmonary edema and CHF develop in the first week of life. Circulatory shock and progressive hypoxemia and acidosis result in death, usually in the first month of life.

Management.
Medical.

1. The patient's trachea is intubated and ventilated appropriately with oxygen, and metabolic acidosis is corrected.

2. Intravenous infusion of prostaglandin E_1 (Prostin VR Pediatric) may temporarily improve the HLHS by reopening the ductus arteriosus (for the dosage, see Appendix D).

3. Balloon atrial septostomy may help decompress the LA and improve oxygenation but will produce only a temporary benefit.

Surgical. Three options are available in the management of these infants: Do nothing or chose one of two surgical options. The two surgical options are the Norwood operation (followed by a Fontan operation) and cardiac transplantation. The surgical procedure of choice remains controversial. The surgical procedures in detail are:

1. Norwood operation is performed initially, and the Fontan-type operation is performed at a later date.

   a. The first-stage Norwood operation is performed in the neonatal period. The reported mortality rate is 35% and higher. Overall, the 12-month survival after the first stage is about 45%, with most deaths occurring within the first 6 months after the operation. The operation consists of the following procedures (Fig. 29-4):

      1) The MPA is divided, the distal stump is closed with a patch, and the ductus arteriosus is ligated.

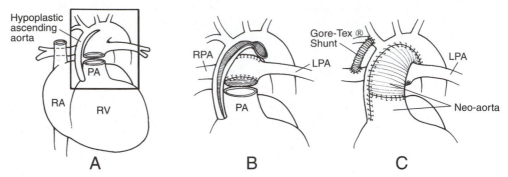

FIG. 29–4.
Schematic diagram of Norwood procedure. **A,** The heart with aortic atresia and a hypoplastic ascending aorta and aortic arch are shown. The MPA is transected. **B,** The distal PA is closed with a patch. An incision that extends around the aortic arch to the level of the ductus is made in the ascending aorta. The ductus is ligated. **C,** A modified right Blalock-Taussig shunt is created between the right subclavian artery and the RPA as the sole source of PBF. By the use of an aortic or PA allograft *(shaded area),* the MPA is anastomosed to the ascending aorta and the aortic arch to create a large arterial trunk. The procedure to widen the atrial communication is not shown.

    2) A right-side Gore-Tex shunt is created (usually with a 4-mm tube) to provide PBF while preventing CHF and pulmonary hypertension.

    3) The atrial septum is excised to allow adequate interatrial mixing.

    4) Using an aortic or PA allograft, one connects the proximal PA and the hypoplastic ascending aorta and aortic arch.

  b. One creates a cavopulmonary shunt (an end-to-side anastomosis of the SVC to the RPA, bidirectional Glenn operation) (see Fig. 14-35, *A*) at 6 months of age in an effort to reduce the volume overload to the systemic RV. The mortality rate for this procedure is less than 5%.

  c. A modified Fontan operation is performed at 1½ years of age (see Fig. 14-35, *B*). To be an optimal candidate for the final Fontan operation, a patient who had the initial cavopulmonary shunt operation should have the following five favorable hemodynamic and anatomic features: (1) unrestrictive interatrial communication, (2) competence of the tricuspid valve, (3) unobstructed PA-to-descending aorta anastomosis (with pressure gradient less than 25 mm Hg), (4) low PVR and undistorted PAs, and (5) preservation of RV function.

    Significant TR appears to be a possible predictor of poor outcome of the Fontan operation. The operative mortality of the third-stage operation (Fontan procedure) is about 15% to 20%. The overall survival rate after the Fontan operation is about 50% at 4 years.

2. Some centers consider cardiac transplantation the procedure of choice (see Chapter 37). If the diameter of the ascending aorta is less than 2.5 mm, cardiac transplantation, rather than the Norwood operation, is believed to provide a better result. The surgical technique of cardiac transplantation is presented in Chapter 37. Donor hearts must be harvested with all the ascending, transverse, and upper descending thoracic aortas intact.

Premature Infants with Patent Ductus Arteriosus

  Prevalence. Clinical evidence of PDA appears in 45% of infants under 1750 g birth weight and in about 80% of infants under 1200 g birth weight. Significant PDA with

CHF occurs in 15% of premature infants with a birth weight less than 1,750 g and in 40% to 50% of those with a birth weight less than 1,500 g.

Pathophysiology.

1. PDA is a special problem in premature infants who are recovering from hyaline membrane disease. With improvement in oxygenation, the PVR drops rapidly, but the ductus remains patent because its responsiveness to oxygen is immature in the premature newborn (see Chapter 8). The resulting large left-to-right shunt makes the lung stiff, and weaning the infant from the ventilator and oxygen therapy becomes difficult.

2. If the infant must remain on ventilator and oxygen therapy for a long time, bronchopulmonary dysplasia develops with resulting pulmonary hypertension (cor pulmonale) and right-sided heart failure. Early recognition and appropriate management are keys to improving the prognosis of these infants.

Clinical manifestations.

1. The history is important in suspecting a significant PDA in a premature neonate. Typically, a premature infant with hyaline membrane disease has made some improvement during the first few days after birth. This is followed by an inability to wean the infant from the ventilator or a need to increase ventilator settings or oxygen levels in 4- to 7-day-old premature infants. Apneic spells or episodes of bradycardia may be the initial signs of PDA in infants who are not on ventilators.

2. The physical examination commonly reveals bounding peripheral pulses, a hyperactive precordium, and tachycardia with or without gallop rhythm. The classic continuous murmur at the left infraclavicular area or ULSB is diagnostic, but the murmur may be only systolic and is difficult to hear in infants who are on ventilators. Premature infants who are fluid overloaded or retaining fluid also may present with hyperdynamic precordiums, heart mumurs (ejection-type systolic murmurs), bounding pulses, and wide pulse pressures.

3. The ECG is not diagnostic. It usually is normal but occasionally shows LVH.

4. Chest x-ray films show the heart to be either of normal size or only mildly enlarged in infants who are intubated and on high ventilator settings. A greater degree of cardiomegaly may be seen in larger premature infants who are not intubated. The infant may have evidence of pulmonary edema or increased PVMs, but these may be difficult to assess in the presence of hyaline membrane disease.

5. Two-dimensional echo and color-flow Doppler studies provide accurate anatomic and functional information.

   a. The two-dimensional echo provides the anatomic information about the diameter, length, and shape of the ductus (Fig. 29-5).

   b. Doppler studies of the ductus (with the sample volume placed at the pulmonary end of the ductus) provide important functional information, such as (1) ductal shunt patterns (pure left-to-right, bidirectional, or predominant right-to-left shunt), (2) pressures in the PA, and (3) magnitude of the ductal shunt or pulmonary perfusion status:

      1) *Ductal shunt pattern.* A continuous positive flow indicates a pure left-to-right shunt with the PA pressure lower than the aortic pressure. In pure right-to-left shunts, flow is continuously negative away from the PA, indicating that the PA pressure is suprasystemic. A bidirectional shunting pattern (with an early negative flow in systole followed by a late positive flow in diastole) is found in infants with a PDA and severe PA hypertension.

      2) *Estimation of PA pressures.* A high ductal flow velocity indicates a low PA pressure, and a low flow velocity indicates a high PA pressure. The pressure

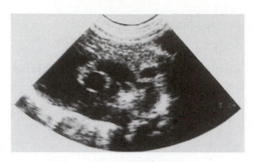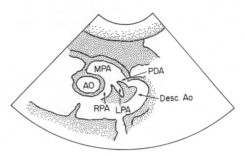

FIG. 29–5.
Parasternal short-axis view demonstrating PDA that connects the MPA and the
descending aorta *(Desc Ao).*

drop may be underestimated in patients with a small pulmonary end of the
ductus, tortuous PDAs, or tunnel-like PDAs with diameters of less than 3 mm
and lengths of more than 10 mm (because of viscous energy loss). However, the
easiest and most accurate estimate of the PA systolic pressure is obtained from
the peak velocity of the TR, when it is present.

3) *Perfusion status.* Increased flow velocity in the left PA suggests a large
left-to-right shunt through the ductus. High PA pressures and a lower flow
velocity (with a pressure drop of less than 5 mm Hg) indicate poor perfusion
of the lungs, which is a bad prognostic sign during the first 24 to 36 hours.

Management.

For symptomatic infants, either pharmacologic or surgical closure of the ductus is
indicated. A small PDA that does not cause symptoms should be followed medically
for 6 months without surgical ligation because of the possibility of spontaneous closure
of the ductus.

Medical.

1. One initially may try fluid restriction to 120 ml/kg/day and a diuretic (such as
furosemide, 1 mg/kg, 2 to 3 times a day) for 24 to 48 hours, but these regimens have
a low success rate. Digoxin is not used because it has little hemodynamic benefit and
a high incidence of digitalis toxicity.

2. One may produce pharmacologic closure of the PDA with indomethacin (a
prostaglandin synthetase inhibitor), 0.2 mg/kg intravenously every 12 hours for up to
three doses, in selected cases. Contraindications to the use of indomethacin include
(1) high blood urea nitrogen (>25 mg/dl) or creatinine levels (>1.8 mg/dl), (2) a low
platelet count ($<80,000/mm^3$), (3) a bleeding tendency (including intracranial
hemorrhage), (4) necrotizing enterocolitis, and (5) hyperbilirubinemia.

Surgical. If the medical treatment described previously is unsuccessful or if the use
of indomethacin is contraindicated, a surgical ligation of the ductus is indicated.

Transient Myocardial Ischemia

Prevalence. Transient myocardial ischemia is a rarely recognized condition; the true
incidence is unknown.

Pathology and pathophysiology.

1. Subendocardial necrosis occurs in the papillary muscles and other areas of the
ventricles in the newborn who had prenatal or perinatal hypoxia and distress.

Hypoxic pulmonary vasoconstriction is believed to be the cause of subendocardial ischemia or necrosis resulting from the imbalance of the oxygen supply and demand.

2. These neonates usually have evidence of pulmonary hypertension, bidirectional shunts at the atrial and/or ductal levels, and TR. Variable degrees of LV dysfunction are demonstrable by echo.

3. A variety of clinical manifestations are seen, depending on the severity of the myocardial dysfunction.

   a. *Transient tachypnea of the newborn* is the mildest form of the condition. Mild LV dysfunction leads to fluid retention, pulmonary edema, and reduced lung compliance, producing tachypnea.

   b. Transient TR/MR results from papillary muscle infarction (indicated by elevated serum levels of creatine phosphokinase MB fraction).

   c. Severe CHF with cardiogenic shock is the most severe form of myocardial dysfunction seen in the newborn.

Clinical manifestations.

1. Full-term neonates with low Apgar scores (<6 at 1 minute) usually develop early respiratory difficulty with tachypnea. Mild cyanosis may be seen, but severe cyanosis is rare.

2. The patient usually has a systolic murmur of TR or MR. CHF with gallop rhythm develops in one third of patients. Rarely, hypotension and vascular collapse result.

3. The ECG may show generalized flat T waves and minor ST-segment depression (a possible reflection of subendocardial ischemia), but these changes also are seen in some normal newborns. Abnormal Q waves suggestive of anterior or inferior infarction may be seen in the limb and precordial leads.

4. Chest x-ray films show varying degrees, sometimes a marked degree, of cardiomegaly. PVMs may be increased by pulmonary venous congestion (described as "wet lung") in severely affected neonates.

5. Echo reveals varying degrees of myocardial dysfunction, including an enlarged LA and/or LV; decreased contractility of the LV, especially of the posterior wall (with resulting decrease in the fractional shortening); and mitral valve regurgitation. All abnormalities tend to improve over 1 to 2 weeks.

6. Laboratory tests may show the following:

   a. Po_2 and pH are mildly reduced but usually without carbon dioxide retention.

   b. Hypoglycemia is seen.

   c. The serum creatine phosphokinase MB fraction may be elevated in patients with significant TR (see Appendix A, Fig. AA-3 for myocardial enzyme changes in myocardial infarction).

   d. A myocardial perfusion scan may show a diffuse impairment of thallium-201 uptake, but this test should be reserved for equivocal cases, such as those in whom myocarditis may be suspected in which myocardial perfusion is normal.

Management.

1. Mild cases require only supportive measures with administration of oxygen, correction of acidosis, and treatment of hypoglycemia because the disease is self-limiting.

2. Ventilatory assistance may be necessary in more severely affected infants.

3. Fluid restriction and diuretics are helpful.

4. Short-acting inotropic agents, such as dopamine, and a vasodilator agent should be considered in severely affected neonates.

   Prognosis.

1. Infants with transient myocardial ischemia usually recover unless the ischemia is associated with severe acidosis, central nervous system damage, or advanced sepsis.

2. Clinical improvement is seen within a few days after initiation of treatment, and TR and ECG abnormalities resolve within a few months. Whether some of these patients will develop arrhythmias, cardiomyopathy, or MVP later in life currently is unclear.

Infants of Diabetic Mothers

Prevalence. At least 1.3% of pregnancies are complicated by diabetes mellitus.

Pathology.

1. The teratogenic action of diabetes mellitus is generalized, affecting multiple organ systems. The prevalence of major congenital malformations in infants of diabetic mothers is as high as 6% to 9% (i.e., 3 to 4 times that found in the general population). Congenital malformations of all types are increased in infants of diabetic mothers, but neural tube defects (anencephaly, myelomeningocele), CHDs, and sacral dysgenesis or agenesis are common. Infants born to insulin-dependent diabetic mothers are the group at highest risk for developing congenital malformations; infants born to mothers with non–insulin-dependent, well-controlled diabetes do not appear to have an increased risk of congenital malformations.

2. Infants of diabetic mothers have a high prevalence of CHDs, cardiomyopathy, and PPHN.

   a. The risk of CHD is 3 to 4 times greater than that in the general population, with VSD, TGA, and COA among the more common defects.

   b. Hypertrophic cardiomyopathy with or without obstruction is seen in 10% to 20% of these infants. The weight of the heart is increased by the increased myocardial fiber size and number (rather than by excess glycogen, as once thought); the hypertrophy is thought to be caused by hyperinsulinemia. Although free walls of both ventricles and the ventricular septum are hypertrophied, the ventricular septum characteristically is more hypertrophied than the LV posterior wall (asymmetric septal hypertrophy) (Fig. 29-6).

   c. Infants of diabetic mothers also are at an increased risk of PPHN. They often are affected by conditions that promote the persistence of pulmonary hypertension,

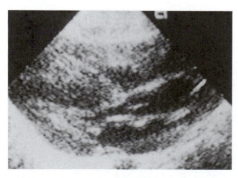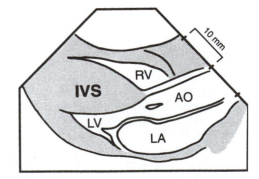

FIG. 29–6.
Parasternal long-axis view of an infant of a diabetic mother. There is an asymmetric hypertrophy of the interventricular septum *(IVS)*, which is at least 2 times as thick as the posterior wall of the LV.

such as hypoglycemia, perinatal asphyxia, respiratory distress, and polycythemia.

Clinical manifestations. The clinical manifestations of only the cardiomyopathy will be presented in this section. CHDs and PPHN are discussed under specific headings.

1. The history usually reveals gestational or insulin-dependent diabetes mellitus in the mother. The patient often has a history of progressive respiratory distress with tachypnea (80 to 100 breaths/min) from birth.

2. These large for gestational age babies often are plethoric and mildly cyanotic and may have tachypnea and tachycardia (> 160 beats/min). Signs of CHF with gallop rhythm may be found in 5% to 10% of these babies. The patient may have a systolic murmur along the LSB, which may be caused by an outflow tract obstruction or an associated CHD.

3. Chest x-ray films may reveal a varying degree of cardiomegaly. Pulmonary vascular markings are normal or mildly increased by pulmonary venous congestion.

4. The ECG usually is nonspecific, but a long QT interval caused by a long ST segment of hypocalcemia may be found. Occasionally, RVH, LVH, or CVH may be seen.

5. Echo may show the following:

   a. The ventricular septum often is disproportionately thicker than the LV posterior wall, but even free walls also are thicker than normal (see Fig. 29-6). The degree of asymmetric septal hypertrophy has no relationship with the severity of the maternal diabetes.

   b. Supernormal contractility of the LV and evidence of LV outflow tract obstruction (systolic anterior motion of the mitral valve and fluttering of the aortic valve) appear in about 50% of the infants.

   c. Rarely, the LV is dilated, and its contractility is decreased.

Treatment.

1. Provide general supportive measures, such as intravenous fluids, correction of hypoglycemia and hypocalcemia, and ventilatory assistance, if indicated.

2. In most cases, the hypertrophy spontaneously resolves within the first 6 to 12 months of life. β-Adrenergic blockers, such as propranolol, may help the LV outflow tract obstruction, but treatment usually is not necessary. Digitalis and other inotropic agents are contraindicated because they may worsen the obstruction.

3. If the LV is dilated with decreased LV contractility, the usual anticongestive measures (e.g., digoxin, diuretics) are indicated.

Bronchopulmonary Dysplasia

Prevalence. Some babies with bronchopulmonary dysplasia develop chronic right-sided heart failure (cor pulmonale); these include 50% of premature infants with birth weights of 500 to 750 g and about 10% of premature infants weighing less than 1500 g who were mechanically ventilated.

Pathophysiology.

1. Severe hyaline membrane disease and its required prolonged endotracheal intubation, mechanical ventilation, and high inspired oxygen concentration result in bronchopulmonary dysplasia. The exact mechanisms by which these factors produce bronchopulmonary dysplasia are not completely understood.

2. Bronchopulmonary dysplasia produces chronic pulmonary hypertension, with gradual dilatation and hypertrophy of the RV. The RV pressure may exceed the level of systemic pressure, and right-sided heart failure may develop if the cause is not eliminated and exacerbating causes persist.

3. The cardiac output may decrease because of right-sided heart failure. In addition, a sudden increase in the PVR by additional factors may decrease pulmonary venous return to the LA, with a further decrease in cardiac output if there is an inadequate right-to-left intracardiac shunt (which will result in arterial desaturation). See Chapter 32 for a detailed discussion of pulmonary hypertension.

Clinical manifestations.

1. The patient usually has a history of premature birth and of respiratory distress syndrome requiring administration of oxygen at a concentration of greater than 60%, mechanical ventilation with high airway pressure, and CHF from a PDA.

2. The patient has retraction of the chest walls and pulmonary rales. Some neonates have systemic hypertension (the mechanisms of which are not clear) with echo evidence of LV wall hypertrophy. Cardiac examination usually is unremarkable, except for an occasional nonspecific systolic ejection murmur or a soft murmur of TR. The liver often is enlarged.

3. Chest x-ray films may reveal diffuse bilateral haziness, sometimes with lacy densities, areas of hyperinflation, increased anteroposterior diameter of the chest, and occasional pectus excavatum. The heart may be of normal size but frequently is enlarged.

4. Echo findings follow:

    a. The RV is dilated, but RV wall thickness is within normal limits (2 to 5 mm).

    b. The LV posterior wall is thickened (7 to 11 mm) in over 80% of infants; this may account for pulmonary edema and systemic hypertension.

Treatment.

1. No specific treatment is available for CHF secondary to bronchopulmonary dysplasia. Sufficient calories, protein, and vitamins for growth and tissue repair are important. Daily sodium intake should be limited to 1 to 2 mEq/kg of body weight.

2. Diuretic therapy decreases airway resistance and improves lung compliance but usually does not affect gas exchange. One of the following may be used.

    a. Hydrochlorothiazide, 2 mg/kg every 12 hours, is administered with or without spironolactone, 1.5 mg/kg every 12 hours.

    b. Furosemide, 2 mg/kg every 12 hours, is administered every other day.

3. Digoxin may be tried, but its beneficial effects are uncertain. Because of intermittent disturbances in serum potassium levels, digoxin may be dangerous.

4. Oxygen inhalation decreases PA pressures and promotes weight gain.

Prognosis.

1. At least 15% of severely affected infants die in the first year. Most surviving infants are asymptomatic by 2 years, and signs or symptoms of lung disease are rare after 5 years.

2. Even years later, some patients have abnormalities of respiratory function and in their exercise tolerance test.

ARRHYTHMIAS AND ATRIOVENTRICULAR CONDUCTION DISTURBANCES

Although once thought to be rare, arrhythmias are not uncommon in healthy full-term and premature newborn infants. Monitoring of the cardiac rhythm in the intensive care setting has allowed detection of many types of arrhythmias and conduction disturbances that are not ordinarily recorded on the routine ECG and rhythm strips. Frequent use of the long-term recording (Holter monitoring) of cardiac rhythm has improved understanding of the frequency and nature of arrhythmias throughout the day (see later discussion).

Continued postnatal development of the conduction system (the SA node, AV node, and bundle of His) and of the sympathetic nervous system of the heart may predispose the newborn to arrhythmias and conduction disturbances that are not seen in older children. In addition, unfavorable environmental factors, such as a maternal disease state (e.g., diabetes mellitus, toxemia), pharmacologic agents given to the mother or neonate, and postnatal difficulties of the newborn (e.g., hypoxia, acidosis, hypothermia, metabolic disturbances, electrolyte imbalance) all can contribute to the rhythm disturbance.

Results of Holter Monitoring in Normal Newborns

Holter monitoring has demonstrated that variations in heart rate and rhythm, previously thought to be uncommon in the newborn, are frequent. Such knowledge is important in planning the management of rhythm disturbances detected on the ECG monitor. Certain rhythm disturbances found frequently in normal newborns may not require treatment.

Full-term newborns.

1. The maximum heart rate was 230 beats/min, the sinus rate in many normal neonates was as low as 75 beats/min, and the lowest rate recorded was 55 beats/min.

2. Benign arrhythmias were common; PAC was the most common arrhythmia, occurring in 10% to 35% of normal infants. Sinus pause was frequent (up to 72%), and 2:1 sinus node exit block was seen in 11%.

3. Nonsinus rhythm was detected in up to 35% of neonates; junctional rhythm was the most common (25%). PVCs were found in 1% to 13% and SVTs in 4%.

Preterm and low-birth-weight newborns.

1. The maximum heart rate was 210 beats/min, and the lowest rate was 75 beats/min.

2. PACs occurred in 2% to 33%, PVCs in 6% to 17%, and junctional rhythm in 18% to 70% of preterm newborns.

3. Bradyarrhythmias are seen more frequently in the preterm than in the term infant. Sudden sinus bradycardia (<90 beats/min) was observed in up to 90% of premature infants. Sinus pause occurred frequently. Sudden sinus arrest of up to 2 seconds' duration was observed in 6% of infants. Sinus arrhythmias were seen in 100% of these infants.

Selected Arrhythmias in the Newborn

This section discusses the significance and management of well-defined arrhythmias that are seen frequently in the newborn. Chapters 24 and 25 explored arrhythmias and AV conduction disturbances. Arrhythmias of the newborn must be interpreted within the context of the long-term ECG monitoring described previously.

The definitions of tachycardia and bradycardia for the adult and older child do not apply to the newborn. The normal resting heart rate of the newborn is 110 to 150 beats/min, but depending on the state of sleep or activity, the rate ranges from 80 to 190 beats/min. Rates persistently above and below this range require investigation.

Sinus tachycardia. The heart rate is faster than 150 beats/min. Transient tachycardia of up to 180 to 190 beats/min is commonly seen in normal newborns, but the maximum sinus rate usually does not exceed 220 beats/min. Persistent tachycardia may be caused by hypovolemia, fever, hyperthyroidism, and drugs, such as catecholamines and xanthines. Treatment should be directed toward the detection and correction of the underlying cause.

Sinus bradycardia. A heart rate persistently below 80 beats/min may be called *bradycardia* in a newborn infant. Transient bradycardia with a heart rate less than 70 beats/min may be seen in normal neonates and requires no treatment. This transient bradycardia may be associated with defecation, yawning, deep sleep, or nasopharyngeal stimulation. Maternal medications or neonatal asphyxia may cause sinus bradycardia in the immediate neonatal period. Treatment should be directed toward correcting or improving underlying causes, when they are known.

Prolonged bradycardia may be related to apnea (either preceding or following the bradycardia) and requires investigation and close monitoring. In premature infants who died suddenly and unexpectedly at home (sudden infant death syndrome), bradycardia was a prominent feature before the advent of apnea. In these cases, bradycardia could be secondary to hypoxemia or obstructive apnea or could be a direct result of impaired brain stem control.

Sinus arrhythmia. The heart rate has a phasic variation while the characteristics of sinus rhythm is maintained. Unlike a similar variation in older children, this variation may or may not be related to respiration. The presence of sinus arrhythmia has no clinical significance. The lack of sinus arrhythmia or the presence of a fixed fast rate may be more serious because it may be observed in asphyxiated newborns. No treatment is needed.

Premature atrial contraction. PACs are common in healthy newborns (up to 35% of full-term neonates and fewer premature newborns). They also are seen in heart defects, after cardiac surgery, and in digitalis toxicity. Many nonconducted PACs may result in a low heart rate. Usually no treatment is indicated, except in infants with digitalis toxicity.

Supraventricular tachycardia. SVT has three different mechanisms. Reciprocating AV tachycardia is the most frequent type of SVT. Nonreciprocating atrial tachycardia and nodal tachycardia are rare forms of SVT (see Chapter 24 for a detailed discussion of SVT).

SVT is characterized by rapid heart rates, usually 200 to 300 beats/min, with a QRS complex of normal duration (Fig. 29-7). The episodes usually start and end abruptly. WPW syndrome is responsible for about 50% of SVT in the neonate. Structural heart diseases (such as Ebstein's anomaly, tricuspid atresia, and cardiac tumors) are less frequent causes of SVT in the neonate. Viral myocarditis and thyrotoxicosis also have been associated with SVT.

Short episodes of tachycardia usually do not harm the patient. Newborns with sustained SVT become restless and tachypneic with feeding difficulties and eventually develop signs of CHF and circulatory shock within 24 to 48 hours after onset. Although rare, SVT diagnosed in utero may present with severe CHF at birth and has a high mortality rate, requiring prenatal treatment (see later discussion).

Adenosine is the treatment of choice, followed by digitalization. Adenosine is given in a rapid intravenous bolus, starting at 50 μg/kg, every 1 to 2 min (maximum, 250 μg/kg). If the patient is unresponsive to adenosine and is in CHF, cardioversion may be performed, followed by digitalization and diuretics. In SVT of short duration without

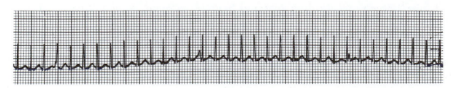

FIG. 29–7.
A rhythm strip showing SVT, with the heart rate of 300 beats/min in a neonate.

signs of CHF, digoxin alone is used. An ice bag applied to the face has been effective in some neonates. Vagal stimulatory maneuvers rarely are effective in neonates. Transesophageal atrial overdrive stimulation may prove effective. Verapamil and propranolol are not the drugs of choice and are tried only when other measures fail. These drugs may produce extreme bradycardia and hypotension in the newborn; one should administer these drugs in a step-by-step dosage, monitor the infant carefully, and be prepared to resuscitate the infant.

One treats fetal SVT by providing digitalization in the mother. Therapy usually is instituted in the mother by intravenous loading of digoxin (8 to 12 μg/kg) over 24 hours, followed by a relatively large oral maintenance dose (0.5 to 0.75 mg/day). Fetal digoxin levels usually are similar to maternal levels, although the ratio of fetal to maternal digoxin ranges from 0.6 to 1.

Atrial flutter/fibrillation. Atrial flutter/fibrillation usually is associated with organic heart disease with dilated atria and with CHDs such as Ebstein's anomaly, MS, tricuspid atresia, myocarditis, or cardiomyopathy. Atrial flutter/defibrillation also is seen with systemic infection and digitalis toxicity. CHF may develop if the ventricular response is fast. Cardioversion is the treatment of choice in infants who are in CHF; the next treatment of choice is digoxin, if the arrhythmia is not caused by digitalis toxicity. In the infant without CHF, digoxin is indicated to prevent CHF by maintaining the ventricular rate within an acceptable range. Propranolol may be added if the patient does not respond to digoxin alone.

Nodal premature beats and nodal escape beats. Nodal (or junctional) premature beats and nodal escape beats usually are idiopathic and are seen in otherwise normal newborn infants. These beats may be a sign of digitalis toxicity. Treatment is not indicated unless the cause is digitalis toxicity.

Nodal (or junctional) rhythm. Nodal rhythm may be seen in otherwise normal neonates, neonates with certain CHDs, and those with increased vagal tone (increased intracranial pressure, pharyngeal stimulation). Nodal rhythm may be a sign of digitalis toxicity. No treatment is indicated if the patient is asymptomatic. Atropine or electrical pacing may be indicated if the patient has symptoms from bradycardia.

Premature ventricular contractions. Many PVCs are idiopathic and frequently are seen in healthy newborns. Occasionally a PVC is associated with CHDs, myocarditis, cardiomyopathy, or cardiac tumors as well as hyperkalemia or asphyxia. Drugs such as catecholamines, theophylline, and caffeine may be the cause. Rarely, a long QT syndrome (Jervell and Lange-Nielsen syndrome and Romano-Ward syndrome) may be responsible for the arrhythmia.

Occasional isolated, uniform PVCs usually are benign. PVCs are more likely to be significant if they are multiform, particularly couplets; they are associated with underlying cardiac conditions, and they appear in runs.

Frequent PVCs require investigation, including an echo examination, and treatment. Lidocaine in an intravenous bolus, followed by an intravenous drip of lidocaine, is a preferred approach. Other antiarrhythmic agents (e.g., phenytoin, propranolol) may be indicated.

Ventricular tachycardia. Ventricular tachycardia is caused by the same conditions as those listed for PVCs, with the exception that ventricular tachycardia does not appear in normal children. Treatment consists of termination of the arrhythmia with lidocaine infusion or cardioversion, correction of the underlying cause when possible, and prevention of recurrence with antiarrhythmic agents (e.g., phenytoin, propranolol).

Ventricular fibrillation. Ventricular fibrillation usually is the terminal arrhythmia, often preceded by ventricular tachycardia, because it results in ineffective circulation. Causes are postoperative states, severe hypoxia, hyperkalemia, myocarditis, myocardial infarction, and drugs (e.g., catecholamines, anesthetics). Immediate cardiopulmonary resuscitation should be performed, including electric defibrillation at the dose of 2 Joules/kg.

Disturbances of Atrioventricular Conduction

A disturbance in conduction from the normal sinus impulse to the eventual ventricular response is assigned to one of three classes, depending on the severity of the conduction disturbance.

First-degree atrioventricular block. The patient has a simple prolongation of the PR interval beyond the upper limits of normal (> 0.12 sec in the newborn). The block produces no hemodynamic disturbance. It may be seen with CHDs (ECD, ASD, and Ebstein's anomaly), digitalis toxicity, or metabolic abnormalities. No treatment is indicated, with the exception of a block caused by digitalis toxicity.

Second-degree atrioventricular block. In second-degree AV block, some, but not all, P waves are followed by QRS complexes.

1. These blocks occur in several types: Mobitz types I and II and higher-grade AV blocks. In Mobitz type I (Wenckebach phenomenon), the PR interval becomes progressively longer until one QRS complex is dropped completely. This type does not progress to complete heart block. In Mobitz type II, the AV conduction is "all or none." The AV conduction is either normal or completely blocked. It is more serious than the type I block, because it may progress to complete heart block. In 2:1 or higher AV block, a QRS complex follows every second, third, or fourth P wave, resulting in 2:1, 3:1, or 4:1 AV block. These blocks occasionally progress to complete heart block.

2. The causes are myocarditis, cardiomyopathy, certain CHDs, postoperative state, and digitalis toxicity.

3. Treatment should be directed toward the underlying cause. Prophylactic pacemaker therapy may be indicated in Mobitz type II or high second-degree AV block.

Third-degree atrioventricular block (complete heart block). In complete heart block, the P wave is completely unrelated to the QRS complex, and each has its own rhythm. The P rate is normal for the newborn, and the QRS rate is slower than the P rate. The QRS duration is normal, because the block is above the bifurcation of the bundle of His. Congenital complete heart block is associated with CHDs in 30% of cases, and this combination may result in CHF. Maternal lupus erythematosus or other connective tissue disease has a frequent association with congenital heart block in the infant.

Patients have a 5% to 10% rate of sudden death in the first year of life. Risk factors for sudden death may include (1) heart rate persistently below 55 beats/min, (2) CHF resulting from associated structural heart defects, (3) presence of significant cardiac anomalies, (4) escape ventricular beats, and (5) long QTc interval. Most newborns without these risk factors do well until late childhood, when they may become symptomatic. One should give pacemaker therapy to the newborn with some or all of these risk factors.

PART VIII

Special Problems

This section explores common pediatric cardiac problems not discussed in previous chapters. The topics include CHF, systemic hypertension, pulmonary hypertension, hyperlipidemia, chest pain, syncope, postoperative syndromes, and cardiac transplantation.

30 / Congestive Heart Failure

DEFINITION

CHF is a clinical syndrome in which the heart is unable to pump enough blood to the body to meet its needs, to dispose of venous return adequately, or a combination of the two.

ETIOLOGY

CHF may result from CHDs or acquired heart diseases with volume and/or pressure overload or from myocardial insufficiency.

Congenital Heart Disease

CHD with volume or pressure overload is the most common cause of CHF in the pediatric age group. Volume overload lesions, such as VSD, PDA, and ECD, are the most common causes of CHF in the first 6 months of life. The time of onset of CHF varies predictably with the type of the defect. Table 30-1 lists common CHDs according to the age at which CHF develops. When using Table 30-1, the following should also be considered:

1. Children with TOF do not develop CHF unless they have received a large aorta–PA shunt procedure (such as Waterston's or Potts' operation), which is no longer performed.

2. ASD rarely causes CHF in the pediatric age group, although it causes CHF in adulthood.

3. Large left-to-right shunt lesions, such as VSD and PDA, do not cause CHF before 6 to 8 weeks of age because the PVR does not fall low enough to cause a large left-to-right shunt until this age. The onset of CHF resulting from left-to-right shunt lesions may be earlier in premature infants (within the first month) because of an earlier fall in the PVR in these infants.

Acquired Heart Disease

Acquired heart disease of various etiologies can cause CHF. The age at onset of CHF caused by acquired heart disease is not as predictable as that of CHD, but the following generalities apply to CHF:

1. Metabolic abnormalities (severe hypoxia and acidosis as well as hypoglycemia and hypocalcemia) can cause CHF in the newborn.

2. Endocardial fibroelastosis, a rare primary myocardial disease, causes CHF in infancy; 90% of cases occur in the first 8 months of life.

3. Viral myocarditis tends to be more common in small children older than 1 year. It occurs occasionally in the newborn period, with a fulminating clinical course.

4. Acute rheumatic carditis is an occasional cause of CHF that primarily occurs in school children.

5. Rheumatic valvular heart diseases, usually volume overload lesions such as MR and/or AR, cause CHF in older children and adults. These diseases are uncommon in industrialized countries.

TABLE 30–1.

Causes of Congestive Heart Failure Resulting from Congenital Heart Disease

Age of Onset	Cause
At birth	HLHS
	Volume overload lesions:
	Severe tricuspid or pulmonary insufficiency
	Large systemic AV fistula
First week	TGA
	PDA in small premature infants
	HLHS (with more favorable anatomy)
	TAPVR, particularly those with pulmonary venous obstruction
	Others:
	Systemic AV fistula
	Critical AS or PS
1-4 wk	COA with associated anomalies
	Critical AS
	Large left-to-right shunt lesions (VSD, PDA) in premature infants
	All other lesions previously listed
4-6 wk	Some left-to-right shunt lesions such as ECD
6 wk-4 mo	Large VSD
	Large PDA
	Others such as anomalous left coronary artery from the PA

6. Dilated cardiomyopathy of the idiopathic type may cause CHF at any age during childhood and adolescence.

7. Cardiomyopathies associated with muscular dystrophy and Friedreich's ataxia may cause CHF in older children and adolescents.

8. Doxorubicin cardiomyopathy may manifest months to years after the completion of chemotherapy for malignancies in children.

Miscellaneous Causes

Miscellaneous causes include the following:

1. SVT causes CHF in early infancy.

2. Complete heart block associated with structural heart defects causes CHF in the newborn period or early infancy.

3. Severe anemia may be a cause of CHF at any age, hydrops fetalis may be a cause in the newborn period, and severe sicklemia may be a cause at a later age.

4. Acute hypertension, as seen in acute postinfectious glomerulonephritis, causes CHF in school-age children. Fluid retention with poor renal function is important as the cause of hypertension in this condition.

5. Bronchopulmonary dysplasia seen in premature infants causes predominantly right-sided heart failure in the first few months of life.

6. Acute cor pulmonale caused by acute airway obstruction (such as seen with large tonsils) can cause CHF at any age but most commonly during early childhood.

CLINICAL MANIFESTATIONS

The diagnosis of CHF relies on several sources of clinical findings, including history, physical examination, and chest-x-ray films. In addition to physical findings discussed here, cardiomegaly on a chest film is nearly a prequisite sign of CHF; an ECG is perhaps the least important test for the diagnosis of CHF. No single test is specific for CHF; the diagnosis is based on several clinical findings.

History

1. Poor feeding of recent onset, tachypnea that worsens during feeding, poor weight gain, and cold sweat on the forehead suggest CHF in infants.

2. Older children may complain of shortness of breath, especially with activities, easy fatigability, puffy eyelids, or swollen feet.

Physical Examination

Physical findings of CHF may be classified as follows depending on their pathophysiologic mechanisms. The more common findings are in italics.

Compensatory response to impaired cardiac function.

1. *Tachycardia, gallop rhythm,* weak and thready pulse are common.

2. *Cardiomegaly* almost always is present. Chest x-ray films are more reliable than physical examination in demonstrating cardiomegaly.

3. Increased sympathetic discharges (e.g., *growth failure, perspiration,* cold wet skin) are common.

Pulmonary venous congestion (left-sided failure).

1. *Tachypnea* is common.

2. Dyspnea on exertion (*poor feeding* in small infants) is common.

3. Orthopnea may be found in older children.

4. Wheezing and pulmonary *rales* may be audible.

Systemic venous congestion (right-sided failure).

1. *Hepatomegaly* is common. It is not always indicative of CHF; a large liver may be palpable in the absence of CHF, such as in conditions with hyperinflated lungs (asthma, bronchiolitis, hypoxic spell) and infiltrative liver disease. On the other hand, the absence of hepatomegaly does not rule out CHF; hepatomegaly may be absent in (early) left-sided failure.

2. *Puffy eyelids* are common in infants.

3. Distended neck veins and ankle edema, which are common in adults, are not seen in infants.

4. Splenomegaly is not indicative of chronic CHF but usually indicates infection.

X-Ray Study

One should demonstrate the presence of cardiomegaly by chest x-ray films. The absence of cardiomegaly almost rules out the diagnosis of CHF. However, the presence of cardiomegaly per se does not mean CHF is present, because some children with large left-to-right shunt lesions have cardiomegaly without heart failure.

Electrocardiography. ECGs help determine the type of the defect but are not helpful in deciding whether CHF is present.

Echocardiography. Echo may confirm an enlarged chamber or impaired LV function (decreased fractional shortening or ejection fraction, increased LPEP/LVET). A more important role of echo may be its ability to determine the cause of CHF. Echo also is useful in serial evaluation of the efficacy of therapy.

TREATMENT

The treatment of CHF consists of elimination of the underlying causes, elimination of the precipitating causes (e.g., infection, arrhythmias, fever), and control of heart failure state. The heart failure state is controlled by the use of multiple drugs, usually inotropic agents, diuretics, and afterload-reducing agents, along with general supportive measures. Eliminating the underlying causes is the most desirable approach whenever possible. Surgical correction of CHDs is such an approach. Every patient with CHF should receive maximal medical treatment, but continuing with long-term anticongestive measures is unwise when the heart defect can be safely repaired through surgery.

General Measures

1. "Cardiac chair" or "infant seat" is used to relieve respiratory distress.

2. Oxygen (40% to 50%) with humidity is administered to infants with respiratory distress.

3. Sedation with morphine sulfate (0.1 to 0.2 mg/kg/dose subcutaneously every 4 hours as needed) or phenobarbital (2 to 3 mg/kg/dose by mouth or intramuscularly every 8 hours as necessary) for 1 to 2 days occasionally is indicated.

4. Salt restriction in the form of a low-salt formula and severe fluid restriction are not indicated in infants. Use of diuretics has replaced these measures. In older children, salt restriction (<0.5 g/day) and avoidance of salty snacks (chips, pretzels) and table salt are recommended.

5. Daily weight measurement is essential in hospitalized patients.

6. Predisposing factors, such as fever (reduction of fever), anemia (packed cell transfusion to raise hematocrit to 35% or higher), and infection, are eliminated.

7. Underlying causes such as hypertension, arrhythmias, and thyrotoxicosis are treated.

Drug Therapy

Three major classes of drugs are used in the treatment of CHF in children: inotropic agents, diuretics, and afterload-reducing agents. Every child with CHF should receive digitalis, unless its use is contraindicated by hypertrophic cardiomyopathy, complete heart block, or cardiac tamponade. Diuretics almost always are used with digitalis glycosides. Afterload-reducing agents have gained popularity in recent years.

Diuretics. Patients with CHF may improve rapidly after a dose of a fast-acting diuretic, such as ethacrynic acid or furosemide, even before digitalization. Table 30-2 shows dosages of commonly available diuretic preparations. There are three major classes of diuretics that are commercially available.

1. Thiazide diuretics (e.g., chlorothiazide, hydrochlorothiazide), which act at the proximal and distal tubules, are less popular.

2. Rapid-acting diuretics, such as furosemide and ethacrynic acid, probably are the drugs of choice. They act primarily at the loop of Henle ("loop diuretics").

3. Aldosterone antagonists (such as spironolactone) are indicated in the treatment of the hyperaldosteronism component of CHF. The serum aldosterone level is significantly increased in patients with persistent CHF, contributing to fluid and salt retention. Patients with an increased level of circulating aldosterone have a diminished response to diuretic agents because aldosterone increases tubular reabsorption of sodium and water at a site distal to the sites of action of other diuretic agents (thiazides or furosemide). In addition, these drugs have value in preventing hypokalemia produced by other diuretics.

TABLE 30–2.

Diuretic Agents and Dosages

Preparation	Route	Dosage
Thiazide Diuretics		
Chlorothiazide (Diuril)	Oral	20-40 mg/kg/day in 2-3 divided doses
Hydrochlorothiazide (HydroDiuril)	Oral	2-4 mg/kg/day in 2-3 divided doses
Loop Diuretics		
Furosemide (Lasix)	IV	1 mg/kg/dose
	Oral	2-3 mg/kg/day in 2-3 divided doses
Ethacrynic acid (Edecrin)	IV	1 mg/kg/dose
	Oral	2-3 mg/kg/day in 2-3 divided doses
Aldosterone Antagonist		
Spironolactone (Aldactone)	Oral	2-3 mg/kg/day in 2-3 divided doses

IV, Intravenous.

TABLE 30–3.

Oral Digoxin Dosage for CHF

Age	TDD* (μg/kg)	Maintenance*† (μg/kg/day)
Prematures	20	5
Newborns	30	8
Under 2 yr	40-50	10-12
Over 2 yr	30-40	8-10

TDD, total digitalizing dose.
*IV dose is 75% of the oral dose.
†Maintenance dose is 25% of the TDD in two divided doses.

Side effects of diuretic therapy. Diuretic therapy alters the serum electrolyte balance and acid-base equilibrium.

1. Hypokalemia is a common problem with diuretic therapy, except with Aldactone. It is more profound with potent loop diuretics. Hypokalemia may increase the likelihood of digitalis toxicity.

2. Hypochloremic alkalosis may result because the loss of chloride ions is greater than the loss of sodium ions through the kidneys, with a resultant increase in bicarbonate levels. Alkalosis also predisposes to digitalis toxicity.

Digitalis glycosides

Dosage of digoxin. Digoxin is the most commonly used digitalis preparation in pediatric patients. The total digitalizing dose and maintenance dosage of digoxin by oral and intravenous routes are shown in Table 30-3. (The dosage of digitoxin appears in Appendix D.) The dosage may be higher in treating SVT, in which the goal of treatment is to delay AV conduction. The maintenance dose is more closely related to the serum digoxin level than is the digitalizing dose, which is given to build a sufficient body store of the drug and to shorten the time required to reach the pharmacokinetic steady state.

The pediatric dosage is relatively larger than that used in adults on the basis of body size. Pharmacokinetic studies indicate that infants and children require a larger dose of digoxin than adults to attain comparable serum levels, primarily because of a large volume of distribution and a more rapid renal clearance, including tubular secretion. The

ECG Changes Associated With Digitalis

Effects

Shortening of QTc, the earliest sign of digitalis effect
Sagging ST segment and diminished amplitude of T wave (the T vector does not change)
Slowing of heart rate

Toxicity

Prolongation of PR interval
  Sometimes a prolonged PR interval is seen in children without digitalis, making a baseline ECG
    mandatory
  The prolongation may progress to second-degree AV block
Profound sinus bradycardia or SA block
Supraventricular arrhythmias, such as atrial or nodal ectopic beats and tachycardias (particularly if ac-
  companied by AV block), which are more common than ventricular arrhythmias in children
Ventricular arrhythmias such as ventricular bigeminy or trigeminy, which are extremely rare in chil-
  dren, although they are common in adults with digitalis toxicity; PVCs, which are not uncommon in
  children as a sign of toxicity.

---

volume of distribution is 7.5 L/kg in neonates, 16 L/kg in infants and children, and 4 L/kg in adults.

How to digitalize. Loading doses of the total digitalizing dose are given in 12 to 18 hours and are followed by maintenance doses. This results in a pharmacokinetic steady state in 3 to 5 days. An intravenous route is preferred over the oral route, particularly when dealing with infants in severe heart failure. An intramuscular route is not recommended, because absorption of the drug from the injection site is unreliable. When an infant is in mild heart failure, the maintenance dose may be administered orally without loading doses; this results in a steady state in 5 to 8 days.

The following is a suggested step-by-step method of digitalization:

1. Obtain a baseline ECG (rhythm and PR interval) and baseline levels of serum electrolytes. Changes in ECG rhythm and PR interval are important signs of digitalis toxicity (see later discussion). Hypokalemia and hypercalcemia predispose to digitoxicity.

2. Calculate the total digitalizing dose (see Table 30-3). Two people should calculate the total digitalizing dose independently and compare figures, because a mistake can be made in the magnitude of a decimal point.

3. Give one half the total digitalizing dose immediately, followed by one fourth and the final one fourth of the total digitalizing dose at 6- to 8-hour intervals.

4. Start the maintenance dose 12 hours after the final total digitalizing dose. Obtain an ECG strip before starting the maintenance dose.

Monitoring for digitalis toxicity by ECG. Digitalis toxicity is best detected by monitoring with ECGs, not serum digoxin levels, during the first 3 to 5 days after digitalization. Box above lists ECG signs of digitalis effects and toxicity. In general, the digitalis effect is confined to *ventricular repolarization,* whereas toxicity involves disturbances in the *formation and conduction of the impulse.* One should assume that any arrhythmia or conduction disturbance occurring *with* digitalis is *caused* by digitalis until proved otherwise.

Serum digoxin levels. Therapeutic ranges of serum digoxin levels for treating CHF are 0.8 to 2.0 ng/ml. Levels obtained during the first 3 to 5 days after digitalization tend to be higher than those obtained when the pharmacokinetic steady state is reached. Serum digoxin levels should be tested at least 6 hours after the last dose or just before a scheduled dose (during the β-phase); samples obtained before 6 hours after the last dose will give a falsely elevated level.

Drug Interactions with Digoxin

Increase in Digoxin Concentration

Quinidine (because of reduced volume of distribution by 30% to 40% and reduced tubular secretion); digoxin concentration increased more than 2 times in adults, 2 times in children; no increase in newborns

Calcium channel blockers (verapamil, nifedipine) (because of decreased tubular secretion of digoxin); 40% rise in adults; similar increase in children

Diuretics (because of diuretic-induced renal insufficiency or hypokalemia and/or hypomagnesemia (no increase with Aldactone)

Indomethacin (because of decreased glomerular filtration); 50% rise in preterm infants

Amiodarone (because of reduced tubular secretion); 65% rise in adults; similar rise in children

Antibiotics (erythromycin, tetracycline) (because of decreased metabolism of digoxin by gut flora)

Reduction in Digoxin Concentration

Vasodilators (e.g., hydralazine, nitroprusside) (because of increased tubular secretion of digoxin as a result of increased renal blood flow)

Cholestyramine, colestipol (because of decreased bioavailability of digoxin)

Antibiotic neomycin (because of decreased intestinal absorption of digoxin by an unknown mechanism)

Frequently determining serum digoxin levels and using those levels for therapeutic goals are neither justified nor practical; occasional determination of the level is adequate. Determination of the serum digoxin level is useful in evaluating possible toxicity (see later discussion), in determining the patient's compliance, detecting abnormalities in absorption and excretion, and the managing accidental overdose.

Endogenous digoxin-like substance or endogenous digoxin-immunoactive factor. Several commonly used radioimmunoassays report false-positive digoxin concentrations in a substantial number of normal full-term and preterm newborns who are not receiving digoxin, with some "apparent digoxin" values falling well into the therapeutic range. The appearance of endogenous digoxin-like substance also has been documented in many clinical situations, including renal failure and hepatic failure, adult patients with heart failure, normal and hypertensive pregnant women, volume expansion or electrolyte imbalance, and healthy adults who exercised on a treadmill. Endogenous digoxin-like substance (EDLS) appears to be secreted from the hypothalamus in conditions with extracellular fluid volume expansion or decreased cardiac output or blood pressure. It was shown to have digitalis-like actions, including inhibition of the sodium–potassium–adenosinetriphosphatase pump and demonstrable cardiotonic effects. Recently, endogenous digoxin-like substance has been shown to be either ouabain or its isomers.

The presence of EDLS has made accurate measurement of digoxin difficult in some newborns and has confused the interpretation of serum digoxin levels. Serum digoxin levels obtained in some newborns may have been affected by endogenous ouabain in the sample. Some authors have suggested that the magnitude of the inotropic effect of endogenous ouabain is similar to that of digoxin. Therefore one should not allow a high serum digoxin level or completely disregard the digoxin level in the newborn on account of a possible contamination of digoxin levels by endogenous ouabain. The full implications of the presence of endogenous digoxin-like substance require further investigation.

Drug interaction with digoxin. Certain drugs when used concomitantly affect serum digoxin levels. Selected drugs that affect the serum digoxin level, and their mechanism(s) of interactions, are summarized in Box above. Quinidine and calcium channel blockers are known to increase serum digoxin levels, and vasodilators decrease the level.

Digitalis toxicity. With the relatively low dosage recommended in Table 30-3, digitalis toxicity is unlikely. However, one should beware of digitalis toxicity with every child receiving digitalis preparations. Patients with conditions listed in Box on p. 408 are more likely to develop toxicity.

Factors That May Predispose to Digitalis Toxicity
_____

High Serum Digoxin Level
High-dose requirement as in treatment of certain arrhythmias
Decreased renal excretion
   Premature infants
   Renal disease
Hypothyroidism
Drug interaction (e.g., quinidine, verapamil, amiodarone)

Increased Sensitivity of Myocardium (Without High Serum Digoxin Level)
Status of myocardium
   Myocardial ischemia
   Myocarditis (rheumatic, viral)
Systemic changes
   Electrolyte imbalance (hypokalemia, hypercalcemia)
   Hypoxia
   Alkalosis
   Adrenergic stimuli or catecholamines
Immediate postoperative period after heart surgery under cardiopulmonary bypass
_____

The diagnosis of digitalis toxicity, again, is a clinical decision and usually is based on the following clinical and laboratory findings:

1. The patient has a history of accidental ingestion.

2. Noncardiac symptoms appear in digitalized children: anorexia, nausea, vomiting, or diarrhea, restlessness, drowsiness, fatigue, and visual disturbances in older children.

3. Heart failure worsens.

4. ECG signs probably are more reliable and appear early (see Box on p. 406).

5. An elevated serum level of digoxin (>2 ng/ml) is likely to be associated with toxicity in a child if the clinical findings suggest digitalis toxicity.

When the diagnosis of digitalis toxicity is established, the following measures are taken:

1. General therapy, including discontinuation of digitalis, discontinuation of diuretics unless absolutely indicated, and continuous ECG monitoring, is provided. Glucose should not be given without potassium. Predisposing factors are evaluated (see Box on p. 408) and eliminated or treated.

2. Specific therapy is provided:

   a. For frequent premature beats or supraventricular arrhythmias, administer potassium chloride. It counteracts arrhythmia-producing effects of digitalis without depressing myocardial contractility. Contraindications for the use of potassium chloride include advanced heart block (second- and third-degree AV block), hyperkalemia, and anuria or oliguria. The dose is: oral, 3 to 5 g/day, diluted in chilled fruit juice; intravenous 0.5 mEq/kg/hr, intravenous drip until arrhythmias disappear or peaked T waves appear (maximum 3 mEq/kg/day).

   b. For tachyarrhythmias:
   Lidocaine: 1 mg/kg intravenous bolus, followed by 1 to 3 mg/kg/hr intravenous drip (maximum total dose, 5 mg/kg).
   Phenytoin (Dilantin): 3 to 5 mg/kg slow intravenous push, repeat in 10 to 15 minutes as necessary (maximum total dose, 500 mg in 4 hours).

TABLE 30–4.

Suggested Starting Dosages of Catecholamines

Drug	Route and Dosage	Side Effects
Epinephrine (Adrenalin)	(IV) 0.1-1.0 µg/kg/min	Hypertension, arrhythmias
Isoproterenol (Isuprel)	(IV) 0.1-0.5 µg/kg/min	Peripheral and pulmonary vasodilatation
Dobutamine (Dobutrex)	(IV) 5-8 µg/kg/min	Little tachycardia and vasodilatation, arrhythmias
Dopamine (Intropin)	(IV) 5-10 µg/kg/min	Tachycardia, arrhythmias, hypertension or hypotension
		Dose-related cardiovascular effects (µg/kg/min):
		Renal vasodilation: 2-5
		Inotropic: 5-8
		Tachycardia: >8
		Mild vasoconstriction: >10
		Vasoconstriction: 15-20

IV, Intravenous.

Propranolol: 0.01 mg/kg, slow intravenous push every 2 minutes (maximum 0.1 mg/kg), followed by 1 to 4 mg/kg/day, by mouth in three or four doses.
Cardioversion: Only if the patient is unresponsive to other measures. Start at 0.5 Joules/kg and increase by a small increment.

c. For heart block:
Atropine: 0.01 to 0.03 mg/kg every 4 to 6 hours, as necessary (maximum 0.4 mg/kg). Transvenous catheter pacing, which is usually indicated.

d. Digibind (Digoxin Immune Fab) may be used in children with an accidental overdose (more than 4 mg of digoxin in children, serum levels >10 ng/ml) or those with life-threatening rhythm disturbances (severe ventricular arrhythmias, progressive bradycardia, or second- or third-degree heart block). When the ingested amount of digoxin is known, the dosage of Digibind is calculated; each vial (40 mg) binds approximately 0.6 mg of digoxin, and 80% of the calculated dose is administered to account for incomplete absorption. In infants and small children (weighing <20 kg), a single vial (40 mg), and for adults, six vials (240 mg) may be adequate. It is administered intravenously over 30 minutes.

Other inotropic agents. In infants in severe CHF with distress, in those with renal dysfunction (such as seen in infants with COA), or in postoperative cardiac patients with heart failure, rapidly acting catecholamines with a short duration of action are preferable to digoxin. Dosages for intravenous drips are suggested in Table 30–4.

Afterload-reducing agents. As a compensatory response to reduced cardiac output seen in CHF, vasoconstriction may be deleterious to the failing ventricle and may worsen CHF. Vasoconstriction is produced by a rise in sympathetic tone and circulating catecholamines and an increase in the activity of the renin-angiotensin system. Reducing afterload tends to augment the stroke volume without changing the contractile state of the heart and therefore without increasing myocardial oxygen consumption.

These agents usually are used with digitalis glycosides and diuretics. Indications for vasodilator therapy include cardiomyopathy, dilated or adriamycin-induced; myocardial ischemia; postoperative cardiac status; severe MR or AR; and systemic hypertension. Recently, some CHDs with large left-to-right shunts (e.g., VSD, AV canal, PDA) have been shown to benefit from hydralazine and captopril, but a deleterious effect was observed with nitroprusside.

Afterload-reducing agents may be divided into three groups based on the site of

TABLE 30–5.

Dosages of Vasodilators

Drug	Route and Dosage	Comments
Hydralazine (Apresoline)	(IV) 1.5 μg/kg/min, or 0.1-0.2 mg/kg/dose, every 4-6 hours (maximum 2 mg/kg every 6 hours) (O) 0.75-3.0 mg/kg/day, in two to four doses (maximum 200 mg/day)	It may cause tachycardia, and it may be used with propranolol. It may cause gastrointestinal symptoms, neutropenia, and lupuslike syndrome.
Nitroglycerin	(IV) 0.5-2.0 μg/kg/min (maximum 6.0 μg/kg/min)	Start with a small dose and titrate based on its effects.
Captopril (Capoten)	(O) Newborn: 0.1-0.4 mg/kg/dose, 1 to 4 times a day Infants: 0.5-6.0 mg/kg/day, 1 to 4 times a day Child: 12.5 mg/dose, 1 to 2 times a day	It may cause hypotension, dizziness, neutropenia and proteinuria. The dose should be reduced in patients with impaired renal function.
Enalapril (Vasotec)	(O) 0.1 mg/kg, once or twice daily	The patient may develop hypotension, dizziness, or syncope.
Nitroprusside (Nipride)	(IV) 0.5-8 μg/kg/min	It may cause thiocyanate or cyanide toxicity (e.g., fatigue, nausea, disorientation), hepatic dysfunction, or light sensitivity.
Prazosine (Minipress)	(O) First dose: 5 μg/kg; increase to 25-150 μg/kg/day, in four doses	It has fewer side effects than hydralazine; orthostatic hypotension or tachyphylaxis may develop.

IV, Intravenous; *O,* oral.

action: arteriolar vasodilators, venodilators, and mixed (or "balanced") vasodilators. Dosages of these agents are presented in Table 30-5.

1. Arteriolar vasodilators (hydralazine) augment cardiac output by acting primarily on the arteriolar bed, with resulting reduction of the afterload. Hydralazine, the most commonly used arteriolar vasodilator, often is administered with propranolol because it activates the baroreceptor reflex, with resulting tachycardia.

2. Venodilators (nitroglycerin, isosorbide dinitrate) act primarily by dilating systemic veins and redistributing blood from the pulmonary to the systemic circuit (with a resulting decrease in pulmonary symptoms). Venodilators are most beneficial in patients with pulmonary congestion but may have adverse effects when preload has been restored to normal by diuretics and/or sodium restriction.

3. "Balanced vasodilators" include angiotensin-converting enzyme inhibitors (such as captopril and enalapril), nitroprusside, and prazosin. These agents act on both arteriolar and venous beds. Nitroprusside frequently is used in postoperative cardiac patients, especially in patients who had pulmonary hypertension and those with postoperative rises in PA pressure. Nitroprusside often is used with dopamine or dobutamine. Blood pressure must be monitored continuously. Angiotensin-converting enzyme inhibitors reduce SVR by inhibiting angiotensin II generation and augmenting production of bradykinin. Prazosin, a postsynaptic α-adrenergic

blocking agent, produces far fewer side effects (less tachycardia) than does hydralazine.

Surgical Management

If medical treatment with the previously mentioned regimen does not improve CHF within a few weeks to months, one should perform either palliative or corrective cardiac surgery for the underlying cardiac defect.

31 / Systemic Hypertension

DEFINITION

Hypertension in children may be defined statistically as systolic and/or diastolic pressure levels greater than the 95th percentile for age and gender on at least three occasions. High normal blood pressure is defined as an average systolic and/or diastolic blood pressure between the 90th and 95th percentiles for age and gender. Values slightly above the 95th percentile may be considered significant hypertension, and values greater than the 95th percentile by 8 to 10 mm Hg may be considered severe hypertension. A prerequisite for these definitions is the availability of reliable normative blood pressure values (see later discussion). For adults, the World Health Organization has defined values (systolic/diastolic) of 140 to 150/90 to 95 mm Hg as borderline hypertension and values above 160/95 mm Hg as hypertension.

Although this definition is widely accepted, hypertension is not defined by specific levels of blood pressure in children because of the lack of reliable sets of normative blood pressure levels for this age group. Many well-conducted epidemiologic studies have provided data on the normal distribution of blood pressure in children by the auscultatory method. A comparison of these observations reveals a wide variation in values. The difference between the highest and lowest mean blood pressure levels (shown in Fig. 31-1) as well as the "95th percentile systolic pressure" is as much as 30 mm Hg for certain age groups. The implication of this is profound. For example, a child who is considered to have a borderline hypertension based on one set of normative values may be in the low normal range but may be in the hypertensive range by other normative values.

The main reason for this discrepancy is likely the methodology used, although the observations are based on different populations. When more than 20 large epidemiologic studies are reviewed, differences in methodology are found in the selection of the occluding cuff (based on the length or the circumference of the arm), position of the patients (supine or sitting), number of measurements made (one to nine), and the level of diastolic pressure (Korotkoff phase IV or V). These epidemiologic studies exhorted physicians to obtain blood pressure measurements in children as part of a routine examination, but these studies also are the source of confusion to practitioners. The size of the cuff used in the studies appears to be an important determinant of the variability.

Normative levels recommended by the National Institute of Health Task Force on Blood Pressure Control in Children (1987) were obtained with a cuff width of three fourths of the length of the arm. However, the selection of this cuff was scientifically unsound because it ignored the basic principle of indirect measurements. Normative levels recommended by the same Task Force in 1977 (that were obtained with a cuff width of two thirds of the length of the arm) were an average 10 mm Hg higher than those found in the most recent study (1987). Both times, the Task Force failed to adopt a scientifically proven method of selecting cuffs based on the thickness of the arm. The thickness-based selection method has been used in adults for several decades. Recently, the American Heart Association correctly recommended that the selection of the occluding cuff be based on the thickness of the arm for children as well. The cuff width should be 40% to 50% of the circumference (or 125% to 155% of the diameter) of the limb on which blood pressure is to be measured, but the American Heart Association has not provided normative blood pressure levels using this method (see Chapter 2 for further discussion). Suggested normative auscultatory blood pressure values for children 6 years and older, based on other studies using the correct blood pressure cuff, are

412

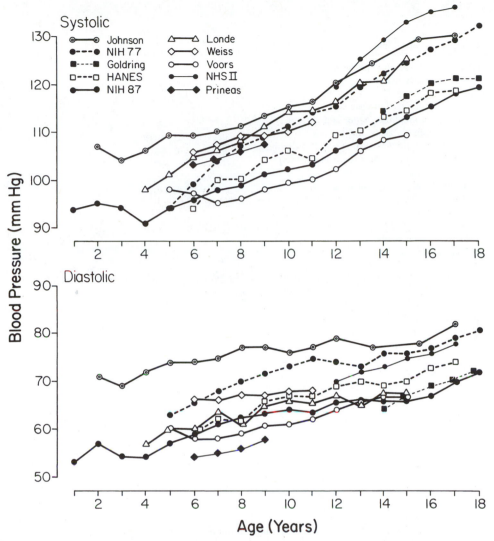

FIG. 31–1.
Comparison of normative blood pressure levels reported by various epidemiologic studies. Mean (or 50th percentile) values of indirect blood pressure measurements of boys from 10 large epidemiologic surveys are shown for comparison. When racial differences are present, values for white children have been illustrated. Selection of the occluding cuff and diastolic signals varies from study to study. Note that a difference of more than 20 mm Hg exists between the highest and the lowest values for certain age groups for both systolic and diastolic pressures. Similar differences are present for 95th percentile values.

presented in Table 2-4. Normative oscillometric blood pressure levels for the first 5 years of life obtained in the office setting are presented in Table 2-5.

ETIOLOGY

Hypertension is classified into two general types: essential (or primary) hypertension, in which a specific etiology cannot be identified, and secondary hypertension, in which a cause can be identified (Box on p. 414). The incidence of essential hypertension in

Causes of Hypertension

Primary (or essential) hypertension: causes unknown
Secondary hypertension
Renal
  Renal parenchymal disease
    Glomerulonephritis, acute and chronic
    Pyelonephritis, acute and chronic
    Congenital anomalies (polycystic or dysplastic kidneys)
    Obstructive uropathies (hydronephrosis)
    Hemolytic-uremic syndrome
    Collagen disease (periarteritis, lupus)
    Renal damage from nephrotoxic medications, trauma, or radiation
  Renovascular diseases
    Renal artery disorders (e.g., stenosis, polyarteritis, thrombosis)
    Renal vein thrombosis
Cardiovascular
  COA
  Conditions with large stroke volume (PDA, aortic insufficiency, systemic AV fistula, complete heart block) (these conditions cause only systolic hypertension)
Endocrine
  Hyperthyroidism (systolic hypertension)
  Excessive catecholamine levels
    Pheochromocytoma
    Neuroblastoma
  Adrenal dysfunction
    Congenital adrenal hyperplasia
      11-β-hydroxylase deficiency
      17-hydroxylase deficiency
    Cushing's syndrome
    Hyperaldosteronism
      Primary
        Conn's syndrome
        Idiopathic nodular hyperplasia
        Dexamethasone-suppressible hyperaldosteronism
      Secondary
        Renovascular hypertension
        Renin-producing tumor (juxtaglomerular cell tumor)
  Hyperparathyroidism (and hypercalcemia)
Neurogenic
  Increased intracranial pressure (any cause, especially tumors, infections, trauma)
  Poliomyelitis
  Guillain-Barré syndrome
  Dysautonomia (Riley-Day syndrome)
Drugs and chemicals
  Sympathomimetic drugs (nose drops, cough medications, cold preparations)
  Amphetamines
  Steroids
  Oral contraceptives
  Heavy-metal poisoning (mercury, lead)
  Cocaine, acute or chronic use
Miscellaneous
  Hypervolemia and hypernatremia
  Stevens-Johnson syndrome
  Bronchopulmonary dysplasia (newborns)

TABLE 31–1.

Most Common Causes of Chronic Sustained Hypertension

Age Group	Causes
Newborns:	Renal artery thrombosis, renal artery stenosis, congenital renal malformation, COA, bronchopulmonary dysplasia
<6 yr:	Renal parenchymal disease, COA, renal artery stenosis
6-10 yr:	Renal artery stenosis, renal parenchymal disease, primary hypertension
>10 yr:	Primary hypertension, renal parenchymal disease

Adapted from Report of the Second Task Force on Blood Pressure Control in Children, *Pediatrics* 79:1-25, 1987.

is not known. However, over 90% of secondary hypertension in children is caused by three conditions: renal parenchymal disease, renal artery disease, and COA.

Table 31-1 lists the common causes of hypertension by age group in children. In general, the younger the child and the more severe the hypertension, the more likely one is to identify an underlying cause.

DIAGNOSIS AND WORK-UP

Many children with mild hypertension are asymptomatic, and hypertension is diagnosed as the result of routine blood pressure measurement. Children with severe hypertension may be symptomatic (headache, dizziness, nausea and vomiting, irritability, personality changes). Occasionally, neurologic manifestations, CHF, renal dysfunction, and stroke may be the presenting symptoms.

Careful evaluation of history, physical findings, and laboratory tests usually point to the cause of hypertension.

History

The past and present medical history and family history, as follows, are gathered:

Past and current history.

1. Neonatal: use of umbilical artery catheters or bronchopulmonary dysplasia

2. Cardiovascular: history of COA or surgery for it. History of palpitation, headache, and excessive sweating (excessive catecholamine levels)

3. Renal: history of obstructive uropathies, urinary tract infection, radiation, trauma, or surgery to the kidney area

4. Endocrine: weakness and muscle cramp (hyperaldosteronism)

5. Medications: e.g., corticosteroids, amphetamines, antiasthmatic drugs, cold medications, oral contraceptives, nephrotoxic antibiotics, cyclosporin

6. Habits: smoking

Family history.

1. Essential hypertension, atherosclerotic heart disease, and stroke

2. Familial or hereditary renal disease (polycystic kidney, cystinuria, familial nephritis)

Physical Examination

1. Accurate measurement of blood pressure is essential.

2. Complete physical examination also is essential, with emphasis on delayed growth (renal disease), bounding peripheral pulse (PDA or AR), weak or absent femoral pulses and/or blood pressure differential between the arms and legs (COA), abdominal bruits (renovascular), and tenderness over the kidney (renal infection).

TABLE 31–2.
Routine and Special Laboratory Tests and Their Significance

Laboratory Tests	Significance of Abnormal Results
Urinalysis, urine culture, blood urea nitrogen, and creatinine levels	Renal parenchymal disease
Serum electrolyte levels (hypokalemia)	Hyperaldosteronism, primary or secondary Adrenogenital syndrome Renin-producing tumors
ECG, chest x-ray studies	Cardiac cause of hypertension, also baseline function
Intravenous pyelography (or ultrasonography, radionuclide studies, computed tomography of the kidneys)	Renal parenchymal diseases Renovascular hypertension Tumors (neuroblastoma, Wilms tumor)

Plasma renin activity, peripheral	High-renin hypertension
	   Renovascular hypertension
	   Renin-producing tumors
	   Some Cushing's syndrome
	   Some essential hypertension
	Low-renin hypertension
	   Adrenogenital syndrome
	   Primary hyperaldosteronism

24-hr urine collection for 17-ketosteroids and 17-hydroxycorticosteroids	Cushing's syndrome Adrenogenital syndrome
24-hr urine collection for catecholamine levels and vanillylmandelic acid	Pheochromocytoma Neuroblastoma
Aldosterone	Hyperladosteronism, primary or secondary Renovascular hypertension Renin-producing tumors
Renal vein plasma renin activity	Unilateral renal parenchymal disease Renovascular hypertension
Abdominal aortogram	Renovascular hypertension Abdominal COA Unilateral renal parenchymal diseases Pheochromocytoma

Routine Laboratory Tests

Initial laboratory tests should be directed toward detecting renal parenchymal disease, renovascular disease, and COA and therefore should include urinalysis; urine culture; serum electrolyte, blood urea nitrogen, creatinine, and uric acid levels; ECG; chest x-ray studies, and possibly echo.

Specialized Studies

More specialized studies may be indicated for the detection of rare causes of secondary hypertension: excretory urography, plasma renin activity, aldosterone levels in serum and urine, 24-hour urine collection for catecholamine levels (norepinephrine, epinephrine) and their metabolites (vanillylmandelic acid levels), renal vein renin, and abdominal aortogram.

Table 31-2 summarizes the applicability of the routine and specialized tests in identifying the cause of secondary hypertension. The decision to undertake special tests and procedures depends on availability and familiarity with the procedure, severity of hypertension, age of the patient, and history and physical findings suggestive of a certain etiology. For example, children under 10 years of age with sustained hypertension require extensive evaluation, because identifiable and potentially curable causes are likely to be found. Adolescents with mild hypertension and a positive family history of essential hypertension are more likely to have essential hypertension, and extensive studies are not indicated.

MANAGEMENT

Essential Hypertension

Nonpharmacologic intervention. Nonpharmacologic intervention should be started as an initial treatment. Counseling should encourage weight reduction, if indicated; low-salt (and potassium-rich) foods; and avoidance of smoking and oral contraceptives.

Drug therapy. Although there are no clear guidelines for identifying those who should be treated with antihypertensive drugs, a family history of early complications of hypertension, the presence of target organ damage (e.g., ocular, cardiac, renal, central nervous system), and the presence of other coronary artery risk factors favor drug therapy. However, the possible adverse effects of long-term drug therapy on growing children have not been evaluated adequately.

The stepped-care approach, using three classes of drugs: diuretics, β-blockers, and vasodilators, is popular. Step 1 is initiated with a small dose of a single antihypertensive drug, either thiazide diuretic or an adrenergic inhibitor, and then proceeds to full dose, if necessary. In black, diabetic, or asthmatic patients, the diuretic is suggested as first-step therapy. (β-Adrenergic blockers may be contraindicated in diabetic patients and asthmatic patients; the diuretic works well in adult black patients. In adolescents with a hyperdynamic-type hypertension (with a rapid pulse) or those associated with hyperthyroidism, a β-blocker is preferable. If the first drug is not effective, a second drug may be added to, or substituted for, the first drug, starting with a small dose and proceeding to full dose (step 2).

If the blood pressure still remains elevated, a third drug, such as a vasodilator, may be added to the regimen (step 3). At this point, the possibility of secondary hypertension should be reconsidered. Table 31-3 shows the dosage of commonly used antihypertensive drugs for children.

Diuretics. Diuretics are the cornerstone of antihypertensive drug therapy, except in patients with renal failure. Their action is related to a decrease in extracellular and plasma volume. The thiazide diuretics (hydrochlorothiazide and chlorothalidone) are

TABLE 31–3.

Recommended Oral Dosages of Selected Antihypertensive Drugs for Children

Drugs	Dose (mg/kg)	Times/day
Diuretics		
Hydrochlorothiazide	1-2	2
Chlorothiazide (Diuril)	0.5-2	1
Furosemide (Lasix)	0.5-2	2
Spironolactone (Aldactone)	1-2	2
Adrenergic Inhibitors		
Propranolol (Inderal)	1-3	3
Methyldopa (Aldomet)	5-10	2
Atenolol (Tenormin)	1-2	1
Vasodilators		
Hydralazine (Apresoline)	1-5	2-3
Minoxidil (Loniten)	0.1-1	2
ACE Inhibitors		
Captopril (Capoten)		
<6 mo	0.05-0.5	3
>6 mo	0.5-2.0	3

Modified from the Second NIH Task Force on Blood Pressure Control in Children, *Pediatrics* 79:1, 1987.

most commonly used. The only important side effect of diuretic therapy in children is hypokalemia, occasionally requiring potassium supplementation in the diet or potassium salt.

Adrenergic inhibitors. If diuretics produce no clinical improvement at the maximum dose and over a sufficient length of time, a sympathetic inhibitor (propranolol, atenolol, methyldopa, or reserpine) should be added to, or substituted for, the diuretic.

1. Propranolol (Inderal), a β-adrenergic blocker, acts at three important locations: on the juxtaglomerular apparatus of the kidney to suppress the renin-angiotensin system, on the central vasomotor center to decrease SVR, and on the myocardium to suppress contractility. One can judge the adequacy of β-adrenergic blockade by noting the suppression of the increase in heart rate when the patient stands up after a few minutes of recumbency. Propranolol is contraindicated in patients with asthma. Atenolol has an advantage of being a longer-acting β-blocker, requiring a single daily dose.

2. Methyldopa (Aldomet) appears to act by reducing SVR by acting directly on the arterioles and by influencing the central nervous system. The major adverse reaction is sedation, occurring in the early stage of therapy. Other side effects include a positive Coombs' tests, lupuslike reaction, hepatitis, and colitis.

Vasodilators. If a diuretic and/or sympathetic inhibitor produce no clinical improvement, a vasodilator agent should be added. Three types of vasodilators are used in the treatment of hypertension: direct-acting arteriolar vasodilators (hydralazine, minoxidil), angiotension-converting enzyme inhibitors (captopril, enalapril, lisinopril), and calcium antagonists (nifedipine, verapamil, diltiazem).

Hydralazine (Apresoline) has been popular in the treatment of hypertension in children (see Table 31-3 for the dosage). When used alone, it produces side effects related to increased cardiac output (flushing, headache, tachycardia, and palpitation) and salt retention. Therefore the concomitant use of a β-adrenergic blocker and a diuretic is recommended. Minoxidil, a vasodilator antihypertensive agent, is less commonly used.

Captopril is an ACE inhibitor widely used in the treatment of pediatric hypertension (see Table 31-3 for the dosage). Enalapril and lisinopril are new and long-acting ACE inhibitors that have been shown to be effective in adult patients with hypertension. A diuretic clearly will enhance the effectiveness of ACE inhibitors.

Calcium antagonists are being used increasingly in the treatment of adult hypertension. They have had limited use in the pediatric age group. Nifedipine has the greatest peripheral vasodilatory action with little effect on cardiac automaticity, conduction, or contractility. Concomitant dietary sodium restriction or the use of a diuretic agent may not be necessary because calcium antagonists cause natriuresis by producing renal vasodilation. The adult dose starts at 10 mg 3 times a day and may be titrated up to 20 to 30 mg 3 times a day.

Secondary Hypertension

Treatment of secondary hypertension should be aimed at removing the cause of hypertension whenever possible. Table 31-4 lists curable causes of systemic hypertension.

Renal parenchymal disease. In nephritides, medical management should be instituted to lower blood pressure in the same manner as has been discussed for essential hypertension. Salt restriction, avoidance of excessive fluid intake, and antihypertensive drug therapy can control hypertension caused by most renal parenchymal diseases. Concomitant antibiotic therapy for infectious processes and general supportive measures may be indicated depending on the nature of the renal disease. If hypertension is difficult to control and the disease is unilateral, unilateral nephrectomy may be considered.

TABLE 31–4.

Curable Forms of Hypertension

Organ/System	Diseases/Conditions
Renal	Unilateral kidney disease (pyelonephritis, hydronephrosis, traumatic damage, radiation nephritis, hypoplastic kidney)
	Wilms' and other kidney tumors
Cardiovascular	COA
	Renal artery abnormalities (e.g., stenosis, aneurysm, fibromuscular dysplasia, thrombosis)
Adrenal	Pheochromocytoma and neuroblastoma
	Adrenogenital syndrome
	Cushing's syndrome
	Primary aldosteronism
Miscellaneous	Glucocorticoid therapy
	Oral contraceptives

Surgical treatment. Renovascular disease may be cured by successful surgery, such as reconstruction of a stenotic renal artery, autotransplantation, or unilateral nephrectomy. Hypertension caused by tumors that secrete vasoactive substances such as pheochromocytoma, neuroblastoma, and juxtaglomerular cell tumor, are treated primarily by surgery.

HYPERTENSIVE CRISIS

A hypertensive emergency is defined as any of the following features:

1. The patient has severe hypertension (>180 mm Hg systolic or 110 mm Hg diastolic) or rapidly increasing blood pressures.

2. The patient has neurologic signs (hypertensive encephalopathy) with severe headache, vomiting, irritability, apathy, seizures, papilledema, retinal hemorrhage, or exudate.

3. The patient has CHF or pulmonary edema.

Aggressive parenteral administration of antihypertensive drugs is indicated to lower blood pressure:

1. Diazoxide (Hyperstat), 3 to 5 mg/kg as an intravenous bolus, or nitroprusside (Nipride), 1 to 3 μg/kg/min as an intravenous drip, is the treatment of choice.

2. If hypertension is less severe, hydralazine (Apresoline), 0.15 mg/kg intravenously or intramuscularly may be used. The onset of action is 10 minutes after an intravenous dose and 20 to 30 minutes after an intramuscular dose. The dose may be repeated at 4- to 6-hour interval.

3. A rapid-acting diuretic, such as furosemide (1 mg/kg), is given intravenously to initiate diuresis.

4. Fluid balance must be controlled carefully, so intake is limited to urine output plus insensible loss.

5. Seizures may be treated with slow intravenous infusion of diazepam (Valium), 0.2 mg/kg, or another anticonvulsant medication.

6. When a hypertensive crisis is under control, oral medications replace the parenteral medications (see Table 31-3 for oral dosages of antihypertensive drugs).

32 / Pulmonary Hypertension

DEFINITION

At sea level, the normal PA pressure (systolic/diastolic) of children and adults is 20/12 mm Hg, and the mean arterial pressure is 15 mm Hg. At 15,000 feet elevation, the PA pressure is 38/14 mm Hg, and the mean arterial pressure is 25 mm Hg. A diagnosis of pulmonary hypertension can be made when the pulmonary mean arterial pressure is 19 to 20 mm Hg in a resting individual at sea level and 25 mm Hg at 15,000 feet elevation.

ETIOLOGY

Pulmonary hypertension is a group of conditions with multiple etiologies rather than a single one. Therefore pathogenesis and management differ among entities. The Box below lists, according to pathogenesis, conditions that cause pulmonary hypertension of a temporary or permanent, acute or chronic nature. Pulmonary hypertension is caused by increased PBF seen in CHDs with large left-to-right shunts (hyperkinetic pulmonary hypertension), alveolar hypoxia, increased pulmonary venous pressure, and primary pulmonary vascular disease. Some oversimplification is inevitable in dividing this diverse group into four categories.

Causes of Pulmonary Hypertension

---

1. Large left-to-right shunt lesions (hyperkinetic pulmonary hypertension): VSD, PDA, ECD
2. Alveolar hypoxia
   Pulmonary parenchymal disease
      Extensive pneumonia
      Hypoplasia of lungs (primary or secondary such as that seen in diaphragmatic hernia)
      Bronchopulmonary dysplasia
      Interstitial lung disease (Hamman-Rich syndrome)
      Wilson-Mikity syndrome
   Airway obstruction
      Upper airway obstruction (large tonsils, macroglossia, micrognathia, laryngotracheomalacia)
      Lower airway obstruction (bronchial asthma, cystic fibrosis)
   Inadequate ventilatory drive (central nervous system diseases)
   Disorders of chest wall or respiratory muscles
      Kyphoscoliosis
      Weakening or paralysis of skeletal muscle
   High altitude (in certain hyperreactors)
3. Pulmonary venous hypertension
   MS, cor triatriatum, TAPVR with obstruction, chronic left heart failure, left-sided obstructive lesions (AS, COA)
4. Primary pulmonary vascular disease
   PPHN
   Primary pulmonary hypertension — rare, fatal form of pulmonary hypertension with obscure etiology
   Thromboembolism
      Ventriculovenous shunt for hydrocephalus, sickle cell anemia, thrombophlebitis
   Collagen disease
      Rheumatoid arthritis, scleroderma, mixed connective tissue disease

---

The term *cor pulmonale* describes RV hypertrophy and/or dilatation secondary to pulmonary hypertension; the latter is caused by diseases of the pulmonary parenchyma or pulmonary vascular system between the origins of the MPA and the entry of the pulmonary veins into the LA. It does not include nonpulmonary causes of RV dysfunction, such as seen with MS or LV failure.

PATHOGENESIS

Pressure *(P)* is related to both flow *(F)* and vascular resistance *(R)*, as shown in the following formula:

$$P \propto F \times R$$

An increase in flow, vascular resistance, or both can result in pulmonary hypertension. Regardless of its etiology, pulmonary hypertension eventually involves constriction of the pulmonary arterioles, resulting in an increase in PVR and hypertrophy of the RV.

The normal RV cannot sustain sudden pressure loads over 40 to 50 mm Hg. Thus acute right-sided heart failure may develop in any condition in which PVR increases abruptly. However, if the RV hypertrophies, it can tolerate mild pulmonary hypertension (with a systolic pressure of about 50 mm Hg) without producing clinical problems. If another burden such as a superimposed lung disease, alveolar hypoxia, or acidosis is added to a mildly hypertrophied RV, requiring generation of higher pressures approximating systemic arterial pressure, the RV will fail.

Hyperkinetic Pulmonary Hypertension

Pulmonary hypertension associated with large left-to-right shunt lesions, such as VSD and PDA, is called *hyperkinetic pulmonary hypertension* and derives from an increase in flow, a direct transmission of the systemic pressure to the PA, and an increase in the PVR by compensatory pulmonary vasoconstriction. If no vasoconstriction occurs, an intractable CHF results. Hyperkinetic pulmonary hypertension is therefore a compensatory response to left-to-right shunt lesions and is usually reversible if the cause is eliminated before permanent changes in the pulmonary arterioles occur (see later section).

Eisenmenger's syndrome (PVOD) occurs in patients who have untreated large left-to-right shunt lesions, such as VSD, PDA, and ECD. The time of onset varies, ranging from infancy to adulthood, but the majority of patients develop PVOD during late childhood or early adolescence. It develops even later in patients with ASD. Many patients with TGA develop PVOD within the first year of life for reasons not entirely clear. Children with Down syndrome with large left-to-right shunt lesions tend to develop PVOD much earlier than normal children with similar lesions.

Alveolar Hypoxia

An acute or chronic reduction in Po_2 in the alveolar capillary region (alveolar hypoxia) elicits a strong pulmonary vasoconstrictor response, which may be augmented by acidosis. It is alveolar hypoxia, not a low Po_2 in the PA or systemic arterial blood, that produces clinically important pulmonary hypertension. Alveolar hypoxia has a much stronger vasoconstrictor effect than a low Po_2 in the PA, suggesting that the oxygen "sensor" is more closely in contact with alveolar space than blood vessels. However, the degree of response varies markedly among species and individuals. The vasoconstriction can be reversed with removal of the cause.

The exact mechanisms of the pulmonary vasoconstrictor response to alveolar hypoxia is not completely understood. The vasoconstriction may be caused by the direct effects of reduced Po_2 on the pulmonary arterioles (with a resulting increase in the plasma membrane permeability to calcium), but it is more likely caused by the indirect actions of humoral agents that are locally released or activated in the lung (see later section). The lung is not just an organ of respiration; it is an organ with active metabolic and endocrine functions. It synthesizes alveolar surfactant and selectively handles circulating vasoactive hormones. The lungs activate certain vasoactive hormones (such as angiotensin I) and inactivate others (such as bradykinin, serotonin, and some prostaglandins). Vasoactive agents implicated in hypoxia-induced pulmonary vasoconstriction include histamine, prostaglandins and related compounds (such as prostaglandin F, thromboxane and endoperoxides), angiotensins, catecholamines, and slow-reacting substances of anaphylaxis. The synthesis and release of biologically active substances in the lung can be provoked by many physiologic and pathologic stimuli, including alveolar hypoxia. Recently, however, decreased synthesis of endothelium-derived relaxing factor, which has been identified as nitric oxide, has become a strong candidate for the mediation of the vasoconstrictor response because the metabolic effects of transient or prolonged hypoxia might alter nitric oxide synthesis and/or release, resulting in pulmonary vasoconstriction.

Pulmonary Venous Hypertension

Increased pressures in the pulmonary veins produce reflex vasoconstriction of the pulmonary arterioles, resulting in PA hypertension. Alveolar hypoxia secondary to pulmonary edema may also contribute to the vasoconstriction. MS, TAPVR with obstruction to pulmonary venous return, and chronic left-sided heart failure are examples of this entity, which causes an elevation of pressure in the LA and thereby the pulmonary veins. Pulmonary hypertension with increased pulmonary venous pressure is usually reversible when the cause is eliminated.

Primary Pulmonary Vascular Disease

The diverse conditions called *primary pulmonary vascular disease* are characterized by a decrease in the cross-sectional area of the pulmonary vascular bed caused by pathologic changes in the vascular tissue itself, thromboembolism, platelet aggregation, or a combination.

Primary pulmonary hypertension is characterized by progressive, irreversible vascular changes similar to those seen in Eisenmenger's syndrome but without intracardiac lesions. This condition is extremely rare in pediatric patients; is a condition of adulthood and is more prevalent in women. It has a poor prognosis. The etiology of primary pulmonary hypertension is not fully understood, but endothelial dysfunction of the pulmonary vascular bed may be an important factor. As in other vascular beds, the endothelium of the pulmonary vascular bed works to maintain normal structure and function. The endothelial cells modulate the tone of vascular smooth muscles by synthesizing prostacyclin and endothelium-derived relaxing factor, which are vasodilators; control the potential proliferation of smooth muscle cells in medial hypertrophy by releasing growth factors and cytokines; and interact with platelets to release anticlotting factors in the blood to maintain a nonthrombotic state by releasing prostacyclin, an inhibitor of platelet function. These delicate functions are themselves influenced by factors such as shear stress, hypoxia, and tissue metabolism. Thus endothelial dysfunction resulting from an external stimulus or the disease process itself is likely to be important in the development and progression of pulmonary hypertension. Some of the histologic patterns seen in this condition (such as plexiform and thrombotic angiopathies) may result from endothelial cell injury, which may lead to smooth muscle proliferation, impaired production of endothelium-derived relaxing factor, and thrombosis in situ. A recent report suggests that local production by the lungs of endothelin-1, a potent vasoconstrictor, may contribute to the vascular abnormalities associated with this disorder: The normal lung may function to clear endothelin-1 from the circulation.

PATHOLOGY

Regardless of the initial events that lead to PA hypertension, elevated PA pressure eventually induces anatomic changes in the pulmonary vessels. Heath and Edwards classify the changes into six grades (Fig. 32-1). Grade 1 consists of hypertrophy of the medial wall of the small muscular arteries; grade 2, hyperplasia of the intima; and grade 3, hyperplasia and fibrosis of the intima with narrowing of the vascular lumen. Changes

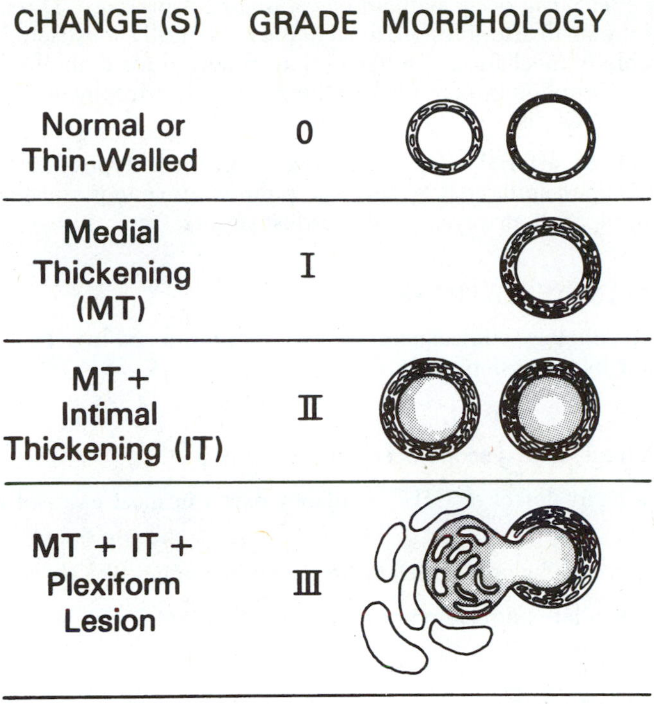

CHANGE (S)   GRADE MORPHOLOGY

Normal or Thin-Walled	0
Medial Thickening (MT)	I
MT + Intimal Thickening (IT)	II
MT + IT + Plexiform Lesion	III

FIG. 32–1.
Heath-Edwards grading of the morphologic changes in the PAs of patients with pulmonary hypertension (see text). (From Roberts WC: *Congenital heart disease in adults,* Philadelphia, 1979, FA Davis.)

up to grade 3 are considered reversible if the cause is eliminated. Changes greater than grade 4 are considered irreversible; they consist of dilatation lesions with saccular formation and fibrinoid necrosis. These advanced changes may augment the hypertension and sustain it even when the original stimulus is removed, especially when the condition is chronic.

PATHOPHYSIOLOGY

1. If severe pulmonary hypertension develops suddenly in the presence of an unprepared (nonhypertrophied) RV, right-sided heart failure develops. This occurs in infants with acute upper airway obstruction or in patients with massive pulmonary thromboembolisms.

2. With chronic pulmonary hypertension, gradual hypertrophy and dilatation of the RV develops. The RV pressure may exceed the systemic pressure.

3. A decrease in cardiac output may result from at least two mechanisms:

   a. A volume and pressure overload of the RV impairs cardiac function, primarily by impaired coronary perfusion of the hypertrophied and dilated RV and decreased LV function, which results from the dramatic leftward shift of the interventricular septum caused by the increasing RV volume. The latter also alters LV structures and decreases the LV's compliance, resulting in increased LV end-diastolic pressure and an increase in LA pressure.

   b. A sudden increase in PVR may decrease pulmonary venous return to the LA, with resulting hypotension and circulatory shock in the absence of a right-to-left intracardiac shunt.

4. Pulmonary edema can occur without elevation of LA pressure. Direct disruption of the walls of the small arterioles proximal to the hypoxically constricted arterioles may be responsible (a mechanism similar to that proposed for high-altitude pulmonary edema). The disruption is more likely if there is no hypertrophy of the muscles in the media of these vessels.

5. Deterioration of arterial blood gas levels occurs. Hypoxemia, acidosis, and occasionally hypercapnia may result from pulmonary venous congestion or edema, compression of small airways, or intracardiac shunts.

CLINICAL MANIFESTATIONS

Regardless of the etiology, clinical manifestations of pulmonary hypertension are similar when significant hypertension exists.

History

1. Dyspnea, fatigue, and syncope occur on exertion.

2. History of a heart defect or CHF in infancy exists in most cases of Eisenmenger's syndrome.

3. Some patients may have histories of headache or angina-like chest pain.

4. Hemoptysis is a late and sometimes fatal development.

Physical Examination

1. Cyanosis with or without clubbing may be present. The neck veins distend, with a prominent *a* wave.

2. An RV lift or tap occurs on palpation.

3. There is a single S2, or it splits narrowly; the P2 is loud. An ejection click and an early diastolic decrescendo murmur of PR are usually present along the MLSB. A regurgitant systolic murmur of TR may be audible at the LLSB.

4. Signs of right-sided heart failure (such as hepatomegaly and ankle edema) may be present.

5. Arrhythmias occur in the late stage.

Electrocardiography

1. RAD and RVH with or without "strain" are seen with severe pulmonary hypertension.

2. RAH is frequently seen late.

X-Ray Studies

1. The heart size is normal or only slightly enlarged, unless CHF supervenes.

2. A prominent MPA segment and dilated hilar vessels with clear lung fields are characteristic.

3. With acute exacerbation, pulmonary edema may be seen.

Echocardiography

Certain changes occur frequently in M-mode and two-dimensional echo and Doppler studies in patients with pulmonary hypertension, but most of these noninvasive studies can not always reliably predict PA pressure. However, these methods can determine whether pulmonary hypertension is mild, moderate, or severe. Several sophisticated methods can be used to estimate systolic, diastolic, or mean pressure in the PA, but a detailed discussion of these methods is beyond the scope of the book. Since a noninvasive estimation of the severity of pulmonary hypertension is important in the

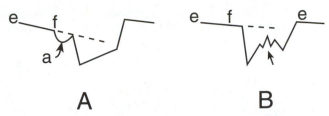

FIG. 32–2.
M-mode echo of the pulmonary valve in pulmonary hypertension. **A,** Normal M-mode echo. **B,** Pulmonary hypertension demonstrating an absent a wave, diminished or negative EF slope, and midsystolic notch or flutter *(arrow).*

management of the patient, relatively simple methods of the estimation are presented here. Semiquantitative estimation of PA pressures can be obtained using various methods such as M-mode or two-dimensional echo, Doppler examination, and systolic time intervals:

1. *Abnormal valve motion on M-mode echo:* An absence or diminished *a* wave, a reduced EF slope, and midsystolic closure (notching) indicate pulmonary hypertension (Fig. 32-2). However, these abnormalities are not always present, and a false-positive result occurs rarely. A *mean* PA pressure of at least 20 mm Hg is necessary before any change in pulmonary valve motion is seen.

2. *Systolic time interval* (see Chapter 6): The ratio of RPEP/RVET (see Chapter 6) has a positive association with PA *diastolic* pressure, but the ratio is not a reliable sign in patients with VSD. The normal ratio is 0.24 with a range of 0.16 to 0.30. Values greater than 0.30 suggest the possibility of elevated PA pressure, and values greater than 0.40 are abnormal.

3. *Two-dimensional echo:* With an elevated RV pressure, the interventricular septum shifts toward the LV and appears flattened at the end of systole. An inspection of the septal curvature at the end of systole provides an estimate of the RV systolic pressure (Fig. 32-3).

4. *Doppler echo:*

   a. Peak TR velocity: The peak TR velocity determined by *continuous wave* Doppler is used to accurately estimate the *systolic* pressure in the PA. The simplified Bernoulli equation ($\Delta P = 4V^2$, see Chapter 6) is used to estimate a systolic pressure drop across the tricuspid valve; a normal central venous pressure of 7 mm Hg is added to the result to estimate *systolic* PA pressure.

   b. With a shunt lesion, such as a VSD, PDA, or a systemic-to-PA shunt, the peak systolic velocity across the shunt can be used for estimating systolic pressure in the RV or PA. In the absence of PS, the systolic pressure in the RV equals that in the PA. The systolic pressure in the LV (which is equal to the aortic pressure estimated by blood pressure measurements taken in the arm) minus the systolic pressure drop across the VSD or the shunt *plus* 7 mm Hg approximates the RV *systolic* pressure. Overestimating the RV pressure can occur if the Doppler examination does not detect the flow jet of highest velocity.

   c. The method of Kitabatake et al may be used to estimate the *mean* PA pressure. A waveform obtained in the RV outflow tract in the parasternal short-axis view is used. The flow velocity in patients with pulmonary hypertension accelerates rapidly and reaches a peak level sooner (decreased acceleration time). A good correlation was found between the mean PA pressure and acceleration time or the ratio of acceleration time to RV ejection time (Fig 32-4). An excellent

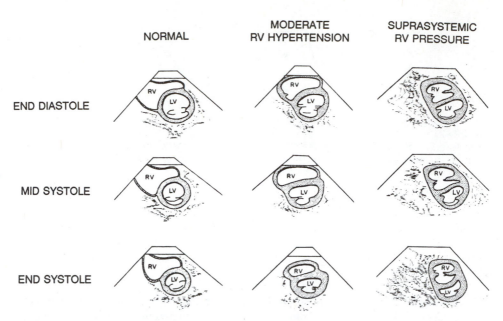

NORMAL   MODERATE   SUPRASYSTEMIC
                RV HYPERTENSION   RV PRESSURE

END DIASTOLE

MID SYSTOLE

END SYSTOLE

FIG. 32–3.
Parasternal short-axis stop-frames of interventricular septal configurations of normal patients and patients with RV hypertension. The top row represents the end-diastolic frames, the middle row represents the midsystolic frames, and the bottom row represents the end-systolic frames. In normal children *(left column),* the typical rounded configuration of the interventricular septum is demonstrated throughout the cardiac cycle. In moderate pulmonary hypertension *(middle column),* the interventricular septum becomes progressively flattened from the end of diastole to the end of systole. When RV pressure is suprasystemic *(right column),* the interventricular septum is flattened at the end of diastole, and at the end of systole, it reverses its curvature to become convex toward the LV. (Modified from King ME, Braun H, Goldblatt A, et al: Interventricular septal configuration as a predictor of right ventricular systolic hypertension in children: a cross-sectional echocardiographic study, *Circulation* 68:68-75, 1983.)

correlation exists between the acceleration time or the ratio of the acceleration time and RV ejection time and the *mean* PA pressures measured by cardiac catheterization.

   d. The end-diastolic velocity of PR can be used to estimate the *diastolic* pressure in the PA. The end-diastolic (not early diastolic) velocity is measured and entered into the modified Bernoulli equation, and a normal central venous pressure of 7 mm Hg is added.

In summary, the following echo techniques provide various parameters of PA pressure:

   1. *Systolic* PA pressures are reliably estimated by the peak TR velocity method if TR is present and by inspection of the interventricular septal curvature at the systole.

   2. The *mean* PA pressure is best estimated by the method of Kitabatake et al (see Fig. 32-4).

   3. *Diastolic* PA pressures are estimated by the end-diastolic velocity of PR and less accurately by systolic time intervals (RPEP/RVET).

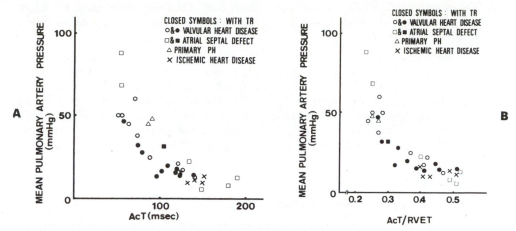

FIG. 32–4.
A, Relationship between mean PA pressure *(MPAP)* and acceleration time *(AcT)* and **B,** between MPAP and AcT/RVET. The relationship for both is curvilinear, with the correlation coefficients of -0.82 and -0.85, respectively. When plotted against $\log_{10}$ (AcT) and $\log_{10}$ (AcT/RVET), a linear relationship was obtained with slightly better correlation coefficients (-0.88 and -0.90, respectively). The linear regression equations were $\log_{10}$ (MPAP) = -0.0068(AcT) + 2.1 and $\log_{10}$ (MPAP) = -2.8 (AcT/RVET) + 2.4. *RVET,* RV ejection time. (From Kitabatake A, Inoue M, Asao M, et al: Noninvasive evaluation of pulmonary hypertension by a pulsed Doppler technique, *Circulation* 68:302-309, 1983.)

4. M-mode echo of the pulmonary valve has some value in detecting pulmonary hypertension.

NATURAL HISTORY

1. Pulmonary hypertension secondary to airway obstruction is usually reversible when the etiology is eliminated.

2. Chronic conditions that produce alveolar hypoxia have a relatively poor prognosis. Pulmonary hypertension of variable degree persists with right-sided heart failure. Superimposed pulmonary infection may be an aggravating factor.

3. Pulmonary hypertension with large left-to-right shunt lesions (hyperkinetic type) or that associated with pulmonary venous hypertension improves or disappears after surgical repair of the cause, if treatment is performed early.

4. Primary pulmonary hypertension is progressive and has a fatal outcome, usually 2 to 3 years after the onset of symptoms.

5. Pulmonary hypertension associated with Eisenmenger's syndrome, collagen disease, and chronic thromboembolism is usually irreversible and has a poor prognosis but may be stable for 2 to 3 decades.

6. Right-sided heart failure is common at the late stage.

7. Chest pain, hemoptysis, and syncope are ominous signs.

8. Atrial and ventricular arrhythmias also occur late.

DIAGNOSIS

1. The history and physical findings suggest pulmonary hypertension.

2. Noninvasive tools (ECG, chest x-ray films, and echo) are often used to detect pulmonary hypertension. Collectively, they are reasonably accurate in assessing severity.

3. Cardiac catheterization demonstrates the presence and severity of pulmonary hypertension. Whether the elevated PVR is due to active vasoconstriction or to permanent changes in the pulmonary arterioles may be assessed by the use of tolazoline (Priscoline) or other vasodilators or the administration of oxygen during cardiac catheterization. Characteristic angiographic findings of advanced pulmonary hypertension secondary to CHD include sparseness of aborization, abrupt tapering of small arteries, and reduced background capillary filling.

MANAGEMENT

1. Acute pulmonary hypertension should be managed:

   a. Arterial Po_2 is improved by intubation and ventilator support with oxygen. Hyperventilation-induced respiratory alkalosis may produce pulmonary vasodilation.

   b. Inotropic agents are used. An ideal inotropic agent should not increase PVR and reduce systemic blood pressure, which is important for coronary perfusion to the RV:

      (1) Digitalis and dopamine are often used but may increase PVR.

      (2) β-Adrenergic agents (dobutamine, isoproterenol) may lower systemic pressure and impair coronary perfusion to the RV. Additional intravascular volume may be needed to maintain the systemic blood pressure.

      (3) Occasionally, norepinephrine or phenylephrine may be used to provide adequate coronary perfusion.

   c. Diuretics are used for pulmonary edema.

   d. Factors that increase pulmonary vasoconstriction (alveolar hypoxia, acidosis, hypercapnia, vasoconstrictor drugs, fat emulsions, hypothermia, and high positive end-expiratory pressure are avoided and eliminated. A high positive end-expiratory pressure reduces the intrapulmonary shunt but increases edema and decreases cardiac output.

   e. Vasodilator drugs are not always salutary because they may decrease SVR more than the PVR. Tolazoline, prazosin, nitroprusside, hydralazine, captopril, and corticosteroids have been tried with beneficial and deleterious effects.

   f. High-dose calcium channel blocking agents (such as nifedipine, 17 mg; diltiazem, 729 mg) with oral anticoagulation have been recommended for adults.

   g. Inhaled nitric oxide is effective in lowering PVR in PPHN (5 to 10 ppm) and in adult respiratory distress syndrome (40 to 80 ppm). Nitric oxide can be used only by inhalation because it is inactivated by hemoglobin.

2. When possible etiologies are removed:

   a. Tonsillectomy and adenoidectomy are performed for upper airway obstruction.

   b. Open heart surgery is performed for large-shunt VSD or PDA.

3. Underlying diseases, such as cystic fibrosis or asthma, are treated.

4. Only symptomatic treatment is available for chronic established or irreversible forms of pulmonary hypertension:

   a. Plasmapheresis is done for polycythemia and severe headache.

   b. CHF is treated with chronic administration of digoxin and diuretics and a low-salt diet.

c. Arrhythmias are treated.

d. Hemoptysis may be treated with bed rest and antitussive medications.

e. The use of nitroglycerin for anginal pain is avoided because it may worsen the pain.

f. Strenuous exertion is avoided.

g. Trips to high altitudes and flights on commercial aircraft are avoided.

h. Oxygen supplement is provided as needed.

i. High-dose calcium channel blocking agents (such as nifedipine, diltiazem) with oral anticoagulation have been recommended for adults, as in acute pulmonary hypertension.

j. Nitric oxide inhalation may be beneficial in patients with primary pulmonary hypertension, at least temporarily.

33 / Hyperlipidemia in Childhood

BY R. GEORGE TROXLER, MD, MPH
MYUNG K. PARK, MD

It is widely believed that atherosclerotic lesions start to develop in childhood and progress to irreversible lesions in adulthood. The following sequence of events, in increasing order of severity, is believed to occur in the American population:

1. Fatty streaks, some of which may resolve, develop in the first and second decades.

2. Fibrous plaque develops in the second and third decades.

3. Complicated fibrotic and calcific lesions are seen after the third decade.

4. Clinical manifestations of atherosclerotic cardiovascular disease then follow (e.g., myocardial infarction, gangrene of extremities, aortic aneurysm).

High levels of total cholesterol, low-density lipoprotein (LDL), and very low-density lipoprotein (VLDL) and low levels of high-density lipoprotein (HDL) are correlated with an increased risk of coronary heart disease in adolescents and young adults. Normal levels of total cholesterol, LDL and HDL, and serum triglyceride in American children and adolescents are presented in Appendix C, Tables C-1 and C-2.

Since substantial and potentially irreversible atherosclerosis may already exist by the fourth decade of life, efforts have been made to lower serum cholesterol levels in children in the hope of preventing or retarding the progress of atherosclerosis. Recently, the National Cholesterol Education Program Expert Panel on Blood Cholesterol Levels in Children and Adolescents (1991, NIH Publication No. 91-2732) has recommended strategies for the prevention and detection of hyperlipidemia in children (see later section).

The reduction of elevated cholesterol levels is only one aspect of the total management plan. Interrelated factors such as genetics, hypertension, diabetes mellitus, obesity, and smoking are risk factors in the development of atherosclerotic cardiovascular disease. The box below lists known cardiovascular risk factors. Physicians should play an increasing role not only in detecting hyperlipidemia, but also in counseling for the prevention of other risk factors.

Other Risk Factors for Early Onset of Coronary Heart Disease

Family history of premature coronary heart disease, cerebrovascular or occlusive peripheral vascular disease (with onset before the age of 55 years for men and before 65 years for women in a sibling, parent, or sibling of a parent)
Cigarette smoking
Hypertension
Low levels of HDL (<35 mg/100 ml)
Diabetes mellitus
Physical inactivity

HDL, High-density lipoprotein.
Adapted from Summary of the Second Report of the National Cholesterol Education Program Expert Panel on Detection, Evaluation, and Treatment of High Blood Cholesterol in Adults (Adult Treatment Panel II), *JAMA* 269:3015-3023, 1993.

LIPIDS AND LIPOPROTEINS

The major lipids of plasma are cholesterol, triglycerides, phospholipids, and free fatty acids. Plasma lipids that are hydrophobic do not circulate freely but rather circulate in the form of lipid-protein macromolecular complexes known as *lipoproteins*. Free fatty acids are bound to albumin. The nonpolar lipids (cholesterol esters and triglycerides) are present in the lipoprotein core surrounded by a monolayer composed of specific proteins (apoproteins) and the polar lipids (unesterified or free cholesterol and phospholipids). This monolayer allows the lipoprotein to remain miscible in plasma.

The plasma lipoproteins have been classified into four major groups based on their density: chylomicrons, VLDL, LDL, and HDL. Electrophoretic techniques permit the separation of the serum lipoproteins based on differences in electrostatic charges; chylomicrons (which remain at the origin), β-lipoproteins (=LDL), pre-β-lipoprotein (=VLDL), and α-lipoproteins (=HDL).

The composition and function of lipoproteins are summarized in Table 33-1. The principal lipid of chylomicrons and VLDL is triglyceride, constituting 90% and 55% of their weight, respectively. LDL is mostly cholesterol (50%) and phospholipids (25%), and HDL is mostly protein (50%) with cholesterol and phospholipid as its major lipids (Table 33-1). The proteins contained in lipoproteins are known as *apoproteins* and serve as enzymatic cofactors and recognition elements in binding to specific receptors.

TABLE 33–1.

Properties and Functions of the Major Plasma Lipoproteins

	Chylomicron	VLDL	LDL	HDL
Hydrated density (g/100 ml)	<0.95	0.95-1.006	1.019-1.063	1.063-1.21
Electrophoresis	Origin	Pre-β	β	α
Major lipid content	Triglycerides (90%) (exogenous)	Triglycerides (55%) Cholesterol (22%) Phospholipid (15%)	Cholesterol (50%) Phospholipid (25%)	Phospholipid (25%) Cholesterol (20%)
Protein content	1%	10%	20%	33%
Apoprotein constituents	B-48 C-I, C-II, C-III A-I, A-II, A-IV, E	B-100 C-I, C-II, C-III E	B-100	A-I, A-II C-I, C-II, C-III E
Origin	Intestine Dietary fat	Liver Endogenous triglyceride	Metabolic product of VLDL catabolism	Liver, intestine Catabolism of VLDLs and chylomicrons
Function	Transports dietary triglycerides	Transports hepatic triglycerides and cholesterol to peripheral tissues to be used as energy or stored as triglycerides	Provides cholesterol to nerve tissues, cell membranes, and other tissues for their metabolic function, including steroid hormone synthesis	Participates in reverse cholesterol transport; provides protection against premature coronary artery disease

VLDL, Very low-density lipoprotein; *LDL*, low-density lipoprotein; *HDL*, high-density lipoprotein.
Modified from Kwieterovich PO Jr: Disorders of lipid and lipoprotein metabolism. In Rudolph AM, editor: *Rudolph's pediatrics*, ed 19, 1991, Appleton & Lange.

LIPID AND LIPOPROTEIN METABOLISM

A simplified review of lipid and lipoprotein metabolism is presented in Fig. 33-1.

Extrahepatic Pathway

In the gastrointestinal tract, dietary fat is degraded into free fatty acids and monoglycerides. They then enter the intestinal villi, where they are reconstructed into a triglyceride particle. Dietary cholesterol absorbed into the intestinal wall is esterified to cholesterol esters by an enzyme. The triglyceride and cholesterol esters are then combined to form *chylomicron* particles with apoproteins (apos) A-I, A-IV, and B-48. Chylomicrons are cleared rapidly from the circulation by the enzyme lipoprotein lipase (LPL), which requires apo C-II as a cofactor (picked up from HDL), leaving a remnant particle rich in cholesterol and apos C, E, and B-48 *(chylomicron remnant)* (see Fig. 33-1). Surface components of chylomicrons, including apo C-II, are transferred to HDL particles. The chylomicron remnants are cleared rapidly from the circulation by remnant

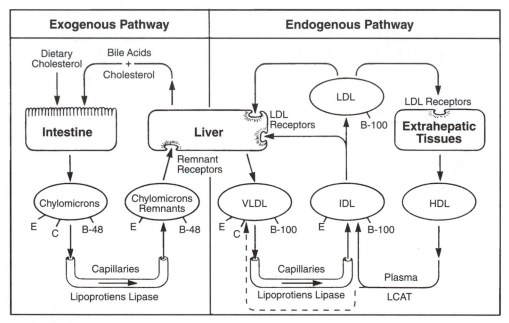

FIG. 33–1.

Endogenous and exogenous pathways of plasma lipid and lipoprotein metabolism. Lipoproteins of chylomicron (intestinal lipoprotein) are hydrolyzed by the enzyme lipoprotein lipase in the capillary beds and produce chylomicron remnants (rich in cholesterol and having apoproteins E and B-48). Chylomicron remnants are cleared rapidly by a remnant receptor in the liver. VLDLs, triglyceride-rich lipoproteins of hepatic origin, are hydrolyzed by lipoprotein lipase in the capillary beds, producing intermediate-density lipoprotein particles. Intermediate-density lipoproteins are taken up by the LDL receptors in the liver or converted into cholesterol ester–rich LDL (with apoprotein B-100 as the only apoprotein) by hepatic triglyceride lipase. LDLs are bound to the LDL receptor and internalized into the liver or extrahepatic tissues. The other major class of lipoproteins, HDL particles, participate in the conversion of free cholesterol from extrahepatic and scavenger cells to cholesterol ester by the action of lecithin-cholesterol acyltransferase *(LCAT)*. Such cholesterol esters are then transferred to VLDL lipoproteins in exchange for triglycerides. The cholesterol esters are ultimately taken up by the liver after conversion to intermediate-density lipoprotein or LDL. The process by which HDLs remove cholesterol from peripheral cells for their ultimate disposal in the liver is called *reverse cholesterol transport.* (Modified from Goldstein JL, Kita T, Brown MS: Defective lipoprotein receptors and atherosclerosis: lessons from an animal counterpart of familial hypercholesterolemia, *N Engl J Med* 309:288-295, 1983.)

receptors that are on the surface of liver cells and that recognize the apo E component of the remnant particle. Chylomicron remnants may be atherogenic. Delayed clearance of chylomicron remnants occurs in inherited deficiency of LPL or its activator, apo C-II (type I hypertriglyceridemia).

Endogenous Pathway

Triglyceride synthesized in the liver is packaged into VLDL with other lipids and apos B-100, C, and E (see Fig. 33-1). The synthesis of VLDL is increased by excess carbohydrate, alcohol, or caloric intake and is suppressed by the chylomicron remnant taken up by the liver. In the capillary beds, triglyceride in the core of the VLDL particle is hydrolyzed by LPL, with a cofactor apo C-II, to produce a remnant *intermediate-density lipoprotein* (IDL). The surface components, except for apos B-100 and E, are transferred to HDL. Compared with VLDL, IDLs have more cholesterol ester and less triglyceride.

IDLs are taken up in the liver by the LDL or remnant receptor or converted into cholesterol-rich LDL by hepatic triglyceride lipase (see Fig. 33-1). Elevation of IDLs is may predispose the patient to premature coronary artery disease and peripheral artery disease (characteristically seen in Frederickson's type III hyperlipoproteinemia).

LDL is usually formed from VLDL breakdown (see Fig. 33-1). Increased LDL synthesis may occur by means of enhanced conversion of VLDL remnants or direct hepatic production of apo B–containing lipoproteins. Apo B-100, the only protein found in LDL, is recognized by a high-affinity LDL receptor on the surfaces of hepatic and certain nonhepatic cells where LDLs are internalized into the cells. About 75% of the LDLs are removed from the bloodstream by the receptor-mediated mechanism, and the remainder is cleared by receptor-independent scavenger cells.

The hepatic and extrahepatic cell can control its own cholesterol content through a feedback-control system in which increased intracellular free cholesterol suppresses endogenous cholesterol production by inhibiting the activity of 3-hydroxy-3-methylglutaryl coenzyme A (HMG-CoA) reductase, the rate-limiting enzyme in cholesterol synthesis, and by suppressing the production of LDL surface receptors through a feedback mechanism. Thus the number of LDL receptors is not fixed and can be modified by genetic defects, decreased by the increased intake of saturated fat and cholesterol, and increased by certain pharmacologic agents. Familial hypercholesterolemia is the prototype disease in which the LDL receptors are absent (homozygotes) or decreased (heterozygotes) (type II hypercholesterolemia).

HDLs are produced by the liver and the gastrointestinal tract and by the peripheral catabolism of chylomicrons and VLDLs (see Fig. 33-1). Cholesterol and phospholipids are the major lipid components of HDLs, with apos A-I and A-II as their major proteins. The HDL secreted by the liver is known as *nascent HDL*. Nascent HDL removes unesterified cholesterol from the tissues and becomes HDL_3 as the cholesterol is esterified and transferred to the lipid core by apo A-I and the enzyme lecithin-cholesterol acyltransferase (LCAT). HDL_3 becomes HDL_2 as more esterified cholesterol is acquired by the lipid core. HDL participates in two important reactions. In the process of lipid and lipoprotein metabolism, apo A-I is transferred from chylomicrons to HDL, and apos C-II and E are transferred from HDL to the triglyceride-rich lipoproteins. Apo A-I is a cofactor for the enzyme LCAT, and apo C-II is a cofactor for lipolysis of triglyceride-rich lipoproteins (see Fig. 33-1). Thus HDL appears to serve as a shuttle for apo C-II. HDL serves as an acceptor for unesterified cholesterol removed from peripheral cells and facilitates the production of esterified cholesterol through the action of LCAT and apo A-I. Cholesterol esters of HDL are transferred directly to the liver or indirectly after transfer to VLDL in exchange for triglycerides. The cholesterol esters from HDL end up in IDL or LDL because the VLDL is subsequently metabolized to IDL or LDL, which is then cleared by the liver receptors. The removal of cholesterol from cells by HDL for ultimate disposal in the liver has been termed *reverse cholesterol transport*. These reactions may explain how HDL and apo A-I can protect against the development of atherosclerosis.

Among the several subtypes of HDL particles, HDL_2 and HDL_3, are clinically important. HDL_2 is closely associated with statistical protection against premature atherosclerosis. Alcohol consumption predominantly increases the HDL_3 subfraction. Lower levels of both subfractions are associated with male gender, hypertriglyceridemia, diabetes mellitus, obesity, uremia, smoking, and the use of androgens and progesterones. Estrogen raises HDL levels.

Cholesterol returning to the liver is converted into bile acids by the enzymatic hydroxylation of cholesterol, or cholesterol and phospholipids are excreted directly into the bile. A large portion of secreted bile acid is reabsorbed in the enterohepatic circulation and recycled. Bile acid sequestrants reduce the reabsorption of secreted bile acids, eventually reducing serum cholesterol levels by increasing the conversion of hepatic cholesterol to bile acids, thus reducing the cholesterol content of the hepatocytes. The reduced hepatic cholesterol stimulates the production of surface receptors for LDL cholesterol, clearing more LDL from the serum.

CLINICAL FEATURES OF HYPERCHOLESTEROLEMIA

Secondary Hypercholesterolemia

All children with LDL levels of at least 130 mg/100 ml should be evaluated for possible secondary hypercholesterolemia. Box below lists causes of secondary hypercholesterolemia. Common causes of secondary hypercholesterolemia in children include obesity, oral contraceptive use, and isotretinoin (Accutane) use or anabolic steroid therapy. In addition to a careful history and physical examination, determination of blood glucose levels and appropriate tests of liver, kidney, and thyroid function may be indicated.

Primary Hypercholesterolemia

If secondary causes of hypercholesterolemia are excluded, primary hypercholesterolemia is present. Screening of all family members is recommended to determine whether

---

Causes of Secondary Hypercholesterolemia

Exogenous Factors

Drugs: Corticosteroids, isotretinoin (Accutane), thiazide, anticonvulsants, β-blockers, anabolic steroids, certain oral contraceptives
Alcohol
Obesity

Endocrine and Metabolic Conditions

Hypothyroidism
Diabetes mellitus
Lipodystrophy
Pregnancy
Idiopathic hypercalcemia
Glycogen storage disease
Sphingolipidosis

Obstructive Liver Disease

Biliary atresia
Biliary cirrhosis

Chronic Renal Disease

Nephrotic syndrome

Miscellaneous

Anorexia nervosa
Progeria
Collagen disease
Klinefelter's syndrome

---

the disorder is familial. Family screening is important not only for detecting hypercholesterolemia in other members of the family, but also in emphasizing the need for the entire family to change their eating patterns. Young patients with elevated LDL levels are more likely to have a familial disorder of LDL metabolism. The two most common familial lipoprotein disorders with elevated LDL levels are familial hypercholesterolemia (FH) and familial combined hyperlipidemia (FCH). However, the

TABLE 33–2.

Clinical Summary of Hyperlipoproteinemia

Fredrickson and Lees Phenotype	Elevated Lipoproteins	Elevated Lipids	Prevalence in Childhood	Symptoms and Signs	Treatment
Type I	Chylomicrons	Triglycerides	Rare	Childhood onset (70%) Abdominal pain due to pancreatitis Eruptive xanthomas Lack of coronary heart disease	Low-fat diet (10-15 g/day)
Type IIa	LDL	Cholesterol	Common	Childhood or adulthood onset Xanthomas of eyelids and palms Tendinitis of Achilles tendon Arcus corneae Coronary heart disease (common in homozygotes)	Low-cholesterol, high-unsaturated-fat diet Bile acid sequestrant, if condition does not respond to diet alone Weight loss if obese
Type IIb	LDL and VLDL	Cholesterol Triglycerides	Uncommon	Late-childhood onset Lack of symptoms and signs (often)	Low-cholesterol, low-fat diet Weight loss if obese
Type III	Chylomicron remnant and IDL	Cholesterol Triglycerides	Very rare	Palmare and tuberosum xanthomas Coronary heart disease ($\pm$)	Low-fat, low-cholesterol diet Weight control
Type IV	VLDL	Triglycerides	Relatively uncommon	Obesity Eruptive xanthomas Abdominal pain	Low-fat, low-cholesterol diet Weight control
Type V	Chylomicron and VLDL	Triglycerides Cholesterol ($\pm$)	Very rare	Obesity Eruptive xanthomas Coronary heart disease (infrequent)	Low-fat diet Weight control

LDL, Low-density cholesterol; *VLDL,* very low-density lipoprotein; *IDL,* intermediate-density lipoprotein.

majority of children with primary elevations of LDL levels have polygenic hypercholesterolemia (i.e., the small effects of a number of different genes influencing the expression). The clinical features of other rare hyperlipoproteinemias are presented in Table 33-2.

Familial hypercholesterolemia. FH, a disorder of lipoprotein metabolism, is due to a lack of or a reduction of LDL receptors. Heterozygotes have about a 50% reduction in LDL receptors, whereas homozygotes have little or no receptor activity. This condition is fairly common, occurring in 1 in every 500 people. It is inherited in an autosomal dominant mode. An evaluation of the family members is important in the diagnosis of this condition. In this condition, one parent and one of two siblings will have elevated total and LDL-cholesterol levels, but the unaffected first-degree relatives will have completely normal levels.

In heterozygotes, total cholesterol and LDL levels are 2 to 3 times higher than normal. Their total cholesterol levels are most often above 240 mg/100 ml, with an average of 300 mg/100 ml, and their LDL levels are above 160 mg/100 ml, with an average of 240 mg/100 ml. Triglyceride levels are usually normal. The presence of xanthomas of the extensor tendon in the parents of such children almost confirm the diagnosis. A heterozygous child or adolescent has normal physical findings; tendon xanthomas are rarely found before the age of 10 years, and they develop in the second decade, primarily in the Achilles tendons and extensor tendons of the hands, in only 10% to 15% of patients. These patients are likely to develop premature cardiovascular disease; rarely angina pectoris develops in the late teenage years.

Homozygosity occurs in children who have inherited two mutant FH genes; it is rare (one in a million). The total cholesterol and LDL levels in these children are 5 to 6 times more than normal. Such children have cholesterol levels that average 700 mg/100 ml but may reach at least 1000 mg/100 ml. Clinical signs such as planar xanthomas, which are flat, orange-colored skin lesions, may be present by the age of 5 years in the webbing of the hands and over the elbows and buttocks. Tendon xanthomas, arcus corneae, and clinically significant coronary heart disease are often present by the age of 10 years. The generalized atherosclerosis often affects the aortic valve with resulting aortic stenosis (AS).

Familial Combined Hyperlipidemia. FCH is more common than FH, possibly occurring in 1 in every 300 people. The characteristic defect in FCH is thought to be an overproduction of apo B-100 by the liver. The dyslipidemia is usually secondary to polygenic factors, rather than primary receptor defects.

Clinically, it may be difficult to separate this entity from FH. In FCH, most patients lack tendon xanthomas, and extreme hyperlipidemia is absent in childhood. FCH is suspected when elevated triglyceride levels are present in parents with hypercholesterolemia; triglyceride levels are moderately elevated in children (average of 120 mg/100 ml for boys and 130 mg/100 ml for girls); levels of total and LDL cholesterol are somewhat lower than in patients with FH; and LDL levels fluctuate from time to time, with triglyceride levels fluctuating in the opposite direction. These children usually have plasma total cholesterol levels between 190 and 220 mg/100 ml. The LDL cholesterol level is usually normal or only mildly elevated. Different lipoprotein phenotypes (IIa, IIb, IV) may be found in children and their parents.

CHOLESTEROL LOWERING STRATEGIES

The Expert Panel (NIH Publication No. 91-2732, September 1991) has recommended two complementary approaches to lower blood cholesterol levels for children and adolescents: a population approach and an individualized approach.

Population Approach

The population approach encourages changes in nutrient intake and eating patterns for

TABLE 33–3.

Nutrient Composition of Step-One and Step-Two Diets

Nutrient	Step-One Diet	Step-Two Diet
Total fat (% total calories)	<30%	<30%
Saturated fatty acids	<10%	<7%
Polyunsaturated fatty acids	Up to 10%	Up to 10%
Monounsaturated fatty acids	10%-15%	10%-15%
Carbohydrates (% total calories)	50%-60%	50%-60%
Protein (% total calories)	10%-20%	10%-20%
Cholesterol (per day)	<300 mg	<200 mg
Total calories	To achieve and maintain desirable weight	To achieve and maintain desirable weight

the entire population of the United States. For children older than 2 years of age, the following are recommended:

1. Nutritional adequacy should be achieved by eating a wide variety of foods.

2. Adequate calories should be provided for normal growth and development.

3. The following pattern of nutrient intake is recommended:

    a. Saturated fatty acids less that 10% of total calories.

    b. Total fat not more than 30% of total calories

    c. Dietary cholesterol less than 300 mg/day

Children younger than 2 years of age may require a higher percentage of calories from fat. The above recommendations are the same as step-one diet (Table 33-3).

Individualized Approach

The individualized approach identifies and treats children and adolescents at risk of having high cholesterol levels. See Appendix C, Tables C-1 and C-2, for normal levels of total cholesterol, LDL, HDL, and serum triglyceride levels in American children and adolescents.

The Expert Panel recommends *selective* screening of children and adolescents with family histories of premature cardiovascular disease or at least one parent with high serum cholesterol levels because of strong evidence demonstrating a familial aggregation of coronary heart disease, high serum cholesterol levels, and other risk factors. Patients who meet the following specific criteria should be screened:

1. Children and adolescents whose parents or grandparents, at 55 years of age or younger, had coronary atherosclerosis after angiography or underwent balloon angioplasty or coronary artery bypass surgery (The new guidelines by the Expert Panel of National Cholesterol Education Program [June 1993] define *positive family history* by gender and age: cardiovascular disease in men 55 years or younger and women 65 years or younger.)

2. Children and adolescents whose parents or grandparents, at 55 years of age or younger, had documented myocardial infarction, angina pectoris, peripheral vascular disease, cerebrovascular disease, or sudden cardiac death

3. The offspring of a parent who had high total cholesterol levels (240 mg/100 ml or higher)

Risk Assessment

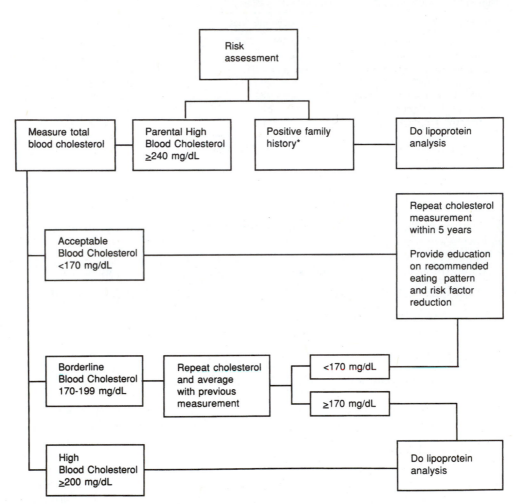

FIG. 33–2.
Risk assessment. (From Expert Panel on Blood Cholesterol Levels in Children and
Adolescents: National Cholesterol Education Program, NIH Publication No. 91-2732,
Sept 1991.)

4. Children and adolescents whose parental or grandparental history is unobtainable,
   particularly those with other risk factors

The recommendations of selective screening are somewhat controversial. Several
recent studies published in the pediatric literature have indicated that about 50% of
children with high LDL levels will be missed if a positive family history of premature
coronary heart disease is used as the screening criteria. Universal cholesterol screening
should theoretically detect all children with high LDL levels, but after considering
several pros and cons of universal screening, the Panel believed that, given the current
state of knowledge, universal screening should not be recommended. However, optional
cholesterol testing by the practicing physician may be appropriate in children judged

to be at higher risk for coronary heart disease (such as those who smoke, have high blood pressure, are obese, or have an excessive fat intake).

The Panel's recommendations are summarized in Fig. 33-2. The screening protocol varies according to the reasons for testing:

1. For young people being tested because they have at least one parent with high blood cholesterol levels, the initial step is a measurement of total cholesterol.

2. For children who have family histories of premature cardiovascular disease, a lipoprotein analysis is recommended because a high proportion of these children have some lipoprotein abnormality.

Depending on total cholesterol and LDL levels, patients' conditions are categorized into *acceptable, borderline,* and *high:*

1. Those who had total cholesterol levels measured (see Fig. 33-2):

   a. If total cholesterol levels are acceptable (<170 mg/100 ml), cholesterol measurement is repeated within 5 years.

   b. If total cholesterol levels are borderline (170 to 199 mg/100 ml), a second measurement is taken, and if the average is borderline or high (>200 mg/100 ml), a lipoprotein analysis is recommended.

2. For those who had lipoprotein analysis done (Fig. 33-3): Regardless of indications, a lipoprotein analysis should be repeated and the average LDL levels determined. The patient's conditions are then categorized into *acceptable* (LDL cholesterol <110 mg/100 ml), *borderline* (110-129 mg/100 ml), and *high* (≥130 mg/100 ml).

   a. If LDL levels are acceptable (<110 mg/100 ml), education about the eating pattern recommended for all children and adolescents and about coronary heart disease risk factors is provided (see Box on p. 430). Lipoprotein analysis is repeated in 5 years.

   b. If LDL levels are in borderline range (110-129 mg/dL), advice about risk factors is provided, the step-one diet is initiated (see Table 33-3), and the patient's status is evaluated in 1 year.

   c. If LDL levels are high (≥130 mg/100 ml), the patient is evaluated for secondary causes and familial disorders, all family members are screened, and the step-one diet is initiated, followed if necessary by the step-two diet (see Table 33-3) and in extreme cases by drug therapy (see later section).

Measurement of Cholesterol and Lipoproteins

1. Total cholesterol and LDL levels are not measured before the age of 2 years, and no treatment is recommended before that age. Cholesterol levels are reasonably consistent thereafter (with some small increment during adolescence).

2. For the measurement of total cholesterol, the child does not have to be fasting for the test.

3. A lipoprotein analysis is obtained by measuring total cholesterol, HDL, and triglyceride levels after an overnight fast of 12 hours. The LDL level is usually estimated by the Friedewald formula:

$$LDL = Total\ cholesterol - HDL - (Triglyceride/5)$$

This formula is not accurate if the child is not fasting, if the triglyceride level is above 400 mg/100 ml, or if chylomicrons or dys-β-lipoproteinemia (type III hyperlipoproteinemia) is present.

Classification, Education, and Followup Based on LDL-Cholesterol

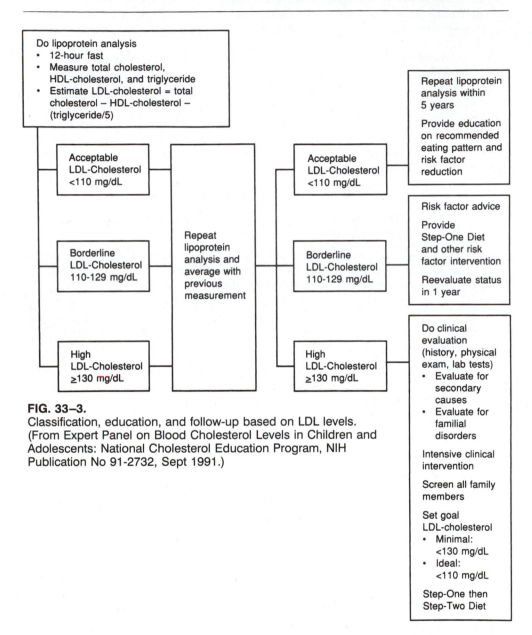

FIG. 33–3.
Classification, education, and follow-up based on LDL levels.
(From Expert Panel on Blood Cholesterol Levels in Children and
Adolescents: National Cholesterol Education Program, NIH
Publication No 91-2732, Sept 1991.)

TREATMENT

Diet Therapy

Diet therapy is prescribed in two steps that progressively reduce the intake of saturated fatty acids and cholesterol. The step-one diet calls for the same nutrient intake recommended in the population approach to lowering cholesterol levels (see Table 33-3): less than 10% of total calories from saturated fatty acids, no more than 30% of calories from total fat, less than 300 mg of cholesterol a day, and adequate calories to support growth and development and to reach or maintain a desirable body weight. Involvement of a registered dietitian or other qualified health professionals is recommended.

If the step-one diet fails to achieve the minimal goals of therapy in 3 months, the step-two diet is prescribed (see Table 33-3). This diet further reduces the saturated fatty acid intake to less than 7% of calories and the cholesterol intake to less than 200 mg a day. Adequate amounts of nutrients, vitamins, and minerals should be provided. A registered dietitian or other qualified nutrition professionals should be consulted. See Appendix C, Table C-3, for detailed information on specific food choices.

Drug Therapy

The Expert Panel recommends drug therapy in children aged 10 years and older if after an adequate trial of diet therapy (6 months to 1 year):

1. The LDL level remains at or above 190 mg/100 ml.

2. The LDL level remains at or above 160 mg/100 ml *plus:*

    a. There is a positive family history of premature cardiovascular disease (before 55 years of age in men and before 65 years in women).

    b. Two or more other cardiovascular disease risk factors (such as low HDL [< 35 mg/100 ml], cigarette smoking, high blood pressure, obesity, or diabetes) are present.

For children and adolescents with hypercholesterolemia, only the bile acid sequestrants (cholestyramine, colestipol) are recommended (see Table 33-4 for the dosage). Nicotinic acid, HMG-CoA reductase inhibitors (lovastatin, pravastatin), probucol, and fibric acid derivatives (gemfibrozil, clofibrate) are not recommended as routine drugs for use in children and adolescents. The mechanism of action, side effects, and adult dosage of lipid-lowering agents are presented in Table 33–5 for the completeness.

TABLE 33–4.

Suggested Initial Dosage of a Bile Acid Sequestrant for Treatment of FH Children and Adolescents

		TC and LDL Levels After Diet (mg/100 ml)	
	Daily Doses*	TC	LDL
	1	< 245	< 195
	2	245-300	195-235
	3	301-345	236-280
	4	345	

* One dose is the equivalent of a 9-g packet of cholestyramine (containing 4 g of cholestyramine and 5 g of filler), one bar of cholestyramine, or 5 g of colestipol.
FH, Familial hypercholesterolemia; *TC,* total cholesterol; *LDL,* low-density lipoprotein.
From National Cholesterol Education Program: Report of the Expert Panel on Blood Cholesterol Levels in Children and Adolescents, NIH Publication No. 91-2732, Sept. 1991.)

TABLE 33–5.

Summary of Lipid-Lowering Drugs

Agents	Mechanisms of Action	Side Effects	Daily Dosage Ranges
Bile acid sequestrants: cholestyramine, colestipol	Increase excretion of bile acids in stool; increase LDL-receptor activity	Constipation, nausea, bloating, flatulence, transient increase in transaminase and alkaline phosphatase levels, increased triglyceride levels ($\pm$), possible prevention of absorption of fat-soluble vitamins	Related to levels of cholesterol, not body weight. For specific dosage, see Table 33-4.
Nicotinic acid (niacin, vitamin B$_3$)	Decreases plasma levels of free fatty acid; possibly inhibits cholesterol synthesis; decreases hepatic VLDL synthesis	Cutaneous flushing, pruritus, gastrointestinal upset, liver function abnormalities, increased uric acid levels, increased glucose intolerance	*Children:* only short-term efficacy reported for homozygous FH, not recommended for routine use. *Adults:* 3-6 g
HMG-CoA reductase inhibitors: lovastatin, pravastatin	Inhibits HMG-CoA reductase, with resulting decrease in cholesterol synthesis; increases LDL-receptor activity	Mild gastrointestinal symptoms, myositis syndrome, elevated transaminase levels, increased CPK levels	*Children:* not recommended. *Adults:* starting dose 20 mg: ranges 40-80 mg.
Probucol	Enhances scavenger pathway removal of LDL	Diarrhea, nausea, flatulence, decreased HDL levels	*Children:* not recommended. *Adults:* 500-100 mg.
Fibric acid derivatives: gemfibrozil, clofibrate	Decrease hepatic VLDL synthesis; increase LPL activity	Increased incidence of gallstones and perhaps gastrointestinal cancer, myositis, diarrhea, nausea, rash, altered liver function, increased CPK levels, potentiation of warfarin	*Children:* not recommended. *Adults:* gemfibrozil: 600-1200 mg; clofibrate: 1-2 g.

LDL, Low-density lipoprotein; *VLDL,* very low-density lipoprotein; *FH,* familial hypercholesterolemia; *HDL,* high-density lipoprotein; *LPL,* lipoprotein lipase; *CPK,* creatine phosphokinase; *HMG-CoA,* 3-hydroxy-3-methylglutaryl coenzyme A.
Adapted from Farmer JA, Gotto AM Jr: *Risk factors for coronary artery disease.* In Braunwald E: *Heart disease,* ed 4, 1992, WB Saunders.)

34 / Child with Chest Pain

Chest pain is frequently encountered in children in the office and emergency room. Although chest pain does not indicate serious disease of the heart or other systems in most pediatric patients, in a society with a high prevalence of atherosclerotic cardiovascular disease, it can be alarming to the child and parents. Physicians should be aware of the differential diagnosis of chest pain in children and should make every effort to find a specific cause before making a referral to a specialist or reassuring the child and the parents of the benign nature of the complaint. Making a routine referral to a cardiologist is not always a good idea; it may increase the family's concern and may result in a prolonged and expensive cardiac evaluation.

ETIOLOGY AND PREVALENCE

According to several reports, the three most common causes of chest pain in children are costochondritis; a pathologic condition of the chest wall (trauma or muscle strain); and respiratory diseases, especially those associated with coughing (Table 34-1). These three conditions account for 45% to 65% of the causes of chest pain in children. Cardiac disease rarely presents with chest pain in children; it accounts for less than 4% of children with chest pain.

Chest pain occurs in children of all ages. Chest pain in children younger than 12 years of age usually has a cardiorespiratory cause such as coughing, asthma, pneumonia, or heart disease. Psychogenic causes are more likely in children older than 12 years of age. Box on p. 444 lists possible causes of noncardiac and cardiac chest pain in children. These causes are also discussed briefly.

TABLE 34–1.

Relative Frequency of Causes of Chest Pain in Children

Cause	Percentage
Idiopathic factors	12-45
Costochondritis	9-22
Musculoskeletal trauma	21
Cough, asthma, pneumonia	15-21
Psychogenic factors	5-9
Gastrointestinal disorders	4-7
Cardiac disorders	0-4
Sickle-cell crisis	2
Miscellaneous	9-21

CLINICAL MANIFESTATIONS

Idiopathic

No etiology can be found in 12% to 45% of patients, even after moderately extensive investigation. Although an organic etiology is less likely in children with chronic chest pain, some of these children are eventually referred for a specialty evaluation.

443

Causes of Chest Pain in Children

Noncardiac Causes

Thoracic cage
   Costochondritis
   Trauma or muscle strain
   Abnormalities of the rib cage or thoracic spine
   Breast tenderness (mastalgia)
Respiratory system
   Severe cough or bronchitis
   Pleural effusion
   Lobar pneumonia
   Exercise-induced asthma
   Spontaneous pneumothorax or pneumomediastinum
Gastrointestinal system
Psychogenic factors
   Hyperventilation
   Conversion symptoms
   Somatization disorders
   Depression
Miscellaneous
   Texidor's twinge
   Herpes zoster
   Pleurodynia

Cardiac Causes

Ischemic ventricular dysfunction
   Structural abnormalities of the heart (Severe AS or PS, HOCM, Eisenmenger's syndrome)
   MVP
   Coronary artery abnormalities (old Kawasaki disease, congenital anomaly, coronary heart disease,
      hypertension, sickle cell disease)
   Cocaine abuse
   Aortic dissection and aortic aneurysm (Turner's, Marfan's, and Noonan's syndromes)
Inflammatory conditions
   Pericarditis (viral, bacterial, or rheumatic)
   Postpericardiotomy syndrome
   Myocarditis, acute or chronic
   Kawasaki disease
Arrhythmias (and palpitation)
   SVT
   Frequent PVCs or ventricular tachycardia (possible)

AS, Aortic stenosis; *PS,* pulmonary stenosis; *HOCM,* hypertrophic obstructive cardiomyopathy; *MVP,* mitral valve prolapse; *SVT,* supraventricular tachycardia; *PVCs,* premature ventricular contractions.

Noncardiac Causes of Chest Pain

Most cases of pediatric chest pain originate in organ systems other than the cardiovascular system. Identifiable noncardiac causes of chest pain are found in 56% to 86% of reported cases.

Costochondritis. Costochondritis causes chest pain in 9% to 22% of children with such pain. It is characterized by mild to moderate anterior chest pain, usually unilateral but occasionally bilateral. The pain may be preceded by exercise, an upper respiratory infection, or physical activity; a specific position may also cause the pain. The pain may radiate to the remainder of the chest, back, and abdomen; it may be exaggerated by breathing, and it may persist for several months. Physical examination (PE) is diagnostic; the clinician finds a reproducible tenderness on palpation over the chondrosternal or costochondral junctions. It is a benign condition.

Tietze's syndrome is a rare form of costochondritis characterized by a large, tender, fusiform (spindle-shaped), nonsuppurative swelling at the chondrosternal junction. It usually affects the upper ribs, particularly the second and third costochondral junctions.

Musculoskeletal. Musculoskeletal chest pain is also common in children. The pain is caused by strains of the pectoral, shoulder, or back muscles after exercise or by trauma to the chest wall from sports, fights, or accidents. A history of vigorous exercise, weight lifting, or direct trauma to the chest and the presence of tenderness of the chest wall or muscles clearly indicate muscle strain or trauma. Abnormalities of the rib cage or thoracic spine can cause mild, chronic chest pain in children.

Respiratory. Respiratory problems are responsible for about 20% of cases of pediatric chest pain, which may result from overused chest wall muscles or from pleural irritation. A history of severe cough, with tenderness of intercostal or abdominal muscles, is usually present. The presence of rales, wheezing, tachypnea, retraction, or fever on examination suggests a respiratory cause of chest pain. Pleural effusion may cause pain that is worsened by deep inspiration. Chest x-ray examination may confirm the diagnosis of pleural effusion, pneumonia, or pneumothorax. In some children, asthma may be the cause of chest pain on exertion, but it may not be suspected until stress tests reveal exercise-induced asthma.

Gastrointestinal. Some gastrointestinal disorders may present as chest pain in children. The onset and relief of pain in relation to eating and diet may help clarify the diagnosis. Esophagitis should be suspected in a child who complains of burning substernal pain that worsens with a reclining posture or abdominal pressure or that worsens after certain foods are eaten. Young children sometimes ingest foreign bodies, such as coins, that lodge in the upper esophagus, or they may ingest caustic substances that burn the entire esophagus. In such cases the history makes the diagnosis obvious.

Psychogenic. Psychogenic disturbances account for about 9% of cases and are seen equally in male and female adolescents. Often a recent stressful situation parallels the onset of the chest pain: a death or separation in the family, a serious illness, a disability, a recent move, failure in school, or sexual molestation. However, a psychologic cause of chest pain should not be lightly assigned without a thorough history taking and a follow-up evaluation. Psychologic or psychiatric consultation may reveal conversion symptoms, a somatization disorder, or even depression.

Miscellaneous.

1. The *precordial catch* (Texidor's twinge or stitch in the side), a one-sided chest pain, lasts a few seconds or minutes and is associated with bending or slouching. The cause is unclear, but the pain is relieved by straightening and taking a few shallow breaths or one deep breath. The pain may recur frequently or remain absent for months.

2. Some male and female adolescents complain of chest pain caused by breast masses *(mastalgia)*. These tender masses may be cysts (in postpubertal girls) or may be part of normal breast development in pubertal boys and girls.

3. *Pleurodynia* (devil's grip), an unusual cause of chest pain caused by coxsackievirus infection, is characterized by sudden episodes of sharp pain in the chest or abdomen.

4. *Herpes zoster* is another unusual cause of chest pain.

5. *Spontaneous pneumothorax or pneumomediastimum* are serious but rare respiratory causes of acute chest pain in children; children with asthma, cystic fibrosis, or Marfan syndrome are at risk. Inhalation of cocaine can provoke pneumomediastinum and pneumothorax with subcutaneous emphysema.

6. *Pulmonary embolism*, although extremely rare in children, has been reported in female adolescents who use oral contraceptives or have had elective abortions. It has also been reported in male adolescents with recent trauma of the lower extremities

and in children with shunted hydrocephalus. Affected patients usually have dyspnea, pleuritic pain, fever, cough, and hemoptysis.

7. *Hyperventilation* can produce chest discomfort and is often associated with paresthesia and lightheadedness.

Cardiovascular Causes of Chest Pain

Cardiovascular disease has been identified as the cause of pediatric chest pain in less than 5% of cases. In other reports, no cardiac cause of chest pain was found. Cardiac chest pain may be caused by ischemic ventricular dysfunction, pericardial or myocardial inflammatory processes, or arrhythmias. A typical *anginal pain* is located in the precordial or substernal area and radiates to the neck, the jaw, either or both arms, the back, or the abdomen. The patient describes the pain as a deep, heavy pressure; the feeling of choking; or a squeezing sensation. Exercise, cold stress, emotional upset, or a large meal typically precipitates anginal pain. Table 34-2 summarizes important clinical findings of cardiac causes of chest pain in children.

Ischemic myocardial dysfunction.

Congenital heart defects. Severe obstructive lesions, such as aortic stenosis (AS), subaortic stenosis, severe pulmonary stenosis (PS), and pulmonary vascular obstructive disease (PVOD) (Eisenmenger complex), may cause chest pain. Mild stenotic lesions do not cause ischemic chest pain. Chest pain from severe obstructive lesions results from increased myocardial oxygen demands from tachycardia and increased blood pressure. Therefore the pain is usually associated with exercise and is a typical anginal pain, as previously discussed. PE often reveals a loud heart murmur best audible at the upper right sternal border (URSB) or upper left sternal border (ULSB), usually with a thrill. The ECG usually shows ventricular hypertrophy with or without "strain" pattern. Chest x-ray films may be abnormal in patients with AS and PS, and definitely abnormal in patients with Eisenmenger's syndrome, with a marked prominence of the main pulmonary artery (MPA) segment. Echocardiography (echo) and Doppler studies permit accurate determination of the type and severity of the obstructive lesions. An exercise electrocardiogram (ECG) may aid in the functional assessment of severity.

Mitral valve prolapse. Chest pain associated with mitral valve prolapse (MVP) has been reported in about 20% of patients. The pain is usually a vague, nonexertional pain of short duration, located at the apex, without a constant relationship to effort or emotion. The pain is presumed to result from papillary muscle or left ventricular (LV) endomyocardial ischemia, but there is increasing doubt as to the causal relationship between chest pain and MVP in children. Occasionally, supraventricular or ventricular arrhythmias may result in cardiac symptoms, including chest discomfort. Thoracoskeletal deformities commonly occur in these children and may cause chest pain. Nearly all patients with Marfan syndrome have MVP.

Cardiac examination reveals a midsystolic click with or without a late systolic murmur. The ECG may show T-wave inversion in the inferior leads. Two-dimensional echo findings of MVP in the adult have recently been revised, but diagnostic echo findings for MVP have not been established in children (see Chapter 21).

Cardiomyopathy. Hypertrophic and dilated cardiomyopathy can cause chest pain from ischemia, with or without exercise, or from rhythm disturbances. PE reveals no diagnostic findings, but the ECG and/or chest x-ray film are abnormal, leading to further studies. Echo studies are diagnostic of the condition (see Chapter 18).

Coronary artery disease. Coronary artery anomalies rarely cause chest pain. They include rare cases of anomalous origin of the left coronary artery from the pulmonary artery (PA) (usually symptomatic during early infancy), coronary artery fistula, aneurysm or stenosis of the coronary arteries as a result of Kawasaki disease, or coronary insufficiency secondary to previous cardiac surgery involving the coronary arteries or the vicinity of these arteries.

The pain caused by coronary artery abnormalities is typical of anginal pain. Cardiac

TABLE 34–2.

Important Clinical Findings of Cardiac Causes of Chest Pain

Conditions	History	PE	ECG	Chest X-ray Film
Severe AS	History of CHD (+)	Loud (>grade 3/6 SEM at URSB with radiation to neck)	LVH with or without strain	Prominent ascending aorta and aortic knob
Severe PS	History of CHD (+)	Loud (grade >3/6) SEM at ULSB	RVH with or without strain	Prominent MPA segment
HOCM	Positive FH in one third of cases	Variable heart murmurs Brisk brachial pulses (±)	LVH Deep Q/small R or QS pattern in LPLs	Mild cardiomegaly with globular-shaped heart
MVP	Positive FH (±)	Midsystolic click with or without late systolic murmur Thin body build Thoracic skeletal anomalies (80%)	Inverted T waves in aVF (±)	Normal heart size Straight back (±) Narrow AP diameter (±)
Eisenmenger's syndrome	History of CHD (+)	Cyanosis and clubbing RV impulse Loud and single S2 Soft or no heart murmur	RVH	Markedly prominent MPA with normal heart size
Anomalous origin of left coronary artery	Symptomatic condition in early infancy, with recurrent episodes of distress	Soft or no heart murmur	Anterolateral MI	Moderate to marked cardiomegaly
Sequelae of Kawasaki or other coronary artery diseases	History of Kawasaki disease (±) Typical exercise-related anginal pain	Usually negative Continuous murmur in coronary fistula	ST-segment elevation (±) Old MI pattern (±)	Normal heart size or mild cardiomegaly
Cocaine abuse	History of substance abuse (±)	Hypertension Nonspecific heart murmur (±)	ST-segment elevation (±)	Normal heart size in acute cases
Pericarditis and myocarditis	History of URI (±) Sharp chest pain	Friction rub Muffled heart sounds Nonspecific heart murmur (±)	Low QRS voltages ST-segment shift Arrhythmias (±)	Cardiomegaly of varying degree
Postpericardiotomy syndrome	History of recent heart surgery Sharp pain Dyspnea	Muffled heart sounds (±) Friction rub	Persistent ST-segment elevation	Cardiomegaly of varying degree
Arrhythmias (and palpitation)	History of WPW syndrome (±) FH of long QT syndrome (±)	May be negative Irregular rhythm (±)	Arrhythmias (±) WPW syndrome (±) Long QTc syndrome (>0.46 sec)	Normal heart size

PE, Physical examination; ECG, electrocardiogram; AS, aortic stenosis; CHD, congenital heart disease; SEM, systolic ejection murmur; FH, family history; URSB, upper right sternal border; LVH, left ventricular hypertrophy; PS, pulmonary stenosis; ULSB, upper left sternal border; RVH, right ventricular hypertrophy; MPA, main pulmonary artery; HOCM, hypertrophic obstructive cardiomyopathy; LPLs, left precordial leads; MVP, mitral valve prolapse; RV, right ventricular; AP, anteroposterior; MI, myocardial infarction; URI, upper respiratory infection; WPW, Wolff-Parkinson-White.

examination may be normal or may reveal a heart murmur (systolic murmur of mitral regurgitation [MR] or continuous murmur of fistulas). The ECG may show myocardial ischemia (ST-segment elevation) or old myocardial infarction. Chest x-ray films may reveal abnormalities suggestive of these conditions. An abnormal exercise ECG further indicates myocardial ischemia. Although echo can be helpful, coronary angiography is usually indicated for the definitive diagnosis.

Cocaine abuse. Even children with normal hearts are at risk of ischemia and myocardial infarction if cocaine is used. Cocaine blocks the reuptake of catecholamines in the central nervous system and peripheral sympathetic nerves. An increase in the sympathetic output and circulating levels of catecholamines causes coronary vasoconstriction. Cocaine also induces the activation of platelets in some but not all patients. The resulting increase in heart rate and blood pressure, increase in myocardial oxygen consumption, possible increase in platelet activation, and myocardial electrical abnormalities may collectively produce anginal pain, infarction, arrhythmias, or sudden death. History and drug screening help physicians in the diagnosis of cocaine-induced chest pain.

Aortic dissection or aortic aneurysm. Aortic dissection or aortic aneurysm rarely cause chest pain. Children with Turner's, Marfan, and Noonan's syndromes are at risk.

Pericardial or myocardial disease.

Pericarditis. Irritation of the pericardium may result from inflammatory pericardial disease; pericarditis may be of a viral, bacterial, or rheumatic origin. In a child who had recent open heart surgery, the cause of the pain may be postpericardiotomy syndrome. Older children with pericarditis may complain of a sharp, stabbing precordial pain that worsens when lying down and improves after sitting and leaning forward. The ECG may reveal low QRS voltages and ST-T changes, and the chest x-ray film may show varying degrees of cardiac enlargement and changes in the cardiac silhouette. Diagnosis of pericardial effusion with or without tamponade can be accurately made by echo examination.

Myocarditis. Acute myocarditis often involves the pericardium to a certain extent and can cause chest pain. Examination may reveal fever, respiratory distress, distant heart sounds, neck vein distention, friction rub, and paradoxical pulse. Chest x-ray films and the ECG may suggest the correct diagnosis, which can be confirmed by echo examination (see Chapter 19).

Arrhythmias.
Chest pain may result from a variety of arrhythmias, especially with sustained tachycardia resulting in myocardial ischemia. Even without ischemia, children may consider palpitation or forceful heartbeats as chest pain. When chest pain is associated with dizziness and palpitation, a resting ECG and a 24-hour ambulatory ECG using a Holter monitor should be obtained. Alternatively, a telephone transmission device may be used to relay the ECG while the patient experiences symptoms.

DIAGNOSTIC APPROACH

A *three-step diagnostic approach* is recommended (Box on p. 449). The *first step* should be directed at detecting the three most common causes of chest pain: costochondritis, musculoskeletal causes, and respiratory diseases; these three account for 45% to 65% of chest pain in children. A thorough history taking and careful physical examination make the diagnosis of these three conditions. The *second step* is to check for cardiac causes, with PE of the cardiovascular system, chest x-ray films, and an ECG. If the cardiac cause of chest pain is not found, the pain is likely due to disease in other systems, including conditions of psychogenic or idiopathic origin; this is the *third diagnostic stage*.

History of Present Illness and the Nature of the Pain

The initial history should be directed at finding the nature of the pain, associated symptoms, and concurrent or precipitating events that may help clarifying the noncardiac or cardiac origin of the pain. Most important, exertion precipites cardiac

Three-Step Approach to Chest Pain

Step 1

The clinician looks for the three most common causes of chest pain in children (45% to 65%): costochondritis, musculoskeletal causes, and respiratory diseases; these are revealed by the history and PE.

Step 2

The physician looks for cardiac causes (0% to 4%); chest x-ray studies and an ECG, in addition to a history and a careful cardiac examination, are needed (see Table 34-2 for differential diagnosis).

Step 3

The physician looks for diseases of other systems including those of psychogenic and idiopathic causes (15% to 45%). Follow-up may clarify the cause.

causes of chest pain, and the quality of pain is described as a pressure or squeezing sensation, not a sharp pain. The following are some examples of questions to ask:

1. What seems to bring out the pain (e.g., exercise, eating, trauma, emotional stress)? Do you get the same type of pain while you watch TV or sit in class?

2. What is the pain like (e.g., sharp, pressure sensation, squeezing)?

3. What is the location (e.g., specific point, localized or diffuse), severity, radiation, and duration (seconds, minutes) of the pain?

4. Does the pain get worse with deep breathing? (If so, the pain may be caused by pleural irritation or chest wall pathology.) Does the pain improve with certain body positions? (This is seen sometimes with pericarditis.)

5. How often and how long have you had similar pain (frequency and chronicity)?

6. Have you been hurt while playing or have you used your arms excessively for any reason?

7. Are there any associated symptoms, such as cough, fever, syncope, dizziness, or palpitation?

8. What treatments for the pain have already been tried?

Past and Family History

After gaining some idea about the nature of the pain, the clinician should focus on important past and family histories. Examples of questions follow:

1. Are there any known medical conditions (e.g., congenital heart disease [CHD] or acquired heart disease, cardiac surgery, infection, asthma), and is the patient on any medications, including birth control pills?

2. Has there been recent heart disease, chest pain, or a cardiac death in the family?

3. Does any disease run in the family?

4. About what is the patient or family member concerned?

5. Has the child been exposed to drugs (cocaine) or cigarettes?

Physical Examination

1. A careful general PE should be performed before the focus turns to the chest. The clinician should note whether the child is in severe distress from pain, is in emotional stress, or is hyperventilating.

2. The skin and extremities should be examined for trauma or chronic disease. Bruising elsewhere on the body may indicate chest trauma that cannot be seen.

3. The abdomen should be carefully examined because it may be the source of pain referred to the chest.

4. The chest should be carefully inspected for trauma or asymmetry. The chest wall should be palpated for signs of tenderness or subcutaneous air. Special attention should be paid to the possibility of costochondritis by palpating each costochondral and chondrosternal junction.

5. The heart and lungs should be auscultated for arrhythmias, heart murmurs, rubs, muffled heart sounds, gallop rhythm, rales, wheezes, or decreased breath sounds.

Examination for Cardiac Causes of Chest Pain

If the three common causes or other identifiable causes of chest pain are not found, the clinician should then direct attention to each of the cardiac causes of chest pain listed in the box on p. 444. By this time, the examiner should have a fairly good idea about the likelihood of the cardiac causes of chest pain. Even though the cardiac causes are not likely, chest x-ray studies and an ECG are usually indicated at this stage. Chest x-ray films should be evaluated for pulmonary pathology, cardiac size and silhouette, and pulmonary vascularity. Arrhythmias, hypertrophy, conduction disturbances (including Wolff-Parkinson-White [WPW] syndrome), abnormal T and Q waves, and an abnormal QT interval are possible findings on the ECG. Table 34-2 summarizes important history information, physical findings, and abnormalities of chest x-ray films and ECGs for cardiac causes of chest pain.

If the family history is negative for hereditary heart disease, if the past history is negative for heart disease or Kawasaki disease, if cardiac examination is unremarkable, and if the ECG and chest x-ray films are normal, the chest pain is not caused by cardiac factors.

Noncardiac Causes of Chest Pain

If no cardiac abnormalities are found, idiopathic or psychogenic causes or an abnormality of another system is the likely cause of chest pain. At this point the clinician can reassure the patient and family of a probable benign nature of the chest pain. Simple follow-up may clarify the cause.

Further Laboratory Investigation

A drug screening for cocaine may be worthwhile in adolescents who have acute, severe chest pain and distress with an unclear etiology.

Referral to Cardiologists

The following are some of the indications for a referral of a child with chest pain for cardiac evaluation:

1. When chest pain suggests anginal pain, when abnormal findings occur in the cardiac examination, or when abnormalities occur in the cardiac x-ray film or ECG, cardiac referral is clearly indicated. The ability of the examiner to recognize common innocent heart murmurs minimizes the frequency of such referrals.

2. When there is a positive family history for cardiomyopathy, long QT syndrome, or another hereditary disease commonly associated with cardiac abnormalities, cardiology referral may be indicated.

3. High levels of anxiety in the family and patient and a chronic, recurring nature of the pain are also important reasons for referrals to a cardiologist.

TREATMENT

When a specific cause of chest pain is identified, treatment is directed at correcting or improving the cause:

1. Costochondritis can be treated by reassurance and occasionally by acetaminophen or nonsteroidal antiinflammatory agents.

2. Most musculoskeletal and nonorganic causes of chest pain can be treated with rest, acetaminophen, or nonsteroidal antiinflammatory agents.

3. If respiratory causes of chest pain are found, treatment is directed at those causes.

4. If serious cardiac anomalies, arrhythmias, or exercise-induced asthma are diagnosed, a referral is made to the cardiology or pulmonary service. Cardiac evaluation requires further specialized studies, such as echo, an exercise stress test, Holter monitoring, or even cardiac catheterization. Depending on the cause, treatment may be surgical or medical.

5. The correct therapy of acute cocaine toxicity has not been established. Calcium channel blockers (nifedipine, nitrendipine), β-adrenergic blockers, nitrates, and thrombolytic agents have resulted in varying levels of success. The use of β-blockers is controversial; they may worsen coronary blood flow.

35 / Syncope

PREVALENCE

The prevalence of syncope and near syncope in children is unknown, but it may be as high as 3% of emergency room visits in some areas.

DEFINITION

Syncope is a transient loss of consciousness and muscle tone that by history does not suggest other altered states of consciousness. In near syncope (i.e., presyncope), premonitory signs and symptoms of imminent syncope occur; these include dizziness with or without blackout, pallor, diaphoresis, thready pulse, and low blood pressure but no loss of consciousness. Recurrent episodes of unexplained syncope may cause functional impairment and possible serious injury to the child and may produce tremendous psychologic stress for the child and the family. Besides, the complaint may represent a serious cardiac condition that can cause sudden death.

ETIOLOGY

The normal function of the brain depends on a constant supply of oxygen and glucose. Significant alterations in the supply of oxygen and glucose may result in a transient loss or near loss of consciousness. Syncope may be caused by circulatory, metabolic, or neuropsychologic problems. The box lists possible causes.

Etiologic Classification of Syncope

Circulatory Causes
  Extracardiac causes
    Common faint or vasodepressor syncope
    Orthostatic hypotension
    Failure of venous return (e.g., increased intrathoracic pressure, decreased venous return, hypovolemia)
    Cerebrovascular occlusive disease
  Intracardiac causes
    Severe obstructive lesions (e.g., AS, PS, HOCM, pulmonary hypertension)
    Myocardial dysfunction (e.g., myocardial ischemia or infarction, Kawasaki disease, coronary artery anomalies)
    Arrhythmias (extreme tachycardia or bradycardia, long QT syndrome)

Metabolic Causes
  Hypoglycemia
  Hyperventilation syndrome
  Hypoxia

Neuropsychiatric Causes
  Epilepsy
  Brain tumor
  Migraine
  Hysteria or nonconvulsive seizures

AS, Aortic stenosis, *PS,* pulmonary stenosis; *HOCM,* Hypertrophic obstructive cardiomyopathy.

In contrast to adults, in whom most cases of syncope are caused by cardiac problems, in children and adolescents, most incidents of syncope are benign, resulting from vasovagal episodes (probably the most common cause), orthostatic syncope, hyperventilation, and breathholding. In this chapter, only circulatory (extracardiac and cardiac) causes of syncope including long QT syndrome, are discussed. Discussion of the metabolic and neuropsychiatric causes of syncope is beyond the scope of this book.

EXTRACARDIAC CAUSES OF SYNCOPE

Vasovagal Syncope

Vasovagal syncope is also called vasodepressor, neurocardiogenic, or common syncope.

Clinical manifestations. Vasovagal syncope is characterized by a prodrome (warning symptoms and signs) lasting a few seconds to a minute; this prodrome consists of dizziness, lightheadedness, pallor, palpitation, nausea, diaphoresis, and hyperventilation followed by the loss of consciousness and muscle tone. The patient usually falls without injury, the unconsciousness does not last more than a minute, and the patient gradually awakens. The syncope usually occurs with anxiety or fright, pain, blood drawing or the sight of blood, fasting, hot and humid conditions, crowded places, and prolonged and motionless standing.

Pathophysiology. A normally erect posture without movement shifts blood to the lower extremities and causes a decrease in venous return and thus decreases in stroke volume and blood pressure. This reduced filling of the ventricle places less stretch on the mechanoreceptor (i.e., C fibers) and causes a decrease in afferent neural output to the brainstem, reflecting hypotension. This decline in neural traffic from the mechanoreceptors and a decreased arterial pressure elicit an increase in sympathetic output, thus resulting in an increase in heart rate and peripheral vasoconstriction to restore blood pressure to the normal range. Thus the normal responses to the assumption of an upright posture are an increase in heart rate, an unchanged or slightly diminished systolic pressure, and an increase in diastolic pressure.

In susceptible individuals, however, a sudden decrease in venous return to the ventricle produces a large increase in the force of ventricular contraction; this causes activation of the left ventricular (LV) mechanoreceptors, which normally respond only to stretch. The resulting paroxysmal increase in neural traffic to the brain stem somehow mimics the conditions seen in hypertension and thereby produces a paradoxic withdrawal of sympathetic activity with a subsequent peripheral vasodilatation, hypotension, and bradycardia. Characteristically, the reduction of blood pressure and especially the heart rate is severe enough to decrease cerebral perfusion and produce loss of consciousness.

Diagnostic tests.

1. Diagnostic tests commonly performed for patients with syncope include electrocardiography (ECG), Holter monitoring, neurologic evaluation with electroencephalography, glucose tolerance test, echocardiography (echo), computed tomography, and magnetic resonance imaging of the head. However, these tests are usually negative and have no value in vasovagal syncope.

2. Tilt testing of various protocols has recently been reported to be useful in diagnosing vasovagal syncope. The angle of the tilt varies from 60 to 80 degrees, and the duration of the tilt varies from 10 to 60 minutes. If the tilt test alone is not positive, the procedure is repeated with an infusion of isoproterenol, starting at 0.02 µg/kg/min and increasing to 1.0µg/kg/min, for 15 minutes. Some believe responses to isoproterenol are nonspecific. If a positive result is obtained within a few minutes and without infusion of isoproterenol, the diagnosis of vasovagal syncope is much clearer, but positive results obtained with a long period of tilting (20 to 30 minutes) and with infusion of a relatively large dose of isoproterenol are questionable. In adults, the

overall reproducibility of syncope by the tilt test was disappointingly low (62%), which causes doubt about the specificity of the test for the diagnosis and the validity of evaluating the effect of an oral drug treatment by a repeat tilt test.

Treatment.

1. Placing the patient in a supine position until the circulatory crisis resolves may be all that is indicated. Inhalation of ammonia is usually effective. If the patient feels the prodrome to a faint, he or she should be told to lie down with the feet raised above the chest: this usually aborts the syncope.

2. Success in preventing syncope has been reported with the following medications:

   a. Fludrocortisone (a mineralocorticoid, through volume expansion)

   b. Metoprolol (a selective beta-1 antagonist, through negative inotropic effects)

   c. Disopyramide (a class 1A antiarrhythmic agent that is an anticholinergic and negative inotropic agent as well as a peripheral vasoconstrictor)

   d. Pseudoephedrine (an alpha-adrenergic stimulant, by preventing venous pooling and hypotension)

   e. Scopolamine (an anticholinergic drug, by lessening vagal tone during syncope), which is given transdermally

Pseudoephedrine (60 mg given orally twice a day for older children and adolescents) or metoprolol (1.5 mg/kg/day given orally in 2 to 3 doses) has been reported to be beneficial in some children. Beneficial effects of an implanted pacemaker by maintaining the heart rate has been reported by some but not by others: Even though the heart rate was maintained, blood pressure dropped, and symptoms still resulted.

Orthostatic Hypotension

The normal response to standing is reflex arterial and venous constriction and a slight increase in heart rate. In orthostatic hypotension, the normal adrenergic vasoconstriction of the arterioles and veins in the upright position is absent or inadequate, resulting in hypotension without a reflex increase in heart rate. In contrast to the prodrome seen with vasovagal syncope, in orthostatic hypotension, patients experience only lightheadedness. Orthostatic hypotension can be precipitated by prolonged bed rest, prolonged standing, and conditions that decrease the circulating blood volume (e.g., bleeding, dehydration). Drugs that interfere with the sympathetic vasomotor response (e.g., calcium channel blockers, antihypertensive drugs, vasodilators, phenothiazines), and diuretics may exacerbate orthostatic hypotension.

In patients suspected of having orthostatic hypotension, blood pressures should be measured in the supine and standing positions. After standing for 5 to 10 minutes without moving their arms or legs, some patients develop hypotension (a drop of 10 to 15 mm Hg) with no increase in the heart rate but do not faint. Patients with orthostatic hypotension also have a positive tilt test but do not display the autonomic nervous system signs of vasovagal syncope, such as pallor, diaphoresis, and hyperventilation.

Elastic stockings, a high-salt diet, sympathomimetic amines, and corticosteroids have been used with varying degrees of success. The patient should be told to move to an upright position slowly.

Micturition syncope is a rare form of orthostatic hypotension. In this condition, rapid bladder decompression results in decreased total peripheral vascular resistance with splanchnic stasis and reduced venous return to the heart, resulting in postural hypotension.

Failure of Systemic Venous Return

Return of the normal amount of venous blood to the heart is necessary to maintain normal LV output and systemic pressure. The pressure in the right atrium (RA) is normally 5 to 10 mm Hg lower than in the venules, and this makes blood flow toward the heart. Decreased venous return may occur as a result of the following:

1. Increased intrathoracic pressure, such as that seen in the straining phase of the Valsalva's maneuver, repetitive coughing, breath-holding, and tracheal obstruction

2. Decreased venous tone, which may be caused by pharmacologic agents that relax vascular smooth muscle (e.g., nitroglycerin) or that eliminate sympathetic tone (e.g., ganglionic blockers, guanethidine)

3. Decreased intravascular volume secondary to hemorrhage or dehydration

Treatment should be directed at eliminating or correcting identifiable causes.

Cerebrovascular Occlusive Disease

Syncope from cerebrovascular occlusive disease is extremely rare in children. Adults with this disease may have syncope with a less significant fall in blood pressure than patients without the disease. Cerebrovascular occlusive disease is often associated with short-term neurologic defects such as hemiparesis, transient blindness, diplopia, speech impairments, confusion, and headache. Bruits may be present over the carotid arteries. Surgical therapy may be advisable in some cases.

Subclavian steal syndrome is a rare type of syncope that occurs when a proximal obstruction of the subclavian artery exists and consequently blood shunts from the brain to the arm via the ipsilateral vertebral artery, especially during exercise. A child who had surgery that sacrificed a subclavian artery, such as Blalock-Taussig shunt and subclavian flap aortoplasty for coarctation repair, may develop the syndrome during adulthood.

CARDIAC CAUSES OF SYNCOPE

Cardiac syncope may be caused by structural heart disease or may be secondary to arrhythmias. A cardiac cause of syncope is suggested by the occurrence of syncope even in the recumbent position, syncope provoked by exercise, chest pain associated with syncope, a history of unoperated or operated heart disease, or a family history of sudden death. Cardiac causes of syncope may include obstructive lesions, coronary insufficiency, and arrhythmias, including long QT syndrome.

Obstructive Lesions

Patients with severe obstructive lesions such as aortic stenosis (AS), pulmonary stenosis (PS), or hypertrophic obstructive cardiomyopathy (HOCM), as well as those with pulmonary hypertension may have syncope. Peripheral vasodilatation secondary to exercise is not accompanied by an adequate increase in cardiac output, thereby resulting in diminished perfusion to the brain. Exercise often precipitates syncope associated with these conditions. Patients may also complain of chest pain, dyspnea, and palpitation.

Obstructive lesions and pulmonary hypertension can be diagnosed by careful physical examination (PE), ECG, chest x-ray studies, and echo. Surgery is indicated for most of these conditions, with the exception of irreversible forms of pulmonary hypertension.

Myocardial Dysfunction

Although rare, myocardial ischemia or infarction secondary to congenital anomalies or acquired disease (Kawasaki disease) of the coronary artery may cause syncope.

Arrhythmias

Either extreme tachycardia or bradycardia can decrease cardiac output and lower the cerebral blood flow below the critical level, causing syncope. Commonly encountered rhythm disturbances include supraventricular tachycardia (SVT), ventricular tachycardia, sick sinus syndrome, and complete heart block. Simple bradycardia is usually well tolerated in children, but the combination of tachycardia followed by bradycardia (overdrive suppression) is more likely to produce syncope. Arrhythmias may be associated with nonidentifiable cardiac causes or structural heart defects.

No identifiable structural defects. Syncope from arrhythmias is rare in children with apparently normal hearts, with the exception of children with the following conditions:

1. Long QT syndrome is characterized by syncope caused by ventricular arrhythmias, prolongation of the QT interval on the ECG, and occasionally a family history of sudden death. Congenital deafness is also a component of Jervell and Lange-Nielsen syndrome but not of Romano-Ward syndrome (see later section).

2. Wolff-Parkinson-White (WPW) syndrome may be associated with SVT.

3. Right ventricular dysplasia (right ventricular cardiomyopathy) is a rare anomaly of the myocardium and is associated with repeated episodes of ventricular tachycardia (see Chapter 18).

Structural heart defects. The following congenital and acquired heart conditions, unoperated or operated, are associated with arrhythmias that may result in syncope:

1. Some preoperative congenital heart defects (CHDs), such as Ebstein's anomaly, mitral stenosis (MS) or mitral regurgitation (MR), and L-transposition of the great arteries (L-TGA), occur.

2. Postoperative CHDs occur, especially after repairs of tetralogy of Fallot (TOF) and transposition of the great arteries (TGA) and after the Fontan operation. These children may have sick sinus syndrome, SVT or ventricular tachycardia, or complete heart block.

3. Dilated cardiomyopathy can cause sinus bradycardia, SVT, or ventricular tachycardia

4. Hypertrophic cardiomyopathy is a common cause of ventricular tachycardia and syncope.

5. Mitral valve prolapse (MVP) is a rare cause of ventricular tachycardia.

The clinician must document a causal relationship between arrhythmias and symptoms by ambulatory ECG recording (Holter monitoring) and/or an exercise tolerance test. Some equivocal cases in which arrhythmias and symptoms are not causally related may require electrophysiologic studies.

Most arrhythmias respond to antiarrhythmic therapy. Long QT syndrome responds well to propranolol. Propranolol or other antiarrhythmic drugs may be indicated in patients with symptomatic MVP syndrome. Occasionally, surgical treatment may be indicated (such as in WPW syndrome causing frequent SVT). Implantation of a pacemaker with a standby mode may be indicated in some patients with sick sinus syndrome.

Differential Diagnosis

A thorough history taking is important when the clinician suspects noncardiovascular syncope; it directs the physician to the correct diagnosis and thereby reduces the number of unnecessary tests.

Epilepsy. Patients with epilepsy may have incontinence, marked confusion in the postictal state, and abnormal EEGs. Patients are rigid rather than limp and may have sustained injuries. Patients do not experience the early symptoms of syncope (e.g., dizziness, pallor, palpitation, diaphoresis). The duration of unconsciousness is longer than that typically seen with syncope (<1 minute).

Convulsive syncope. Some children may exhibit tonic-clonic movement during loss of consciousness from vasovagal syncope. These children have normal EEGs and do not respond to antiseizure medications. They often have positive tilt tests. During the tonic-clonic seizure activity, the EEG may demonstrate diffuse slowing of the brain wave rather than the hypersynchronous spike wave activity seen during epilepsy.

Hypoglycemia. Hypoglycemia has characteristics similar to syncope, such as pallor, perspiration, abdominal discomfort, lightheadedness, confusion, unconsciousness, and possible subsequent occurrence of seizures. However, hypoglycemic attacks differ from syncope in that the onset and recovery occurs more gradually, they do not occur during or shortly after meals, and the presyncopal symptoms do not improve in the supine position.

Hyperventilation. Hyperventilation spells produce hypocapnia, resulting in an intense cerebral vasoconstriction. A typical spell usually begins with an apprehensive feeling with "deep sighing respirations" that the patient rarely notices. The patient often experiences abdominal discomfort, palpitations, lightheadedness and rarely loss of consciousness. The supine position may help the patient relax and may stop the anxiety-hyperventilation cycle. The syncopal episode can be reproduced in the office when the patient hyperventilates.

Hysteria. Syncope resulting from hysteria is not associated with injury and occurs only in the presence of an audience. A teenager may be able to give an accurate presyncopal history but during these attacks does not experience the pallor and hypotension that characterize true syncope. The attacks may last longer (up to an hour) than a brief syncopal spell. Episodes usually occur during an emotionally charged setting and are rare before 10 years of age. Spells are not consistently related to postural changes and are not improved by the supine position.

Diagnostic Work-Up
History. A thorough and accurate history is more important than a PE and is essential in determining a cost-effective diagnostic work-up for each patient.

1. The precipitating factors, suddenness of the onset, progression and duration of the syncope, presyncopal symptoms, presence and duration of unconsciousness, and recovery period are all important.

2. Accompanying signs and symptoms, such as pallor, diaphoresis, palpitation, and nausea, are also important aspects of history taking.

3. The presence of associated diseases and sequelae, medications, past medical history, recent illness, metabolic disease, social interactions, and family history should also be obtained.

Physical examination. Since the patient visits the office after the event, the results of the PE are usually normal. However, complete PE should always be performed, focusing on the patient's cardiac, pulmonary and neurologic status. In the absence of abnormal cardiac and other systems' examination, the focus should be placed on the three common noncardiac causes of syncope: vasovagal syncope, orthostatic hypotension, and hyperventilation syncope.

Vasovagal syncope. The diagnosis of vasovagal syncope is made by elicitation of a typical history and by exclusion of other causes of syncope. Patients with diagnoses of probable vasovagal syncope do not require extensive work-up. The tilt test has been recommended by some in the evaluation of syncope of unknown origin, but it has not been well standardized, and its specificity and reproducibility are questionable (see previous section).

Orthostatic hypotension. If orthostatic hypotension is suspected, the pulse rate and blood pressure are measured in the supine and standing positions (after the patient stands 5 to 10 minutes). A 10 to 15 mm Hg drop in systolic pressure is abnormal, especially if the heart rate does not compensate by increasing.

Hyperventilation syncope. If hyperventilation syncope is suspected, the patient may be made to hyperventilate to reproduce the syncope.

Laboratory studies. Laboratory studies should be appropriately guided by results of the history and PE.

1. An ECG (with emphasis on the QT interval) may be all that is needed in an otherwise healthy patient who faints immediately after an emotional shock.

2. Futher investigation is required if any of the following applies:

    a. The faint is exercise induced.

    b. The faint is preceded by chest pain.

    c. There is evidence of seizure activity or loss of bowel or bladder control.

    d. The faint is atypical of vasovagal syncope.

    e. The syncope is recurrent (more than 2 or 3 times).

    f. PE suggests a cardiovascular abnormality.

    g. There is family history of unexplained death.

3. Initial laboratory studies may include ECG, chest x-ray studies, serum electrolyte levels, fasting blood glucose levels, hemoglobin levels, and an EEG.

Further studies. Further studies will probably be directed by the cardiology or neurology service and may include some or all of the following: echo and color-flow Doppler studies, 24-hour ambulatory ECG monitoring, treadmill exercise test for cardiovascular abnormalities, and a computed tomographic scan of the brain for neurologic evaluation. A tilt test may be indicated in some patients with unexplained syncope.

LONG QT SYNDROME

Patients with long QT syndrome may have syncope, seizures, or rapid palpitation during exercise or with emotion. This syndrome is characterized by prolongation of the QT interval on the ECG and a high incidence of lethal ventricular arrhythmias. The QT prolongation is not due to factors known to prolong the interval (see Chapter 3).

There are three groups of patients in this syndrome: patients with Jervell and Lange-Nielsen syndrome, patients with Romano-Ward syndrome, and patients with the sporadic form:

1. Jervell and Lange-Nielsen (1957) first described families in Norway in whom a long QT interval occurred on ECG and in whom congenital deafness, syncopal spells, and a history of sudden death in the family occurred. Syncopal attacks are due to ventricular arrhythmias. This syndrome is transmitted as an autosomal recessive pattern.

2. Romano-Ward syndrome, subsequently reported independently by Romano et al in Italy (1963) and Ward in Ireland (1964), has all the features of the Jervell and Lange-Nielsen syndrome but without deafness. This syndrome transmits in an autosomal dominant mode.

3. A significant number of affected individuals with normal hearing appears to represent sporadic cases, with a negative family history of the syndrome.

Pathophysiology

Congenital sympathetic imbalance, with excessive or unopposed activity of the left stellate ganglion, subnormal activity of the right stellate ganglion, or both, is believed to be the most likely cause of long QT syndrome. Left cardiac sympathetic denervation surgeries and right stellate ganglion stimulation produce some shortening of the QT interval. Left cardiac sympathetic nerve stimulation exerts a very high arrhythmogenic potential by inducing delayed afterdepolarization, which is known to cause ventricular arrhythmias.

Clinical Manifestations

1. The family history is positive in about 60% of patients, and deafness is present in 5% of patients with the syndrome.

2. Presenting symptoms may be syncope (26%), seizure (10%), cardiac arrest (9%), or presyncope or palpitation (6%). The majority of these symptoms occur during exercise or with emotion. Symptoms of long QT syndrome are related to ventricular arrhythmias and are usually manifested by the end of the second decade of life.

3. The ECG shows a prolonged QT interval with a corrected QT (QTc) interval greater than 0.44 second (Fig. 35–1). In addition, bradycardia (20%), second-degree atrioventricular (AV) block, multiform premature ventricular contractions (PVCs), monomorphic or polymorphic ventricular tachycardia (10% to 20%), and abnormal T-wave morphology (bifid, diphasic, or notched) are frequently found; all of these are considered to be risk factors of sudden death.

4. A treadmill exercise test results in highly significant prolongation of the QTc interval in response to exercise, with the maximal prolongation present after 2 minutes of recovery. Ventricular arrhythmias may develop during the test in up to 30% of patients.

5. Holter monitoring reveals prolongation of the QT interval, major changes in the T-wave configuration (T-wave alternation), and ventricular arrhythmias. The QTc interval on Holter monitor may be longer than that recorded on standard ECG (see later section).

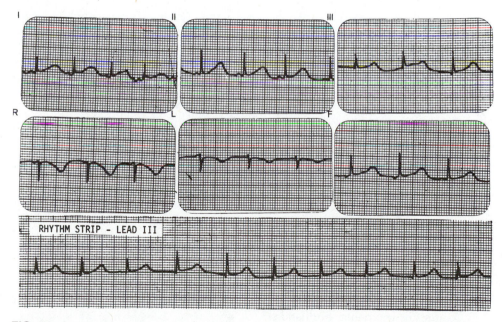

FIG. 35–1.
ECG of a patient with the Romano-Ward syndrome at age 6 demonstrates the longest QTc interval (0.56 second). The precordial leads are not shown. Two negative P waves in a VF suggest a junctional mechanism. This child received 10 mg of propranolol 4 times a day until the age of 13, with complete cessation of syncopal attacks; the dose was smaller than the usual antiarrhythmic dose. There were seven cases of sudden death associated with syncopal attacks on the maternal side of the family. His mother (age 27) and sister (age 5) had moderate prolongation of QTc intervals but experienced no syncopal attacks.

Diagnosis

The potential high risk of sudden death in undiagnosed and untreated patients requires a correct diagnosis so that proper and effective treatment can be instituted. On the other hand, the diagnosis of this disease with a poor prognosis should not be made lightly because the diagnosis may imply a lifelong commitment to treatment.

Because the onset of the QRS complex, the end of the T wave, or both may be difficult to define, the clinician cannot always obtain an accurate measurement of the QT interval. Lead II is the preferred lead to measure the QT interval. The QTc interval is calculated by using Bazett's formula (see Chapter 3). The QTc interval represents the QT interval normalized for a heart rate of 60 beats/min. The longest QTc interval follows the shortest R-R interval. The QTc interval is longer during sleep; therefore Holter monitoring may show the QTc interval to be 0.05 second longer than the interval on a standard ECG, and the uncorrected QT interval may vary as much as 0.03 second. Accordingly, comparison of the Holter with a standard ECG for the QTc interval may be inaccurate.

Controversies exist as to the diagnostic criteria for the condition. The Pediatric Electrophysiology Society (Garson, 1993) used the following "intentionally wide" criteria in the diagnosis of the syndrome:

1. The presence of a prolonged QTc interval of longer than 0.44 second in the absence of other underlying causes such as prematurity, electrolyte disturbance, or central nervous system abnormality. (This criterion is debatable; see later section.)

2. A positive family history of long QT syndrome *plus* unexplained syncope, seizure, or cardiac arrest associated with typical inciting events such as exercise or emotion, even if the QTc interval is normal (<0.44 second). (The QTc interval can vary over time.)

Inclusion of the first criterion of the diagnosis with a QT interval only slightly longer than 0.44 second without symptoms or a positive family history is debatable (Guntheroth, 1993), since as many as 1% to 4% of normal children have QTc intervals of longer than 0.46. Such an inclusion becomes important when one considers a lifelong prophylactic treatment of children with asymptomatic conditions. Therefore in children with borderline prolongation of the QTc interval, the clinician should obtain another ECG and a treadmill test or a Holter monitoring before assigning the diagnosis, starting the patients on a beta-blocker, and using the first ECG as a guide to the adequacy of beta-blocker therapy. Subsequent ECGs may show a more convincing prolongation of the QT interval, and a treadmill exercise test and Holter monitoring may also help confirm the diagnosis of long QT syndrome.

Treatment

1. Long QT syndrome is a serious disease that can result in sudden death, but treatment is at best only partially effective. The knowledge of risk factors should be considered in making the treatment plan.

   a. Risk factors for sudden death include bradycardia for age (sinus bradycardia, junctional escape rhythm, or second-degree AV block), an extremely long QTc interval (>0.55 second), symptoms at presentation (syncope, seizure, cardiac arrest), younger age at presentation (<1 month), and documented torsades de pointes or ventricular fibrillation.

   b. T-wave alternation (major changes in T-wave morphology) is a relative risk factor.

   c. Noncompliance with medication is an important risk factor for sudden death.

   d. Low risk is found for children with normal QTc intervals, no symptoms, and only a positive family history.

2. The following are three major treatments for the long QT syndrome: beta-adrenergic blockers, left cardiac sympathetic denervation, and a demand cardiac pacemaker.

a. *Beta-blockers.* The present therapy of choice is treatment with beta-blockers. There is a concensus that all symptomatic children with long QT syndrome should be treated with propranolol or other beta-blockers. Propranolol and other beta-blockers (e.g., atenolol, metoprolol) are equally effective in reducing symptoms, but the QTc interval usually remains prolonged. Moderate doses of beta-blockers may be better than larger doses because moderate doses lessen the trend toward bradycardia, a known risk factor for sudden death, especially in patients with sinus or AV nodal disorders. Even with treatment with beta-blockers, sudden death can occur: Over 80% of cases of sudden death occurred while patients were on medications; some of these cases of sudden death were caused by noncompliance. Age, gender, QT interval, type of symptoms, and type of ventricular arrhythmias are not predictors of the effectiveness of treatment.

Whether to treat asymptomatic children with QTc intervals of 0.44 second or slightly longer and a positive family history of long QT syndrome is controversial (Garson, 1993; Guntheroth, 1993). The Society recommends treatment with beta-blockers because 9% of these children may have cardiac arrest as the first symptom. However, the Society's report indicates that 5% of "effectively treated" patients suffered sudden death while on medications. In addition, 96% of the Society's patients had QTc intervals longer than 0.46 second, and only 4% of control subjects had QTc intervals greater than 0.46 second, suggesting that children with QTc intervals of less than 0.46 second are at relatively low risk, although some of them developed QTc intervals longer than 0.46 second or whose conditions became symptomatic on follow-up. Symptoms are more likely to occur in patients with QTc intervals longer than 0.48 second. In view of the relatively low risk in these children, lifelong treatment with beta-blockers is debatable (Guntheroth, 1993). Beta-blocker treatment may be dangerous to some patients with the syndrome because treatment tends to produce bradycardia, one of the important risk factors. As an alternative to treatment with beta-blockers, these children may be followed closely for the development of QTc interval longer than 0.46 seconds or symptoms. If these occur, treatment is clearly indicated.

b. *Left cardiac sympathetic denervation.* For patients who continue to have syncope or ventricular tachycardia, a left cardiac sympathetic denervation, preferably a high thoracic left sympathectomy, may be effective. The high thoracic left sympathectomy involves the lower part of the left stellate ganglion and removal of the first four or five thoracic ganglia, with almost no risk for Horner's syndrome. Other denervation surgeries, such as left stellectomy and left cervicothoracic sympathectomy, almost always result in Horner's syndrome and often provide inadequate cardiac sympathetic denervation. After a high thoracic sympathectomy, there is a dramatic reduction in the incidence of major cardiac events, although sudden death still occurs (8%); the procedure has a 5-year survival rate of 94%. Whether beta-blockers should be continued despite their incomplete efficacy or slowly withdrawn after the surgery is unclear.

c. *Demand cardiac pacemaker.* Implantation of a pacemaker and defibrillator may be considered for high-risk patients, especially those with QTc intervals longer than 0.60 second. Patients should be kept on beta-blockers. Permanent demand cardiac pacing is associated with a significant reduction in recurrent syncopal events, but it does not provide complete protection from sudden death, which occurs in 16% of patients. In the adult, the rate of the demand pacemaker is set at 70 to 80 beats/min. The beneficial effects of demand pacemakers are probably related to the prevention of bradycardia and the shortening of long QT intervals.

Prognosis

The prognosis is very poor in untreated patients; the mortality rate is 75% to 80%. Beta-blockers may reduce the mortality rate to some extent but not completely protect patients from sudden death. The adjusted annual mortality rate is 4.5% during treatment.

36 / Postoperative Syndromes

Four well-recognized syndromes are seen in the period after heart surgery in children; these include postcoarctectomy hypertension, postpericardiotomy syndrome, postperfusion syndrome, and hemolytic anemia syndrome.

POSTCOARCTECTOMY HYPERTENSION

Classic postcoarctectomy syndrome is rare, but paradoxical hypertension is commonly seen after coarctation surgery.

Paradoxic Hypertension

A mild degree of systolic hypertension develops within 36 hours after coarctation surgery, and this may be followed by a more delayed diastolic hypertension developing 48 hours after surgery and lasting 7 to 14 days. The sympathetic nervous system and the renin-angiotensin system may be responsible for the early systolic hypertension, and the renin-angiotensin system may play a major role in the diastolic hypertension. The so-called paradoxic hypertension may be the rule after coarctation surgery rather than the hallmark of a special syndrome. In about 10% to 20% of cases, mild abdominal discomfort and distention are noted during the first 5 or 6 postoperative days.

Postcoarctectomy Syndrome

First described in the 1950s, postcoarctectomy syndrome is characterized by severe, intermittent abdominal pain beginning 4 to 8 days after surgery, with accompanying fever and leukocytosis. In severe cases, abdominal distention, ileus, melena, and gangrenous bowel were reported. Persistent paradoxic hypertension may be present. The fully developed syndrome was present in about 5% of cases. Abdominal findings may be caused by arteritis resulting from a sudden increase in pulsatile pressures in the arteries distal to the coarctation; hypertension may be caused by an altered baroreceptor response plus increased excretion of epinephrine or norepinephrine.

Management.

1. Blood pressure should be monitored carefully in the postoperative period to detect rebound hypertension. The clinician must ensure that the hypertension in the arm is not due to a residual coarctation or to improper blood pressure measurement.

2. The feeding of solid foods is delayed in patients with postcoarctectomy syndrome.

3. The reduction of rebound hypertension may be accomplished by the following:

   a. Beta-adrenergic blockers such as propranolol (0.01 to 0.05 mg/kg intravenously over 10 minutes every 6 to 8 hours)

   b. Vasodilators such as hydralazine (0.15 mg/kg intramuscularly or intravenously every 4 to 6 hours) or nitroprusside (starting at 0.5 to 1.0 μg/kg/min intravenous infusion that may be increased to 5 μg/kg/min to achieve desired effects)

   c. Angiotensin-converting enzyme inhibitors, such as captopril, which are effective and well tolerated

   d. Sympatholytic agents such as reserpine (0.07 mg/kg intramuscularly every 6-8 hours)

462

POSTPERICARDIOTOMY SYNDROME

A febrile illness with pericardial and pleural reaction, postpericardiotomy syndrome, develops after surgery involving pericardiotomy. It is believed to be an autoimmune response in association with a recent or remote viral infection. There is a high titer of antiheart antibodies in patients who develop the syndrome, along with high antibody titers against adenovirus, coxsackievirus B1-6, and cytomegalovirus. A nonsurgical example of this syndrome is seen after myocardial infarction (Dressler's syndrome) and traumatic hemopericardium. The prevalence is about 25% to 30% of patients who receive pericardiotomy.

Clinical Manifestation.

1. The onset of the syndrome is a few weeks to a few months (median 4 weeks) after cardiac surgery that involves pericardiotomy. It is rare in infants younger than 2 years of age.

2. The syndrome is characterized by fever (sustained or spiking up to 40° C) and chest pain. Chest pain may be severe, caused by both pericarditis and pleuritis. Chest pain resulting from pericardial effusion radiates to the left side of the chest and shoulder and worsens in a supine position. Pleural pain worsens on deep inspiration. On physical examination (PE), pericardial and pleural friction rubs and hepatomegaly are usually present. Tachycardia, tachypnea, rising venous pressure, and falling arterial pressure with a paradoxical pulse are signs of cardiac tamponade.

3. Chest x-ray films show an enlarged cardiac silhouette and pleural effusion, especially on the left. The electrocardiogram (ECG) shows persistent ST-segment elevation and flat or inverted T waves in the limb leads and left precordial leads (LPLs).

4. Echocardiography (echo) is the most reliable test in confirming the presence and amount of pericardial effusion and evaluating evidence of cardiac tamponade (see Chapter 19).

5. Leukocytosis with shift to the left and an elevated erythrocyte sedimentation rate are present.

6. Although the disease is self-limiting, its duration is highly variable; the median duration is 2 to 3 weeks. Recurrences are common, appearing in 21% of patients.

Management.

1. Bed rest is all that is needed for a mild case.

2. Nonsteroidal antiinflammatory agents, such as ibuprofen or indomethacin, may be effective in most cases.

3. In severe cases, moderate doses of corticosteroids may be indicated for a few days if the diagnosis is secure and infection has been ruled out. A more prompt response is seen with steroid therapy, but a serious drawback is the tendency for the condition to rebound after withdrawal of the drug, with some patients becoming steroid-bound.

4. Emergency pericardiocentesis may be required if signs of cardiac tamponade are present.

5. Diuretics may be used for pleural effusion.

POSTPERFUSION SYNDROME

Postperfusion syndrome, which occurs only after open heart surgery using a pump oxygenator, is due to a cytomegalovirus infection. The virus may be transmitted to the patient from a viremia from healthy donors. The syndrome has almost disappeared since freshly drawn blood is no longer used, except in patients with severe cyanotic heart defects.

Clinical Manifestations.

1. The onset is 4 to 6 weeks after cardiac surgery using cardiopulmonary bypass.

2. The syndrome is characterized by the triad of fever, splenomegaly, and atypical lymphocytosis. Hepatomegaly is also common. Low-grade fever, with elevations to 38° to 39° C, occur. Malaise and anorexia are commonly present.

3. The fever and atypical lymphocytosis are short-term manifestations (lasting about 2 weeks), but splenomegaly usually lasts 3 to 4 weeks to 3 to 4 months. No recurrence has been reported.

4. The white blood cell count may be normal, but atypical lymphocytes are seen in the peripheral smears. Cytomegalovirus may be demonstrated in the urine, or a changing titer to the virus may be demonstrated in the serum.

Management.

1. No specific treatment is available.

2. The syndrome is self-limiting, lasting for a week to a few months.

HEMOLYTIC ANEMIA SYNDROME

Hemolytic anemia may occur after cardiac surgery, especially after the repair of endocardial cushion defect (ECD) and other congenital heart defects (CHDs) using synthetic patch material or aortic or mitral valve replacements. Hemolysis is due to unusual intracardiac turbulence with fragmentation of red cells. Iron deficiency anemia is superimposed.

Clinical Manifestations.

1. The onset occurs 1 to 2 weeks after surgery with the placement or insertion of synthetic and prosthetic materials.

2. The syndrome is characterized by low-grade fever, anemia, jaundice, dark urine, hepatomegaly, and reticulocytosis. Iron deficiency anemia may develop because of excessive loss of iron in the urine in chronic cases.

3. Peripheral smears reveal abnormal crenated and fragmented red blood cells and reticulocytosis. Hemoglobinemia, methemalbuminemia, and hemosiderinuria are also present.

Management.

1. The anemia is treated medically, by iron replacement therapy or blood transfusion. Most patients respond to oral iron therapy.

2. Surgical correction of turbulence is indicated if the anemia is severe and the correction is technically possible.

37 / Cardiac Transplantation

Lower and Shumway at Stanford University performed the first successful orthotopic heart transplantation in a dog in 1960. Barnard in South Africa unexpectedly performed the first successful human heart transplantation in 1966. This was followed by an explosive interest in heart transplantation but almost uniformly poor results because of organ rejection. Introduction of cyclosporine in 1980 markedly improved the results of adult heart transplantation. This success has extended to pediatric patients, including the newborn. Cardiac transplantation is considered standard therapy for children with certain end-stage heart diseases in many cardiac centers and for selected complex congenital heart defects (CHDs) in some centers. Although many ethical issues and questions exist and simple answers are not likely to be found in the near future, cardiac transplantation will find wider applications and contribute substantially to the treatment of children's heart disease. Pediatricians will have an increasing chance to participate in the care of cardiac transplant recipients. This chapter describes an overview of the steps involved in donor and recipient selection, postoperative management, immuno-suppressive therapy, long-term complications, and prognosis. With rapid advances being made in this field, important changes are expected to occur rapidly in many areas of cardiac transplantation.

PREVALENCE AND INDICATIONS

Pediatric heart transplantations comprise over 10% of heart transplantations performed each year. In the past, cardiomyopathy was the most common indication for cardiac transplantation, accounting for 70% to 80% of pediatric transplants. In recent years, an increasing number of pediatric patients with severe CHDs and those with doxorubicin cardiomyopathy are becoming candidates.

In infants younger than 12 months of age, hypoplastic left heart syndrome (HLHS) is the most common indication (63%). Other indications include complex congenital anomalies other than HLHS (29%), cardiomyopathy (6.5%), and unresectable cardiac tumors (1.5%).

SELECTION OF THE RECIPIENT

Careful selection of appropriate recipients remain the most important determinant of a favorable outcome. In general, the recipient should satisfy the following selection criteria:

1. Terminal heart disease with death expected within 6 to 12 months

2. Normal function or reversible dysfunction of the kidneys and liver

3. Lack of systemic infection

4. Malignancy under complete remission for longer than 1 year

5. Pulmonary vascular resistance (PVR) less than 8 Wood units/m^2 and presence of adequate dimension of hilar pulmonary arteries (PAs) (if the PVR is high or, if severe hypoplasia or stenosis of PAs is present, then the patient may be a candidate for heart and lung transplantation)

6. Lack of systemic disease that would limit recovery or survival, including diabetes mellitus and degenerative neuromuscular disease

7. Lack of drug addiction

8. Lack of mental deficiency

Equally important for successful pediatric heart transplantation are a family history of stability, past history of compliance, and evidence of strong motivation for the transplant as assessed by physicians and social workers. The child and parents should demonstrate sufficient responsibility, resources, and psychologic strength to cope with multiple outpatient clinic visits, routine endomyocardial biopsy, and a lifetime of vigilance in the immunosuppressed state. Unique to pediatric transplantation is the demonstration of a reliable caregiver for the recipient child. The caregiver identified need not be a parent but must have legal responsibility for total care to deal with the strict medical regimen required.

EVALUATION AND MANAGEMENT OF THE CARDIAC DONOR

Brain Death

The cardiac donor must meet the legal definition of *brain death*. The specific application of brain death criteria must conform to individual state laws, which may contain minor variations from state to state. The clinical diagnosis of brain death requires that there be loss of function of the entire brain, including the cortex and brain stem, and that the loss of brain function be irreversible.

Screening

The screening of potential donors is accomplished in three phases:

1. *Primary screening* is done by organ-procurement specialists to obtain information on the body size, ABO blood type, serologic data on hepatitis B and human immunodeficiency virus (HIV), cause of death, clinical course, and routine laboratory data.

2. *Secondary screening* is performed by cardiac surgeons or cardiologists, who pay attention to the extent of other (especially thoracic) injuries, the extent of treatment required to sustain acceptable hemodynamic status, electrocardiography (ECG), chest x-ray films, arterial blood gas analysis, and echocardiogram (echo).

3. *Tertiary screen* is inspection of the heart by a "harvesting" surgeon to make sure there is no evidence of a palpable thrill over the heart and great arteries, obvious arteriosclerotic heart disease, or myocardial contusion.

General Requirements

The donor should meet the following general requirements:

1. No history of previous intravenous drug abuse, sexual practices associated with high risk of acquired immunodeficiency syndrome (AIDS), HIV-positive status, known heart disease, active infection, documented cardiac arrest or myocardial infarction, or prolonged hypotension

2. No evidence of cardiac abnormalities by physical examination (PE), echo, ECG, or myocardial enzyme tests

3. Left ventricular (LV) fractional shortening greater than 28%, regardless of inotropic support

4. Specific compatibility should exist between the donor and recipient in three aspects.
   a. The donor and recipient should have ABO blood group compatibility. (Unlike

renal transplantation, histocompatibility typing and matching does not predict success in heart transplantation.)

   b. The donor and recipient should be approximately the same size. The donor's body weight should be within 20% of the recipient's weight; a larger donor heart is better tolerated than a smaller one. A donor-recipient weight ratio of 4.0 or less is acceptable for infant heart transplantation.

   c. The donor should be within close geographic range so that the donor heart can be harvested, transported, and implanted within 4 hours. For infant transplantation, a longer duration is acceptable (up to 9 hours).

Medical Management of Donor Heart Before Transplantation

The donor should be managed in the intensive care unit with routine monitoring. The systolic blood pressure should be maintained in the normal range (> 100 mg Hg for adults). Fluid resuscitation may be necessary initially on patients for whom fluid were restricted (to prevent brain edema, for example). Hypotension despite adequate filling pressure is treated with dopamine. Normal serum electrolyte levels, acid-base balance, and oxygenation should be maintained. The hematocrit should be above 30%.

INFORMED CONSENT FROM THE FAMILY AND PATIENT

The public usually misunderstands what the transplantation can accomplish. The patient and parents must fully understand the short- and long-term implications of the transplantation by knowing the following facts that are not well publicized:

1. Unlike most cardiac surgeries, the cardiac transplantation is not a cure for the condition for which it is being considered. It can be viewed as another medical problem that will require *lifelong* medical attention, including frequent hospital visits or admissions for noninvasive and invasive procedures, frequent adjustments of immunosuppressive and antibiotic medications, varying degrees of limitations in activity, and adjustments in lifestyle.

2. There is always a threat of rejection and infection throughout the patient's life. Even with full compliance, rejection can occur; even death or a need for retransplantation occur.

3. The heart received will not last for an indefinite period; it will eventually develop allograft coronary artery disease, requiring consideration of retransplantation.

4. Immunosuppressive therapy may cause malignancies (especially lymphoma in children) and an increased risk of infection (see later section for further discussion).

5. Lifelong medical attention will place a tremendous financial, emotional, and social burden on the family for a lifetime. As a result, a dysfunctional family could result.

OPERATIVE TECHNIQUE

Surgical techniques similar to those described by Lower and Shumway in 1960 (Fig. 37-1) are still used today. When the native heart is explanted, the posterior walls of both atria of the recipient heart are left in place and anastomosed to the donor heart. End-to-end anastomoses are also made between the donor and recipient aortas and PAs. The donor heart is harvested in such a way to avoid injury to the sinoatrial (SA) node. The hospital mortality rate is 10% to 15%.

For most babies with HLHS, certain modifications to this technique are necessary to augment the ascending aorta and aortic arch, such as those shown in Fig. 37-2. Such an aortic arch reconstruction, which causes an increased mortality rate, may be considered unnecessary in some patients with "adequately sized ascending aortas." The aorta is considered adequate in size when the ratio of the diameter of the ascending aorta just

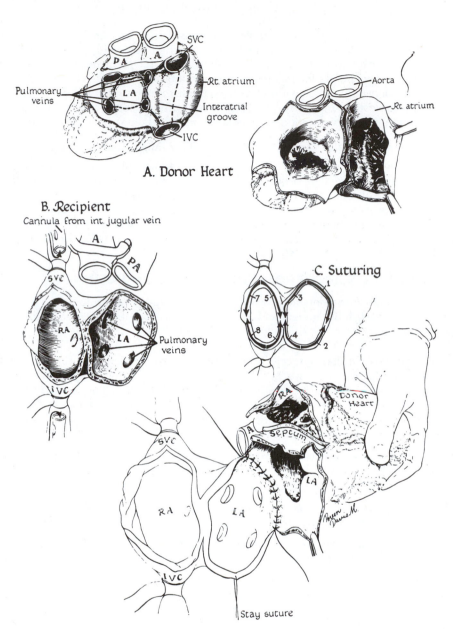

FIG. 37–1.
Original surgical technique developed by Shumway and co-workers. **A,** The donor heart is excised by division of the venae cavae and pulmonary veins at their respective atrial junction and by division of the great arteries several centimeters beyond the semilunar valves. The heart is further prepared by removing the posterior wall of the left atrium *(LA)* and longitudinally opening the posterior wall of the right atrium *(RA)*. The sinoatrial nodal area and atrial septum remain intact in the donor heart. **B,** The recipient bed is prepared by excising the recipient heart, including the atrial appendages, leaving generous cuffs of the aorta *(A)* and PA. **C,** The left atrial, right atrial, and aortic and pulmonary anastomoses are performed sequentially. *IVC,* Inferior vena cava; *Rt,* right; *SVC,* superior vena cava. (From Stinson EB, Dong E, Schroeder JS, et al: Initial clinical experience with heart transplantation, *Am J Cardiol,* 22:791-803, 1968.)

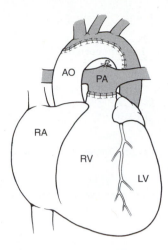

FIG. 37–2.
Modification of heart transplantation surgery for HLHS.

proximal to the innominate takeoff to that of the descending aorta just distal to the ductus arteriosus is 0.8 or greater.

POSTOPERATIVE MANAGEMENT

Postoperative management is directed toward the detection and treatment of three major causes of death after heart transplantations: acute cardiac failure (22%), infection (22%), and rejection (15%). This section includes the principles of postoperative management; each institution has a detailed management plan established by the transplantation team.

General Care

1. Postoperative care is similar to that of most patients who have had cardiac surgery; exception is immunosuppression. Inotropic support with isoproterenol, dobutamine, or amrinone for 2 or 3 days is usually needed.

2. The patient is in a total reverse isolation for 1 week, and then mask and hand-washing protocols are maintained until discharge. Vascular lines and various tubes are removed as soon as possible to minimize the risk of infection.

3. Antibiotics (usually vancomycin and ceftazimide) are administered intravenously during the first 48 hours after transplant.

Immunosuppressive Therapy

Immunosuppressive therapy is begun 4 to 12 hours before surgery and continued throughout the patient's life. Successful immunosuppression depends on a delicate balance between suppression of the host mechanisms that would reject the foreign graft and preservation of the mechanisms of the immune response that protect against bacterial, fungal, and viral invasion. The so-called triple-drug therapy consists of cyclosporine, adrenocortical steroids, and azathioprine (see Table 37-1 for the dosage).

Cyclosporine. Cyclosporine is the most commonly used agent of maintenance therapy. It is a fungal metabolite that inhibits the production and release of the lymphokines interleukin-1 from the activated macrophage and interleukin-2 (T-cell growth factor) from the activated T-helper cells, thus preventing the formation of cytotoxic T cells without affecting suppressor T cells. The first dose of oral cyclosporine is administered before surgery because it may be the most effective when given before the antigenic challenge. Peak blood levels are achieved at about 3.5 hours after an oral dose. The dosage is 5 to 10 mg/kg/day given orally in 2 to 3 doses to produce therapeutic

TABLE 37–1.

Dosages of Immunosuppressive Agents

Drug	Preoperative	Early Postoperative	Late Postoperative
Cyclosporine	6 mg/kg PO	5-10 mg/kg/day PO 0.5-2 mg/kg/day IV	4-6 mg/kg/day PO
Methylprednisolone		8 mg/kg IV for children 250 mg IV for adults, given before and after cardiopulmonary bypass	–
Prednisone		1 mg/kg/day PO tapered to 0.4 mg/kg/day	0.2 mg/kg/day PO (or discontinued)
Azathioprine		2 mg/kg/day PO	1-2 mg/kg/day PO

Adapted from Reitz BA: *Heart and heart-lung transplantation.* In Braunwald E, *Heart disease: a textbook of cardiovascular medicine,* ed 4, Philadelphia, 1992, WB Saunders. *PO,* By mouth; *IV,* intravenous

whole blood trough levels of 300 to 400 ng/ml for the first 3 postoperative weeks. The dose is then reduced to 4 to 6 mg/kg/day by mouth to produce blood levels of 100 to 200 ng/ml. Cyclosporine is eliminated primarily by the liver. Children who are on phenobarbital, phenytoin, or carbamazepine require higher doses of cyclosporine because these drugs increase cyclosporine metabolism. The drug's primary toxic effect is on renal function. When renal function is impaired, this dose is reduced to as low as 1 mg/kg. Cyclosporine is continued for as long as the patient lives.

Adrenocortical steroids. Methylprednisolone (8 mg/kg for children, 250 mg for adults) is administered intravenously as the sternotomy is made, and the same dose is repeated after cardiopulmonary bypass has been discontinued. After 24 hours, prednisone is administered in high doses (1 mg/kg/day by mouth). After about 3 weeks, the dose is tapered to 0.2 to 0.4 mg/kg/day. Further tapering or discontinuation depends on the institution's protocol and the presence or absence of rejection. Some centers discontinue it after 6 to 12 months, particularly in neonates and infants, but in many centers, this regimen continues as long as the patient lives.

Azathioprine (Imuran). Azathioprine (Imuran) is added as an immunosuppressive agent in most protocols. Azathioprine is a purine analogue antimetabolite with some selective anti-T-cell activity. It is first given orally to the patient just before the transplantation operation. The starting dose is 2 mg/kg/day given orally to produce a peripheral white blood cell count around 5,000/mm^3. If the count falls below 4,000/mm^3, the drug is reduced, or it is stopped if the reduction is severe. The drug is generally continued indefinitely.

Identification of Acute Rejection

Endomyocardial biopsy remains the most important method for the identification of acute rejection and is performed once a week for the first 4 to 6 weeks after surgery in older children and adults. Thereafter biopsies are performed every 3 to 4 months. For newborns and small infants, a routine endomyocardial biopsy is not performed; these patients are followed primarily by echo and other noninvasive means.

1. Subtle symptoms may be the only indication of the beginning of a rejection episode. These symptoms include unexplained fever, tachycardia, fatigue, shortness of breath, joint pain, and personality changes.

2. Echo techniques rely on a physiologic abnormality of the rejecting heart (myocardial edema or decreased LV contractility) (see section on monitoring for rejection).

TABLE 37–2.

Standardized Endomyocardial Biopsy Grading (ISHLT Scale)

Grade	"New" Nomenclature	"Old" Nomenclature
0	No rejection	No rejection
1	1A, focal (perivascular or interstitial) infiltrate without necrosis	Mild rejection
	1B, diffuse but sparse infiltrate without necrosis	
2	One focus only, with aggressive infiltration and/or focal myocyte damage	"Focal" moderate rejection
3	3A, multifocal aggressive infiltrates and/or myocyte damage	"Low" moderate rejection
	3B, diffuse inflammatory process with necrosis	"Borderline/severe" rejection
4	Diffuse aggressive polymorphous infiltrate ± edema, ± hemorrhage, ± vasculitis, with necrosis	"Severe acute" rejection

ISHLT, International Society of Heart and Lung Transplantation.
Adapted from Billingham ME, et al: A working formulation for the standardization of nomenclature in the diagnosis of heart and lung rejection: Heart Rejection Study Group, *J Heart Transpl* 9:587-593, 1990.

3. The endomyocardial biopsy is graded according to the International Society of Heart and Lung Transplantation scale (1990) (Table 37-2).

Treatment of Acute Rejection

Generally, mild rejection (grade 1) is not believed to warrant acute treatment, although about 25% of patients may progress to a higher grade of rejection. With moderate or severe rejection (grade 3 or 4), specific antirejection therapy is initiated.

1. Methylprednisolone given intravenously or prednisone given orally for 3 days are followed by prednisone given orally, which is tapered to the baseline dose over the next 2 weeks. The doses of methylprednisolone are 1,000 mg for adults, 15 mg/kg for children weighing less than 50 kg, and those for prednisone are 100 mg for adults.

2. If rejection does not respond to steroids or if hemodynamic compromise occurs, antithymocyte sera, such as antithymocyte globulin (ATG) or the monoclonal antibody to T3 lymphocytes (OKT3), are used for 5 and 10 days, respectively.

3. If all measures prove ineffective, retransplantation is considered.

Infection

Immunosuppressive medications used to prevent allograft rejection increase the risk of infection. Although cyclosporine has reduced the severity and frequency of infection, infection remains a leading cause of death after heart transplantation. There are two peak incidences for infections after transplantation. The "early" infection, occurring within the first month of transplantation, is dominated by nosocomial, often catheter-related, infection caused by *Staphylococcus* species and gram-negative organisms. In contrast, the "late" infection, occurring within 2 to 5 months, is caused by opportunistic infections from organisms such as cytomegalovirus (CMV), pneumocystis, and fungal pathogens (see later section). The lung has been the most common site of infection in heart transplant recipients, followed by the blood, urine, gastrointestinal tract, and sternal wound.

POSTTRANSPLANTATION FOLLOW-UP

Follow-up examinations are intended to detect rejection, infection, and the side effects of immunosuppression. Infection and rejection remain the most common causes of death after heart transplantation. Graft failure, lymphoma, and coronary artery disease are responsible for the remaining deaths. Physicians must also be aware of the unique physiology of the transplanted heart, which responds differently to exercise and to certain medications.

Outpatient Examinations and Endomyocardial Biopsy

Outpatient examinations and endomyocardial biopsy are performed frequently in the first months after transplant and less frequently thereafter (see later section), according to the individual institution's practice.

Monitoring for Side Effects of Immunosuppression

1. Hypertension and renal toxicity are common side effects of cyclosporine therapy. Less severe adverse side effects include reversible hepatotoxicity, fluid retention, hirsutism, gum hypertrophy, and gastrointestinal symptoms. Rarely, lymphoma develops with a larger dose of the drug (10%).

   a. The mechanism of cyclosporine-associated nephrotoxicity is probably related to the vasoconstrictor effect of the drug with decreased renal blood flow. The vasoconstriction may be mediated through prostaglandins and endothelin as well as a direct effect of cyclosporine.

   b. Hypertension occurs in 50% to 90% of heart transplant recipients who receive cyclosporine. The mechanisms of cyclosporine-associated hypertension include nephrotoxicity, increased sympathetic tone, volume expansion, increased endothelin levels, and stimulation of the renin-angiotensin system. Calcium channel blockers, angiotension-converting enzyme inhibitors, and β- and α-blockers have been used with varying levels of success.

2. Growth retardation may occur with large doses of steroids. The dosage of steroids is kept at a minimum, or steroids are not given at all.

3. Azathioprine may produce bone marrow depression (e.g., thrombocytopenia, leukocytopenia, anemia), alopecia, and gastrointestinal symptoms.

Monitoring of and Treatment for Rejection

Approximately 70% of patients experience rejection within the first 3 months after transplantation; however, lethal rejection is low in infants (6%). A high index of suspicion is necessary to detect rejection, particularly in the early months after transplantation because many rejections occur without symptoms.

1. Clinically evident cardiac dysfunction or congestive heart failure (CHF) is usually absent. Nonspecific clinical signs and symptoms (e.g., fever, tachycardia, malaise, personality changes, gallop rhythm, arrhythmias, hypotension) may be the only indications of rejection. These symptoms are often due to infection rather than rejection. Decreased ECG voltages and decreased ventricular function (by echo) are late signs of acute rejection.

2. Recently, the Loma Linda group reported echo changes in infant heart transplantation recipients during rejection. Rejection was associated with an increase in LV posterior wall thickness at the end of diastole, a tendency for a decrease in LV dimension and volume, an increase in LV mass, an increase in the LV volume/mass ratio, and a fall in the LV posterior wall-thickening fraction. The two most consistent changes were LV mass and the posterior wall-thickening fraction. LV fractional shortening did not change significantly.

3. The endomyocardial biopsy provides the earliest detectable indication. On endomyocardial biopsy, cardiac rejection is characterized by cellular infiltration of the myocardium, particularly around blood vessels, with or without damage or destruction of the myocytes. In so-called *chronic rejection*, endothelial cells are

also damaged or destroyed. This is believed to be the basis for accelerated coronary artery disease (see later section).

4. Patients with no or mild rejection (grade 0 or 1) on the biopsy receive no change in the dosage. Moderate rejection (grade 3) is treated with higher doses of steroids, whereas severe rejection (grade 4) is treated with higher doses of steroids and/or antithymocyte sera, with hospitalization and hemodynamic monitoring (see previous section).

Monitoring for Infection

Infection after the immediate posttransplantation period is caused by opportunistic infective agents, such as CMV, *Pneumocystis* organisms, and fungus. Infection is a common cause of death and is probably related to the immunosuppressive therapy. The average mortality rate from infection is about 12%; that of fungal infection is about 36%. The lung is the most commonly infected organ; the mortality rate of patients with infected lungs is 22%. CMV remains the most common single infection, but the specific agent for CMV, gancyclovir, does not appear to reduce the incidence of primary CMV infection. Pediatric patients have a higher incidence of otitis media and sinusitis as well as the gastrointestinal manifestations of many childhood illnesses. The efficacy of pyrimethamine and trimethoprim-sulfamethoxazole has been proved for the prophylaxis of toxoplasmosis and pneumocystis infection, respectively. The risk/benefit ratio of using influenza vaccines after transplantation remains controversial; most researchers agree that all live vaccines should be avoided. Children receiving immunosuppressive therapy, as well as their siblings, should not receive the oral polio vaccine or other live vaccines.

Allograft Coronary Artery Disease

An unusual accelerated form of coronary artery disease, probably an immune mediated disease, is the third most common cause of death, following only by infection and rejection. Coronary artery disease is the major determinant of long-term survival. Virtually all patients have some histopathologic evidence of coronary artery disease by 1 year after transplantation. It may occur in up to 40% of transplanted hearts in 3 years and in more than 50% of patients in 5 years. This disease also occurs in pediatric patients, perhaps to a lesser degree, but 28% of pediatric patients surviving 6 months to 6 years after transplantation develop coronary artery disease.

Coronary angiography is necessary to make the diagnosis of the disease: The unique angiographic hallmark of this disease is diffuse, concentric, longitudinal and rapid pruning and obliteration of distal branch vessels. Many centers recommend performing the first coronary angiography within 2 to 4 weeks of the transplantation to obtain a baseline; centers also recommend performing an exercise stress test, if appropriate for the patient's age, and coronary angiography 1 year after the transplantation to evaluate graft function and to detect premature and aggressive coronary atherosclerosis.

Most patients with transplanted, denervated hearts fail to experience typical chest pain. Life-threatening ventricular arrhythmias, CHF, silent myocardial infarction, and sudden death may result. The only effective treatment is retransplantation.

Malignancy

Another side effect of chronic immunosuppressive treatment may be the development of malignant neoplasm, occurring in 1% to 2% of patients each year or 12.5% during a mean follow-up period of 50 months. A unique form of lymphoma, *posttransplant lymphoproliferative disease,* is the most common tumor reported (80%) with cyclosporine-based immunosuppression; it occurs more frequently in young patients. Most of these tumors are thought to be the result of the Epstein-Barr virus infection. The use of OKT3 and ATG, as well as higher initial doses of cyclosporine and prednisone, appear to increase the risk of posttransplant lymphoproliferative disease. About 40% of the patients respond to a reduction in immunotherapy, but chemotherapy and radiation therapy may be needed.

Cutaneous malignancy (squamous cell and basal cell carcinomas) is the most common tumor associated with the use of azathioprine, perhaps related to the drug's enhanced photosensitivity. The mortality rate from posttransplant tumors is high (38%).

Physiology of the Transplanted Heart

The transplanted heart remains largely, but not entirely, denervated throughout the life of the recipient.

1. The response of the transplanted heart to exercise or stress is less than normal but adequate for most activities. With exercise, the heart rate accelerates slowly, and it parallels the rise in circulating catecholamine levels.

2. Most patients with denervated hearts experience no chest pain, even with significant coronary artery disease.

3. Transplant recipients are supersensitive to catecholamines, in part because of the upregulation of β-receptors and in part because of a loss of norepinephrine uptake in sympathetic neurons.

4. Coronary vasodilator response may be abnormal if coronary artery disease has developed.

PROGNOSIS

The pediatric survival rate is 70% to 80% at 1 year, 65% to 75% at 3 years, and 60% to 70% at 5 years. Newborns and infants appear to have better survival rates after the transplantation; the 5-year actuarial survival rate is 80%. The survival rate among newborn recipients at 5 years is 84%, with no subsequent deaths occurring in a 5-year follow-up.

Appendix A: Miscellaneous

TABLE A–1.

Reccurence Risks Given One Sibling who has a Cardiovascular Anomaly

Anomaly	Suggested Risk (%)
Ventricular septal defect	3.0
Patent ductus arteriosus	3.0
Atrial septal defect	2.5
Tetralogy of Fallot	2.5
Pulmonary stenosis	2.0
Coarctation of the aorta	2.0
Aortic stenosis	2.0
Transposition of the great arteries	1.5
AV canal (complete endocardial cushion defect)	2.0
Endocardial fibroelastosis	4.0
Tricuspid atresia	1.0
Ebstein's anomaly	1.0
Persistent truncus arteriosus	1.0
Pulmonary atresia	1.0
Hypoplastc left heart syndrome	2.0

Modified from Nora JJ, Nora AH: The evaluation of specific genetic and environmental counseling in congenital heart diseases, *Circulation* 57:205-213, 1978.)

TABLE A–2.

Affected Offspring Given One Parent with a Congenital Heart Defect

Defect	Mother Affected (%)	Father Affected (%)
Aortic stenosis	13.0-18.0	3.0
Atrial septal defect	4.0-4.5	1.5
AV canal (Complete endocardial cushion defect)	14.0	1.0
Coarctation of the aorta	4.0	2.0
Patent ductus arteriosus	3.5-4.0	2.5
Pulmonary stenosis	4.0-6.5	2.0
Tetralogy of Fallot	6.0-10.0	1.5
Ventricular septal defect	6.0	2.0

From Nora JJ, Nora AH: Maternal transmission of congenital heart disease: new recurrence risk figures and the questions of cytoplasmic inheritance and vulnerability to teratogens, *Am J Cardiol* 59:459-463, 1987.)

TABLE A–3.

Classification of Antiarrhythmic Drugs According to Their Mechanism of Action

Class	Action	Drugs
I	*Sodium channel blockade*	
A	Moderate phase-0 depression and slow conduction (2+)*; prolonged repolarization	Quinidine, procainamide, disopyramide
B	Minimal phase-0 depression and slow conduction (0 to 1+); shorten repolarization	Lidocaine, phenytoin, tocainide, mexiletine
C	Marked phase-0 depression and slow conduction (4+); little effect on repolarization	Encainide, lorcainide, flecainide
II	*Beta-adrenergic blockers*	Propranolol, others
III	*Prolong repolarization*	Amiodarone, bretylium
IV	*Calcium channel blockade*	Diltiazem, verapamil

*Relative magnitude of effect on conduction velocity is indicated on a scale of 1+ to 4+.
Adapted from Gilman AG, Goodman LS, Rall TW, Murad F, eds: *Goodman and Gilman's the pharmacological basis of therapeutics,* ed 7, New York, 1985, Macmillan.

TABLE A–4.

New York Heart Association Functional Classification

Class	Impairment
I	The patient has the disease, but the condition is asymptomatic.
II	The patient experiences symptoms with moderate activity.
III	The patient has symptoms with mild activity.
IV	The patient's condition is symptomatic at rest.

This is a classification of functional impairment in exercise capacity based on symptoms of dyspnea and fatigue. It is simple and useful in the evaluation of cardiac patients.

TABLE A–5.

Oxygen Consumption Per Body Surface Area*

	Heart Rate (beats/min)												
Age (yr)	50	60	70	80	90	100	110	120	130	140	150	160	170
Male Patients													
3				155	159	163	167	171	175	178	182	186	190
4			149	152	156	160	163	168	171	175	179	182	186
6		141	144	148	151	155	159	162	167	171	174	178	181
8		136	141	145	148	152	156	159	163	167	171	175	178
10	130	134	139	142	146	149	153	157	160	165	169	172	176
12	128	132	136	140	144	147	151	155	158	162	167	170	174
14	127	130	134	137	142	146	149	153	157	160	165	169	172
16	125	129	132	136	141	144	148	152	155	159	162	167	
18	124	127	131	135	139	143	147	150	154	157	161	166	
20	123	126	130	134	137	142	145	149	153	156	160	165	
25	120	124	127	131	135	139	143	147	150	154	157		
30	118	122	125	129	133	136	141	145	148	152	155		
35	116	120	124	127	131	135	139	143	147	150			
40	115	119	122	126	130	133	137	141	145	149			

TABLE A–5. *Continued*

Age (yr)	Heart Rate (beats/min)												
	50	60	70	80	90	100	110	120	130	140	150	160	170
Female Patients													
3				150	153	157	161	165	169	172	176	180	183
4			141	145	149	152	156	159	163	168	171	175	179
6		130	134	137	142	146	149	153	156	160	165	168	172
8		125	129	133	136	141	144	148	152	155	159	163	167
10	118	122	125	129	133	136	141	144	148	152	155	159	163
12	115	119	122	126	130	133	137	141	145	149	152	156	160
14	112	116	120	123	127	131	134	133	143	146	150	153	157
16	109	114	118	121	125	128	132	136	140	144	148	151	
18	107	111	116	119	123	127	130	134	137	142	146	149	
20	106	109	114	118	121	125	128	132	136	140	144	148	
25	102	106	109	114	118	121	125	128	132	136	140		
30	99	103	106	110	115	118	122	125	129	133	136		
35	97	100	104	107	111	116	119	123	127	130			
50	94	98	102	105	109	112	117	121	124	128			

*In (ml/min)/m². From LaFarge CG, Miettinen OS: The estimation of oxygen consumption, *Cardiovasc Res* 4:23, 1970.

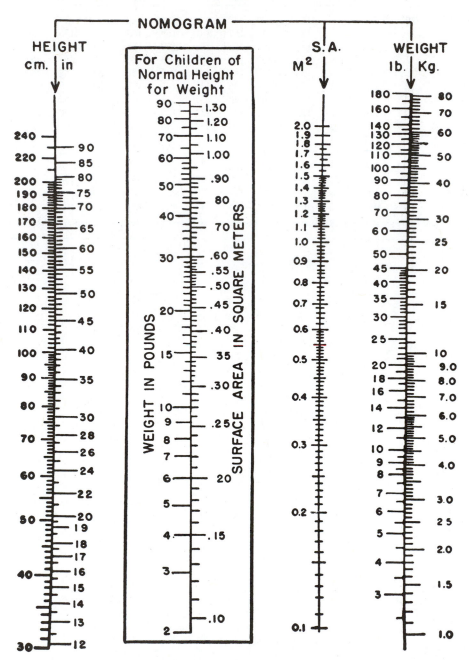

FIG. A–1.
Body surface area nomogram.

Name: _____

needs protection from
BACTERIAL ENDOCARDITIS
because of an existing
HEART CONDITION

Diagnosis: _____

Prescribed by: _____

Date: _____

For Dental/Oral/Upper Respiratory Tract Procedures

I. Standard Regimen In Patients At Risk (includes those with prosthetic heart valves and other high risk patients):

Amoxicillin 3.0 g orally one hour before procedure, then 1.5 g six hours after initial dose.*

For amoxicillin/penicillin-allergic patients:

Erythromycin ethylsuccinate 800 mg or erythromycin stearate 1.0 g orally 2 hours before a procedure, then one-half the dose 6 hours after the initial administration.*

—OR—

Clindamycin 300 mg orally 1 hour before a procedure and 150 mg 6 hours after initial dose.*

II. Alternate Prophylactic Regimens For Dental/Oral/Upper Respiratory Tract Procedures In Patients At Risk:

A. For patients unable to take oral medications:

Ampicillin 2.0 g IV (or IM) 30 minutes before procedure, then ampicillin 1.0 g IV (or IM) OR amoxicillin 1.5 g orally 6 hours after initial dose.*

—OR—

For ampicillin/amoxicillin/penicillin-allergic patients unable to take oral medications:

Clindamycin 300 mg IV 30 minutes before a procedure and 150 mg IV (or orally) 6 hours after initial dose.*

B. For patients considered to be at high risk who are not candidates for the standard regimen:

Ampicillin 2.0 g IV (or IM) plus gentamicin 1.5 mg/kg IV (or IM) (not to exceed 80 mg) 30 minutes before procedure, followed by amoxicillin 1.5 g orally 6 hours after the initial dose. Alternatively, the parenteral regimen may be repeated 8 hours after the initial dose.*

For amoxicillin/ampicillin/penicillin-allergic patients considered to be at high risk:

Vancomycin 1.0 g IV administered over one hour, starting one hour before the procedure. No repeat dose is necessary.*

*Note: Initial pediatric dosages are listed below. Follow-up oral dose should be one-half the inital dose. Total pediatric dose should not exceed total adult dose.

Amoxicillin:†	50 mg/kg	Vancomycin:	20 mg/kg
Clindamycin:	10 mg/kg	Ampicillin:	50 mg/kg
Erythromycin ethylsuccinate or stearate:	20 mg/kg	Gentamicin:	2.0 mg/kg

† The following weight ranges may also be used for the initial pediatric dose of amoxicillin:
< 15 kg (33 lbs), 750 mg
15–30 kg (33–66 lbs), 1500 mg
> 30 kg (66 lbs), 3000 mg (full adult dose)

Kilogram to pound conversion chart: (1 kg = 2.2 lb)

Kg	Lb
5	11.0
10	22.0
20	44.0
30	66.0
40	88.0
50	110.0

For Genitourinary/Gastrointestinal Procedures

I. Standard regimen:

Ampicillin 2.0 g IV (or IM) plus gentamicin 1.5 mg/kg IV (or IM) (not to exceed 80 mg) 30 minutes before procedure, followed by amoxicillin 1.5 g orally 6 hours after the initial dose. Alternatively, the parenteral regimen may be repeated once 8 hours after the initial dose.*

For amoxicillin/ampicillin/penicillin-allergic patients:

Vancomycin 1.0 g IV administered over 1 hour plus gentamicin 1.5 mg/kg IV (or IM) (not to exceed 80 mg) one hour before the procedure. May be repeated once 8 hours after initial dose.**

II. Alternate oral regimen for low-risk patients:

Amoxicillin 3.0 g orally one hour before the procedure, then 1.5 g 6 hours after the initial dose.**

**Note: Initial pediatric dosages are listed below. Follow-up oral dose should be one-half the initial dose. Total pediatric dose should not exceed total adult dose.

Ampicillin:	50 mg/kg	Gentamicin:	2.0 mg/kg
Amoxicillin:	50 mg/kg	Vancomycin:	20 mg/kg

Note: Antibiotic regimens used to prevent recurrences of acute rheumatic fever are inadequate for the prevention of bacterial endocarditis. In patients with markedly compromised renal function, it may be necessary to modify or omit the second dose of gentamicin or vancomycin. Intramuscular injections may be contraindicated in patients receiving anticoagulants.

Adapted from *Prevention of Bacterial Endocarditis: Recommendations by the American Heart Association* by the Committee on Rheumatic Fever, Endocarditis, and Kawasaki Disease. *JAMA* 1990;264:2919–2922, © 1990 American Medical Association (also excerpted in *J Am Dent Assoc* 1991;122:87–92).

Please refer to these joint American Heart Association–American Dental Association recommendations for more complete information as to which patients and which procedures require prophylaxis.

 American Heart Association

National Center
7320 Greenville Avenue
Dallas, Texas 75231

78-1003 (CP)
90-100M
4-91-511.2M
90 06 19 B

The Council on Dental Therapeutics of the American Dental Association has approved this statement as it relates to dentistry.

FIG. A–2.

Antibiotic prophylaxis against bacterial endocarditis. (From Dajani AS et al: Prevention of bacterial endocarditis. Recommendation by the American Heart Association, *JAMA* 264:2919-2922, 1990.)

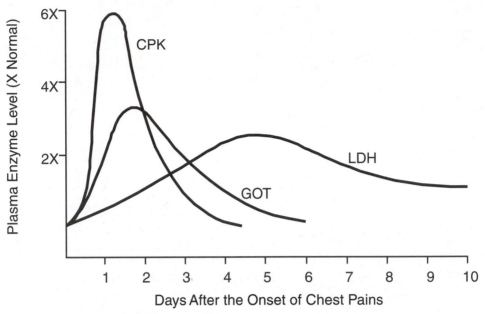

Cardiac Enzymes in Acute Myocardial Infarction

FIG. A–3.
Typical plasma profile for the MB isoenzyme of creatine phosphokinase *(CPK),* serum glutamic oxaloacetic acid transferase *(SGOT),* and lactic dehydrogenase *(LDH)* activities after the onset of acute myocardial infarction. False elevation of CPK levels occurs in 15% of patients with disease of other systems, such as muscle disease, alcoholic intoxication, diabetes mellitus, skeletal muscle trauma, vigorous exercise, convulsions, intramuscular injections, and pulmonary embolism. Elevated levels of the CPK-MB isoenzyme are more specific for myocardial infarction. Brain and kidney tissues contain predominantly the BB isoenzyme, skeletal muscle contains principally the MM isoenzyme, and cardiac muscle contains both MM and MB isoenzymes. False-positive elevations of LDH occur in patients with hemolysis, leukemia, liver disease or congestion, renal disease, pulmonary embolism, skeletal muscle disease, shock, and myocarditis. The heart contains principally the LDH_1 isoenzyme, whereas liver and skeletal muscle contain primarily LDH_4 and LDH_5. Elevations of LDH and the ratio of LDH_1 to total LDH occur in more than 95% of patients with myocardial infarction. Because false elevations of SGOT occur frequently and because the time that it takes for SGOT levels to become elevated is intermediate between that of CPK and LDH, the diagnostic benefit of SGOT is negligible.

Appendix B: Normal Electrocardiographic Values and Images

TABLE B–1.

Normal M-Mode Echocardiographic Measurements*

BW (kg)	3	5	8	10	15
BSA	0.24	0.34	0.45	0.52	0.68
IVS (mm)	4.5 (3.5-5)	4.5 (4-5.5)	5 (4.5-6)	5.5 (4.5-6.5)	6 (5-7)
LVPW (mm)	4 (3.5-5)	4.5 (4-5)	5 (4-6)	5 (4.5-6)	6 (5-7)
AO (mm)	12 (10-14)	13 (11-16)	15 (12-17)	16 (13-18)	18 (15-22)
LA (mm)	18 (15-21)	20 (16-23)	21 (17-25)	22 (18-26)	25 (21-29)
LVDD (mm)	21 (18-23)	25 (22-27)	28 (24-31)	29 (25-32)	33 (29-36)
LVSD (mm)	14 (12-17)	16 (13-19)	17 (14-21)	18 (15-22)	21 (17-24)
LV Mass (g)	17 (13-22)	27 (19-35)	37 (27-48)	46 (32-63)	62 (42-82)

*Mean (95% prediction interval).
BW, Body weight; *BSA,* body surface area; *IVS,* interventricular septum; *LVPW,* left ventricular posterior wall; *AO,* aorta; *LA,* left atrium; *LVDD,* left ventricular diastolic dimension; *LVSD,* left ventricular systolic dimension; *LV,* left ventricular.

TABLE B–2.

Dimensions of Aorta and Pulmonary Arteries by 2D Echo*†

Echo Views	BSA (m²)	0.25	0.3	0.4	0.5
	BW (kg)	3	4	7	10
	AA	10 (7-13)‡	11 (7.5-15)	13 (9-16)	14 (10-18)
	MPA	9 (5-12)	10 (6-13)	11 (7-14)	12 (8-16)
	RPA	5.5 (3.5-8)	6 (4-8.5)	6.5 (4.5-9)	7.5 (5-10)
	AA	7.5 (4-10)	8 (4.5-11)	9 (6-12)	10 (6.5-13)
	TA	6 (4-8.5)	7 (4.5-9)	8 (5.5-11)	9 (6.5-11)
	RPA	6 (4-8)	6.5 (4.5-9)	7.5 (5-10)	8.5 (6-11)
	TA	9 (6-11)	10 (7-12.5)	11 (8-14)	12 (9.5-15)
	RPA	6 (4-8)	6.5 (4.5-9)	7 (5-10)	8 (6-10)

* Values are rounded off to the nearest 0.5 mm for measurements less than 10 mm and to the nearest 1.0 mm for measurements 10 mm and greater.
† Measurements are made at the end of diastole (the Q wave), using a leading-edge technique.
‡ Figures in parentheses are the tolerance limits weighed for body surface area for prediction of normal values for 80% of the future population with 50% confidence.

20	25	30	40	50	60	70
0.82	0.94	1.06	1.27	1.47	1.65	1.82
7 (5.5-8.5)	7 (5.5-9)	7.5 (6-9)	8.5 (6.5-10)	8.5 (7-10)	9 (8-10.5)	9.5 (7.5-11)
6.5 (5.5-8)	7 (6-8)	7 (6-8.5)	8 (6.5-9)	8.5 (7-9.5)	8.5 (7.5-10)	9 (7.5-11)
19 (16-23)	21 (17-24)	22 (18-26)	23 (19-27)	25 (20-29)	26 (21-30)	27 (23-32)
27 (22-32)	28 (23-33)	30 (24-35)	32 (26-37)	33 (37-38)	34 (28-41)	36 (29-42)
35 (31-39)	37 (33-41)	39 (34-43)	42 (37-47)	44 (39-49)	46 (41-51)	48 (42-53)
23 (18-27)	24 (19-28)	25 (21-29)	27 (22-32)	28 (23-33)	29 (24-34)	31 (25-36)
78 (55-100)	92 (65-115)	102 (74-134)	126 (88-164)	148 (104-192)	167 (120-220)	186 (132-244)

Data from Henry WL, Ware J, Gardin JM, Hepner SI, McKay K, Weidner M: Echocardiographic measurements in normal subjects: growth-related changes that occur between infancy and early adulthood, *Circulation* 57: 278-285, 1987.

0.6	0.7	0.8	0.9	1.0	1.2	1.4
13	16	19	23	28	37	46
15 (11-19)	16 (12-20)	17 (12-21)	17 (13-22)	18 (14-23)	20 (15-25)	22 (16-27)
13 (9-17)	14 (9-18)	15 (11-19)	15 (11-20)	16 (12-21)	17 (13-23)	19 (14-24)
8 (5.5-10)	8.5 (6-11)	9 (7-11)	9 (7-12)	10 (7-12)	10 (8-14)	11 (8-15)
11 (7.5-14)	12 (8.5-15)	12 (9-16)	13 (9.5-13)	14 (11-18)	15 (12-19)	17 (14-21)
10 (7.5-12)	11 (8-13)	11 (8.5-14)	12 (9.5-15)	13 (10-16)	14 (11-17)	15 (12-18)
9 (6.5-11)	9.5 (7-12)	10 (8-13)	11 (9-14)	12 (9-15)	13 (10-16)	14 (11-17)
13 (10.5-16)	14 (11-17)	15 (13-18)	16 (13-20)	17 (14-20)	19 (15-22)	20 (17-24)
9 (6.5-11)	9.5 (7.5-11)	10 (8-12)	11 (9-13)	11 (9-14)	12 (10-15)	13 (11-16)

2D, Two-dimensional; *echo,* echocardiography; *BSA,* body surface area; *BW,* body weight; *AA,* ascending aorta; *MPA,* main pulmonary artery; *RPA,* right pulmonary artery; *TA,* transverse aorta.
Data from Snider AR, Enderlein MA, Teitel DJ, Juster RP: Two-dimensional echocardiographic determination of aortic and pulmonary artery sizes from infancy to adulthood in normal subjects, *Am J Cardiol* 53:218-224, 1984.

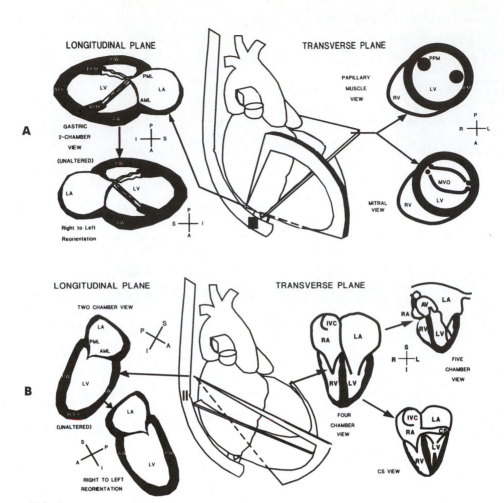

FIG. B–1.
A, Biplane transesophageal echocardiographic views from transgastric position III.
B, Biplane transesophageal echocardiographic views at midesophageal position II.

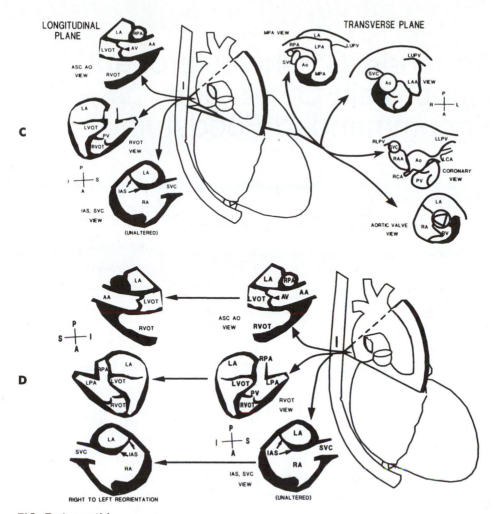

FIG. B–1. cont'd
C, Biplane transesophageal echocardiography views from the base of the heart at position I. **D,** Basal views of the heart and great vessels with use of the longitudinal plane probe at position I. (From Bansal RC et al: Biplane transesophageal echocardiography: technique, image orientation, and preliminary experience in 131 patients, *J Am Soc Echo* 3:348-366, 1990.)

Appendix C: Cholesterol and Lipoprotein Levels and Recommended Foodstuff

TABLE C–1.

Reference Values for Serum Total Cholesterol and Low-Density Lipoprotein in American Children and Adolescents (mg/100 ml)

	Serum Total Cholesterol					Serum Low-Density Lipoprotein				
	Males					**White Males**				
			Percentiles					Percentiles		
Age	5	50	75	90	95	5	50	75	90	95
0-4	117	156	176	192	209					
5-9	125	164	180	197	209	65	93	106	121	133
10-14	123	160	178	196	208	66	97	112	126	136
15-19	116	150	170	188	203	64	96	112	127	134
	Females					**White Females**				
			Percentiles					Percentiles		
Age	5	50	75	90	95	5	50	75	90	95
0-4	115	161	177	195	206					
5-9	130	168	184	201	211	70	101	118	129	144
10-14	128	163	179	196	207	70	97	113	130	140
15-19	124	160	177	197	209	61	96	114	133	141

From The LRC Prevalence Study (North America), NIH Publication No. 80-1527, July 1980.

TABLE C–2.

Reference Values for Serum High-Density Lipoprotein and Triglyceride in American Children and Adolescents (mg/100 ml)

	Serum High-Density Lipoprotein					Serum Triglyceride				
	White Males					**Males**				
			Percentiles					Percentiles		
Age	5	50	75	90	95	5	50	75	90	95
0-4						30	53	69	87	102
5-9	39	56	65	72	76	31	53	67	88	104
10-14	38	57	63	73	76	33	61	80	105	129
15-19	31	47	54	61	65	38	71	94	124	152
	White Females					**Females**				
			Percentiles					Percentiles		
Age	5	50	75	90	95	5	50	75	90	95
0-4						35	61	79	99	115
5-9	37	54	63	69	75	33	57	73	93	108
10-14	38	54	60	66	72	38	72	93	117	135
15-19	36	53	63	70	76	40	70	90	117	136

From The LRC Prevalence Study (North America), NIH Publication No. 80-1527, July 1980).

TABLE C–3.

Food To Choose and Decrease for the Step-One* and Step-Two Diets

Choose	Decrease
Meat, Poultry, and Fish	
Beef, pork, lamb—lean cuts well trimmed before cooking	Beef, pork, lamb—regular ground beef, fatty cuts, spare ribs, organ meats, sausage, regular luncheon meats, wieners, bacon
Poultry without skin	Poultry with skin, dried chicken
Fish, shellfish	Fried fish, fried shellfish
Processed meat—prepared from lean meat (for example, turkey, ham, tuna wieners)	Regular luncheon meats (for example, bologna, salami, sausage, wieners)
Eggs	
Egg whites (two whites equal one whole egg in recipes), cholesterol-free egg substitute	Egg yolk (if more than four per week on Step-One or if more than two per week on Step-Two); includes egg used in cooking
Dairy Products	
Milk—skim or 1% fat (fluid, powdered, evaporated), buttermilk	Whole milk (fluid, evaporated, condensed), 2% low-fat milk, imitation milk
Yogurt—nonfat or low-fat yogurt or yogurt beverages	Whole-milk yogurt, whole-milk yogurt beverages
Cheese—low-fat natural or processed cheese (part-skim mozzarella, ricotta) with no more than 6 g of fat per ounce on Step-One, or 2 g of fat per ounce on Step Two	Regular cheese (American, blue, Brie, cheddar, Colby, Edam, Monterey jack, whole-milk mozzarella, Parmesan, Swiss), cream cheese, Neufchâtel cheese
Cottage cheese—low fat, nonfat, or dry curd (0 to 2% fat)	Cottage cheese (4% fat)
Frozen dairy dessert—ice milk, frozen yogurt (low fat or nonfat)	Ice cream
	Cream, half-and-half, whipping cream, nondairy creamer, whipped topping, sour cream
Fats and Oils	
Unsaturated oils—safflower, sunflower, corn, soybean, cottonseed, canola, olive, peanut	Coconut oil, palm kernel oil, palm oil
Margarine—made from unsaturated oils previously listed, light or diet margarine	Butter, lard, shortening, bacon fat
Salad dressings—made with unsaturated oils previously listed, low fat or oil free	Dressing made with egg yolk, cheese, sour cream, whole milk
Seeds and nuts—peanut butter, other nut butters	Coconut
Cocoa powder	Chocolate
Breads and Cereals	
Breads—whole-grain bread, hamburger and hot dog buns, corn tortilla	Bread in which eggs are a major ingredient, croissants
Cereals—oat, wheat, corn, multigrain	Granola made with coconut
Pasta	Egg noodles and pasta containing egg yolk
Rice	
Dry beans and peas	
Crackers—low fat animal-type, graham, saltine	High fat crackers
Homemade baked goods using unsaturated oil, skim or 1% milk, and egg substitute—quick breads, biscuits, cornbread muffins, bran muffins, pancakes, waffles	Commercially baked pastries, muffins, biscuits
Soup—chicken or beef noodle, minestrone, tomato, vegetarian, potato	Soup containing whole milk, cream, meat fat, poultry fat, or poultry skin

* The Step-One Diet has the same nutrient recommendations as the eating pattern recommended for the general population.
From National Cholesterol Education Program: *Report of the Expert Panel on Blood Cholesterol Levels in Children and Adolescents,* NIH Publication No 91-2732, September, 1991.

TABLE C–3.

Food To Choose and Decrease for the Step-One* and Step-Two Diets—cont'd

Choose	Decrease
Vegetables	
Fresh, frozen or canned vegetables	Vegetables prepared with butter, cheese, or cream sauce
Fruits	
Fruit—fresh, frozen, canned or dried	Fried fruit or fruit served with butter or cream sauce
Fruit juice—fresh, frozen, or canned	
Sweets and Modified Fat Desserts	
Beverages—fruit-flavored drinks, lemonade, fruit punch	
Sweets—sugar, syrup, honey, jam, preserves, candy made without fat (candy corn, gumdrops, hard candy), fruit-flavored gelatin	Candy made with chocolate, coconut oil, palm kernel oil, palm oil
Frozen desserts—sherbet, sorbet, fruit ice, popsicles	Ice cream and frozen treats made with ice cream
Cookies, cake, pie, pudding—prepared with egg whites, egg substitute, skim milk or 1% milk, and unsaturated oil or margarine; gingersnaps; fig bar cookies; angel food cake	Commercially baked pies, cakes, doughnuts, high-fat cookies, cream pies

Appendix D: Pediatric Cardiovascular Drug Dosages

Pediatric Cardiovascular Drug Dosages

Drug	Route and Dosage	Toxicity or Side Effects	How Supplied
Adenosine (Adenocard) (antiarrhythmic)	*Children and adults:* IV: 50 μg/kg Repeat q1-2 min, increasing to 250 μg/kg	Transient bradycardia and tachycardia Transient AV block in atrial flutter/fibrillation (±)	Inj: 3 mg/ml
Amiodarone (Cordarone) (class III antiarrhythmic agent)	*Children:* PO: 5-10 mg/kg/day in two doses for 10 days If responsive, 3-5 mg/kg once a day May be reduced to 2.5 mg/kg for 5 of 7 days thereafter *Adults:* PO: *Loading:* 800-1600 mg/day for 1-3 wk, then reduce to 600-800 mg/day for 1 mo *Maintenance:* 400 mg/day	Progressive dyspnea and cough, worsening of arrhythmias, hepatotoxicity, nausea and vomiting, corneal microdeposits, hypotension and heart block, ataxia, hypothyroidism or hyperthyroidism, photosensitivity.	Tab: 200 mg
Amrinone (Inocor) (noncatecholamine inotropic agent with vasodilator effects)	*Children:* IV: *Loading:* 0.5 mg/kg over 2-3 min in ½NS (not D5W) *Maintenance:* 5-20 μg/kg/min *Adults:* IV: *Loading:* 0.75 mg/kg over 2-3 min *Maintenance:* 5-10 μg/kg/min	Thrombocytopenia, hypotension, tachyarrhythmias, hepatotoxicity, nausea and vomiting, fever	Inj: 5 mg/ml (20 ml)
Atenolol (Tenormin) (β₁-adrenoceptor blocker, antihypertensive, antiarrhythmic)	*Children:* PO: 1-2 mg/kg/day *Adults:* PO: 50 mg once a day for 1-2 week (alone or with diuretic for hypertension) May increase to 100 mg once a day	CNS symptoms (dizziness, tiredness, depression), bradycardia, postural hypotension, nausea and vomiting, rash, blood dyscrasias (agranulocytosis, purpura)	Tab: 25, 50, 100 mg Inj: 0.5 mg/ml

IV, Intravenous; *q,* every; *AV,* atrioventricular; *inj,* injection; *PO,* by mouth; *tab,* tablet; *NS,* normal saline; *CNS,* central nervous system; *WBC,* white blood cell; *PR,* per rectum; *IM,* intramuscular; *caps,* capsules; *GI,* gastrointestinal; *supp,* suppositories; *susp,* suspension; *prn,* as necessary; *sol,* solution; *CHF,* congestive heart failure; *TDD,* total digitalizing dose; *ECG,* electrocardiographic; *CR,* controlled-release; *IHSS,* idiopathic hypertrophic subaortic stenosis; *RBF,* renal blood flow; *ACE,* angiotensin-converting enzyme; *SC,* subcutaneous; *LFT,* liver function test; *APTT,* activated partial thromboplastin time; *PDA,* patent ductus arteriosus; *BP,* blood pressure; *NE,* norepinephrine; *NG,* nasogastric; *PT,* prothrombin time; *INR,* International Normalized Ratio; *TT,* thrombin time.

Drug	Route and Dosage	Toxicity or Side Effects	How Supplied
Azathioprine (Imuran) (immunosuppressive agent)	*Children:* PO: Starting dose—2 mg/kg/day (to produce WBC count around 5,000/mm^3), may be reduced if WBC count falls below 4,000/mm^3	Leukopenia, thrombocytopenia, nausea and vomiting	Tab: 50 mg Inj: 5 mg/ml
Bretylium tosylate (Bretylol) (class III antiarrhythmic agent)	***For ventricular fibrillation or tachycardia:*** *Children:* IV: 5 mg/kg/dose over 8 min, then 10 mg/kg/dose q15-30 min (maximum 30 mg/kg) *Adults:* IV: 5-10 mg/kg bolus over 8 min q6hr or 1-2 mg/min IV infusion	Hypotension, worsening of arrhythmias, aggravation of digitoxicity, nausea and vomiting	Inj: 50 mg/ml (10 ml ampule)
Captopril (Capoten) (angiotensin I converting enzyme inhibitor, antihypertensive, vasodilator)	*Children:* PO: Newborn—0.1-1.4 mg/kg/dose 1-4 times/day Infants—0.5-0.6 mg/kg/day in 1-4 doses Child—12.5 mg/dose 1-2 times/day Smaller dose in renal impairment *Adults:* PO: 25 mg 2-3 times/day initially Increase to the usual dose of 50 mg 3 times/day for 1-2 weeks Increase 25 mg/dose q1-2 wk to maximum 150 mg 3 times/day (Usually used with diuretic) Smaller dose in renal impairment	Neutropenia/agranulocytosis, proteinuria, hypotension and tachycardia rash, taste impairment, small increase in serum potassium levels ($\pm$)	Tab: 12.5, 25, 50, 100 mg
Chloral hydrate (Noctec) (sedative, hypnotic)	*Children:* Sedative (PO, PR): 25 mg/kg/dose q8hr Hypnotic (PO, PR): 50-75 mg/kg/dose *Adults:* Sedative (PO, PR): 250 mg/dose 3 times/day Hypnotic (PO, PR): 500-2,000 mg/dose	Mucous membrane irritation (laryngospasm if aspirated), GI irritation, excitement/delirium. (Contraindicated in hepatic and renal impairment)	Syrup: 250, 500 mg/5 ml Supp: 324, 500, 648 mg
Chlorothiazide (Diuril) (diuretic)	*Children:* PO: 20-40 mg/kg/day in two doses *Adults:* PO: 250-500 mg/dose once a day or intermittently	Hypokalemia, hyponatremia, hypochloremic alkalosis, prerenal azotemia, hyperuricemia, hyperglycemia, rarely blood dyscrasias, allergic reactions	PO susp 250 mg/5 ml (237 ml) Tab: 250, 500 mg Inj: 500 mg (vial, for reconstruction with 18 ml sterile water)

Drug	Route and Dosage	Toxicity or Side Effects	How Supplied
Chlorpromazine (Thorazine) (sedative, anti-emetic)	*For sedation or nausea:* *Children >6 mo:* IM: 0.5 mg/kg/dose q6-8hr prn PO: 0.5 mg/kg/dose q4-6hr prn PR: 1-2 mg/kg/dose q6-8hr prn *Adults:* IM: 25-mg test dose, then 25-50 mg q3-4hr PO: 10-25 mg q4-6hr PR: 100 mg q6-8hr	Hypotension, arrhythmias, first-degree AV block, ST-T changes, hepatotoxicity, leukopenia or agranulocytosis	Inj: 25 mg/ml Syrup: 10 mg/5 ml (120 ml) Tab: 10, 25, 50, 100, 200 mg Supp: 25, 100 mg
Cholestyramine (Questran) (cholesterol-lowering agent)	*Children:* PO: 250-1,500 mg/kg/day in 2-4 doses *Adults:* PO: *Starting*—1 packet (or scoopful) of Questran Powder or Light 1-2 times/day *Maintenance:* 2-4 packets or scoopfuls/day in 2 doses (or 1-6 doses) Maximum: 6 packets/day	Constipation and other GI symptoms, hyperchloremic acidosis, bleeding	Packet of 9-g Questran Powder or 5-g Questran Light, each packet containing 4 g anhydrous cholestyramine resin)
Clofibrate (Atromid-S) (antilipidemic, triglyceride-lowering agent)	*Children:* PO: 0.5-1.5 mg/day in 2-3 doses *Adults:* PO: *Initial and maintenance*—2 g/day in 2-3 doses	Nausea and other GI symptoms (vomiting, diarrhea, flatulence), headache, dizziness, fatigue, rash, blood dyscrasias, myalgia, arthralgia, hepatic dysfunction	Caps: 500 mg
Colestipol (Colestid) (lipid lowering agent)	*Children:* PO: 300-1,500 mg/day in 2-4 doses *Adults:* PO: Starting dose: 5 g 1-2 times/day, increment of 5 g q1-2 mo Maintenance: 5-30 g/day in 2-4 doses (mix with 3-6 oz water or another fluid)	Constipation and other GI symptoms (abdominal distention, flatulence, nausea and vomiting, diarrhea), rarely rash, muscle and joint pain, headache, dizziness	Packet: 5 g
Cyclosporine (Sandimmune) (immunosuppressive agent)	*Children:* PO: 5-10 mg/kg/day in 2-3 doses for 3 postoperative wks (blood level 300-400 ng/ml) Reduce to 4-6 mg/kg/day thereafter (blood level 100-200 ng/ml)	Nephrotoxicity, tremor, hypertension, less commonly hepatotoxicity, hirsutism, gum hypertrophy, rarely lymphoma, hypomagnesemia	Oral sol: 100 mg/ml Gelatin caps: 25, 100 mg
Diazepam (Valium) (sedative, antianxiety, antiseizure agent)	*For sedation:* *Children >6 mos:* IM, IV: 0.1-0.3 mg/kg/dose q2-4hr (max 0.6 mg/kg in 8 hr) PO: 0.2-0.8 mg/kg/day in 3-4 doses, or 1-2.5 mg 3-4 times/day initially and increase prn	Apnea, drowsiness, ataxia, rash, hypotension, bradycardia, hyperexcited state	Inj: 5 mg/ml Tab: 2, 5, 10 mg

Drug	Route and Dosage	Toxicity or Side Effects	How Supplied
Diazepam (Valium) (sedative, antianxiety, antiseizure agent)—cont'd	*Adults:* IM, IV: 2-10 mg/dose q3-4hr prn PO: 2-10 mg/dose q6-8hr prn		
Diazoxide (Hyperstat) (peripheral vasodilator)	*For emergency use only:* *Children and Adults:* IV: 1-3 mg/kg (maximum 150-mg single dose), repeat q5-15min, titrate to desired effects	Hypotension, transient hyperglycemia, nausea and vomiting, sodium retention (CHF±)	Inj: 15 mg/ml
Digitoxin (Crystodigin, Purodigin) (cardiac glycoside)	*Children:* *TDD:* PO: Premature and full-term newborn—20 μg/kg; child 1 mo-2 yr old—30 μg/kg; child >2 yr old—20 μg/kg IV, IM: Same as PO TDD *Maintenance:* PO, IV, IM: 15% (10%-20%) of TDD once a day *Adults:* PO: *Loading:* 0.6 mg initially, then 0.4 mg and 0.2 mg q4-6hr *Maintenance:* 0.15 mg once a day (ranges 0.05-0.3 mg/day)	Same as for digoxin	Elixer: 50 μg/ml Tab: 0.05, 0.1 mg Inj: 0.2 mg/ml
Digoxin (Lanoxin) (cardiac glycoside)	*Children:* *TDD:* PO: Premature infant—20 μg/kg; full-term newborn—30 μg/kg; child 1 mo-2 yr old—40-50 μg/kg; child >2 yr—30-40 μg/kg IV: 75%-80% of PO dose *Maintenance:* PO: 25%-30% of TDD/day in 2 doses *Adults:* PO: *Loading:* 8-12 μg/kg *Maintenance:* 0.10-0.25 mg/day	AV conduction disturbances, arrhythmias, nausea and vomiting (see Box on p. 406 for ECG changes)	Elixir: 50 μg/ml (60 ml) Tab: 0.125, 0.25 0.5 mg Inj: 100, 250 μg/ml Lanoxicaps: 0.05, 0.1, 0.2 mg
Digoxin immune Fab (Digibind) (digoxin antidote)	*Infants and children:* IV: 1 vial (40 mg) dissolved in 4 ml H₂O, over 30 min *Adults:* IV: 4 vials (240 mg)	Allergic reaction (rare), hypokalemia, rapid AV conduction in atrial flutter	Vial (40 mg)

Drug	Route and Dosage	Toxicity or Side Effects	How Supplied
Disopyramide (Norpace) (class IA anti-arrhythmic agent)	*Children:* PO: child <1 yr old—10-30 mg/kg/day q6hr; child 1-4 yr old—10-20 mg/kg/day q6hr; child 4-12 yr old—10-15 mg/kg/day q6hr; child 12-18 yr old—6-15 mg/kg/day q6hr (q4hr dosing when given regular caps) *Adults:* PO: 600 mg/day (400-800 mg/day) in four doses of caps or 2 doses of CR caps Initially use regular caps and later switch to CR caps (twice a day)	Heart failure or hypotension, anticholinergic effects (urinary retention, dry mouth, constipation), nausea and vomiting, hypoglycemia	Caps: 100, 150 mg CR caps: 100, 150 mg
Dobutamine (Dobutrex) (β_1-adrenergic stimulator)	*Children:* IV: 2-15 µg/kg/min in D5W or NS (incompatible with alkali solution) *Adults:* IV: 2.5-10.0 µg/kg/min (maximum 40 µg/kg/min)	Tachyarrhythmias, hypertension, nausea and vomiting, headache (Contraindicated in IHSS and atrial flutter/fibrillation)	Inj: 12.5 mg/ml (20-ml vial)
Dopamine (Intropin, Dopastat) (natural catecholamine inotropic agent)	*Children:* IV: Effects are dose dependent: 2-5 µg/kg/min—increased RBF and urine output 5-15 µg/kg/min—increased RBF, increased heart rate, increased cardiac contractility and cardiac output 20 µg/kg/min—α-adrenergic effects with decreased RBF ($\pm$) (Incompatible with alkali solution)	Tachyarrhythmias, nausea and vomiting, hypotension or hypertension, extravasation (tissue necrosis [treat with local infiltration of phentolamine])	Inj: 40 mg/ml (5 ml), 80 mg/ml (5 ml), 160 mg/ml (5 ml)
Enalapril (Vasotec) (ACE inhibitor, vasodilator)	*Children:* PO: 0.1 mg/kg once or twice daily (maximum 0.5 mg/kg/day) *Adults:* **For CHF** PO: Start with 2.5 mg once or twice daily (usual range 5-20 mg/day) **For hypertension** PO: Start with 5.0 mg once a day (usual dose 10-40 mg/day)	Hypotension, dizziness, fatigue, headache	Tab: 2.5, 5, 10, 20 mg

Drug	Route and Dosage	Toxicity or Side Effects	How Supplied
Ephedrine sulfate (α- and β-adrenoceptor stimulant)	*Children:* IV, IM: 0.2-0.3 mg/kg/dose q4-6hr prn *Adults:* IV: 5-25 mg/dose q3-4hr IM, SC: 25-50 mg/dose q4-6hr	Similar to epinephrine	Inj: 25, 50 mg/ml
Epinephrine (Adrenalin) (α-, β_1, and β_2-adrenergic stimilator)	*Children:* IV: 1:10,000 sol — Begin with 0.1 μg/kg/min; Increase to 1 μg/kg/min to achieve desired effects	Tachyarrhythmias, hypertension, nausea and vomiting, headache, tissue necrosis (±)	Inj: 0.01 mg/ml (1:100,000 sol, 5 ml) 0.1 mg/ml (1:10,000 sol, 10 ml) 1 mg/ml (1:1,000 sol, 1 ml)
Ethacrynic acid (Edecrine) (loop diuretic)	*Children:* PO: 25 mg/dose once a day (maximum 2-3 mg/kg/day) IV: 1 mg/kg/dose *Adults:* PO: 50-100 mg once a day (maximum 400 mg) IV: 0.5-1 mg/kg/dose or 50 mg/dose	Dehydration, hypokalemia, prerenal azotemia, hyperuricemia, eighth cranial nerve damage (deafness), abnormal LFT, agranulocytosis or thrombocytopenia, GI irritation, rash	Tab: 25, 50 mg Inj: 50 mg (vial for reconstruction with 50 ml D5W)
Fentanyl (Sublimaze) (narcotic analgesic)	*For sedation:* *Children:* IV: child 1-3 yr old — 2-3 μg/kg/dose; child 3-12 yr old — 1-2 μg/kg/dose; child >12 yr old — 0.5-1.0 μg/kg/dose; may repeat q30-60 min *Adults:* IV: 50-100 μg/dose	Respiratory depression, apnea, rigidity, bradycardia	Inj: 50 μg/ml
Furosemide (Lasix) (loop diuretic)	*Children:* IV: 0.5-2 mg/kg/dose 2-4 times/day PO: 1-2 mg/kg/dose 1-3 times/day prn (max 6 mg/kg/dose) *Adults:* IV: 20-40 mg/dose 2-4 times/day PO: 20-80 mg/dose 1-4 times/day prn	Hypokalemia, hyperuricemia, prerenal azotemia, ototoxicity, rarely bloody dyscrasias, rash	PO sol: 10 mg/ml (60 ml) Tab: 20, 40, 80 mg Inj: 10 mg/ml (2, 4, 10 ml)
Heparin (anticoagulant)	*Children:* IV: *Initial:* 50 U/kg IV inj *Maintenance:* 100 U/kg q4hr IV drip: 20,000 U/m²/24 hr Keep whole-blood clotting time 2.5-3 times control or APTT 1.5-2 times control	Bleeding (antidote protamine sulfate)	Inj: 1,000, 2,500, 5,000, 7,500, 10,000 U/ml

Drug	Route and Dosage	Toxicity or Side Effects	How Supplied
Heparin (anticoagulant)—cont'd	*Adults:* IV: *Initial:* 10,000 U IV inj *Maintenance:* 5,000-10,000 U q4-6hr IV drip: Initial dose: 5,000 U followed by 20,000-40,000 U/day		
Hydralazine (Apresoline) (peripheral vasodilator, antihypertensive)	*Children:* IM, IV: 0.15-0.2 mg/kg/dose (for emergency) May be repeated q4-6hr PO: 0.75-3 mg/kg/day in 2-4 doses *Adults:* IM, IV: 20-40 mg/dose (for emergency), repeat prn PO: Start with 10 mg 4 times/day for 3-4 days, increase to 25 mg 4 times/day for 3-4 days, then up to 50 mg 4 times/day	Hypotension, tachycardia and palpitation, lupus-like syndrome with prolonged use (fever, arthralgia, splenomegaly and positive LE-cell preparation), blood dyscrasias	Inj: 20 mg/ml Tab: 10, 25, 50, 100 mg
Hydrochlorothiazide (Hydrodiuril) (diuretic)	*Children:* PO: 2-4 mg/kg/day in 2 doses *Adults:* PO: 25-100 mg/day, single or divided doses May be given intermittently	Same as for chlorothizide	Tab: 25, 50, 100 mg
Hydroxyzine (Vistaril, Atarax) (sedative)	*Children:* IM: 1 mg/kg/dose q4-6hr prn PO: child <6 yr old—50 mg/day in 4 doses; child >6 yr old—50-100 mg/day in 4 doses *Adults:* IM: 25-100 mg q4-6hr (maximum 600 mg/day) PO: 50-100 mg/dose q6hr	CNS symptoms (drowsiness, tremor, convulsion), anticholinergic effects (dry mouth, blurred vision, palpitations, hypotension, urinary frequency)	Inj: 25, 50 mg/ml PO susp: 25 mg/5 ml Tab: 10, 25, 50, 100 mg Caps: 25, 50, 100 mg
Indomethacin (Indocin) (nonsteroidal antiinflammatory, antipyretic agent)	*For PDA closure in premature infants:* IV: 0.2 mg/kg initially, then 0.1 mg/kg (for age >48hr), 0.2 mg/kg (for age 2-7 days), 0.25 mg/kg (for age >7 days), may be given up to 2 doses q12hr (total up to 3 doses)	GI or other bleeding, GI disturbances, renal impairment, electrolyte disturbances (decreased sodium and increased potassium levels)	Vial: 1 mg

Drug	Route and Dosage	Toxicity or Side Effects	How Supplied
Isoproterenol (Isuprel) (β1- and β2-adrenergic stimulator)	*Children:* IV: 0.1-0.5 μg/kg/min, titrate to desired effect *Adults:* IV: 2-20 μg/min, titrate to desired effect (incompatible with alkali solution)	Similar to epinephrine	Inj: 0.2 mg/ml (1:5,000 solution: 1.5 ml)
Ketamine (Ketalar) (dissociate anesthetic)	*Children:* IM: 8-12 mg/kg Repeat smaller doses q30min prn IV: 2-3 mg/kg/dose Repeat smaller dose q30min prn	Hypertension/tachycardia, respiratory depression or apnea, CNS symptoms (dreamlike state, confusion, agitation)	Inj: 10, 50, 100 mg/ml
Lidocaine (Xylocaine) (class IB antiarrhythmic agent)	*Children:* IV: *Loading:* 1 mg/kg/dose q5-10min prn *Maintenance:* 30 μg/kg/min IV drip (range 20-50 μg/kg/min) *Adults:* IV: *Loading:* 1 mg/kg/dose q5min *Maintenance:* 1-4 mg/min IV drip	Seizure, respiratory depression, CNS symptoms (anxiety, euphoria or drowsiness), arrhythmias, hypotension or shock	Inj: 10 mg/ml (5-ml amp), 20 mg/ml (5, 10 ml-ampule)
Meperidine (Demerol) (narcotic analgesic)	*Children:* IM, IV, PO: 1-1.5 mg/kg/dose q3-4hr prn *Adults:* IM, IV, PO: 50-100 mg/dose q3-4hr prn	Respiratory depression, hypotension, bradycardia, nausea and vomiting	Inj: 25, 50, 75, 100 mg/ml Tab: 50, 100 mg Syrup: 50 mg/5 ml
Metaraminol (Aramine) (α- and β-adrenoceptor stimulant)	*Children:* IV: 0.01 mg/kg/dose IV bolus 5 μg/kg/min IV infusion initially, titrate to achieve desired effects *Adults:* IV: 0.5-5 mg IV bolus q5-10min prn 1-4 μg/kg/min IV infusion	Similar to norepinephrine	Inj: 10 mg/ml
Methyldopa (Aldomet) (antihypertensive)	*Children:* IV: 5-10 mg/kg/dose over 30-60 min, then 20-40 mg/kg/day in 4 doses (maximum 65 mg/kg/day or 3 g/day) PO: 10 mg/kg/day in 2-4 doses May be increased or decreased (maximum 65 mg/kg/day or 3 g/day)	Sedation, orthostatic hypotension and bradycardia, lupus-like syndrome, Coombs (+) hemolytic anemia and leukopenia, hepatitis or cirrhosis, colitis, impotence	Inj: 50 mg/ml PO susp: 250 mg/ml (16 oz) Tab: 125, 250, 500 mg

Drug	Route and Dosage	Toxicity or Side Effects	How Supplied
Methyldopa (Aldomet) (antihypertensive)—cont'd	*Adults:* IV: 250-500 mg q6hr (maximum 1 g q6h) PO: 250 mg 2-3 times/day for 2 days May be increased or decreased q2 days Usual dose: 0.5-2 g/day in 2-4 doses (maximum 3 g/day)		
Metoprolol (Lopressor) (β-adrenoceptor blocker)	*Children >2 yr:* PO: 1-5 mg/kg/day in 2 doses *Adults:* PO: 100 mg/day in 1-3 doses initially May increase to 450 mg/day in 2-3 doses Usual dose 100-450 mg/day (Usually used with hydrochlorothiazide 25-100 mg/day)	CNS symptoms (dizziness, tiredness, depression), bronchospasm, bradycardia, diarrhea, nausea and vomiting, abdominal pain	Tab: 50, 100 mg
Mexiletine (Mexitil) (class 1B antiarrhythmic agent)	*Children:* PO: 6-8 mg/kg/day initially, then 2-5 mg/kg/dose q6-8hr Increase 1-2 mg/kg/dose q2-3days until desired effects achieved (with food or antacid) *Adults:* PO: 200 mg q8hr for 2-3 days Increase to 300-400 mg q8hr (Usual dose 200-300 mg q8hr) Therapeutic level: 0.75-2.0 μg/ml	Nausea and vomiting, CNS symptoms (headache, dizziness, tremor, paresthesia, mood changes), rash, hepatic dysfunction (±)	Caps: 150, 200, 250 mg
Milrinone (Primacor) (Phosphodiesterase inhibitor, non-catecholamine inotropic, vasodilator agent)	*Children:* IV: Loading: 10-50 μg/kg over min, then 0.1-1.0 μg/kg/min IV drip *Adults:* IV: Loading: 50 μg/kg over 10 min 0.5 μg/kg/min IV drip (ranges 0.375-0.75 μg/kg/min)	Arrhythmias, hypotension, hypokalemia, thrombocytopenia	Inj: 1 mg/ml
Minoxidil (Loniten) (peripheral vasodilator)	*Children <12 yr:* PO: 0.2 mg/kg/day in 1-2 doses initially Increase 0.1-0.2 mg/kg/day q3days until desired effects achieved (Usual dose 0.25-1.0 mg/kg/day in 1-2 doses) (maximum 50 mg/day)	Reflex tachycardia and fluid retention (used with a β-blocker and diuretic), pericardial effusion, hypertrichosis, rarely blood dyscrasias (leukopenia, thrombocytopenia)	Tab: 2.5, 10 mg

Drug	Route and Dosage	Toxicity or Side Effects	How Supplied
Minoxidil (Loniten) (peripheral vasodilator)—cont'd	*Children >12 yr and adults:* PO: 5 mg once a day initially May be increased to 10, 20, 40 mg in single or divided doses (Usual dose 10-40 mg/day in 1-2 doses) (maximum 100 mg/day)		
Morphine sulfate (narcotic analgesic)	*Children:* SC, IM, IV: 0.1-0.2 mg/kg/dose q2-4hr (maximum 15 mg/dose) *Adults:* SC, IM, IV: 2.5-20 mg/dose q2-6hr prn	CNS depression, respiratory depression, nausea and vomiting, hypotension, bradycardia	Inj: 8, 10, 15 mg/ml
Naloxone (Narcan) (narcotic antagonist)	*Children:* IM, IV: 5-10 μg/kg/dose q2-3min for 1-3 doses prn (may need 5-10 doses) *Adults:* IM, IV: 0.4-2 mg/dose q2-3min for 1-3 doses prn	Ventricular arrhythmia, pulmonary edema ($\pm$), nausea and vomiting, seizure	Inj: 0.4, 10 mg/ml Neonatal Narcan: 0.02 mg/ml
Nifedipine (Procardia, Adalat) (calcium channel blocker)	*Children:* **For hypertrophic cardiomyopathy:** PO: 0.6-0.9 mg/kg/day in 3-4 doses *Adults:* PO: 10 mg 3 times/day initially Titrate up to 20 or 30 mg 3-4 times/day over 7-14 days Usual dose 10-20 mg 3 times/day (maximum 180 mg/day)	Hypotension, peripheral edema, CNS symptoms (headache, dizziness, weakness), nausea	Caps: 10 mg
Nitroglycerine (Nitro-Bid IV) (peripheral vasodilator)	*Children:* IV: 0.5-1.0 μg/kg/min Increase 1.0 μg/kg/min q20 min to tritrate to effect (maximum 6.0 μg/kg/min) (Dilute in D5W or NS with final concentration <400 μg/ml, light sensitive) *Adults:* IV: Initial dose: 5 μg/min through infusion pump Increase 5 μg/min q3-5min until desired effects achieved.	Hypotension, tachycardia, headache, nausea and vomiting	Inj: 5 mg/ml

Drug	Route and Dosage	Toxicity or Side Effects	How Supplied
Nitroprusside (Nipride) (peripheral vasodilator)	*Children:* IV: 0.5-8 µg/kg/min, with BP monitoring Usual dose 2-3 µg/kg/min (Dilute stock solution [50 mg] in 250-2000 ml D5W, light sensitive)	Hypotension, sweating and palpitation, nausea and vomiting, cyanide toxicity (metabolic acidosis earliest and most reliable evidence; monitor thiocyanate level when used >48hr and in renal failure)	Inj: 50 mg (vial for reconstruction with 2-3 ml D5W)
Norepinephrine (Levophed, Levarterenol) (α- and β-adrenoceptor stimulant)	*Children:* IV: 0.1 µg/kg/min initially, increase dose to attain desired effects *Adults:* IV: Add 4 ml Levarterenol to 1,000 ml D5W, start at 2-3 ml/min (8-12 µg/min) and adjust rate	Hypertension, bradycardia (reflex), arrhythmias, tissue necrosis (treat with phentolamine infiltration)	Inj: 1 mg/ml
Phentolamine (Regitine) (α-adrenoceptor blocker)	*For phenochromocytoma:* *Children:* IM, IV: 0.05-0.1 mg/kg/dose Repeat q5min until hypertension is controlled, then q2-4hr prn *Adults:* IM, IV: 2.5-5.0 mg/dose Repeat q5min until hypertension is controlled, then q2-4hr prn *For treatment of extravasated α-adrenergic drugs:* SC: 0.1-0.2 mg/kg locally within 12hr (maximum 10 mg)	Hypotension, tachycardia or arrhythmias, nausea and vomiting	Inj: 5 mg/ml
Phenylephrine (Neo-Synephrine) (α-adrenoceptor stimulant)	*For hypotension:* *Children:* IM, SC: 0.1 mg/kg/dose q1-2hr prn IV: 5-10 µg/kg/dose IV bolus q10-15min or 0.1-0.5 µg/kg/min IV infusion *Adults:* IM, SC: 2-5 mg/dose q1-2hr prn IV: 0.1-0.5 mg/dose IV bolus q10-15min prn Start IV infusion at 100-180 µg/min; maintain at 40-60 µg/min	Arrhythmias, hypertension, angina	Inj: 10 mg/ml

Drug	Route and Dosage	Toxicity or Side Effects	How Supplied
Phenytoin (Dilantin) (class IB antiarrhythmic agent)	*Children:* IV: 2-4 mg/kg/dose over 5-10 min followed by: PO: 2-5 mg/kg/day in 2-3 doses (Therapeutic level: 5-18 µg/ml for arrhythmias, 10-20 µg/ml for seizure) *Adults:* IV: 100 mg q5min (total 500 mg) PO: 250 mg 4 times for 1 day, 250 mg twice for 2 days, and 300-400 mg/day in 1-4 doses	Rash, Stevens-Johnson syndrome, CNS symptoms (ataxia, dysarthria), lupus-like syndrome, blood dyscrasias, peripheral neuropathy, gingival hypertrophy	Inj: 50 mg/ml PO susp: 30, 125 mg/5 ml (240 ml) Infatab: 50 mg (chewable) Caps: 30, 100 mg
Potassium chloride	***Supplement in diuretic therapy:*** *Children:* PO: 1-2 mEq/kg/day in 3-4 doses, 0.8-1.5 ml 10% potassium chloride/kg/day, or 0.4-0.7 ml 20% potassium chloride/kg/day in 3-4 doses	GI disturbances, ulcerations, hyperkalemia	10% sol: 1.3 mEq/ml 20% sol:2.7 mEq/ml
Potassium gluconate	***Supplement in diuretic therapy:*** *Children:* PO: 1-2 mEq/kg/day in 3-4 doses or 0.8-1.5 ml/kg/day in 3-4 doses	Same as for potassium chloride	Elixir: 1.3 mEq/ml
Potassium triplex (acetate-bicarbonate-citrate)	***Supplement in diuretic therapy:*** *Children:* PO: 1-2 mEq/kg/day in 3-4 doses or 0.3-0.6 ml/kg/day in 3-4 doses	Same as for potassium chloride	PO sol: 3 mEq/ml
Prazosin (Minipress) (postsynaptic α-adrenergic blocker; antihypertensive)	*Children:* PO: 5 µg/kg as a test dose, then 25-150 µg/kg/day in 4 doses *Adults:* PO: 1 mg 2-3 times/day initially Increase to 20 mg/day in 2-4 doses Usual dose 6-15 mg/day	CNS symptoms (dizziness, headache, drowsiness), palpitation, nausea	Caps: 1, 2, 5 mg
Procainamide (Pronestyl) (class IA antiarrhythmic agent)	*Children:* IV: *Loading:* 3-6 mg/kg/dose over 5 min repeated q10-30 min (maximum 100 mg) *Maintenance:* 20-80 µg/kg/min by IV infusion (maximum 2 g/24hr) PO: 15-50 mg/kg/day q3-6hr (maximum 4 g/24hr)	Nausea and vomiting, blood dyscrasias, rash, lupus-like syndrome, hypotension, confusion or disorientation	Inj: 100, 500 mg/ml Tab: 250, 375, 500 mg Tab, sustained release: 250, 500, 750, 1,000 mg Caps: 250, 375, 500 mg

Drug	Route and Dosage	Toxicity or Side Effects	How Supplied
Procainamide (Pronestyl) (class IA anti- arrhythmic agent)—cont'd	*Adults:* IV: *Loading:* 50-100 mg/ dose q5min prn *Maintenance:* 1-6 mg/ min by IV infusion PO: 250-500 mg/dose q3-6hr (usual dose: 2-4 g/day) Therapeutic level: 4-10 μg/ml		
Promethazine (Phenergan) (sedative, anti- emetic)	*For nausea and vomiting:* *Children:* IM, PR: 0.25-0.5 mg/kg q4- 6hr prn *Adults:* IM, PR: 12.5-25 mg q6hr prn *For sedation before surgery:* *Children:* IM, PO, PR: 0.5-1 mg/kg/ dose q6hr prn *Adults:* IM, PO, PR: 25-50 mg q4- 6hr prn	CNS stimulation, anticholin- ergic effects	Inj: 25, 50 mg/ml Tab: 12.5, 25, 50 mg Syrup: 6.25 mg/5 ml Supp: 12.5, 25, 50 mg
Propranolol (In- deral) (β- adrenoceptor blocker, class II antiarrhyth- mic agent)	*For hypertension:* *Children:* PO: 2-4 mg/kg/day in 2-4 doses (maximum 16 mg/kg/day) *For arrhythmias:* *Children:* IV: 0.01-0.15 mg/kg/dose over 10 min (maxi- mum 1 mg/dose) PO: 2-4 mg/kg/day in 3-4 doses (maximum 16 mg/kg/day) *Adults:* IV: 1 mg/dose q5min (maxi- mum 5 mg) PO: 40-320 mg/day in 3-4 doses	Hypotension, syncope, bron- chospasms, nausea and vomiting, hypoglycemia, lethargy or depression, heart block	Tab: 10, 20, 40, 60, 80, 90 mg
Prostaglandin E$_1$ or Alprostadil (Prostin VR)	*For patency of ductus arteriosus:* IV: Begin infusion at 0.05- 0.1 μg/kg/min When desired effects achieved, reduce to 0.05, 0.025, and 0.01 μg/kg/min If unresponsive, dose may be increased to 0.4 μg/kg/min	Apnea, flushing, bradycar- dia, hypotension, fever	Ampule: 500 μg
Protamine sul- fate	*Antidote to heparin overdose:* IV: Each 1-mg protamine neutralizes approx 100 U heparin given in proceding 3-4 hr Slow IV infusion at rate not exceeding 20 mg/ min or 50 mg/10 min Check APTT	Hypotension, bradycardia, dyspnea, flushing, coagu- lation problem	Inj: 10 mg/ml

Drug	Route and Dosage	Toxicity or Side Effects	How Supplied

Quinidine gluconate (class IA antiarrhythmic agent)	*Children:*
	PO: Test for idiosyncracy with 2 mg/kg
	    10-30 mg/kg/day in 2-3 doses
	    Usual dose 160-660 mg q12hr
	Adults:
	PO: 25 mg test dose
	    200-400 mg q4-6hr
		Nausea and vomiting, ventricular arrhythmias, prolonged QRS complex, depressed myocardial contractility, blood dyscrasias, symptoms of cinchonism	Tab, sustained release: 330 mg
			Inj: 80 mg/ml

Quinidine sulfate (class IA antiarrhythmic agent)	*Children:* PO: Initial: 3-6 mg/kg q2-3hr for 5 doses May increase to 12 mg/kg q2-3hr for 5 doses *Maintenance:* 7-12 mg/kg/day in 4 doses	Same as for quinidine gluconate	Caps: 200, 300 mg Tab: 100, 200, 300 mg Tab, sustained release: 300 mg
Reserpine (Serpasil) (depletion of NE store antihypertensive)	*Children:* **For acute hypertension:** IM: 0.02-0.07 mg/kg q8-24hr (maximum 2.5 mg/day) (May be used with hydralazine) PO: 0.02 mg/kg/day in 2 doses *Adults:* PO: 0.5 mg/day in 2 doses for 1-2 wk *Maintenance dose:* 0.1-0.25 mg/day	Mental depression, nasal stuffiness, bradycardia, hypotension	Inj: 2.5 mg/ml Tab: 0.1, 0.25 mg
Sodium polystyrene sulfonate (Kayexalate) (potassium lowing agent)	**For hyperkalemia (slowly effective, taking hours to days)** *Children:* PO, NG: 1 g/kg/dose q6hr PR: 1 g/kg/dose q2-6hr *Adults:* PO, NG, PR: 15 g (4 level tsp) 1-4 times/day	(Cation exchange resin with practical exchange rates of 1 mEq potassium per 1 g resin) NOTE: Delivers 1 mEq sodium for each mEq of potassium removed.) Nausea and vomiting, constipation, severe hypokalemia (monitor serum potassium levels, ECG, muscle weakness, confusion), hypocalcemia or hypernatremia (edema)	Powder: 454 g/lb Susp: 15 g/60 ml
Spironolactone (Aldactone) (aldosterone antagonist)	*Children:* PO: 3 mg/kg/day in 1-3 doses *Adults:* PO: 50-100 mg/day in 1-3 doses (maximum 200 mg/day)	Hyperkalemia (when given with potassium supplements), gynecomastia, agranulocytosis	Tab: 25, 50, 100 mg

Drug	Route and Dosage	Toxicity or Side Effects	How Supplied
Streptokinase (Streptase) (thrombolytic agent)	*Children:* IV: *Loading:* 10,000 U/kg over 20-30 min (maximum 250,000 U) *Maintenance:* 1000 U/kg/hr in NS Obtain fibrinogen level in 4hr (normal 2-4 g/L) Fibrinogen 1.0-1.4 g/L indicates effectiveness of therapy If no decrease in 4hr, increase to 2000 U/kg/hr in 500 U/kg/hr increments If no decrease in fibrinogen level, switch to urokinase *Adults:* IV: Loading: 250,000 U over 30 min Maintenance: 100,000 U/hr for 24-72 hr Obtain tests at baseline and q4hr: APTT, TT, fibrinogen, PT, hematocrit, platelet count APTT and TT should be <2 times control	Potential for allergic reaction to repeated use, premedicate with acetaminophen and antihistamine, and repeat q4-6hr	Inj: 250,000, 750,000, 1,500,000 U/6.5 ml vial
Tocainide (Tonocard) (class IB antiarrhythmic agent)	*Children:* PO: 20-40 mg/kg/day in 3 doses *Adults:* PO: 400 mg q8hr May increase to 600 mg q8hr Usual dose 400-600 mg q8hr	Dizziness and vertigo, nausea and vomiting, blood dyscrasias ($\pm$)	Tab: 400, 600 mg
Tolazoline (Priscoline) (α-adrenoceptor blocker)	***For neonatal pulmonary hypertension:*** IV: *Loading:* 1-2 mg/kg over 10 min *Maintenance:* 1-2 mg/ kg/hr IV infusion	Hypotension and tachycardia, pulmonary hemorrhage, GI bleeding, arrhythmias, thrombocytopenia, leukopenia	Inj: 25 mg/ml
Triamterene (Dyrenium) (potassium-conserving diuretic)	*Children:* PO: 2-4 mg/kg/day in 1-2 doses *Adults:* PO: 100-300 mg/day in 1-2 doses (maximum 300 mg)	Nausea and vomiting, leg cramps, dizziness, hyperuricemia, rash, prerenal azotemia	Caps: 50, 100 mg

Drug	Route and Dosage	Toxicity or Side Effects	How Supplied
Urokinase (Abbokinase) (thrombolytic agent)	*Children:* **For clot lysis:** IV: *Loading:* 4000 U/kg/ dose IV over 10 min *Maintenance:* 4000-6000 U/kg/hr (continue until clot is dissolved, usually 24-74 hr) Monitor same laboratoty tests as for streptokinase **For catheter clearance:** IV: Infuse 1 ml (containing 5000 U/ml) into catheter, aspirate with 5 ml syringe q5min 6 times; may repeat urokinase infusion prn *Adults:* **For pulmonary embolism:** IV: Priming dose: 4,400 U/kg IV infusion 4,400 U/kg/hr for 12 hr by infusion pump	Bleeding, allergic reactions, rash, fever and chills, bronchospasm	Inj: 250,000 U/vial
Verapamil (Isoptin, Calan) (class IV anti-arrhythmic agent)	*Children:* IV: child 0-1 yr old — 0.1-0.2 mg/kg over 2 min Usual single dose 0.75-2 mg May repeat same dose in 30 min (should be used with extreme caution only when other drugs fail) Child 1-15 yr — 0.1 mg/kg over 2 min (single maximum dose 2-5 mg) May repeat same dose in 15 min PO: 3-5 mg/kg/day in 3 doses *Adults:* IV: 5-10 mg over 2 min May repeat 10 mg in 30 min prn PO: 240-480 mg/day in 3 doses	Hypotension, bradycardia, cardiac depression	Inj: 2.5 mg/ml Tab: 40, 80, 120 mg
Vitamin K	**Antidote to dicumarol or warfarin:** PO: 2.5-10 mg in 1 dose for correction of excessive PT from dicumarol or warfarin overdose		Tab: 5 mg

Drug	Route and Dosage	Toxicity or Side Effects	How Supplied
Warfarin (Coumadin) (anticoagulant)	*Children:* PO: *Initial:* 1-3 mg/day qday for 2-4 days in evening (large loading dose not recommended). Daily PT determination *Maintenance:* 1-5 mg/day once a day Keep INR at 2.5-3.5 Heparin preferred initially for rapid anticoagulation, warfarin may be started concomitantly with heparin or may be delayed 3-6 days *Adults:* PO: *Initial:* 2-5 mg/day qday for 2-4 days (large loading dose not recommended); adjust dosage based on INR *Maintenance:* 2-10 mg/day qday	Bleeding (antidote: vitamin K or fresh-frozen plasma) *Increased PT response:* Salicylates, acetaminophen, alcohol, lipid-lowering agents, phenytoin, ibuprofen, some antibiotics *Decreased PT response:* Antihistamines, barbiturates, oral contraceptives, vitamin C, diet high in vitamin K	Tab: 1, 2, 2.5, 5, 7.5, 10 mg

Suggested Readings

GENERAL REFERENCES

Adams FH, Emmanouilides GC, Riemenschneider TA: *Moss' heart disease in infants, children, and adolescents,* ed 4, Baltimore, 1989, Williams & Wilkins.

Fyler DC: *Nadas' pediatric cardiology,* St Louis, 1992, Mosby.

Gillette PC, Garson A Jr: *Pediatric arrhythmias: electrophysiology and pacing,* Philadelphia, 1990, Saunders.

Kirklin JW, Barratt-Boyes BG: *Cardiac surgery: morphology, diagnostic criteria, natural history, techniques, results, and indications,* ed 2, New York, 1993, Churchill Livingstone.

Park MK, Guntheroth WG: *How to read pediatric ECGs,* ed 3, St Louis, 1992, Mosby.

Silverman NH: *Pediatric echocardiography,* Baltimore, 1993, Williams & Wilkins.

Snider AR, Serwer GA: *Echocardiography in pediatric heart disease,* St Louis, 1990, Mosby.

CHAPTER 1: HISTORY TAKING

Copel JA, Kleinman CS: Congenital heart disease and extracardiac anomalies: association and indications for fetal echocardiography, *Am J Obstet Gynecol* 154:1121-1132, 1986.

Greenwood RD, Rosenthal A, Nadas AS: Cardiovascular malformations associated with congenital diaphragmatic hernia, *Pediatrics* 57:92-97, 1976.

Nora JJ: *Etiologic aspects of heart disease.* In Adams FH, Emmadouilides GC, Reimenschnieder TA, eds: *Moss' heart disease in infants, children, and adolescents,* ed 4, Baltimore, 1989, Williams & Wilkins.

Smith DW: *Recognizable patterns of human malformation,* ed 3, Philadelphia, 1982, Saunders.

CHAPTER 2: PHYSICAL EXAMINATION

Fyler DC, Nadas AS: *History, physical examination, and laboratory tests.* In Fyler DC, ed: *Nadas' pediatric cardiology,* St Louis, 1992, Mosby.

Guntheroth WG: Initial evaluation of the child for heart disease, *Pediatr Clin North Am* 25:657-675, 1978.

Park MK, Guntheroth WG: Accurate blood pressure measurement in children: a review, *Am J Noninvas Cardiol* 3:297-309, 1989.

Park MK, Lee D-H, Johnson GA: Oscillometric blood pressure in the arm, thigh and calf in healthy children and those with aortic coarctation, *Pediatrics* 91:761-765, 1993.

Report of the Second Task Force on Blood Pressure Control in Children, *Pediatrics* 79:1-25, 1987.

Rosenthal A: How to distinguish between innocent and pathologic murmurs in childhood, *Pediatr Clin North Am* 31:1229-1240, 1984.

CHAPTER 3: ELECTROCARDIOGRAPHY

Park MK, Guntheroth WG: *How to read pediatric ECGs,* ed 3, St Louis, 1992, Mosby.

CHAPTER 4: CHEST ROENTGENOGRAPHY

Elliott LP: *Radiologic differentiation of the common congenital heart and great vessels.* In Roberts WC, ed: *Congenital heart disease in adults,* Philadelphia, 1979, FA Davis.

Gedgaudas E, Knight L: Plain-film diagnosis of heart disease: a physiologic approach, *JAMA* 232:63-67, 1975.

CHAPTER 5: FLOW DIAGRAM

Kawabori I: Cyanotic congenital heart defects with decreased pulmonary blood flow, *Pediatr Clin North Am* 25:759-776, 1978.

Kawabori I: Cyanotic congenital heart defects with increased pulmonary blood flow, *Pediatr Clin North Am* 25:777-795, 1978.

Stevenson JG: Acyanotic lesions with normal pulmonary blood flow, *Pediatr Clin North Am* 25:725-742, 1978.

Stevenson JG: Acyanotic lesions with increased pulmonary blood flow, *Pediatr Clin North Am* 25:743-758, 1978.

CHAPTER 6: NONINVASIVE TECHNIQUES

Beder SD: *Ambulatory electrocardiography.* In Adams FH, Emmanouilides GC, Riemenschneider TA, eds: *Moss' heart disease in infants, children, and adolescents,* ed 4, Baltimore, 1989, Williams & Wilkins.

Cumming GR, Everatt D, Hartman L: Bruce treadmill test in children: normal values in a clinic population, *Am J Cardiol* 41:69-75, 1978.

Nishimura RA, Abel MD, Hatle LK, et al: Assessment of diastolic function of the heart: background and current applications of Doppler echocardiography. II. Clinical studies. *Mayo Clin Proc* 64:181-204, 1989.

Porter CJ, Gillette PC, McNamara DG: Twenty-four hour ambulatory ECGs in the detection and management of cardiac arrhythmias in infants and children, *Pediatr Cardiol* 1:203-208, 1980.

CHAPTER 7: INVASIVE PROCEDURES

Allen HD, Driscoll DJ, Fricker FJ, et al: Guidelines for pediatric therapeutic cardiac catheterization: a statement for professionals from the Committee on Congenital Cardiac Defects of the Council on Cardiovascular Disease in the Young, the American Heart Association, *Circulation* 84:2248-2258, 1991.

Cassidy SC, Schmidt KG, Van Hare GF, et al: Complications of pediatric cardiac catheterization: a 3-year study, *J Am Coll Cardiol* 19:1285-1293, 1992.

Lock JE, Keane JF, Mandell VS, et al: *Cardiac catheterization.* In Fyler DC, ed: *Nadas' pediatric cardiology,* St Louis, 1992, Mosby.

Rome JJ, Keane JF, Perry SB, et al: Double-umbrella closure of atrial defects: initial clinical applications, *Circulation* 82:751-758, 1990.

Ruckman RN, Keane JF, Freed MD, et al: Sedation for cardiac catheterization: A controlled study, *Pediatr Cardiol* 1:263-268, 1980.

CHAPTER 8: FETAL AND PERINATAL CIRCULATION

Guntheroth WG, Kawabori I, Stevenson JG: *Physiology of the circulation: fetus, neonate, and child.* In Kelly VC, ed: *Practice of pediatrics,* vol 8, Philadelphia, 1982-1983, Harper & Row.

Rudolph AM: *Congenital diseases of the heart: clinical-physiologic considerations in diagnosis and management,* Chicago, 1974, Mosby.

CHAPTERS 9, 10, AND 11: PATHOPHYSIOLOGY OF LEFT-TO-RIGHT SHUNT LESIONS, PATHOPHYSIOLOGY OBSTRUCTIVE AND VALVULAR REGURGITANT LESIONS, AND PATHOPHYSIOLOGY CYANOTIC CONGENITAL HEART DEFECTS

Guntheroth WG, Morgan BC, Mullins GL: Physiologic studies of paroxysmal hyperpnea in cyanotic congenital heart disease, *Circulation* 31:66-76, 1965.

Heath D, Edwards JE: The pathology of hypertensive pulmonary vascular disease, *Circulation* 18:533-547, 1958.

King SB, Franch RH: Production of increased right-to-left shunting by rapid heart rates in patients with tetralogy of Fallot, *Circulation* 44:265-271, 1971.

Moller JH, Amplatz K, Edwards JE: *Congenital heart disease,* Kalamazoo, Mich, 1971, Upjohn.

Rudolph AM: *Congenital diseases of the heart,* Chicago, 1974, Mosby.

CHAPTER 12: LEFT-TO-RIGHT SHUNT LESIONS
ASD:

Lock JE, Rome JJ, Davis R, et al: Transcatheter closure of atrial septal defect, *Circulation* 79:1091-1099, 1989.

Radzik D, Davignon A, van Doesburg N, et al: Predictive factors for spontaneous closure of atrial septal defects diagnosed in the first 3 months of life, *J Am Coll Cardiol* 22:851-853, 1993.

Sideris EB, Sideris SE, Thampoulos BD, et al: Transvenous atrial septal defect occlusion by the buttoned device, *Am J Cardiol* 66:1524-1526, 1990.

VSD:

Graham TP Jr, Bender HW, Spach MS: *Ventricular septal defect.* In Adams FH, Emmanouilides GC, Riemenschneider TA, eds: *Moss' heart disease in infants, children and adolescents,* ed 4, Baltimore, 1989, Williams & Wilkins.

Soto B, Becker AE, Moulaezt AH, et al: Classification of ventricular septal defects, *Br Heart J* 43:332-363, 1980.

Van Mill GJ, Moulaert AJ, Harinck E: *Atlas of two-dimensional echocardiography in congenital cardiac defects,* Boston, 1983, Martinus Nijhoff.

PDA:

Musewe NN, Smallhorn JF, Benson LN, et al: Validation of Doppler-derived pulmonary arterial pressure in patients with ductus arteriosus under different hemodynamic states, *Circulation* 76:1081-1091, 1987.

Rao PS, Sideris EB, Haddad J, et al: Transcatheter occlusion of patent ductus arteriosus with adjustable buttoned device: initial clinical experience, *Circulation* 88:1119-1126, 1993.

ECD, Complete and Partial:

Anderson RH, Macartney FJ, Shinebourne EA, et al: *Atrioventricular septal defects.* In Anderson RH, Macartney FJ, Shinebourne EA, et al, eds: *Pediatric cardiology,* New York, 1987, Churchill Livingstone.

Piccoli GP, Gerlis LM, Wilkinson JL, et al: Morphology and classification of atrioventricular defects, *Br Heart J* 42:621-632, 1979.

Rastelli GC, Kirklin JW, Titus JL: Anatomic observation on complete form of persistent common atrioventricular canal with special reference to atrioventricular valves, *Mayo Clin Proc* 41:296-308, 1966.

PAPVR:

Ward KE, Mullins CE: *Anomalous pulmonary venous connections; pulmonary vein stenosis; atresia of the common pulmonary vein.* In Garson A Jr, Bricker JT, McNamara DG, eds: *The science and practice of pediatric cardiology,* Philadelphia, 1990, Lea & Febiger.

CHAPTER 13: OBSTRUCTIVE LESIONS

Pulmonary Stenosis:

Stanger P, Cassidy SC, Dried DA, et al: Balloon pulmonary valvuloplasty: results of the valvuloplasty and angioplasty of congenital anomalies registry, *Am J Cardiol* 65:775-783, 1990.

Aortic Stenosis:

Kouchoukos NT, Davila-Roman VG, Spray TL, et al: Replacement of the aortic root with a pulmonary autograft in children and young adults with aortic valve disease, *N Engl J Med* 330:1-6, 1994.

Van Son JAM, Schaff HV, Danielson GK, et al: Surgical treatment of discrete and tunnel subaortic stenosis. II. Late survival and risk of reoperation, *Circulation* 88:159-169, 1993.

COA:

Hellenbrand WE, Allen HD, Golinko RJ, et al: Balloon angioplasty for aortic recoarctation: results of valvuloplasty and angioplasty of congenital anomalies registry, *Am J Cardiol* 65:793-797, 1990.

Tynan M, Finley JP, Fontes V, et al: Balloon angioplasty for the treatment of native coarctation: results of valvuloplasty and angioplasty of congenital anomalies registry, *Am J Cardiol* 65:790-793, 1990.

CHAPTER 14: CYANOTIC CONGENITAL HEART DEFECTS

D-TGA:

Jex RK, Puga FJ, Julsrud PR, et al: Repair of transposition of the great arteries with intact ventricular septum and left ventricular outflow tract obstruction, *J Thorac Cardiovasc Surg* 100:682-686, 1990.

Jones RA, Giglia TM, Sanders SP, et al: Rapid, two-stage arterial switch for transposition of the great arteries and intact ventricular septum beyond the neonatal period, *Circulation* 80 (suppl I):I-203-I-208, 1989.

Kovalchin JP, Allen HD, Cassidy SC, et al: Pulmonary valve eccentricity in D-transposition of the great arteries and implications for the arterial switch operation, *Am J Cardiol* 73:186-190, 1994.

Lupinetti FM, Bove EL, Minich LL, et al: Intermediate-term survival and functional results after arterial repair for transposition of the great arteries, *J Thorac Cardiovasc Surg* 103:421-427, 1992.

Waldeman JD, Lamberti JJ, George L, et al: Experience with Damus procedure, *Circulation* 78(suppl III):III-32-III-39, 1988.

Yacoub M, Bernhard A, Lange P, et al: Clinical and hemodynamic results of the two-stage anatomic correction of simple transposition of the great arteries, *Circulation* 62(suppl I):I-190-I-196, 1980.

L-TGA:

Dabizzi RP, Barletta GA, Caprioli G, et al: Coronary artery anatomy in corrected transposition of the great arteries, *J Am Coll Cardiol* 12:486-491, 1988.

Lundstrom U, Bull C, Wyse RKH, et al: The natural and "unnatural" history of congenitally corrected transposition, *Am J Cardiol* 65:1222-1229, 1990.

TOF:

Di Donato RM, Jonas RA, Lang P, et al: Neonatal repair of tetralogy of Fallot with and without pulmonary atresia, *J Thorac Cardiovasc Surg* 101:126-137, 1991.

Kirklin JW, Blackstone EH, Jonas RA, et al: Morphologic and surgical determinant of outcome events after repair of tetralogy of Fallot and pulmonary stenosis, a two-institution study, *J Thorac Cardiovasc Surg* 103:706-723, 1992.

Lakier JB, Stanger P, Heymann MA, et al: Tetralogy of Fallot with absent pulmonary valve: natural history and hemodynamic considerations, *Circulation* 50:167-175, 1974.

Park MK, Trinkle JK: Absent pulmonary valve syndrome: a two-stage operation, *Ann Thorac Surg* 41:669-671, 1986.

Puga FJ, Leoni FE, Julsrud PR, et al: Complete repair of pulmonary atresia, ventricular septal defect, and severe peripheral arborization abnormalities of the central pulmonary arteries, *J Thorac Cardiovasc Surg* 98:1018-1029, 1989.

Sawatari K, Imai Y, Kurosawa H, et al: Staged operation for pulmonary atresia and ventricular septal defect with major aortopulmonary collateral arteries, *J Thorac Cardiovasc Surg* 98:738-750, 1989.

Touati GD, Vouhe PR, Amodeo A, et al: Primary repair of tetralogy of Fallot in infancy, *J Thorac Cardiovasc Surg* 99:396-403, 1990.

TAPVR:

Lupinetti FM, Kulik TJ, Beekman RH, et al: Correction of total anomalous pulmonary venous connection in infancy, *J Thorac Cardiovasc Surg* 106:880-885, 1993.

Van der Velde ME, Parness IA, Colan SD, et al: Two-dimensional echocardiography in pre- and postoperative management of totally anomalous pulmonary venous connection, *J Am Coll Cardiol* 18:1746-1751, 1991.

Tricuspid Atresia:

Bridges ND, Mayer JE, Lock JE, et al: Effects of baffle fenestration on outcome of the modified Fontan operation, *Circulation* 86:1762-1769, 1992.

Castaneda AR: From Glenn to Fontan: a continuing evolution, *Circulation* 86(suppl II):II-80-II-84, 1992.

Driscoll DJ, Offord KP, Feldt RH, et al: Five- to fifteen-year follow-up after Fontan operation, *Circulation* 85:469-496, 1992.

Giannico S, Corno A, Marino B, et al: Total extracardiac right heart bypass, *Circulation* 86(suppl II):II-110-II-117, 1992.

Pearl JM, Laks H, Drinkwater DC, et al: Modified Fontan procedure in patients less than 4 years of age, *Circulation* 86(suppl II):II-100-II-105, 1992.

Pulmonary Atresia:

Bull C, de Leval MR, Mercanti C, et al: Pulmonary atresia and intact ventricular septum: a revised classification, *Circulation* 66:266-280, 1982.

Hanley FL, Sade RM, Blackstone EH, et al: Outcomes in neonatal pulmonary atresia with intact ventricular septum: a multiinstitutional study, *J Thorac Cardiovasc Surg* 105:406-427, 1993.

Ebstein's Anomaly

Carpentier A, Chauvaud S, Mace L, et al: A new reconstructive operation for Ebstein's anomaly of the tricuspid valve, *J Thorac Cardiovasc Surg* 96:92-101, 1988.

Danielson GK, Driscoll DJ, Mair DD, et al: Operative treatment of Ebstein's anomaly, *J Thorac Cardiovasc Surg* 104:1195-1202, 1992.

Shiina A, Sewer JB, Edwards WD, et al: Two-dimensional echocardiographic spectrum of Ebstein's anomaly: detailed anatomic assessment, *J Am Coll Cardiol* 3:356-370, 1984.

Truncus Arteriosus:

Lenox CC, Debich DE, Zuberbuhler JR: The role of coronary artery abnormalities in the prognosis of truncus arteriosus, *J Thorac Cardiovasc Surg* 104:1724-1742, 1992.

Spicer RL, Behrendt D, Crowley DC, et al: Repair of truncus arteriosus in neonates with the use of a valveless conduit, *Circulation* 70(suppl I):I-26-I-29, 1984.

Single Ventricle:

Freedom RM, Benson LN, Smallhorn JF, et al: Subaortic stenosis, the univentricular heart, and banding of the pulmonary artery: an analysis of the courses of 43 patients with univentricular heart palliated by pulmonary artery banding, *Circulation* 73:758-764, 1986.

Newfeld EA, Niakidoh H: Surgical management of subaortic stenosis in patients with a single ventricle and transposition of the great vessels, *Circulation* 76(suppl III): III-29-III-33, 1987.

Stein DG, Laks H, Drinkwater DC, et al: Results of total cavopulmonary connection in the treatment of patients with a functional single ventricle, *J Thorac Cardiovasc Surg* 102:280-287, 1991.

DORV:

Kirklin JW, Pacifico AD, Blackstone EH, et al: Current risks and protocols for operation for double-outlet right ventricle: derivation from an 18 year experience, *J Thorac Cardiovasc Surg* 92:913-930, 1986.

Sridaromont S, Feldt RH, Ritter DG, et al: Double outlet right ventricle: hemodynamic and anatomic correlation, *Am J Cardiol* 38:85-94, 1976.

Splenic Syndromes:

Lamberti JJ, Waldman JD, Mathewson JW, et al: Repair of subdiaphragmatic total anomalous pulmonary venous connection without cardiopulmonary bypass, *J Thorac Cardiovasc Surg* 88:627-630, 1984.

Sapire DW, Ho SY, Anderson RH, et al: Diagnosis and significance of atrial isomerism, *Am J Cardiol* 58:342-346, 1986.

Van Mierop LHS, Gessner IH, Schiebler GL: Asplenia and polysplenia syndrome, *Birth Defects: Original Article Series* 8:36-44, 1972.

CHAPTER 15: VASCULAR RING

Huhta J, Gutgesell H, Latson L, et al: Two-dimensional echocardiographic assessment of the aorta in infants and children with congenital heart disease, *Circulation* 70:417-424, 1984.

Shuford WH, Sybers RG: *The aortic arch and its malformation with emphasis on the angiographic features,* Springfield, Ill, 1974, Charles C Thomas.

CHAPTER 16: CHAMBER LOCALIZATION AND CARDIAC MALPOSITION

Huhta JC, Smallhorn JF, Macartney FJ: Two dimensional echocardiographic diagnosis of situs, *Br Heart J* 48:97-108, 1982.

Van Praagh R, Weinberg PM, Foran RB, et al: *Malposition of the heart.* In Adams FH, Emmanouilides GC, Riemenschneider TH, eds: *Moss' heart disease in infants, children, and adolescents,* ed 4, Baltimore, 1989, Williams & Wilkins.

CHAPTER 17: MISCELLANEOUS CONGENITAL HEART DEFECTS

Gao Y, Burrows PE, Benson LN, et al: Scimitar syndrome in infancy, *J Am Coll Cardiol* 22:873-882, 1993.

Grifka RG, O'Laughlin MP, Nihill MR, et al: Double-transseptal, double-balloon valvuloplasty for congenital mitral stenosis, *Circulation* 88:123-129, 1992.

Lucas RV, Jr, Krabill KA: *Anomalous venous connections, pulmonary and systemic.* In Adams FH, Emmanouilides GC, Riemenschneider TA, eds: *Moss' heart disease in infants, children, and adolescents,* ed 4, Baltimore, 1989, Williams & Wilkins.

Takeuchi S, Imamura H, Katsumoto K, et al: New surgical method for repair of anomalous left coronary artery from pulmonary artery, *J Thorac Cardiovasc Surg* 89:7-11, 1979.

Tashiro T, Todo K, Haruta Y, et al: Anomalous origin of the left coronary artery from the pulmonary artery, *J Thorac Cardiovasc Surg* 106:718-722, 1993.

Van Son JAM, Danielson GK, Schaff HV, et al: Congenital partial and complete absence of the pericardium, *Mayo Clin Proc* 68:743-747, 1993.

CHAPTER 18: PRIMARY MYOCARDIAL DISEASE

Anderson JL, Gilbert EM, O'Connell JB, et al: Long-term (2 year) beneficial effects of beta-adrenergic blockage with bunindolol in patients with idiopathic dilated cardiomyopathy, *J Am Coll Cardiol* 17:1373-1381, 1991.

Friedman RA, Moak JP, Garson A Jr: Clinical course of idiopathic dilated cardiomyopathy in children, *J Am Coll Cardiol* 18:152-156, 1991.

Ino T, Benson LN, Freedom RM, et al: Endocardial fibroelastosis: natural history and prognostic risk factors, *Am J Cardiol* 62:431-434, 1988.

Katritsis D, Wilmshurst PT, Wendon JA, et al: Primary restrictive cardiomyopathy: clinical and pathologic characteristics, *J Am Coll Cardiol* 18:1230-1235, 1991.

Lipshultz SE, Sanders SP, Goorin AM, et al: Monitoring for anthracycline cardiotoxicity, *Pediatrics* 93:433-437, 1994.

Marcus FI, Fontaine GH, Guiraudon G, et al: Right ventricular dysplasia: a report of 24 adult cases, *Circulation* 65:384-398, 1982.

Maron BJ, Bonow RO, Cannon RO III, et al: Hypertrophic cardiomyopathy. Interrelations of clinical manifestations, pathophysiology, and therapy. I. *N Engl J Med* 316:780-789, 1987.

Maron BJ, Bonow RO, Cannon RO III, et al: Hypertrophic cardiomyopathy. Interrelations of clinical manifestations, pathophysiology, and therapy. II. *N Engl J Med* 316:843-852, 1987.

Steinherz LJ, Graham T, Hurwitz R, et al: Guidelines for cardiac monitoring of children during and after anthracycline therapy: report of the Cardiology Committee of the Children's Cancer Study Group, *Pediatrics* 89:942-949, 1992.

CHAPTER 19: CARDIOVASCULAR INFECTIONS

Akagi T, Kato H, Inoue O, et al: Valvular heart disease in Kawasaki syndrome: incidence and natural history, *Am Heart J* 120:366-372, 1990.

American Heart Association Committee on Rheumatic Fever, Endocarditis, and Kawasaki Disease: Diagnostic guidelines for Kawasaki disease, *Am J Dis Child* 144:1218-1219, 1990.

Dajani AS, Bisno AL, Chung KJ, et al: Prevention of bacterial endocarditis: recommendation by the American Heart Association, *JAMA* 264:2919-2922, 1990.

Dajani AS, Taubert KA, Takahashi M, et al: Guidelines for long-term management of patients with Kawasaki disease: report from the Committee on Rheumatic Fever, Endocarditis, and Kawasaki disease, Council on Cardiovascular Disease in the Young, American Heart Association, *Circulation* 89:916-922, 1994.

Drucker NA, Colan SD, Lewis AB, et al: γ globulin treatment of acute myocarditis in the pediatric population, *Circulation* 89:251-257, 1994.

Kato H, Ichinose E, Yoshioka F, et al: Fate of coronary aneurysms in Kawasaki disease: serial coronary angiography and long-term follow-up study, *Am J Cardiol* 49:1758-1766, 1982.

Koren G, Schaffer F, Silverman E, et al: Determinants of low serum concentrations of salicylates in patients with Kawasaki disease, *J Pediatr* 112:663-667, 1988.

Newburger JW, Takahashi M, Beiser AS, et al: A single intravenous infusion of gamma globulin as compared with four infusions in the treatment of acute Kawasaki syndrome, *N Engl J Med* 324:1633-1639, 1991.

Nocton JJ, Dressler F, Rutledge BJ, et al: Detection of Borrelia Burgdorferi DNA by polymerase chain reaction in synovial fluid from patients with Lyme arthritis, *N Engl J Med* 330:229-234, 1994.

Steere AC: Lyme disease, *N Engl J Med* 321:586-596, 1989.

CHAPTER 20: ACUTE RHEUMATIC FEVER

Committee on Rheumatic Fever and Infective Endocarditis of the Council on Cardiovascular Disease of the Young, American Heart Association: Prevention of rheumatic fever, *Circulation* 70:1118A-1122A, 1985.

Dajani AS, Ayoub E, Bierman FZ, et al: Guidelines for the diagnosis of rheumatic fever: Jones criteria, updated 1992, *Circulation* 87:302-307, 1993.

Markowitz M, Gordis L: *Rheumatic fever*, Philadelphia, 1972, Saunders.

Swedo SE, Leonard HL, Shapiro MB, et al: Sydenham's chorea: physical and psychological symptoms of St. Vitus dance, *Pediatrics* 91:706-713, 1993.

CHAPTER 21: VALVULAR HEART DISEASE

Bisset GS III, Schwartz DC, Meyer RA, et al: Clinical spectrum and long-term follow-up of isolated mitral valve prolapse in 119 children, *Circulation* 62:423-429, 1980.

Levine RA, Triulzi MO, Harrigan P, et al: The relationship of mitral annular shape to the diagnosis of mitral valve prolapse, *Circulation* 75:756-767, 1987.

Levine RA, Stathogiannis E, Newell JB, et al: Reconsideration of echocardiographic standards for mitral valve prolapse: lack of association between leaflet displacement isolated to the apical four chamber view and independent echocardiographic evidence of abnormality, *J Am Coll Cardiol* 11:1010-1019, 1988.

Lock JE, Khalilullah M, Shrivastava S, et al: Percutaneous catheter commissurotomy in rheumatic mitral stenosis, *N Engl J Med* 313:1515-1518, 1985.

Smith MS, Doroshow C, Womack WM, et al: Symptomatic mitral valve prolapse in children and adolescents: catecholamines, anxiety, and biofeedback, *Pediatrics* 84:290-298, 1989.

Warth DC, King ME, Cohen JM, et al: Prevalence of mitral valve prolapse in normal children, *J Am Coll Cardiol* 5:1173-1177, 1985.

CHAPTER 22: CARDIAC TUMORS

Ludomirsky A: *Cardiac tumors.* In Garson A Jr, Bricker JT, McNamara DG, eds: *The science and practice of pediatric cardiology,* Philadelphia, 1990, Lea & Febiger.

McAllister HA, Fenoglio JJ Jr: *Tumors of the cardiovascular system: atlas of tumor pathology,* second series, Washington, DC, 1978, Armed Forces Institute of Pathology.

CHAPTER 23: CARDIAC INVOLVEMENT IN SYSTEMIC DISEASES

Caddell JL: *Metabolic and nutritional diseases.* In Adams FH, Emmanouilides GC, Riemenschneider TA, eds: *Moss' heart disease in infants, children, and adolescents,* ed 4, Baltimore, 1989, Williams & Wilkins.

Pierpoint MEM, Moller JH: *Cardiac manifestations of systemic disease.* In Adams FH, Emmanouilides GC, Riemenschneider TA, eds: *Moss' heart disease in infants, children, and adolescents,* ed 4, Baltimore, 1989, Williams & Wilkins.

Shores J, Berger KR, Murphy EA, et al: Progression of aortic and the benefit of long-term β-adrenergic blockade in Marfan's syndrome, *N Engl J Med* 330:1335-1341, 1994.

CHAPTER 24: CARDIAC ARRHYTHMIAS

Lerman BB, Belardinelli L: Cardiac electrophysiology of adenosine: basic and clinical concepts, *Circulation* 83:1499-1509, 1991.

Rocchini AP, Chun PO, Dick M: Ventricular tachycardia in children, *Am J Cardiol* 47:1091-1097, 1981.

Yabek SM: Ventricular arrhythmias in children with an apparently normal heart, *J Pediatr* 119:1-11, 1991.

CHAPTER 25: DISTURBANCES IN ATRIOVENTRICULAR CONDUCTION

Ross BA: *Atrioventricular block.* In Garson A, Jr, Bricker JT, McNamara DG, eds: *The science and practice of pediatric cardiology,* Philadephia, 1990, Lea & Febiger.

CHAPTER 26: PACEMAKERS IN CHILDREN

Dreifus LS, Fisch C, Griffin JC, et al: Guidelines for implantation of cardiac pacemakers and antiarrhythmia devices: a report of the American College of Cardiology/American Heart Association Task Force on Assessment of Diagnostic and Therapeutic Cardiovascular Procedures (Committee on Pacemaker Implantation), *J Am Coll Cardiol* 18:1-13, 1991.

Friedman RA: Pacemakers in children: medical and surgical aspects, *Texas Heart Institute J* 19:178-184, 1992.

CHAPTER 27: ST SEGMENT AND T WAVE CHANGES

Towbin JA, Bricker JT, Garson A: Electrocardiographic criteria for diagnosis of acute myocardial infarction in childhood, *Am J Cardiol* 69:1545-1548, 1992.

CHAPTER 28: SPECIAL FEATURES IN CARDIAC EVALUATION OF THE NEWBORN

Rudolph AM: *Congenital diseases of the heart: clinical-physiologic considerations in diagnosis and management,* St Louis, 1974, Mosby.

CHAPTER 29: CARDIAC PROBLEMS OF THE NEWBORN

Albersheim SG, Solimanu AJ, Sharma AK, et al: Randomized, double-blind, controlled trial of long-term diuretic therapy for bronchopulmonary dysplasia, *J Pediatr* 115:615-6:0, 1989.

Chang AC, Farrell PE Jr, Murdison KA, et al: Hypoplastic left heart syndrome: hemodynamic and angiographic assessment after initial reconstructive surgery and relevance to modified Fontan procedure, *Pediatr Cardiol* 17:1143-1149, 1991.

Duc G: Assessment of hypoxia in the newborn: suggestions for a practical approach, *Pediatrics* 48:469-481, 1971.

Kinsella JP, Neish SR, Shaffer E, et al: Low-dose inhalational nitric oxide in persistent pulmonary hypertension of the newborn, *Lancet* 340:819-820, 1992.

Mills JL: Congenital malformations in diabetes: report of the Ross Conference on Pediatric Research, 93:12-19, 1987.

Musewe NN, Poppe D, Smallhorn JF, et al: Doppler echocardiographic measurement of pulmonary artery pressure from ductal Doppler velocities in the newborn, *J Am Coll Cardiol* 15:446-456, 1990.

Norwood WI, Lang P, Castaneda AR, et al: Experience with operations for hypoplastic left heart syndrome, *J Thorac Cardiovasc Surg* 82:511-519, 1981.

Reimenschneider TA, Emmanouilides GC: *Persistent pulmonary hypertension in the newborn.* In Adams FH, Emmanouilides GC, Reimenschneider TA, eds: *Moss' heart disease in infants, children, and adolescents,* ed 4, Baltimore, 1989, Williams & Wilkins.

Rudolph AM: High pulmonary vascular resistance after birth. I. Pathophysiologic considerations and etiologic classification, *Clin Pediatr* 19:585-590, 1980.

Southall DP, Richards J, Mitchell P, et al: Study of cardiac rhythm in healthy newborn infants, *Br Heart J* 43:14-20, 1980.

Starnes VA, Griffin ML, Pitlick PT, et al: Current approach to hypoplastic hypoplastic left heart syndrome: palliation, transplantation, or both, *J Thorac Cardiovasc Surg* 104:189-195, 1992.

Southall DP, Johnson AM, Shinebourne EA, et al: Frequency and outcome of disorder of cardiac rhythm and conduction in a population of newborn infants, *Pediatrics* 68:58-66, 1981.

Walther FJ, Bender MJ, Leighton JO: Persistent pulmonary hypertension in premature neonates with severe respiratory distress syndrome, *Pediatrics* 90:899-904, 1992.

CHAPTER 30: CONGESTIVE HEART FAILURE

Artman M, Graham TP Jr: Guidelines for vasodilator therapy of congestive heart failure in infants and children, *Am J Cardiol* 113:994-1005, 1987.

Ebara H, Suzuki S, Nagashima K, et al: Digoxin-like immuno-reactive substances in urine and serum from preterm and term infants: relationships to renal excretion of sodium, *J Pediatr* 108:760-762, 1986.

Friedman WF: New concepts and drugs in the treatment of congestive heart failure, *Pediatr Clin North Amer* 31:1197-1227, 1984.

Ludens JH, Clark M, DuCharme DW, et al: Purification of an endogenous digitalislike factor from human plasma for structural analysis, *Hypertension* 17:923-929, 1991.

Montigny M, Davignon A, Fouron J-C, et al: Captopril in infants for congestive heart failure secondary to a large ventricular left-to-right shunt, *Am J Cardiol* 63:631-633, 1989.

Park MK: The use of digoxin in infants and children with specific emphasis on dosage, *J Pediatr* 108:871-877, 1986.

CHAPTER 31: SYSTEMIC HYPERTENSION

Park MK, Guntheroth WG: Accurate blood pressure measurement in children: Review article, *Am J Noninvas Cardiol* 3:297-309, 1989.

Report of the Second Task Force on Blood Pressure Control in Children, *Pediatrics* 79:1-25, 1987.

CHAPTER 32: PULMONARY HYPERTENSION

Din-Xuan AT: Disorders of endothelium-dependent relation in pulmonary disease, *Circulation* 38(suppl V):V-81-V-87, 1993.

Harned HS Jr: *Pediatric pulmonary heart disease,* Boston, 1990, Little, Brown.

King ME, Braun H, Goldblatt A, et al: Interventricular septal configuration as a predictor of right ventricular systolic hypertension in children: a cross-sectional echocardiographic study, *Circulation* 68:68-75, 1983.

Kitabatake A, Inoue M, Asao M, et al: Noninvasive evaluation of pulmonary hypertension by a pulsed Doppler technique, *Circulation* 68:302-309, 1983.

McMurtry IF, Rounds S, Stanbrook HS: Studies of the mechanism of hypoxic pulmonary vasoconstriction, *Adv Shock Res* 8:21-29, 1982.

Perkin RM, Anas NG: Pulmonary hypertension in pediatric patients, *J Pediatr* 105:511-522, 1984.

Stevenson JG: Comparison of several noninvasive methods for estimation of pulmonary artery pressure, *J Am Soc Echo* 2:157-171, 1989.

CHAPTER 33: HYPERLIPIDEMIA IN CHILDHOOD

Farmer JA, Gotto AM Jr: *Risk factors for coronary artery disease.* In Braunwald E, ed: *Heart disease: a textbook of cardiovascular medicine,* ed 4, Philadelphia, 1992, Saunders.

Kwiterovich PO Jr: *Disorders of lipid and lipoprotein metabolism.* In Rudolph AM, ed: *Rudolph's pediatrics,* ed 19, Norwalk, Conn, 1991, Appleton & Lange.

National Cholesterol Education Program: *Report of the Expert Panel on Blood Cholesterol Levels in Children and Adolescents,* U.S. Department of Health and Human Services. NIH Publication No 91-2732, September, 1991.

Summary of the Second Report on the National Cholesterol Education Program (NCEP) Expert Panel on Detection, Evaluation, and Treatment of High Blood Cholesterol in Adults (Adult Treatment Panel II), *JAMA* 269:3015-3023, 1993.

CHAPTER 34: CHILD WITH CHEST PAIN

Brenner JI, Ringel RE, Berman MA: Cardiologic perspectives of chest pain in childhood: a referral problem? to whom? *Pediatr Clin North Am* 31:1241-1258, 1984.

Driscoll DJ, Glichlich LB, Gallen WJ: Chest pain in children: a prospective study, *Pediatrics* 57:648-651, 1976.

Klone RA, Hale S, Alker K, Rezkalla S: The effects of acute and chronic cocaine use on the heart, *Circulation* 85:407-418, 1992.

Middleton D: Evaluating the child with chest pain, *Emerg Med* 22:23-27, 1990.

Rowe BH, Dulburg CS, Peterson RG, et al: Characteristics of children presenting with chest pain to a pediatric emergency department, *Can Med Assoc J* 143:388-394, 1990.

Selbst SM, Ruddy RM, Clark BJ: Pediatric chest pain: a prospective study, *Pediatrics* 82:319-323, 1988.

CHAPTER 35: SYNCOPE

Blanc JJ, Mansourati J, Maheu B, et al: Reproducibility of a positive passive upright tilt test at a seven-day interval in patients with syncope, *Am J Cardiol* 72:467-471, 1993.

Leramn-Sagie T, Rechavia E, Strasberg B, et al: Head-up tilt for the evaluation of syncope of unknown origin in children, *J Pediatr* 118:676-679, 1991.

O'Marcaigh AS, MacLellan-Tobert SG, Perter CP: Tilt-table testing and oral metoprolol therapy in young patients with unexplained syncope, *Pediatrics* 93:278-283, 1994.

Samoil D, Grubb BP, Kip K, et al: Head-upright tilt table testing in children with unexplained syncope, *Pediatrics* 92:426-430, 1993.

Sra JS, Jazayeri MR, Avitall B, et al: Comparison of cardiac pacing with drug therapy in the treatment of neurocardiogenic (vasovagal) syncope with bradycardia or asystole, *N Engl J Med* 328:1117-1121, 1993.

Steiper MJ, Campbell RM: Efficacy of alpha-adrenergic agonist therapy for prevention of pediatric neurocardiogenic syncope, *J Am Coll Cardiol* 22:594-597, 1993.

Long QT Syndrome

Garson A Jr, Dick M II, Fournier A, et al: The long QT syndrome in children: an international study of 287 patients, *Circulation* 87:1866-1872, 1993.

Garson A Jr: How to measure the QT interval: what is normal? *Am J Cardiol* 72:14B-16B, 1993.

Guntheroth WG: Long QT syndrome in children, *Circulation* 87:2058-2059, 1993 (editorial).

Moss AJ, Schwartz PJ, Crampton RS, et al: The long QT syndrome: prospective longitudinal study of 328 families, *Circulation* 84:1136-1144, 1991.

Moss AJ, Liu JE, Gottlieb S, et al: Efficacy of permanent pacing in the management of high-risk patients with long QT syndrome, *Circulation* 84:1524-1529, 1991.

Schwartz PJ, Locati EH, Moss AJ, et al: Left cardiac sympathetic enervation in the therapy of congenital long QT syndrome: a worldwide report, *Circulation* 84:503-511, 1991.

Weintraub RG, Gow RM, Wilkinson JL: The congenital long QT syndromes in childhood, *J Am Coll Cardiol* 16:674-680, 1990.

CHAPTER 36: POSTOPERATIVE SYNDROMES

Engle MA: *Postoperative problems.* In Adams FH, Emmanouilides GC, Riemenschneider TA, eds: *Moss' heart disease in infants, children, and adolescents,* ed 4, Baltimore, 1989, Williams & Wilkins.

CHAPTER 37: CARDIAC TRANSPLANTATION

Bailey L, Concepcion W, Shattuck H, et al: Method of heart transplantation for treatment of hypoplastic left heart syndrome, *J Thorac Cardiovasc Surg* 92:1-5, 1986.

Bailey LL, Gundry SR, Razzouk AJ, et al: Bless the babies: one hundred fifteen late survivors of heart transplantation during the first year of life, *J Thorac Cardiovasc Surg* 105:805-815, 1993.

Baum D, Bernstein D, Starnes VA, et al: Pediatric heart transplantation at Stanford: results of a 15-year experience, *Pediatrics* 88:203-214, 1991.

Bernstein D, Baum D, Berry G, et al: Neoplastic disorders after pediatric heart transplantation. II. *Circulation* 88:230-237, 1993.

24th Bethesda Conference (chaired by Hunt SA): *J Am Coll Cardiol* 199322:1-64.

Boucek MM, Mathis CM, Kanakriyeh MS, et al: Serial echocardiographic evaluation of cardiac graft rejection after infant heart transplantation, *J Heart Lung Transplant* 12:824-831, 1993.

Pahl E, Fricker FJ, Armitage J, et al: Coronary arteriosclerosis in pediatric heart transplant survivors: limitation of long-term survival, *J Pediatr* 116:177-183, 1990.

Reitz BA: *Heart and heart-lung transplantation.* In Braunwald E, ed: *Heart disease: a textbook of cardiovascular medicine,* ed 4, Philadelphia, 1992, Saunders.

Index

---

t indicates tables; *f* indicates figures.